I0787597

NUTRITIONAL HEALTH

NUTRITION ◊ AND ◊ HEALTH
Adrianne Bendich, Series Editor

Nutritional Health: Strategies for Disease Prevention, Second Edition, edited by
Norman J. Temple, Ted Wilson, and David R. Jacobs, Jr., 2006

Nutrients, Stress, and Medical Disorders, edited by **Shlomo Yehuda and David I.
Mostofsky,** 2006

Calcium in Human Health, edited by **Connie M. Weaver and Robert P. Heaney,** 2006

Preventive Nutrition: The Comprehensive Guide for Health Professionals, Third Edition,
edited by **Adrianne Bendich and Richard J. Deckelbaum,** 2005

The Management of Eating Disorders and Obesity, Second Edition, edited by **David J.
Goldstein,** 2005

Nutrition and Oral Medicine, edited by **Riva Touger-Decker, David A. Sirois,
and Connie C. Mobley,** 2005

IGF and Nutrition in Health and Disease, edited by **M. Sue Houston, Jeffrey M. P.
Holly, and Eva L. Feldman,** 2005

Epilepsy and the Ketogenic Diet, edited by **Carl E. Stafstrom and Jong M. Rho,** 2004

Handbook of Drug–Nutrient Interactions, edited by **Joseph I. Boullata and Vincent T.
Armenti,** 2004

Nutrition and Bone Health, edited by **Michael F. Holick and Bess Dawson-Hughes,**
2004

Diet and Human Immune Function, edited by **David A. Hughes, L. Gail Darlington,
and Adrianne Bendich,** 2004

Beverages in Nutrition and Health, edited by **Ted Wilson and Norman J. Temple,** 2004

Handbook of Clinical Nutrition and Aging, edited by **Connie Watkins Bales
and Christine Seel Ritchie,** 2004

Fatty Acids: Physiological and Behavioral Functions, edited by **David I. Mostofsky,
Shlomo Yehuda, and Norman Salem, Jr.,** 2001

Nutrition and Health in Developing Countries, edited by **Richard D. Semba and
Martin W. Bloem,** 2001

Preventive Nutrition: The Comprehensive Guide for Health Professionals, Second Edition,
edited by **Adrianne Bendich and Richard J. Deckelbaum,** 2001

Nutritional Health: Strategies for Disease Prevention, edited by **Ted Wilson
and Norman J. Temple,** 2001

*Clinical Nutrition of the Essential Trace Elements and Minerals: The Guide for Health
Professionals,* edited by **John D. Bogden and Leslie M. Klevey,** 2000

Primary and Secondary Preventive Nutrition, edited by **Adrianne Bendich
and Richard J. Deckelbaum,** 2000

The Management of Eating Disorders and Obesity, edited by **David J. Goldstein,** 1999

Vitamin D: Physiology, Molecular Biology, and Clinical Applications, edited by
Michael F. Holick, 1999

Preventive Nutrition: The Comprehensive Guide for Health Professionals,
edited by **Adrianne Bendich and Richard J. Deckelbaum,** 1997

NUTRITIONAL HEALTH

Strategies for Disease Prevention

SECOND EDITION

Edited by

NORMAN J. TEMPLE, PhD

*Centre for Science, Athabasca University, Athabasca
Alberta, Canada*

TED WILSON, PhD

*Department of Biology, Winona State University
Winona, MN*

DAVID R. JACOBS, JR., PhD

*School of Public Health, University of Minnesota
Minneapolis, MN*

Foreword by

DAVID S. LUDWIG, MD, PhD

*Director, Obesity Program, and the Division of Endocrinology,
Children's Hospital Boston,
and Associate Professor, Pediatrics, Harvard Medical School
Boston, MA*

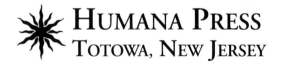

HUMANA PRESS
TOTOWA, NEW JERSEY

Cover design by Patricia F. Cleary.

Production Editor: Amy Thau

For additional copies, pricing for bulk purchases, and/or information about other Humana titles, contact Humana at the above
address or at any of the following numbers: Tel.: 973-256-1699; Fax: 973-256-8341; E-mail: orders@humanapr.com or visit
our website at http://humanapress.com

This publication is printed on acid-free paper. ∞
ANSI Z39.48-1984 (American National Standards Institute) Permanence of Paper for Printed Library Materials.

Printed in the United States of America. 10 9 8 7 6 5 4 3 2 1
eISBN: 1-59259-980-X
Library of Congress Cataloging-in-Publication Data

Nutritional health : strategies for disease prevention / edited by
  Norman J. Temple, Ted Wilson, David R. Jacobs. -- 2nd ed.
    p. ; cm. -- (Nutrition and health)
  Includes bibliographical references and index.
  ISBN 1-58829-454-4 (alk. paper)
  1. Diet in disease. 2. Nutrition. 3. Diet therapy. 4. Medicine,
Preventive.   I. Temple, Norman J. II. Wilson, Ted. III. Jacobs,
David R. IV. Seris: Nutrition and health (Totowa, N.J.)
  [DNLM: 1. Nutrition. 2. Chronic Disease. 3. Diabetes Mellitus
--prevention & control. 4. Heart Diseases--prevention & control.
5. Hypertension--prevention & control. 6. Neoplasms--prevention
& control.   WB 400 F935 2006]
  RM216.N8628 2006
  614.5'939--dc22

                                                    2005013116

Dedication

To Anthony, my son, with pride.

—Norman

To my patient and loving wife, Karen: we are what we eat—organic.

—Ted

To my granddaughter Maya Sylvia Abeni Jacobs: eat well and live long.

—David

Series Editor's Introduction

The *Nutrition and Health Series* of books has had great success because each volume has the consistent overriding mission of providing health professionals with texts that are considered essential because each includes: (1) a synthesis of the state of the science; (2) timely, in-depth reviews by the leading researchers in their respective fields; (3) extensive, up-to-date fully annotated reference lists; (4) a detailed index; (5) relevant tables and figures; (6) identification of paradigm shifts and the consequences; (7) virtually no overlap of information between chapters, but targeted, interchapter referrals; (8) suggestions of areas for future research; and (9) balanced, data-driven answers to patient, as well as health professional's questions that are based on the totality of evidence rather than the findings of any single study.

The series volumes are not the outcome of a symposium. Rather, each editor has the potential to examine a chosen area with a broad perspective, both in subject matter, as well as in the choice of chapter authors. The international perspective, especially with regard to public health initiatives, is emphasized where appropriate. The editors, whose trainings are both research- and practice-oriented, have the opportunity to develop a primary objective for their book, define its scope and focus, and then invite the leading authorities to be part of their initiative. The authors are encouraged to provide an overview of the field, discuss their own research, and relate the research findings to potential human health consequences. Because each book is developed *de novo*, the chapters are coordinated so that the resulting volume imparts greater knowledge than the sum of the information contained in the individual chapters.

Nutritional Health: Strategies for Disease Prevention, Second Edition, edited by Drs. Norman J. Temple, Ted Wilson, and David R. Jacobs, is a very welcome addition to the *Nutrition and Health Series* and fully exemplifies the series' goals. The first volume of *Nutritional Health*, which was edited by Ted Wilson and Norman Temple, was published in 2001 and contained 20 chapters. In the intervening 5 years, there have been many important research papers published that are now reviewed and put in perspective in this updated volume. The 26 chapters included in this expanded new edition examine the current clinical findings and put these into historic perspective, as well as point the way to future research opportunities. The editors are internationally recognized leaders in the field of nutrition, excellent communicators, and have worked tirelessly to develop a book that is destined to be the benchmark in the field because of its extensive, in-depth chapters covering the most important aspects of the complex interactions between diet and its nutrient components and their impacts on disease states and health conditions that increase the risk of chronic disease. Given the growing concern regarding the increase in adult and childhood obesity, it is not surprising to find an emphasis on obesity, weight control, diabetes, and other chronic diseases associated with obesity in *Nutritional Health: Strategies for Disease Prevention, Second Edition*. However, as in the first edition, there are introductory chapters that provide readers with the basics so that the more clinically related chapters can be easily understood. The first chapter, for instance, provides a mini-course on the basics of nutritional epidemiology, which is then followed by the related chapter that outlines the major challenges encountered in nutritional epidemiological research. These two chapters are very helpful to the readers of *Nutritional Health: Strategies for Disease Prevention, Second Edition* as they can continue through the volume with excellent information and perspective to evaluate the synthesis of the data provided in the subsequent chapters.

The editors have chosen 37 of the most well-recognized and respected authors from around the world to contribute the 26 informative chapters in the volume. Key features of this comprehensive volume include the bulleted Key Points that are at the beginning of each chapter, the detailed tables and informative figures, the extensive, detailed index, and the more than 1000 up-to-date references that provide the reader with excellent sources of worthwhile information about stress–nutrient interactions. Additionally, many of the chapters provide practitioners with clear guidelines and diet information that can be easily used with clients and/or patients.

Hallmarks of all of the chapters include complete definitions of terms with the abbreviations fully defined for the reader and consistent use of terms between chapters. In addition to the Key Points section at the beginning of each chapter, there is also a summary section at the conclusion of each chapter that provides the highlights of major findings. The volume contains a highly annotated index, and within chapters, readers are referred to relevant information in other chapters.

This important reference text provides practical, data-driven integrated resources based on the totality of the evidence to help the reader evaluate the critical role of nutrition, especially in at-risk populations, in optimizing health and preventing chronic illnesses. The overarching goal of the editors is to provide fully referenced information to health professionals so they may have a balanced perspective on the value of foods and nutrients that are routinely consumed and how these help to maintain mental, as well as physical, health. Of added value to academic discussions, especially in classrooms, are the diverse perspectives of the chapter authors. As an example, some authors indicate that certain dietary supplements have no value, whereas other authors suggest that certain supplements are of value and each author provides the evidence for his or her position. Similarly, within a chapter, there may be positive data concerning one bioactive molecule and evidence that a related molecule may not be efficacious. These discussions are critical to sharpen the development of the scientific, data-driven interactions, and in this volume, it is the totality of the evidence that is used to defend a perspective.

The volume is also of great value when students, clients, patients, or the media inquire about novel substances, such as long-chain fatty acids, flavonoids, carotenoids, herbs, vitamins, minerals, carbohydrates, amino acids, and other dietary components. The major diets are compared and their effects on weight loss, as well as lipids, are discussed. The major chronic diseases are all reviewed, including cancer, cardiovascular disease, diabetes, Alzheimer's, and age-related eye diseases. Unique to this volume are the chapters that take a global perspective and examine the dietary recommendations between countries. The important interaction of diet and exercise is reviewed in depth. Nutrition is more than simply diet, and the factors that can impact the availability of the dietary factors to reach the human circulatory system are also discussed in several chapters, including those that review novel foods and functional foods and the way that biotechnology has influenced the food industry globally. Another novel chapter reviews the area of nutritional anthropology and includes the example of pica as a determinant of economic and social interactions that can impact nutritional status. A critical factor that has increased greatly in importance during the last five years is the Internet—and the original chapter in the first edition has been extensively updated for this volume. This final chapter contains close to 100 website addresses to help readers identify excellent sources of information.

In conclusion, *Nutritional Health: Strategies for Disease Prevention, Second Edition* provides health professionals in many areas of research and practice with the most up-to-date, well-referenced, and easy-to-understand volume on the importance of nutrition in reducing chronic diseases and optimizing health. This volume will serve the reader as the benchmark in this complex area of interrelationships between diet, specific nutrients, health, and disease. As stated in the Foreword written by Dr. David S. Ludwig from Harvard Medical School, "Altogether, *Nutritional Health: Strategies for Disease Prevention, Second Edition* is a remarkable achievement and a fascinating read..." The editors are applauded for their efforts to develop the most authoritative resource in the field to date and this excellent text is a very welcome addition to the *Nutrition and Health Series*.

Adrianne Bendich, PhD, FACN

Foreword

In their pursuit of improved health, Americans receive 3 billion prescriptions for medicines and undergo about 50 million surgical procedures annually, each with financial cost and safety risk. During this same year, they consume about half a trillion meals. One wonders how many of those prescriptions and procedures might be unnecessary with increased attention to the quality of those meals. Judging from the 26 chapters in *Nutritional Health: Strategies for Disease Prevention, Second Edition*, the answer may be many.

As I write this foreword, the media remains abuzz with revised estimates from the Centers for Disease Control and Prevention (CDC) that obesity causes "only" 100,000—not 300,000—excess deaths per year in the United States. However, none of these projections take into account the looming impact of the pediatric obesity epidemic. Never before have so many children been so heavy from such an early age. As these children age, they will carry the cumulative effects of excessive weight for many years. Chapter 5 emphasizes the point that a diagnosis of type 2 diabetes in adulthood shortens life expectancy by 10 years or more. What will happen to an overweight 4-year-old who develops type 2 diabetes at 14 years old?

Obesity does not result, for the most part, from inherent metabolic or anatomical defects requiring pharmacological or surgical intervention. Although genetic factors indisputably affect body-weight regulation, progressive weight gain does not invariably occur over time among relatively sedentary populations living amidst plenty (take, for example, Western Europe or Japan through most of the last half of the 20th century). Clearly, changes in diet quality, physical activity level, and the social environment underlie the obesity epidemic. And at any body weight, the likelihood of developing diabetes, heart disease, cancer, and other life-threatening conditions is strongly influenced by dietary quality. These topics are considered from many different perspectives by the authors of *Nutritional Health: Strategies for Disease Prevention, Second Edition*.

So, what is the optimal diet for the treatment of obesity, the prevention of chronic disease, and the maintenance of optimal health? Readers will not receive a definitive answer to this question, which should come as no surprise. Indeed, premature conclusions based on inadequate evidence may do more harm than good to public health.

Controversy exists within these pages on several issues, such as whether the relative amount of fat in the diet or glycemic index/load importantly affects risk for obesity, diabetes, or heart disease. Other points remain unresolved: does the ratio of n-3:n-6 fatty acids in the diet play a role in the development of diabetes, atherosclerosis, cancer, or neurodegenerative disease? Should every adult be encouraged to consume less salt and, barring contraindications, have one or two alcoholic drinks each day? Do vitamin supplements, herbal extracts, or "functional foods" improve health for individuals without nutrient deficiencies? Fortunately, Chapters 1 and 2 provide a useful roadmap for how answers to these and other questions can be found with modern nutritional research methods.

However, in our pursuit of the mechanisms relating diet to disease, we must avoid the temptation to be overly reductionist, as eloquently argued by Dr. Liu in Chapter 10. Plant foods contain hundreds or thousands of nutrients, phytochemicals, and indigestible substances that interact in a complex and potentially synergistic fashion. No purified supplements could ever provide the benefit and safety (let alone appeal) of a nutritious diet. Indeed, a broad consensus does exist among the authors regarding the benefits of a plant-based diet, with particular emphasis on macronutrient quality. I also expect unanimity on one recommendation: drink tea, coffee, or water instead of sugar-sweetened drinks.

However, even a complete understanding of the dietary determinants of disease will have little practical significance if efforts by nutrition experts and clinicians are systematically undermined by policies that place the interests of private profit over public health. Chapters 22 and 23 take a sober look at the corrosive effects of junk food advertising to young children, unregulated political contributions from the food industry, and agricultural policies that favor high-calorie, low-quality commodities, such as sugar, refined grain products, and cheap oils. These policies and practices disproportionately affect poor and minority populations, exacerbating the preexisting health discrepancies described in Chapter 24.

The last century has brought us a long way from the family farm as the foundation of our food supply, and Chapter 21 considers the effects of continuing biotechnological development on the methods of food production. Genetically modified foods have the potential to provide considerable benefit in developing nations, the treatment of vitamin A deficiency with golden rice being one example. However, I am concerned that a single-minded focus on increasing production efficiency through biotechnology may have a darker side: control of the food supply by a few multinational corporations, loss of genetic diversity, deterioration of animal welfare, environmental disruption, and unexpected adverse health effects. Regarding information technology, Chapter 26 discusses how the internet offers unprecedented opportunities for the empowerment of people worldwide through instant access to nutritional information.

Altogether, *Nutritional Health: Strategies for Disease Prevention, Second Edition* is a remarkable achievement and a fascinating read, and I congratulate the editors on the publication of their opus magnum, and recommend it to all health care professionals, researchers, and students interested in the promotion of optimal health.

David S. Ludwig, MD, PhD

Preface

Five years have elapsed since the first edition of *Nutritional Health: Strategies for Disease Prevention,* was written. Yet during that time, much water has flowed under the bridge of the advancing river that is nutrition research and practice. Three developments illustrate this dynamic change: the fierce debate, especially in Europe, over the acceptability of genetically modified foods; the vast numbers of new foods appearing in supermarkets (and none perhaps more controversial than low-carbohydrate foods); and the development of the Internet as an indispensable research tool. With the great accumulation of developments in the field of nutrition, the need for a new edition of this book was obvious.

During the last century of nutritional advancement, we have frequently been faced with great opportunities that were brilliantly disguised as insoluble problems. Perhaps we are biased, but in our eyes, problems associated with nutrition are among the most exciting of those in the life sciences. How many other branches of the life sciences offer the promise of slashing the burden of human disease by one-third or more?

With a smattering of brilliant exceptions, until the 1970s, few people gave serious consideration to the notion that our diet plays an important role in chronic diseases, such as heart disease and cancer. Today, we have a vastly greater understanding of the role of diet in disease. We know, for example, how fruits and vegetables affect cancer, how fats affect heart disease, and how calcium affects osteoporosis. Now, in the early years of the 21st century, our vastly improved knowledge of nutrition gives us the capability to prevent a sizable fraction of the chronic diseases that afflict the people of our world, but only if we can fully inform its populace about these discoveries.

Ironically, despite overwhelming evidence that nutrition has enormous potential to improve human well-being—at modest cost and using the knowledge we already have—it still fails to receive the resources it merits. Growth in funding for nutrition research and education remains stunted. By contrast, countless millions of dollars are spent on the glamor areas of biomedical research, such as genetic engineering and gene therapy. But we already know that our genes can only explain a fraction of our disease burden. Even if gene therapy reaches its full potential, it seems most improbable that it will ever achieve one-quarter of what nutrition can do for us today.

In the words of Confucius: "The essence of knowledge is that, having acquired it, one must apply it." However, a major barrier is that information concerning nutrition often fails to reach the health professionals who most need to apply it, namely the physicians, dietitians, and nurses who represent the front-line workers in health care. How do we bring this information to others who also need this information, such as the nutrition professors who lack the time to read more than a tiny portion of the literature outside of their main area of interest?

Nutritional Health: Strategies for Disease Prevention, Second Edition endeavors to address the needs of those who would benefit most from up-to-date information on recent advances in the field of nutrition. Accordingly, our book contains a series of chapters by experts in a diverse range of nutritional areas. Our aim is not so much to cover all the leading edges of nutrition, as it is to discuss recent thinking and discoveries that have the greatest capacity to improve human health and nutritional implementation.

Some readers may disagree with the opinions presented, but in nutrition, differences of opinion are often unavoidable. Owing to the constant changes in our diet, nutrition is by nature in constant dynamic flow, as are our opinions of what constitutes the best nutritional habits. The views expressed in *Nutritional Health: Strategies for Disease Prevention, Second Edition* are in many cases particular interpretations by the authors of each chapter on their areas of specialization.

Norman J. Temple, PhD
Ted Wilson, PhD
David R. Jacobs, Jr., PhD

Contents

Dedication v

Series Editor's Introduction vii

Foreword xi

Preface xiii

Contributors xvii

1. Impact of Nutritional Epidemiology 1
   Barrie M. Margetts

2. Challenges in Research in Nutritional Epidemiology 25
   David R. Jacobs, Jr.

3. The Nutrition Transition is Speeding Up: *A Global Perspective* 37
   Barry M. Popkin

4. Medical Nutrition Therapy for Diabetes: *Prioritizing Recommendations
   Based on Evidence* 49
   Marion J. Franz

5. Diet and the Prevention of Type 2 Diabetes 77
   Norman J. Temple and Nelia P. Steyn

6. Diet and the Control of Blood Lipids 91
   **Tricia L. Psota, Sarah K. Gebauer, Gigi Meyer,
   and Penny M. Kris-Etherton**

7. Diet and Blood Pressure: *Moving Beyond Preoccupation With Salt
   to Composite Dietary Patterns* 111
   Karen E. Charlton

8. Fish, n-3 Polyunsaturated Fatty Acids, and Cardiovascular Disease 133
   Jayne V. Woodside and Ian S. Young

9. Diet and Cancer Prevention 151
   Cindy D. Davis and John A. Milner

10. Health Benefits of Phytochemicals in Whole Foods 173
    Rui Hai Liu

11. Herbs as Useful Adjuncts to Manage Chronic Diseases 189
    Winston J. Craig

12. What Are the Health Implications of Alcohol Consumption? 211
    Eric Rimm and Norman J. Temple

13. Diet in the Prevention and Treatment of Obesity 223
    Sahaspahorn Paeratakul, George A. Bray, and Barry M. Popkin

14. Diets and Exercise Programs for Weight Loss 239
    Lisa Sanders, Kathleen Page, Dena Bravata, and Marguerite Brainerd

15. The Developmental Origins of Chronic Disease in Adult Life 261
    David J. P. Barker

16. Trends in Dietary Guidelines Around the Global Village 285
    Jayne V. Woodside, Geraldine Cuskelly, and Norman J. Temple

17. Marketing Dietary Supplements for Health and Profit 299
    Norman J. Temple and Diane H. Morris

18. Optimizing Nutrition for Exercise and Sports..313
    Richard B. Kreider and Brian Leutholtz

19. Novel Foods: *Today's Functional Foods Marketplace* 347
    Jill K. Rippe

20. Functional Foods: *A Critical Appraisal* 363
    Ted Wilson and David R. Jacobs, Jr.

21. Use of Biotechnology to Improve Food Production and Quality 373
    Travis J. Knight and Donald C. Beitz

22. Food Industry and Political Influences on American Nutrition.....................387
    Marion Nestle, Ted Wilson, and Audrey Balay-Karperien

23. Population Nutrition, Health Promotion, and Government Policy 397
    Norman J. Temple and Marion Nestle

24. Dietary Intake, Cardiovascular Disease,
    and Sociodemographic Characteristics 413
    Lyn M. Steffen

25. Core Concepts in Nutritional Anthropology 425
    Sera L. Young and Gretel H. Pelto

26. Nutrition on the Internet 439
    Tony Helman

Index 453

Contributors

AUDREY BALAY-KARPERIEN, BS • *School of Community Health, Charles Sturt University, Australia*

DAVID J. P. BARKER, PhD, MD, FRCP, FRCOG, FRS • *Division of Developmental Origins of Adult Health and Disease, School of Medicine, University of Southampton, Southampton, UK*

DONALD C. BEITZ, PhD • *Department of Animal Science, Iowa State University, Ames, IA*

MARGUERITE BRAINERD, RD, CD-N • *Waterbury Hospital, Waterbury, CT*

DENA BRAVATA, MD, MS • *Center for Primary Care and Outcomes Research, Stanford University, Stanford, CA*

GEORGE A. BRAY, MD • *Pennington Biomedical Research Center, Louisiana State University System, Baton Rouge, LA*

KAREN E. CHARLTON, Mphil, MSc • *Chronic Diseases of Lifestyle Unit, Medical Research Council, Cape Town, South Africa*

WINSTON J. CRAIG, PhD, RD • *Department of Nutrition, Andrews University, Berrien Springs, MI*

GERALDINE CUSKELLY, PhD • *Department of Medicine, Queen's University Belfast, Belfast, Northern Ireland*

CINDY D. DAVIS, PhD • *Division of Cancer Prevention, Nutritional Science Research Group, National Cancer Institute, Rockville, MD*

MARION J. FRANZ, MS, RD, CDE • *Nutrition Concepts by Franz, Minneapolis, MN*

SARAH K. GEBAUER, BS • *Department of Nutritional Sciences, The College of Health and Human Development, Pennsylvania State University, University Park, PA*

TONY HELMAN, MB, BS, Dip Obst RCOG, Mast Med, Gr D Hum Nutr, MRACGP • *Faculty of Health and Behavioural Sciences, Deakin University, Victoria, Australia*

DAVID R. JACOBS, JR., PhD • *Division of Epidemiology, School of Public Health, University of Minnesota, Minneapolis, MN*

TRAVIS J. KNIGHT, PhD • *Department of Animal Science, Iowa State University, Ames, IA*

RICHARD B. KREIDER, PhD, FACSM • *Center for Exercise, Nutrition, and Preventive Health Research, Baylor University, Waco, TX*

PENNY M. KRIS-ETHERTON, PhD, RD • *Department of Nutritional Sciences, The College of Health and Human Development, Pennsylvania State University, University Park, PA*

BRIAN LEUTHOLTZ, PhD, FACSM • *Center for Exercise, Nutrition, and Preventive Health Research, Baylor University, Waco, TX*

RUI HAI LIU, MD, PhD • *Department of Food Science, Cornell University, Ithaca, NY*

DAVID S. LUDWIG, MD, PhD • *Director, Obesity Program, and the Division of Endocrinology, Children's Hospital Boston; and Associate Professor, Pediatrics, Harvard Medical School, Boston, MA*

BARRIE M. MARGETTS, PhD, RPHNutr, FFPH • *Institute of Human Nutrition, University of Southampton, Southampton, UK*

GIGI MEYER, BS • *Department of Nutritional Sciences, The College of Health and Human Development, Pennsylvania State University, University Park, PA*

JOHN A. MILNER, PhD • *Division of Cancer Prevention, Nutritional Science Research Group, National Cancer Institute, Rockville, MD*

DIANE H. MORRIS, PhD, RD • *Mainstream Nutrition, Tokyo, Japan*

MARION NESTLE, PhD, MPH • *Department of Nutrition, Food Studies, and Public Health, New York University, New York, NY*

SAHASPAHORN PAERATAKUL, PhD (DECEASED) • *Pennington Biomedical Research Center, Louisiana State University System, Baton Rouge, LA*

KATHLEEN PAGE, MD • *Yale Primary Care Residency Program, New Haven, CT*

GRETEL H. PELTO, PhD • *Division of Nutritional Sciences, Cornell University, Ithaca, NY*

BARRY M. POPKIN, PhD • *School of Public Health, Carolina Population Center, University of North Carolina at Chapel Hill, Chapel Hill, NC*

TRICIA L. PSOTA, BS • *Department of Nutritional Sciences, The College of Health and Human Development, Pennsylvania State University, University Park, PA*

ERIC RIMM, ScD • *Department of Nutrition, Harvard School of Public Health, Boston, MA*

JILL K. RIPPE, MS • *Main Street Ingredients, La Crosse, WI*

LISA SANDERS, MD • *Yale Primary Care Residency Program, New Haven, CT*

LYN M. STEFFEN, PhD, MPH • *Division of Epidemiology, School of Public Health, University of Minnesota, Minneapolis, MN*

NELIA P. STEYN, PhD • *Chronic Diseases of Lifestyle Unit, Medical Research Council, Cape Town, South Africa*

NORMAN J. TEMPLE, PhD • *Centre for Science, Athabasca University, Athabasca, Alberta, Canada*

TED WILSON, PhD • *Department of Biology, Winona State University, Winona, MN*

JAYNE V. WOODSIDE, PhD • *Department of Medicine, Queen's University Belfast, Belfast, Northern Ireland*

IAN S. YOUNG, MD • *Department of Medicine, Queen's University Belfast, Belfast, Northern Ireland*

SERA L. YOUNG, MA • *Division of Nutritional Sciences, Cornell University, Ithaca, NY*

1

Impact of Nutritional Epidemiology

Barrie M. Margetts

KEY POINTS

- Nutritional epidemiology provides a toolkit for asking questions about how nutrition affects health, to define the causes, and therefore guide ways to prevent nutrition-related health problems.
- The approach is population based, but the way exposure is defined and measured needs to take into account the underlying biology.
- Dietary behavior is intrinsically variable, and a key aspect to designing useful studies is to differentiate error from true underlying variation.
- The methods used to derive measures need to be checked before use to ensure that the measures are sufficiently accurate and free from bias.
- Clever analyses can never compensate for poor study design; the key concern must be to design the study as well as possible to reduce the effects of chance, bias, and confounding on the observed measure of effect.

1. INTRODUCTION

Nutritional epidemiology is concerned with exploring the relationship between nutrition and health in human populations *(1)*. It has developed out of an epidemiological approach, classically defined as the study of the *distribution* and *determinants* of health-related conditions or events in defined populations, and the application of this study to the control of health problems *(2)*. *Distribution* refers to analysis of time, place, and classes of persons affected; *determinants* are all the physiological, biological, social, cultural, and behavioral factors that influence health. Why nutritional epidemiology? Nutritional epidemiology is the only method in nutritional science that provides direct information on nutrition and health in human populations consuming normal amounts of foods and nutrients.

Why nutritional epidemiology and not dietary epidemiology? Nutrition is more than what people eat. When trying to understand causal mechanisms, what is ideally required is a measure of what is eaten; what happens to the components of the food (absorption, interaction with other components); how what is eaten adds to, and interacts with, body pools of the nutrient; and how that body pool meets (or does not meet) the metabolic

From: *Nutritional Health: Strategies for Disease Prevention, Second Edition*
Edited by: N. J. Temple, T. Wilson, and D. R. Jacobs © Humana Press Inc., Totowa, NJ

demands for substrates and cofactors to maintain optimal function (from a cellular to whole body sense), which may be called health. Health is a broad concept that can be summarized as being the ability to function optimally, to grow, think, and be well; it is more than the absence of illness. From a nutritional point of view, what is of interest is understanding how dietary intake meets the demands for substrates and cofactors required for maintaining functional capacity. It may be misleading to measure the dietary supply without a sense of what the metabolic demands are. For example, the demands for nutrients in a child with an infection are different from a child without an infection; at the same level of dietary intake, the infected child will direct nutrients (substrates and cofactors) toward fighting the infection and not toward growth and activity. The child's behavior may change to alter the balance between supply and demand, and thus not reflect what would normally happen when the child was well. Ideally, nutritional epidemiology measures the functional availability of nutrients, not simply the dietary supply. When dietary intake alone, or anthropometry alone, is used as a proxy for nutritional status, and related to measures of health, the results may be misleading. In practice, it is often difficult to measure demands in large-scale epidemiological studies, but it is important to consider how well the measure of dietary intake used reflects functional availability of the substrates and cofactors required to maintain function. At the very least it may be helpful to know if someone is gaining or losing weight, and if they have any infections or health problems that may alter metabolic demands that alter the needs for substrates and cofactors. Optimal function can only be maintained when the dietary supply, plus body pools, balance demands. Reductive adaptation in function may occur undetected for some time, perhaps until body pools are used up, and then it may appear that suddenly there is a problem. Nutritional epidemiological studies are also helpful in identifying how current behavior compares with some standard or guideline for the purposes of monitoring and surveillance.

Whenever information on nutrition is being collected, there are important methodological issues that need to be considered to minimize the likelihood of obtaining biased, and therefore unhelpful, information. The underlying objective of all nutritional epidemiological research should be to maintain and improve health. Poor-quality information does not help achieve this objective.

The impact of nutritional epidemiology is to provide an insight into the nutritional factors that may cause and prevent nutrition-related health problems; used properly it should guide metabolic research that can explore causal mechanisms in more depth. Metabolic studies can highlight the clues that can be further assessed in epidemiological studies to explore whether the proposed mechanism may have some relevance in human health. Much metabolic research is undertaken on the justification of the impact the research will have on human health, but often with little consideration as to how the work fits in with epidemiological research. For example, the effects of specific carcinogens or phytochemicals in the potential food supply are studied in animal models in vivo in doses that are not relevant to human exposure, or based on assumptions about bioavailability in humans that are not tested or justified. Researchers across the breadth of nutrition have a responsibility to work together to provide information in a coherent manner that can be used to inform those responsible for making decisions about what we should or should not eat or about the risk/harm of foods we are exposed to. Nutritional epidemiology helps provide an evidence-based approach to the solution of important public health problems.

The purpose of this chapter is to provide some guidance as to how to design and interpret nutritional epidemiological studies; to help the nonspecialist in nutritional epidemiology to make sense of work in this area. It seems almost a rule of nature that "experts" in a field develop language and jargon to describe their field of work in such a way as to exclude others. Further reading is recommended *(3,4)*.

2. EXPOSURE, OUTCOME, AND OTHER VARIABLES

Before starting any nutritional epidemiological studies it is essential to be clear about what factors you want to measure and how accurately you need to measure them. The research should begin with a sound review of the relevant literature that identifies the key factors, and likely strength of associations, being investigated. Without this information it will not be possible to design a sound study. A clear research question (hypothesis) will identify the relevant measures of exposure, outcome, and also other factors or variables that may influence the relationship between exposure and outcome.

2.1. Exposure

Exposure is a generic term to describe factors (variables or measures) to which a person or group of people come into contact and that may be relevant to their health *(5)*. This could include food and the constituents of foods (nutrients and nonnutrients), smoking, alcohol, air pollution, noise, dietary advice, or health promotion via advertisements, etc., or the social environment; in other words, any factor that has an impact on a person or group may be defined as an exposure. If the desired exposure is the nutritional status of a particular nutrient, it should measure food intake and the metabolic fate of the constituents that affect function. A biochemical measure may be used as a measure of exposure, but if it is used as a proxy for dietary behavior, the relationship between the dietary and biochemical measure must be established to ensure that it is a relevant measure of diet.

2.2. Outcome

Outcome is another generic term used to describe factors (variables and measures) that are being studied in relation to the effects of an exposure; often these outcome measures are disease states, but they may also be anthropometric or physiological measures. Depending on the study, these outcome measures may be expressed as continuous or discrete variables. Often, an outcome with a continuous distribution will be divided into categories and a measure of effect assessed across these categories. For example, blood pressure may be analyzed as a continuous outcome measure or subjects may be categorized as those with or without hypertension on the basis of whether they fall above or below an agreed cutoff point. Even for nominally discrete outcome measures, such as disease states, it should be recognized that there is no clear distinction between presence and absence of disease, that diseases progress, and at some point in that progression the disease may become diagnosed.

2.3. Other Variables: Confounding and Effect Modification

A major issue to consider in interpreting epidemiological research is the possibility that variables other than the exposure of interest have influenced the true relationship between exposure and outcome. These other variables need to be measured so that their effects on the exposure–outcome relationship can be properly investigated. It is common practice to adjust the relationship between exposure and outcome for these other variables using regression or some other statistical approach. However, this approach may be misleading. If a variable that has been adjusted for is in the causal pathway, then the adjusted estimate of the effect of the exposure on the outcome will be weakened; however, this smaller estimate would reflect information about the causal pathway, whereas the unadjusted estimate would reflect the magnitude of the causal phenomenon. If the relationship between exposure and outcome differs at different levels of the other variable, an adjusted effect will mask important biological interaction. It is, therefore, important to consider the way in which the other variables that are being adjusted for may relate to the exposure, the outcome, and the relationship between exposure and outcome.

Confounders are associated with both exposure and outcome and distort the relationship under investigation. For a variable to be a confounder, the following qualifications must me met:

1. It must be associated with, but not causally dependent on, the exposure of interest.
2. It must be a risk factor for outcome, independent of its association with the exposure of interest.
3. The foregoing must apply within the population under study.

A confounder cannot lie in the causal pathway. However, it is acknowledged that it is often difficult to tell whether a given covariate is or is not on the causal pathway.

Effect modifiers are variables where the effect of the exposure on the outcome operates differently at different levels of the other variable. Such an effect is referred to as an "interaction." An effect modifier will lie in the causal pathway that relates the exposure of interest to the outcome.

It is never possible to eliminate the effects of all potential confounders (this is referred to as "residual confounding"), and it is therefore important to measure known or suspected confounders so that they can be considered in the analysis. Where variables are known to be confounders, the investigator can control for them either in the design (by randomization, restriction, e.g., exclude smokers, or matching) or in the analysis (by stratification and/or multiple regression), provided sufficient valid information is available on the confounding factor. It will not be possible to control for the confounder if it has not been measured or has been measured poorly.

It is not always easy to disentangle the effects of other variables. Always check before statistically adjusting as to whether the other variables are likely to be confounders or effect modifiers. It is optimal to do this before the study starts, so that the study can be designed accordingly, but if this is not possible it can be done during the analysis. The best approach is to undertake a series of analyses stratified by the variable of interest. Confounding can be adjusted for in an analysis. When there is effect modification, the results for each stratum of the variable should be presented separately and the variable should not be adjusted for. The need for undertaking stratum-specific analyses should be considered in the way the study is designed to ensure that there are sufficient subjects in each stratum of analysis. If the sample size is too small, stratum-specific estimates of effect may have wide confidence intervals that may suggest no statistically significant effect when in fact there is one. Figure 1 summarizes these differences.

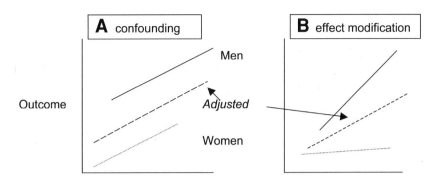

Fig. 1. Relationship between exposure and outcome. (**A**) with gender as a confounder and (**B**) with gender as effect modifier. The adjusted slope in (**B**) does not reflect the underlying difference in the relationship between exposure and outcome by gender.

Diet is a most complex exposure to measure where there may be both confounding and effect modification between aspects of diet, and between socio-demographic factors, and other biological variables, such as body mass. One of the major challenges over the next few years will be to understand the effects of dietary patterns where higher consumption of "protective" factors may simply reflect lower consumption of "harmful" factors. For example, in Europe and North America people who eat more fruit and vegetable tend to eat less meat and animal fat. Is the apparent protective effect of fruit and vegetable intake owing to increased intake of substances in these foods, or to the lower consumption of other harmful substances in meat and animal fats? Does it relate to the way the meat is cooked? How should this be dealt with? If the exposure of interest is fruit intake, the researchers should stratify subjects by level of meat consumption and assess whether the relationship between fruit and cancer differs at different levels of meat intake. If this is indeed the case, then it would suggest an interaction between meat and fruit. In that case stratum-specific, rather than meat-adjusted, results should be presented. If the effect of fruit does not interact with the effect of meat, but meat consumers have a higher risk of cancer independently of fruit and they also eat less fruit, then meat will be a confounder and should be adjusted for in the analysis. Gender is often considered to be a confounder, because intake differs by gender, and disease rates are usually higher in men. However, gender may be an effect modifier in some circumstances, for example, where there may be some hormone-related effect with gender acting as a proxy for an underlying etiological difference.

As chronic diseases become more common in countries of the Southern Hemisphere (the terms Northern and Southern Hemisphere are used instead of developed and developing as they convey less of a hierarchical sense of development), there is growing evidence that early nutrition interacts with later nutrition to increase risk. For example, a child with a low birth-weight, who subsequently becomes a heavy adolescent, has an increased risk of heart disease, compared with a person who had the same body mass index (BMI) as an adolescent, but with a higher birth-weight.

3. MEASUREMENT OF NUTRITIONAL EXPOSURE, OUTCOME, AND OTHER VARIABLES

Whenever information is obtained from any source about exposure, outcome, or other variables of interest, it is important to consider whether the information that is collected measures what is required, with an appropriate level of accuracy. In this chapter the emphasis is placed on measures of nutritional exposure, but it is essential to have some indication of the validity of the measures of outcome (e.g., accuracy and completeness in an unbiased sample) *and* potential confounders and effect modifiers. There is no one right way to make any of these measures, the method used must be appropriate for the study being undertaken. It is important to be able to check the assumptions that the measures used are valid (consider also whether the measures are able to differentiate between subjects above and below cutoff points—sensitivity and specificity) before the study begins, because it may not be possible to adjust for measurement error appropriately in the analysis.

3.1. Nutritional Exposure

Nutritional exposure may cover individual foods or dietary patterns, as well as the substances added to foods. It may include the following:

1. The components found in foods (either nutrients or nonnutrients, such as phytochemicals).
2. Substances added to food during the growing, manufacturing, and processing of the food (additives, preservatives, and pesticides).
3. Chemical alterations that occur during cooking.
4. Markers of the dietary intake measured in body tissues or in bodily excretions.

In some situations nutritional exposure is inferred from anthropometric measurements or clinical signs of deficiency. Depending on which of these measures is the intended exposure, different approaches will be required, and different assumptions need to be made (and checked) about the validity and quality of the measures used to approximate the exposure.

The exposure needs to be measured with sufficient accuracy to enable the primary question of the research to be answered with reasonable confidence.

4. METHODS USED TO MEASURE DIET

The selection of an appropriate method to measure exposure and the correct use of that method must be considered before the study proper begins. Other texts have covered the different approaches that can be used to measure diet *(6,7)*.

Broadly, the appropriate methods may be described in terms of:
- The sample:
  - Individual
  - Group
  - Population
- Time frame
  - Current or past intake
  - Usual intake

- Critical period (biologically relevant)
- Unit of interest:
  - Food
  - Food patterns
  - Nutrients
  - Nonnutrients (as currently defined)
- Unit of expression:
  - Absolute or relative intake (grams of fat or percent energy from fat)
  - Cumulative exposure over time (e.g., total lifetime calcium intake)
  - The average exposure over time (e.g., amount of fat per day)
  - Peak exposure at a critical time (e.g., folate intake in first trimester of pregnancy)
- Level of accuracy required: study-specific based on question being addressed

5. UNDERSTANDING AND ASSESSING ERROR IN DIETARY DATA: IMPLICATIONS

Most nutritional epidemiological studies seek to explore the association between diet and health. To establish whether diet protects or harms health (increases or decreases risk), it is important to obtain the correct estimate of effect (measure of association) between what is eaten and outcome measure. For this relationship to be believed it must be assumed that the method used to assess diet is unbiased, and that the measurement error can be assessed and taken into account in the measure of the diet–health association. It is *never* possible to measure exposure without error, or to separate error from true within-person variation. Bias may lead to either exaggeration or attenuation of the measure of effect; it is often assumed that measurement error is random and that this will lead to an attenuation of effect. The level of attenuation also affects the statistical power of the study. If the measure of association is attenuated, it may be wrongly concluded that there is no association when there truly is one. It is important to first understand the sources of error so that these can be differentiated from the within-person variation in diet, and then it may be possible to consider how best to assess and then adjust for this error.

It may be difficult to separate the normal variation that exists in dietary habits from the error in measuring that variation. Part of the difficulty is defining the truth, usually through a validation study, the estimate of which is itself subject to error. Even if a correct estimate of the error can be obtained, it is not clear how to "adjust" for that in the analysis. It is increasingly clear that there is bias in dietary reporting; that is, those who under- or overreport their true consumption are not the same as those that report their true intake more accurately. Unless this source of "variation" in the overall measure of association is taken into account, the correct measure of association will be obscured (biased). It may be possible to explore the potential for bias by stratified analysis, but it is better to understand and eliminate the bias in the first place by consideration of the best methods to use for the target population under study. Kipnis et al. *(8)* and Freedman et al. *(9)* have discussed these issues in more detail, as well as providing the statistical approaches they have developed to deal with bias and error in the use of dietary assessment methods. There is still a great deal of debate in this area *(10–12)*. In this chapter, the underlying concepts and principles are summarized without the detail of the mathematical models. Figure 2

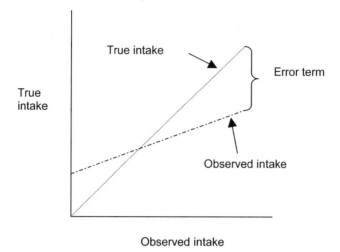

Observed intake

Fig. 2. Schematic of relationship between true intake and observed intake.
True intake = *observed intake* + *error term* (includes within-person variation in diet plus systematic and random error components associated with the instrument).
Attenuation factor (error term) = correlation between the true and observed intake X
Ratio of variance of true to observed intake

is a simplified schematic of the relationship between true and observed measures, and the way attenuation may be visualized.

In most epidemiological studies the aim is to assess the impact of long-term or usual intake. If we assume (not necessarily a valid assumption) that a 7-d weighed record is the best and most accurate assessment of a person's intake, and if subjects were asked to record their diet using this method on two separate occasions, and if the aim is to estimate fat intake, then it would be expected that there will be some difference between the means of fat intake for the two measures of fat intake. Part of this difference would be a reflection of the true difference in foods eaten between the two 7-d recordings, and part of it would be because people misreported (either accidentally or deliberately) what they ate during each recording, and that there were some differences in which foods or what amount was misreported. It may be that people accurately reported what they ate, but that they changed their diet during the period of recording. If the misreporting was exactly the same (or if there was none) for each assessment, then the difference between the two recordings would be the differences in what people ate over the two recording periods. This latter source of variation is not error. A food frequency questionnaire (FFQ) when repeated may give different answers for the same reasons, although it is assumed that the FFQ does not reflect what is eaten during any single week, but is a summary measure of usual intake, and may therefore have a smaller component of within-subject variation, because of real changes in diet. It is a good idea, however, to ask people if their diet has changed from the first to the second period of assessment.

Although in theory it is easy to visualize the attenuation factor (error term), in practice it is difficult to calculate, and it must be assumed that the error is nondifferential (unbiased) with respect to health outcome that is the being explored in the diet–health study.

6. VALIDATION

Whenever any information is being collected, it is important to assess whether it is *fit for purpose*, i.e., whether the measure used is valid. A measure is valid if it measures what it purports to measure. The purpose of the validation study is to assess the attenuation factor (as Kipnis et al. *[8]* describe it). In most situations it is not possible to have an absolute measure of the true exposure, and the new or *test measure* of exposure is usually compared with another measure, which is considered from previous research to be more accurate (the *reference measure*) than the new measure. A study that compares these measures is a validation study, but should be referred to as a study of the relative validity (sometimes called concurrent validity) of the test compared with the reference measure. Many prefer to call this a calibration study as it reflects the reality that one measure is calibrated against another.

If a test measure is compared with a reference measure, it is assumed that the reporting errors in the test measure are not related to the errors in the reference measure. It is assumed that the reference measure only contains within-person random error, and that this error is uncorrelated with the error in the reference measure *(8)*. Ideally, what is required is some measure of the following: person-specific biases, intake-related biases, and a measure of within-person random errors (or true within-person variation in intake). It is further assumed that both intake-related and person-specific biases are zero. It will be difficult to establish whether all these assumptions are true. It may be that certain biomarkers are good estimates of the true intake, for example for energy assessed as expenditure with doubly labeled water and urinary nitrogen, but there are few other biomarkers that can, with confidence, be shown to be a better estimate of the truth than multiple days of dietary recording estimate. It should be remembered that although a biochemical parameter may be measured with more technical accuracy, it cannot be assumed that it is a better measure of dietary behavior.

Given that it is unlikely that there will be perfect agreement between a test and a reference measure, and given that no reference measure can be considered a perfect measure, it is reasonable to ask what level of agreement may be acceptable to decide whether the test measure is useful. As a check on the accuracy of the reference measure some workers now use two reference measures *(10)*. It is assumed that one of the reference measures is able to measure the true exposure more accurately. For example, urinary nitrogen and a 7-d weighed record will be used as the reference measures to assess relative validity of a questionnaire. It is assumed the errors of the two reference measures are unrelated and independent from the errors of the test method. It would be expected that the two reference measures should be highly correlated with each other, and, if they are not, it may suggest that the reference measure (7-d weighed record) is not a good measure of the underlying truth. If the correlation between the test and reference measures is then calculated, it may be that the lack of agreement between them is not because the test measure does not measure the truth, but because the reference measure does not. It would be unreasonable to expect the test and reference measure to be more highly correlated than the two reference measures, so it is also possible, therefore, to judge the expected realistic maximum correlation.

The correct way to express the results from a validation study depends on how the measures are going to be used in the main study. If absolute intakes are required, then the validation must assess how well the test measure assesses absolute intake. If the purpose is to rank subjects and assess change in risk across levels of exposure (say fourths or fifths), then the validation study must assess the degree of misclassification likely between fourths or fifths of the distribution. Simply expressing the association between a test and reference measure using a correlation coefficient may be misleading and unhelpful. Ideally, the required level of accuracy of the test measure should be established before the study begins. The measure of validity can then be used in the design, analysis, and interpretation of the main study. Where the measure of validity is assessed during, rather than before, the main study, careful thought needs to be given as to how the results will be analyzed and used in the interpretation of the main study.

It is very useful to present plots of data. This has the benefit of showing the actual data, identifies the impact that potential outliers may have, and gives a clearer sense of the agreement between test and reference measure across the range of values in the population. Figure 3B presents the scatterplot for a 4-d weighed intake estimate of folate with the red blood cell (RBC) folate level in the same population of the elderly in the United Kingdom. This example may be used to illustrate some general points; here we assume the weighed intake is the test measure, and the RBC folate is the reference measure. The overall Spearman correlation was 0.31, which was highly statistically significant. The scatterplot shows that for both measures there are a few high values, particularly for RBC folate, which occur across a range of lower dietary folate levels. The plot shows that the R-squared value is about 7%, which suggests that relatively little of the variation in RBC folate is explained by the dietary folate measure. It would not be easy to predict a person's dietary intake from the blood level. When each variable is categorized into thirds, 43% of subjects are allocated to the same third using both measures, and 13% are grossly misclassified into opposite thirds (*see* Fig. 3A). If we assume that the RBC folate level was correct (the reference measure), then the 4-d weighed intake estimates this truth reasonably well, but even so, more than half the sample would be misclassified.

7. UNDERREPORTING AND OVERREPORTING

Underreporting and, to a lesser extent, overreporting are potentially important aspects of measurement error. The primary concern with misreporting is that it leads to bias, based on the assumption that those people who misreport their diet do so deliberately or, for various reasons, truthfully but uniformly underestimate or overestimate their actual intake. It is therefore necessary to assess the likely size and effect of under- or overreporting. This can be done by comparison of measured intakes with true intakes or proxy measures. Most work has been done on energy intake, using measures of energy expenditure as a check. If energy intake is less than measured energy expenditure, then it may be concluded that energy intake is underreported if subjects are not losing weight or are in an unstable metabolic condition. Black and colleagues (*13*) have shown that

A Number of subjects in each third

		Thirds of red blood cell folate			
		1	2	3	Total
Thirds of dietary folate	1	166+	114	79*	359
	2	132	127+	110	369
	3	75*	145	194+	414
Total		373	386	383	1142

B Scatter plot

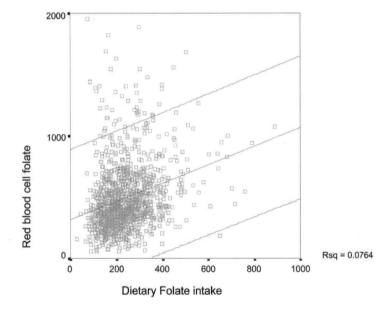

Fig. 3. Relationship between dietary intake of folate and red blood cell folate. **(A)** Number of subjects in each third. Each variable divided into thirds cross-tabulated. Plus signs (+) represent where exact agreement in allocation, asterisks (*) where allocation in opposite thirds. **(B)** Scatter plot (regression line with 95% confidence intervals); Rsq R-squared. (Spearman correlation 0.31; $p < 0.001$). Data extracted from the National Diet and Nutrition Survey: people aged 65 yr and over (*see* ref. *20* for more details).

underreporting can occur across the whole range of intakes, and that it may be misleading to use an arbitrary cut-off to define underreporting. Recently, however, Subar et al. *(14)* have defined underreporting as reported energy intake lower than the 95% confidence interval of the log ratio of reported intakes to biomarker measurements.

For epidemiological purposes, energy expenditure can be estimated using a regression equation that only requires information on the age, gender, and weight of the subject *(15)*. This simple measure of basal metabolic rate (BMR) relates well to measured energy expenditure and can be used to compare energy expenditure with a measure of dietary intake. If the estimated energy intake is less than the BMR (or a bit more to allow for some level of activity—often $1.2 \times$ BMR, *see* ref. *13* for more details), it suggests that the estimated energy intake is unrealistically low.

There are a number of ways that this measure of underreporting should be used in the analysis and interpretation of the study. It is often assumed that all subjects below an agreed level of the energy/BMR (E/BMR) ratio should simply be excluded from the study. However, before doing this, and thereby losing considerable statistical power, it is worth exploring whether the underreporting has led to a biased estimate of effect (altered the relationship between the measured exposure estimate and outcome). Ideally, the relationship between exposure and outcome should be explored separately in people with E/BMR ratios above and below the agreed cut-off. If the relationship found within each stratum of E/BMR is different, then there is a suggestion of bias and the results from the two strata should not be combined because the estimated measure of effect would be incorrect. If, however, the relationship is similar in each stratum, it may suggest that there is no bias and that the estimate of effect would not be distorted by leaving all the subjects in the analysis. It is also worth checking whether the E/BMR ratio is different in different levels of other potentially confounding factors such as age, gender, and BMI. If over-weight people underestimate their intake more than average-weight people, and BMI is associated with the exposure–outcome relationship, then it will be important to take account of the differential underreporting of energy intake in overweight subjects.

Tooze et al. *(16)* have recently explored the psychosocial predictors of energy underreporting for both a FFQ and a 24-h recall, using doubly labeled water in the OPEN study. They found that the predictors of underreporting were different in men and women. Among women, underreporting was more common using the FFQ among those with a fear of negative evaluation and a history of weight loss, as well among those women with a higher percentage energy from fat. For men, BMI, comparison of activity level with that of others, and eating frequency were the best predictors of underreporting based on the FFQ. However, it should be noted that for the FFQ in both men and women, the variables described above accounted for only a small proportion (about 10%) of the variation in the estimate of energy intake. A key question was to identify the sources of the remaining 90% of the variation. In the 24-h recalls, where the models explained more of the variation (about 25%), the factors that predicted underreporting in women were social desirability, fear of negative evaluation, BMI, percentage of energy from fat, usual activity, and variability in number of meals, whereas in men it was social desirability, dietary restraint, BMI, eating frequency, dieting history, and education.

Intakes of other nutrients or foods may also be under- or overreported. The direction of effect may depend on a host of factors related to the perception of subjects and the methods used. It is often assumed that vegetable and fruit consumption is overestimated and that fat intake is underestimated. However, the analysis of recalled fat intake in women with breast cancer, when compared to actual intake 10 yr before, suggested that cases overestimated their past intake *(4)*. The reason put forward was that women who had breast cancer and "knew fat caused breast cancer" overestimated their true past exposure. Apart from a reasonably accurate biological marker of energy expenditure and perhaps protein intake (multiple 24-h urinary nitrogen excretion), there are few measures of true dietary exposure that can be used to check the accuracy of reported intakes.

There are few studies that have assessed measurement error in populations from the Southern Hemisphere, and without evidence it should not be assumed that the errors in reporting intake in these populations will be the same as in Northern Hemisphere countries. The same applies to economically deprived areas of Europe or North America.

8. ENERGY ADJUSTMENT

The concept of energy density and the optimal approach to expressing the levels of intakes, particularly of macronutrients (protein, fat, and carbohydrate), has been debated for many years. The prevailing view suggests that the relevant measure of exposure for macronutrients is the intake relative to energy intake, rather than a simple measure of absolute intake. One reason for expressing macronutrient intake relative to energy intake is that it makes it easier to compare intakes across different levels of energy intake, for example, men and women and different ages. In judging whether it is appropriate to adjust for energy intake, it is important to consider whether it is logical from a biological or mechanistic perspective. Data should be analyzed with and without adjusting for energy to assess the impact that adjusting may have on the interpretation of results. It may be that for some situations the absolute level of intake is a more relevant measure of exposure.

Energy adjustment is most useful when the following conditions hold true (after Flegal [17]):

- The exposure of interest is not the absolute amount of the nutrient but the amount relative to energy.
- Energy over- or underreporting is proportionally the same for all foods, so that the correct proportion of the nutrient to energy intake is reported.

If these conditions do not apply, energy adjustment may be misleading.

9. BIOLOGICAL SAMPLES

Samples may be taken from a wide range of body tissues and fluids and are potentially useful markers or indicators of exposure and outcome. The use of biological markers of dietary intake is attractive because they appear to be more objective measurements of exposure than measures of intake derived by questioning the subjects themselves. This assumption should always be tested before using biological markers to infer dietary intake. A particular issue to consider is that most markers do not provide a measure of absolute intake, only the relative ranking of intakes. Although the technical errors of measurement (repeatability) of markers may be smaller, the marker may not be a relevant measure of the dietary exposure of interest. For a biological marker to be a useful indicator of exposure it must be sensitively and specifically related to dietary intake across the range of intakes in the population under study. Ideally, as the level of dietary exposure increases or decreases, so should the level of the biological marker. That is, there should be a time-related relationship between the marker and the dietary intake of interest. This may be the case, for example, between urinary nitrogen excretion and dietary protein intake, but for most other readily available markers this is not the case. Most markers used at present are concentrations in blood, which may not accurately reflect the intake over the time frame required. There are a complex series of steps involved in the absorption, transport, and distribution of a nutrient found in food and subsequently measured as a

Table 1
Summary of Study Designs Used in Nutritional Epidemiological Research

Study design	Populations	Study group individuals
Experimental	Community trials or Community Intervention studies	Clinical trials (therapeutic or secondary or tertiary prevention) Field trials (primary prevention). Field intervention studies.
Observational	Ecological studies	Cross-sectional (prevalence) studies. Case–control (referent) studies. Cohort (longitudinal) studies.

biological sample. The circulating level may be dependent on a range of other potentially rate-limiting factors. It may be, therefore, that there is only a weak relationship between dietary intake and a marker because the level measured in blood, for example, is dependent on a transport protein or other coenzymes. Other texts have discussed these issues further *(3,4)*.

Although the potential benefits of biomarkers are attractive, they should not be used uncritically. The following should be considered:

- Most markers can generally only be used as indicators of the relative ranking of individual dietary intakes in a group and do not generally provide a measure that is indicative of absolute dietary intake.
- Most markers are measured as a concentration that may not reflect the amount of the substance available at the site of biological function; blood levels may be regulated by the body and may not truly reflect the availability of the substance; removal or addition of a substance to the measure used in the blood may be limited by the availability of other related limiting substances (e.g., retinol binding protein).
- Correlations between true intake levels and markers tend not be any better than between true intake and more traditional dietary methods (such as recalls and questionnaires). This may be partly explained by the relatively fast turnover rates in many markers and large intraindividual variation in true intake.
- The level of a marker, such as plasma β-carotene, may only be partly determined by the dietary intake of carotene. The marker may be a proxy or indicator of a dietary pattern.
- The level of the marker may be affected by other factors, such as smoking or drugs.

10. TYPES OF EPIDEMIOLOGICAL STUDIES

Broadly, epidemiological studies can be divided into experimental and observational investigations (*see* **Table 1**). The main study designs will be briefly summarized; further texts provide more detail *(3)*. For all studies where data are collected from individuals, some *a priori* information is required about how common the exposure and outcome are likely to be in the study population, and what effect the exposure is expected to have on outcome. Without this information, it will not be possible to ascertain how many subjects to include in a study, or how accurately exposure must be able to be measured. In *all* studies, a thorough literature review should be conducted as a first step to help in the design of the study.

10.1. Ecological Studies

In ecological studies of the association between nutrition and health, population or group indices of dietary intake or nutritional status (exposure) are related to population or group indices of health status (outcome). The unit of analysis is not an individual but a group defined by time (e.g., calendar year or birth cohort), geography (e.g., country, province, or city), or socio-demographic characteristics (e.g., ethnicity, religion, or socio-economic status). For example, national dietary fat intake for each country in Europe (from Food and Agriculture Organization food balance sheet data) can be plotted against rates of heart disease for each country. Within a country, national trends for consumption of foods may be plotted against trends for morbidity or mortality. Ecological studies are helpful when within-group (country or region) variation in exposure is small compared with between-group variation. It is often difficult in ecological studies to control for other potentially confounding factors and to explore interactions. When comparing national levels of exposure and outcome, it is important to consider the relevant time frame for comparison; there is likely to be some lag time between exposure and its effect on outcome.

Ecological studies are ideal for exploring newly proposed hypotheses; this serves as a basis for developing more detailed individual level studies in the future. Ecological studies are weak in terms of drawing causal inferences about the effects of factors operating at an individual level. In some situations, individual level data are not available and an ecological approach is all that is available. Ecological studies may be very useful for monitoring national trends in health indicators and the wider social, cultural, economic, and environmental factors that influence health that cannot be measured at an individual level.

10.2. Cross-Sectional Studies

Cross-sectional studies (sometimes described as "prevalence surveys") measure both exposure and outcome in the present and at the same point in time in individuals. Generally, cross-sectional studies sample from the population in such a way as to reflect the population characteristics for both exposure and outcome and thus can be used to describe the prevalence of nutrition problems in a community. If information on population characteristics (e.g., age, gender, income, and education) is also collected, it can be used to assess the influence these factors may have on the exposure–outcome relationship. When repeated in the same population, a cross-sectional survey can be used for surveillance and monitoring.

The sampling frame, number of subjects (sample size and power), response rate, and potential information bias may all influence the validity of the prevalence estimates derived. If a particular sector of the sample is excluded (e.g., malnourished children too sick to participate), the prevalence estimate and reported associations may be misleading. The optimal sample size should be calculated before the study starts to ensure that enough subjects are included. Sample size is determined by the prevalence of the measures of interest, differences expected in the estimates of prevalence between groups in the study, the accuracy of the measures, and the required level of statistical power. Failure to detect statistically significant differences between groups may be a function of sample size. If exposure and outcome measures are rare in a general population sample, a very large sample size will be required to estimate the prevalence of these measures with any accuracy.

In a cross-sectional study the measure of interest is often expressed at a group level such as the average intake or proportion above a cutoff. As long as the distribution of the population can be correctly described to ensure that the measure of central tendency (such as the average) is correct, assuming a sufficiently large sample and that the errors of reporting exposure are random (rather than systematic that may lead to bias), it does not matter if each individual's actual intake is not measured exactly. This means that a 24-h dietary recall could be used, which does not estimate within-person variation. The researcher cannot describe individual intakes using this approach, and the identification of individuals at risk (of being too high or too low) cannot be made; what can be said is that a certain proportion of the population may be above or below a cutoff.

The main disadvantage of cross-sectional studies is that it is not possible to determine temporality in an attempt to disentangle cause from effect because the exposure is not measured before the onset of the outcome. It may be that, for example, the outcome or illness may have altered the dietary patterns, rather than the other way around (for example, someone starts drinking milk to relieve symptoms after they get an ulcer). Nevertheless, cross-sectional studies can take into account other potentially confounding factors.

10.3. Case–Control Studies

Case–control studies (sometimes termed case–referent studies) start with subjects defined in some way as cases and controls (or outcome plus, outcome minus) and assess past exposure to assess risk of past exposure on outcome status. The estimate of risk is the odds ratio, as true risk cannot be assessed because of the different ways cases are selected. The odds ratio is calculated as the odds of being exposed in the cases compared with the odds of being exposed in the controls; if the odds are higher in cases than controls, it can be inferred that the exposure increases risk. Case–control designs are efficient where the outcome (e.g., ovarian or liver cancer) is rare (in an absolute sense) and all available cases can be recruited from the population of interest, where the range of exposure is sufficient to reflect some important potential for impact on outcome, and where the exposure is common.

Ideally, a population is defined (e.g., the catchment area of a hospital or the walking distance for mothers to bring malnourished children to a clinic) from which all cases of interest are identified over a specified period of time. This population must be sufficiently large to generate a statistically viable number of cases. Controls are then drawn at random from the same population from which the cases are drawn. All noncases could be recruited for comparison, but it is more statistically efficient to take a sample of the population. Controls are often selected at random and matched on certain characteristics that are known to influence outcome, but that of themselves are of no direct interest in the study (e.g., age and gender). It is necessary to consider how exposure is defined. Usually exposure is categorized into groups, in the simplest form as exposed and not exposed. For smoking, this may be clear. For diet, it is less obvious as to what level is defined as exposed; is it those above the median, or in the highest third, or above some biologically determined threshold? Obviously, the way the exposed group is defined will have a direct effect on the way the unexposed group is defined. It is clear that in defining risk it should always be stated as to how exposed and unexposed have been defined, and the interpretation of risk needs to reflect this. It is statistically most efficient to use a continuous measure of exposure, and assess risk per unit change of exposure. Where exposure is categorized, it is statistically most efficient to define the exposed as above the median.

The decision as to what level is defined as exposed has implications for sample size and power of the study. If, for example, the study asks the question as to whether vegetarians have a lower risk of cancer than omnivores, then it is important to know how common vegetarianism is (and how it is defined) in the population. Remember that in a case–control study subjects are recruited based on outcome status, without knowledge of their exposure status. In the United Kingdom, about 5% of the general population are vegetarians. This prevalence estimate is required to estimate how many subjects need to be recruited to detect a desired level of effect with reasonable confidence (say 80% power at the 5% level of statistical significance). Let us say that 200 exposed subjects (vegetarians) are required, then to have this number, 4000 cases and 4000 controls will be required; this means that there will be 3800 subjects in each of the unexposed groups. For such an uncommon exposure a case–control study may not be the ideal design. Case–control studies are most efficient for common exposures.

For chronic diseases, the dietary exposure of interest is usually some time in the past nearer to the time when diet may have been "causing" the disease to develop. Subjects are usually asked to recall their exposure, or it is assumed that current exposure reflects past exposure. The wrong estimate of effect occurs when cases and controls misreport their exposure differently. If both cases and controls misreport their diet in the same way, then (perhaps counterintuitively) the odds ratio will actually reflect the true effect of differences in exposure. Differential misreporting may occur when cases reflect back as to why they got the disease, and embellish their true exposure, whereas controls have not reflected as to their past behavior. This has been suggested as the main reason why case–control studies overestimate the effect of fat intake on risk of breast cancer in US studies, compared with findings from cohort studies (4).

When comparing results from different studies, it is important to check how exposure is defined; it may be that there are differences in the results between studies, not because of any underlying differences in effect, but simply in the way the risk was assessed. For example, if one study defined exposed as having a processed meat intake above three times per day, and another study defined it as once a day, and let us say that the true threshold of effect is two times per day, then in the study that used once a day as a definition of exposed, the exposed group will contain people who are truly not exposed, leading to a dilution of the estimate of effect. Caution is required in pooling estimates of effect from different studies without first checking that the range of exposure in the group defined as exposed is comparable across studies.

10.4. Cohort Studies

Cohort studies (sometimes called "prospective studies") measure exposure in the present, whereas outcome is assessed at some point in the future. They start by defining levels of exposure and following people forward in time to see how exposure affects the outcome. At the start of the study outcome status is unknown, unlike in case–control studies that select participants with known outcome status. As in the discussion above for case–control studies, it is important to consider how exposure status is defined. Cohort studies are ideal when the exposure of interest is relatively rare or uncommon (such as for being a vegetarian), as it is possible to preselect subjects from a wider population that satisfy the required level of exposure for inclusion. The power of a cohort study is determined by the projected incidence of the outcome, as the estimate of risk is the ratio of the incidence of outcome in exposed compared with unexposed. Unlike cross-sectional surveys, a cohort study can assess temporality of a putative cause (exposure) and its effect (outcome), as the exposure is measured before the outcome is known, and therefore not influenced by knowledge of the outcome status.

The sample for a cohort study is not always selected to represent the distribution within the whole population. The sample may be weighted to maximize heterogeneity of exposure, or it might be selected to minimize loss to follow-up; both of these factors may be considered to be of more importance than the representativeness of the sample. For both cohort and experimental studies, the primary concern is to select a sample that is not going to be lost in the follow-up period. For example, a number of large cohort studies follow up health professionals who have to be registered to maintain their practice, and so can be traced through these registers.

Cohort designs can be an efficient way of sampling rare exposures from the population; the benefit here is that it is possible to maximize the range of dietary exposure that can be studied. For example, vegetarians with very different dietary habits from the general population can be recruited and compared with a sample of omnivores to explore the effects of the dietary differences on health outcomes. If one was to take a random sample of the population, only about 5% are vegetarians, and so the sample would need to be very large to recruit sufficient vegetarians to have a statistically viable sample. It is important to consider how many people are required to be followed over what length of time to have sufficient disease endpoints to calculate an estimate of the risk of disease in the vegetarian group compared with the omnivore group.

In a cohort study, the exposure measure is often divided into thirds or fourths of the distribution and the change of risk assessed across these categories (logistic regression). The requirement for the measure of exposure in this type of analysis is that the measured intakes of subjects can accurately rank the true intake of the population (i.e., so that people with high and low intakes can be differentiated). The selection of the cut-off points used to define groups may critically affect the estimate of risk obtained. Some authors prefer to use a regression approach where instead of grouping data, each individual observation contributes to the regression equation (multiple regression); what is then described is the change in outcome per unit change in exposure. Both approaches, multiple logistic and linear regression, allow for the adjustment of the effects of other factors.

Cohort studies are often very large, may take many years to be conducted, and are usually expensive. As with other study designs, where confounding factors need to be considered, so does the accuracy of the measures of exposure used. Measurement error and misclassification may lead to nonstatistically significant associations that may not reflect the true underlying associations.

10.5. Experimental Studies

Experimental studies are the most robust test of a causal hypothesis. An experiment is the only study design where the exposure ("treatment") is actually manipulated by the researcher and the effect that manipulation has on outcome can be assessed. The most important aspect of experimental studies is that allocation to different treatment groups is random and not influenced either by the observer or the participant. In other respects, apart from random allocation of treatment, experimental studies may be considered to be similar to cohort studies. Experimental studies sometimes select representative samples of the whole population (community interventions), or sometimes samples of people from selected outcome groups (clinical trials). The primary questions to answer in designing an experiment are: what is the required length of follow-up to ensure that the treatment has time to alter metabolic processes necessary to affect outcome?; how should compliance with the treatment regime be checked?; how should observer and participant effects be minimized?; and is the sample size adequate to measure the hypothesized effect with reasonable statistical confidence?

11. DEVELOPING CULTURALLY SENSITIVE AND SPECIFIC MEASURES OF EXPOSURE

Considerable effort has been expended in identifying optimal approaches to measuring dietary exposure in North American and European populations. Most approaches that have been developed assume a certain degree of literacy and numeracy. Extrapolating methods from one social group to another within a country is likely to lead to problems; these are magnified many times when extrapolating from one country and culture to another. The following list summarizes a number of key points to consider when developing methods, particularly where the researcher may not be familiar with the local situation. Wherever the research is conducted, the best possible approach should be used, and where some compromise must be made, the effect this has on the validity of the study should be considered before the study begins. A poorly conducted study will not help address major public health problems because it will not answer the key questions. Lack of resources, although being a real constraint for research and development in many parts of the world, should not be used as an excuse for poorly thought-out research. Priority must be given to addressing issues that are of major public health concern. It is also patronizing to suggest that a cheaper, secondhand approach is good enough in poorer countries, in many ways the opposite could be argued. Greatest effort and attention to detail should be directed to places of greatest need and potential impact. An important part of research should be to develop the human resources and skills base in each country in which the work is done.

- General issues
  - ○ If things can go wrong, they probably will, so assume this as a starting point and (based on your previous experience) check assumptions you are tempted to make.
  - ○ When undertaking fieldwork, consider the local infrastructure required to do the work. Consider the effect your presence will have on local coworkers' responsibilities and consider their needs, just as you would expect to be treated yourself. Consider what local colleagues will get out of the work you are doing.
  - ○ If you use equipment in remote areas, consider what might happen if it goes wrong (and halfway through your study!). Always consider robust, simple, accurate methods and have a backup strategy.
  - ○ Decide what you really need to know and what level of support you require to gather that level of information (i.e., can individuals do what you want, do you have to use observational techniques or other approaches not dependent on numeracy or literacy).
  - ○ Check whether your proposed fieldworkers are acceptable to the local community (in some communities women do not like strangers either watching them cook, or touching their food, but may be quite happy for a locally known person to do this).
  - ○ How do you get informed consent from subjects? If the community elders approve, is this adequate?
- Specific dietary issues
  - ○ Start the process by talking to the target group (focus group discussion) to identify how they describe foods and their preparation (and names used); this will help clarify whether your concepts are similar to those of the target group.
  - ○ Consider how to check the accuracy (validity) of the method to be used; if the population is illiterate, different reference measures may be required; if a biological measure is used, consider impact of infection or poor nutritional status on sensitivity of measure to range of dietary intake.
  - ○ Some foods may be taboo at certain times in certain groups of people—check this before you start. Check also fasting or festival days—in many cultures these occur very often and should be considered as part of a normal or usual diet (i.e., they should not always simply be excluded).
  - ○ Check when, where, and how people access their food; assessing diet just after payday may give very different results from just before payday.
  - ○ If people grow their own food, they may consider and report this differently from purchased food.
  - ○ Consider the impact of social and family dynamic on what individuals within a group might eat—men may eat before women, boys are sometimes fed before girls, and mothers may simply eat what, if anything, is left.
  - ○ Consider the possibility that people are telling you what they think you want to hear. How can this be checked? Think of cross-checking questions and perhaps ways to unobtrusively observe behavior.
  - ○ Do not make assumptions about what appears to be a simple diet. Consider the role of rarely eaten but rich sources of nutrients (or foods gathered in the field while working, as well as those cooked at home).
  - ○ Consider using complementary methods, such as 24-h recalls and FFQs, together in cross-sectional or cohort study. This combination of approaches may allow an estimate of gram weights of foods, as well as an estimate of the frequency of consumption of rarely eaten foods that may be rich in nutrients.

- o Assess whether you need to use an observational approach or whether you can rely on self-reported intakes (consider literacy, but also social desirability bias leading to dietary change).
- o Where families eat from a communal pot, observational techniques may be required (if the research requires individual level assessment).
- o Pretest and pilot different approaches before you start actual data collection; it is likely your preconceived ideas are not appropriate.
- o If you want to determine amounts of foods consider all options; portion size estimation and assumptions may not be valid (e.g., in our study in India, within-household variation in roti [local type of unleavened bread] size was very small from day to day, but between- household variation was great; our approach was to weigh a series of rotis in each family before the study and use that as the portion size for that family).
- o Where a staple is the main source of energy (or a single food item is the main source of a vitamin or mineral), estimating the correct portion size may be more important for that staple or food item than where there is a wider variety of foods contributing to the nutrient of interest.
- o Consider potential seasonal variation and other sources of foods not immediately obvious (such as food sent by friends or relatives in a city).
- o When planning interventions to change dietary patterns, consider income that may be sent from abroad and other family responsibilities.
- • Physical activity
  - o Check concepts of distance and time before asking simple questions about length of time engaged in different activities. Proxy measures may be required, and the validity of these measures will need to be checked.

12. SUMMARY OF KEY POINTS TO CONSIDER IN DESIGNING A NUTRITIONAL EPIDEMIOLOGICAL STUDY

The following list summarizes key points that may help the reader in either designing or critically reading a report of original research in nutritional epidemiology. The information has been modified after Sempos et al. *(19)*.

- • The goal is to assess how dietary exposure relates to health risk; different epidemiological approaches can be used, with strengths and weaknesses that need to be considered.
- • The relationship between dietary exposure and health risk is complex. The link between what is eaten, absorbed, and incorporated into cell function, and the effect this has on biological processes that may affect "health" (i.e., the host's ability to maintain optimal function at the cellular, organ, and whole-body level) may be modulated by other factors that need to be considered at the same time.
- • Before using a method, it is essential to check whether it provides a measure that is appropriately accurate. This assumes that a validation study is undertaken before the proper study begins—the development of the method needs to take into account the social and cultural context in which it will be used.
- • Covariates (dietary and other factors) related to the exposure of interest need to be measured with minimal and known error (same issues as applied to measurement error and impact for exposure of interest).
- • Check that the nutrient database used is complete for the foods and nutrients you are interested in.

- The method used to assess exposure must reflect the above complexity.
- Exposure can be measured using traditional dietary survey methodology, but may also include measures of nutritional status (biochemical, anthropometric, and clinical); biomarkers of intake; and biological intermediaries, concentrations of which are influenced by diet.
- All dietary survey methods have flaws. For whatever purpose the dietary data are collected, the measure derived from the method will have some error and will not be a perfect measure of the true required exposure.
- Measures derived from biological samples are likely to have less technical error (no underreporting or information bias) than dietary measures, and where it is possible to establish a dose–response relationship with dietary exposure, this may be the preferred method from which to derive the measure of exposure. It is important to consider whether the biological measure is related to the relevant exposure of interest (in terms of time frame and dose); concentrations in blood may not indicate the true functional dynamic state of the availability of the measure being made.
- Prospective studies must be able to capture changes in dietary patterns over time with sufficient accuracy to determine whether that change is related to the change in outcome; this is related to sample size and the variability of the measure used, and assumes nondifferential errors in reporting exposure.
- It is always good practice to check for differential reporting errors in subjects in the study; this can be done by age, gender, BMI, or energy expenditure.
- Statistical modeling cannot adjust for or eliminate the effects of bias, nor can it eliminate the effects of the complex biological interaction between different aspects of diet (and in some cases it should not be used where dietary patterns interact as discussed in Section 5).
- It may not be appropriate to use the estimates of the errors of dietary measures derived from validation studies to "adjust or correct" the measure of exposure–outcome relationship. The assumption about the direction, specificity, and effects of the error need to be carefully considered before assuming that the effect of the error is to lead to attenuation of effect; it is possible that differential error may lead to an exaggeration of effect.
- Evaluation of causal relationships generally requires the integration of information from the basic, clinical, and population sciences, including epidemiology.
- Causal inferences should be drawn with caution and only after considering the possible effects of chance, bias, and confounding, and the effects of study design (particularly in observational studies) and measurement error on the size and direction of measures of effect reported.

ACKNOWLEDGMENTS

I would like to thank my colleagues Michael Nelson, Alan Jackson, Shobha Rao, Este Vorster, Rachel Thompson, and Daniel Warm for helpful discussions that have shaped this chapter. Any errors or omissions are the sole responsibility of the author.

REFERENCES

1. Byers T. The role of epidemiology in developing nutritional recommendations: past, present and future. Am J Clin Nutr 1999; 69:1340S–1348S.
2. Last JM, ed. A Dictionary of Epidemiology. Third Edition. Oxford University Press, New York, 1995.

3. Margetts BM, Nelson M, eds. Design Concepts in Nutritional Epidemiology. Second Edition. Oxford University Press, Oxford, 1997.

4. Willett W. Nutritional Epidemiology. Second Edition. Oxford University Press, New York, 1998.

5. Armstrong BK, White E, Saracci R. Principles of Exposure Measurement in Epidemiology. Oxford University Press, Oxford, 1992.

6. Cameron ME, van Staveren WA, eds. Manual on Methodology for Food Consumption Studies. Oxford University Press, Oxford, 1988.

7. Margetts BM, Nelson M. Measuring dietary exposure in nutritional epidemiological studies. Nutr Res Rev 1995; 5:165–178.

8. Kipnis V, Midthune D, Freedman L, et al. Bias in dietary-report instruments and its implications for nutritional epidemiology. Public Health Nutr 2002; 5:915–923.

9. Freedman LS, Fainberg V, Kipnis V, Midthune D, Carroll RJ. A new method for dealing with measurement error in explanatory variables of regression models. Biometrics 2004; 60:172–181.

10. Kipnis V, Subar AF, Midthune D, et al. Structure of dietary measurement error: results of the OPEN biomarker study. Am J Epidemiol 2003; 158:14–21.

11. Willett W. Invited commentary: OPEN Questions. Am J Epidemiol 2003; 158:22–24.

12. Kipnis V, Subar AF, Schatzkin A, et al. Kipnis et al. respond to "OPEN Questions." Am J Epidemiol 2003; 158:25–26.

13. Black, AE, Prentice AM, Goldberg GR, et al. Measurements of total energy expenditure provide insights into the validity of dietary measurements of energy intake. J Am Diet Assoc 1993; 93:572–579.

14. Subar AF, Kipnis V, Troiano RP, et al. Using intake biomarkers to evaluate the extent of dietary misreporting in a large sample of adults: The OPEN Study. Am J Epidemiol 2003; 158:1–13.

15. Food and Agricultural Organization/World Health Organization/United Nations University. Energy and protein requirements. Report of a joint expert consultation. WHO Technical Report Series no. 724. World Health Organization, Geneva, 1985.

16. Tooze JA, Subar AF, Thompson FE, Troiano R, Schatzkin A, Kipnis V. Psychosocial predictors of energy underreporting in a large doubly labeled water study. Am J Clin Nutr 2004; 79:795–804.

17. Flegal KM. Evaluating epidemiologic evidence of the effects of food and nutrient exposures. Am J Clin Nutr 1999; 69:1339S–1344S.

18. Kaaks R, Riboli E, Sinha R. Biochemical markers of dietary intake. In: Toniolo P, B11offetta P, Shuker DEG, Tothman N, Hulka B, Pearce N, eds. Application of Biomarkers in Cancer Epidemiology. IARC (International Agency for Research on Cancer) Scientific Publications No. 142. Oxford University Press, Oxford, 1997, pp. 7103–7126.

19. Sempos CT, Liu K, Ernst ND. Food and nutrient exposures: what to consider when evaluating epidemiologic evidence. Am J Clin Nutr 1999; 69:1330S–1338S.

20. Finch S, Doyle W, Lowe C, et al. National Diet and Nutrition Survey: People Aged 65 Years and Over. The Stationary Office, London, 1998.

2

Challenges in Research in Nutritional Epidemiology

David R. Jacobs, Jr.

KEY POINTS

- Diet is a complex aggregate of foods and behaviors. The food is comprised of a wide variety of intended and unintended chemicals that may act singly on human metabolism, but more likely act as a group in a synergistic fashion.
- The study of nutrition and disease in aggregates of human beings—nutritional epidemiology—is hampered by the difficulty in accurately characterizing this complex aggregate, that is, in stating what people are eating. Part of this difficulty is inherent in the large day-to-day variability in what is eaten. Another part of the difficulty relates to finding efficient and accurate ways to collect dietary information, minimizing participant burden, and maximizing utility of the data for investigators.
- Much progress has been made in nutritional epidemiology in recent years owing to the use of food frequency questionnaires, which pose little participant burden and are relatively easy to analyze. However, such data collection instruments are still characterized by high within-person variation and at the same time, severely limit collection of important details about diet.
- The author speculates on protocol changes and computer technology advances that might allow more complete and accurate diet data collection.
- It is important to study foods, food groups, and food patterns, as well as nutrients and other chemicals contained in food. Food is what people eat. Where many chemical constituents of a food act synergistically, an association will be found with the food but none will be found with individual constituents. The association of food patterns with risk provides feedback to policy makers on the likely success of nutritional pronouncements.

1. INTRODUCTION

Much has been written about the practice and challenges of research in nutritional epidemiology. For general details concerning this topic, the reader is referred to existing and extensive source materials, including *Design Concepts in Epidemiology*, edited by Margetts and Nelson (ref. *1*; *see also* Chapter 1) and *Nutritional Epidemiology* by Willett *(2)*. These books provide myriad technical details on the goals of nutritional epidemiol-

From: *Nutritional Health: Strategies for Disease Prevention, Second Edition*
Edited by: N. J. Temple, T. Wilson, and D. R. Jacobs © Humana Press Inc., Totowa, NJ

ogy and the conduct and interpretation of studies, with discussion of potential pitfalls. This chapter focuses on two issues that are particularly challenging in nutritional epidemiology: (1) how to find out what people eat, and (2) how to think about the effect of diet on health.

2. HOW TO FIND OUT WHAT PEOPLE EAT

2.1. The Nature of Dietary Information

A full characterization of a person's diet would consist of a large number of discrete pieces of information. There are thousands of foods, prepared in myriad ways, and eaten in various amounts and combinations. Even a single "food," such as a carrot *(2)* or an onion *(3)*, presents a challenge, as there are many varieties and genetic variation; growing conditions are influential in food composition. The timing and context of eating, as well as the number of meals eaten, all contribute to metabolism of food. Willett *(2)* spends an entire chapter demonstrating that actual consumption varies widely from day to day. It may take months for individual diets to settle down to a steady-state average.

Each food supplies myriad chemicals. Among these chemicals, Willett *(2)* lists essential nutrients (vitamins, minerals, lipids, and amino acids), major energy sources (fat, protein, carbohydrate, and alcohol), additives (preservatives and flavorings), agricultural contaminants (pesticides and growth hormones), microbial toxins (aflatoxins), inorganic contaminants (cadmium and lead), chemicals formed in the cooking or processing of food (nitrosamines), natural toxins (natural pesticides), and other natural compounds (including DNA, enzymes, and enzyme inhibitors, many of which he says are thought of as "incidental to the human diet"). Energy content and nutrients, along with a few natural compounds, are readily available in a variety of food tables, whereas assessment of the remaining categories requires specialized databases. All of these chemicals pertain to each food eaten and can be summarized over the entire diet. The complete characterization of diet, foods, and the chemicals eaten, is clearly formidable. At some point in the research process, this large volume of information must be synthesized to be used in data analysis, that is statistical variables, such as food groups and nutrients, must be defined based on the available information.

2.2. Methods of Dietary Assessment

Two primary classes of methods have been used historically to assemble individual dietary information and synthesize it into something usable in data analysis, described in detail by Willett *(2)*. The first method includes dietary recalls and records. Dietary recalls are obtained by an interviewer assisting the participant to remember precisely what was eaten, usually over the past 24 h. Dietary records, on the other hand, are obtained by having the participant write down what was eaten, shortly after it was consumed; in practice, participants often wait until the end of the day to do their recording, so that the record easily transmutes to a self-administered recall. Variations in these methods include weighing foods before eating; collecting a duplicate portion of the food for subsequent chemical analysis; and recording onto partially precoded forms. Dietary recalls may differ in how intensively they inquire about different aspects of diet; for example, an interviewer may inquire deeply and pointedly, to a greater or lesser extent, for hard-to-obtain full information on such topics as alcoholic beverages drunk, salt-containing condiments used, or brand names of products eaten. Timing of eating may be obtained so that the integrity of individual meals can be maintained in the database. In both recalls and records, the data consist of a description of the food eaten and its portion size, perhaps with notes on brand names and preparation methods. The fact that a hamburger and a bun were eaten will generally be maintained in the database, but it is common not to maintain whether the two were eaten as a sandwich.

The second method is a food frequency questionnaire (FFQ), characterized by asking the participant general questions about diet. A typical question would be: "Do you eat hamburgers, and if so, how often and in what portion size?" Other kinds of general questions are also common. For example, one might ask: "When you eat a hamburger, is it usually a low-fat variety?" The scope of questions may include related aspects, for example: "Do you prefer white bread or whole wheat bread?" An important aspect is that foods are often grouped: "How often do you eat apples or pears?" FFQs come in several varieties, e.g., from 12 to 250 questions, with and without information about portion size. Those that ask about portion size are called semiquantitative FFQs. In a popular variant, the Willett-style questionnaire, a portion size is given for each food and frequency of portions is queried. In the other popular variant, the Block-style questionnaire, frequency of eating occasions is queried for each food, with a separate question about portion size. Additional variants exist, for example, in which pictures or food models are provided to facilitate food recognition and portion size estimation.

The dietary history method is closely related to the FFQ. Here, time is spent in general discussion of the diet prior to recording answers to the formal questions; this discussion is thought to improve the context of the interview and help the participant to put together the information needed. In the diet history, the close-ended questions may be general, e.g., "Do you eat red meat?," with an open-ended elicitation of foods eaten for those who answer affirmatively. The Coronary Artery Risk Development in Young Adults (CARDIA) Diet History *(4–6)* follows this form; 1609 food codes or recipes were endorsed by at least one of more than 5000 participants in one of two administrations of this questionnaire.

It is probably a coincidence of history that the primary approach to dietary assessment used in cardiovascular disease epidemiology in important studies through the early 1980s was the 24-h recall; used for example in the Lipid Research Clinics *(7,8)* and Multiple Risk-Factor Intervention Studies *(9,10)*. Special attention was paid to translating the myriad pieces of information into energy and nutrient intake. The synthesis of the data proved otherwise quite difficult and relatively little work was done with the influence of individual foods or food groups on long-term health outcomes. Where food grouping was done, it was done inflexibly, so only certain combinations of foods could be examined. Examination of nutrients within food groups (e.g., monounsaturated fat from plant vs animal foods) has received little attention. In principle, the data are available for such analyses, but it is unlikely that anyone will ever have the time, money, and study connections for such purposes. In contrast, cancer epidemiologists have long used FFQs *(11)*. This choice may be related to the traditional use of the case–control design for rare cancers. The desired information was the diet before diagnosis, and this would not be obtainable by recording or recalling current diet. In the cancer epidemiology field much more has been written about foods and food groups than in the cardiovascular disease epidemiology field. In contrast to analyses of dietary recall data, nutrient analyses within food groups are fairly common. On the other hand, the FFQ obtains much less information than does the recall/record method. For example, information about "yellow and green leafy vegetables" may be all that is collected; which of these vegetables was eaten may not be asked.

2.3. Ability to Represent Usual Diet

Two major conceptual differences exist between the recall/record and FFQ methods. The first relates to representativeness of usual diet. The strength of the recall/record method is that it can collect accurate and detailed information about actual consumption of particular meals. However, the particular day or meal is rarely of interest in nutritional epidemiology. It is well agreed that a single day's recall or record is inadequate as a representation of typical intake *(2)*. The general experience has been that the recall/record method has not worked well in studies of diet and chronic disease outcomes. Nevertheless, multiple days of recalls or records can represent typical diet quite well, as is well-illustrated by clear epidemiological relationships seen in only 95 children in the Framingham Children's Study *(12,13)*. However, it is rare for large studies to undertake more than one or possibly two days of recalls.

The FFQ class of methods, in contrast, asks about typical dietary pattern during a longer time frame, typically the past year. Many studies have found associations of nutrients and/or food groups with chronic disease outcomes using this method *(14)*. An even more powerful method uses repeated FFQ assessments during follow-up in a cohort study *(15)*. When typical diet is not changing greatly over several years, averaging results from repeated FFQ assessments can be quite powerful.

2.4. Who Synthesizes Dietary Information?

The second major conceptual difference between the recall/record and FFQ methods relates to how the myriad dietary details get synthesized into data analytic variables. In the recall/record method, a huge database is created with near infinite flexibility. The researcher is responsible for putting this information together in a manner that is usable in data analysis. In practice, this synthesis is often limited to energy and nutrient intake analysis; however, it is well within reason that the inherent flexibility in this method may be realized in the next years as computer technology continues to improve.

In the FFQ class of methods, the participant synthesizes the information. Much potential detail and therefore flexibility is lost, but the vastly reduced amount of information collected tends to make it a small job to create arbitrary combinations of food and nutrient variables. It seems likely that the investigators' formal synthesis of multiple recalls or records would be more accurate than the participant's informal synthesis. However, especially if the investigators' synthesis never gets done, the participant's synthesis is not without merit, despite variability in synthetic capability across participants and difficulty in defining typical patterns. For example, if a person actually drank 20 glasses of milk in a month, including one stretch of 5 d in which 10 of the glasses were drunk, one might say that the typical pattern is two-thirds of a glass per day. A recall could easily be done on a day when no milk or two glasses were drunk, thus getting the wrong answer, but it is easy for a person to synthesize their pattern into something like a glass every other day.

Some cleverness may be needed in the FFQ mode to get at nutritional concepts with which the public is less familiar, such as whole grain bread. A prime example is the use by Willett of the term "dark bread" to elicit breads that were most likely to have at least moderate whole grain content. Although "dark bread" is a somewhat oblique reference, asking directly about whole grain bread might not have been well understood by participants, and most breads containing a substantial amount of whole grain are darker than American white bread. Dark bread is oblique owing to exceptions popular in the United States, including pumpernickel cooked with molasses and rye bread made with refined rye. Despite these potential problems, the reference to "dark bread" succeeded in eliciting breads that were inversely associated with coronary heart disease mortality in the Iowa Women's Health Study *(14)*. Another interesting Willett innovation in an attempt to get at an important detail, and also used in the Iowa Women's Health Study, was the additional query of the brand name of the usual breakfast cereal eaten *(14)*. Despite the fact that many people eat more than one breakfast cereal, this detail provided the ability to categorize brands, a great boon in the study of whole grains and health. Similarly, the CARDIA Diet History was innovative in that it intended to blend recall and synthesis. It asked for the last 30 d of typical intake, recent enough for some level of recall to assist the participant in synthesizing. It also allowed tremendous detail in the participant's self-assessment of typical intake by prompting the participant with 100 general food categories (e.g., eggs), then asking the participant to name all foods consumed within each category.

2.5. Can Accurate Dietary Information be Obtained?

A great deal of progress has been made in understanding the relation of diet to chronic disease, based mainly on FFQs. Nevertheless, validation studies of FFQs against 1 to 4 wk of food diaries are somewhat discouraging. It is difficult for most people to summarize their diet accurately. There are several reasons for this including: that such summarization requires considerable quantitative ability; that most people simply eat, without making habitual summaries of what they are eating; that diet varies considerably and what is typical for the past month might be different from what is typical for the past year; and that the researchers' questions might not be the optimal formulation for eliciting particular dietary facts. Criterion measures have revealed correlations in the range of 0.3 to 0.6 between the two methods *(5,16–18)*. The resulting within-person error leads to serious problems in interpretation of dietary data *(1,2,19,20)*.

Certain analytic and interpretive approaches to data can be helpful. Cautious statements and consistency checks are called for. For example, an assertion that a nutrient is related to incident disease will be stronger if all the foods that contain the nutrient are individually also related to that disease, given that different foods contain different mixes of nutrients *(2)*. Conversely, if an apparent relationship of disease with a nutrient exists only for a single food that was eaten often and is high in the nutrient, then that would be more consistent with the concept that the food, not the nutrient, is causally related to incident disease. In that case, the causal pathway might rely on a synergy of the components of the food or on a different single nutrient. Meta-analysis showing consistency of findings across studies can also be helpful *(21,22)*. Nevertheless, the FFQ method appears to have intrinsic limitations in how precisely it can define individual intake. Among possibilities for improvement of the FFQ method are increasing precision and innovation of questions; repeated administrations of the questionnaire with averaging to reduce the influence of within-person variation in intake; and enhancing dietary awareness of participants, for example by encouraging or requiring the participant to keep informal dietary records for a few days prior to filling out the questionnaire or by giving advance instruction in portion size determination.

A single recall or record does not accurately represent typical dietary information because of intrinsic day-to-day variation *(2)*. In contrast, in the Framingham Children's Study the clarity of findings in only 95 children with repeated diet assessments is impressive *(12,13)*, but they obtained many more diet records than is typical of studies in nutritional epidemiology. The detail obtained from many dietary records is seductive from the research perspective. This approach far outstrips the flexibility of the already successful studies, at Harvard and the University of Minnesota for example, which have relied on FFQs. It is a powerful cohort study design indeed that obtains unlimited accurate dietary characterization and follow-up for many different chronic disease outcomes. However, even with added power from such a large number of diet records, it is probable that thousands of participants would be needed in studies of remote and rare chronic disease outcomes. In most practical epidemiological situations, the possibilities are limited for obtaining 4 to 12 24-h diet records per year in the assembly line fashion that would be needed for a cohort study of a chronic disease.

Given present methodologies it is unlikely that many studies will achieve this standard. Nevertheless, we can dream. Given the success of the internet and the surge in computer power, one might hope for better methods in the future. In particular, one could imagine widespread collection of self-administered dietary information on the internet, with full software including help and dialog boxes that would simulate the support currently given by an interviewer. Thus, the dietary collection instrument could even be a mixture of recall and synthesis. The open-ended methods of the CARDIA Diet History might be helpful, combined with some aspects of artificial intelligence. Branching logic for finding food codes could be employed, similar to that currently used by the Nutrition Data System for Research (NDS-R), a "Windows-based software package incorporating a time-tested, highly accurate database with an up-to-date interface," released in 1998 by the Nutrition Coordinating Center of the University of Minnesota *(23)*. One could even envision questionnaires filled out over the telephone, with automated voice prompts to assist in accuracy. As questionnaires accrued, the foods database could automatically expand in line with what was reported by participants. Thus, a participant could repeatedly and at their convenience do a 24-h recall or report typical intake over the past week with verbal or online prompts that helps find correct food codes and pointed questions to help improve the quality of the information obtained.

A requisite for exploiting this type of ambitious scheme would be correspondingly simple-to-use programs to extract nutrients, foods, food groups, and food group-specific nutrients. The researcher would require package programs to assemble the data, to formulate and reformulate food groups, and to compute nutrient values. As new information comes along, it could be added to the food table to simplify study of novel compounds.

These schemes are perhaps dream-like, but may not be completely out of the question. Who would have imagined only a few years ago the internet or, to cite one important application, millions of journal abstracts and articles themselves would be available at the touch of a few computer keystrokes? In the near term, however, it is most likely that nutritional studies of chronic disease outcomes will continue to be based on the FFQ class of methodologies, bolstered by findings in short-term human and animal studies and the native ingenuity of the scientists doing the research.

Willett *(2)* comments on another method that has promise but also pitfalls: correlation of food intake with biomarkers. A biomarker is a chemical measured in some biological sample, commonly blood or urine, but others as well, for example feces, hair, toenails, cheek cells, adipocytes, and skin scrapings. Minerals reside in toenails, which grow over several months; therefore this measure represents an average intake over several months. Urinary nitrogen is discussed in the chapter by Margetts as a marker of nitrogen and therefore protein intake. Sodium and potassium intake are mirrored quite rapidly (e.g., more than 2 d) in urinary sodium and potassium. Serum carotenoids and ascorbic acid are highly responsive to both dietary and supplemental intake of the same substances. Nevertheless, biomarkers are not perfect as indicators of dietary intake. Each tissue and substance has its own half-life and metabolism. Some tissues store substances, and some use them rapidly. The amount of a substance in blood may not be representative of its occurrence throughout the body. Substances may be maintained homeostatically, or may be partially under dietary and partially under homeostatic control. There may be changes in nutrients consumed prior to storage, for example, elongation of fatty acids. For all these reasons, biomarkers are rarely perfect representations of intake. An example is the imperfect relation between serum carotenoids and total antioxidant intake *(24)*. Furthermore, biomarkers tell nothing about dietary behaviors. Still, biomarkers have a future in dietary assessment. Research should continue to identify and better understand biomarkers in relation to dietary intake.

3. WHAT ELEMENT OF DIET SHOULD BE STUDIED?

In Subheading 2.1, following Willett *(2)*, the kinds of chemicals that are dietary components was cited. The number and kind of such components present a very complex picture. Diet can also be described in terms of food, food groups, or dietary patterns. The early history of nutrition research focused primarily on chemicals, with some justification according to Willett. The existence of deficiency diseases such as scurvy (ascorbic acid), rickets (vitamin D), beri-beri, pellagra, and neural tube defects (B vitamins) points to one class of nutritional problems. Willett cites a model of Mertz *(25)* that begins with death and deficiency disease at sufficiently low level of a nutrient, complemented by similarly severely reduced function at levels that are sufficiently high. Also in the model is reduced function at modestly reduced or elevated levels of the nutrient. Willett calls this "subclinical dysfunction," a view much in line with the slow, mostly subclinical development of diseases, such as cancer and cardiovascular disease. There is also a broad plateau at highest function across a wide range of intake of the nutrient.

Willett *(2)* further thinks that focus on major energy sources is justified because they are quantitatively important in our diets and manifestly vary markedly across human populations. These focuses on nutrients have led to the development of extensive tables of energy and these dietary chemicals. Furthermore, there is a strong tendency among basic scientists towards reductionism: the belief that worthwhile knowledge consists of simple pathways linking single nutrients to bodily function and pathogenesis *(26,27)*, what Willett calls "linkage to our fundamental knowledge of biology." An excellent example is the protective association of folate with neural tube defects *(28)*, as is improvement in insulin function and metabolic control in diabetics with supplemental magnesium *(29)*. Much remains to be studied regarding the composition of foods. The tabulated nutrient composition of a food does not fully describe the physiological effect of that food, whether because of differential bioavailability or unknown constituents. There are thousands of untabulated or unidentified compounds in foods. Additionally, a relatively undeveloped aspect of diet characterization is that of food function. For example, Blomhoff and colleagues *(24,30)* analyzed thousands of food samples for their total antioxidant content, measured as the molar content of donatable electrons using the ferric reducing ability of plasma; those data are available as a dietary exposure measure. A similar functional assessment in the idea stage is the ability of a given food to prevent cell proliferation in in vitro incubation with cancer cells, as in the work by Eberhardt et al. *(31)*.

Foods themselves should also be studied even if that does not immediately lead to additional knowledge of specific biological pathways. Foods are what people eat; findings regarding foods are directly applicable to people's diets. Most importantly, it is quite likely that there are synergies among food constituents and between foods *(26,27)*; studies of individual chemical constituents may never find the relevant pathways because they are more complex than the researchers imagined. In a nondeficiency state, despite findings that foods containing antioxidants are associated with better long-term health, consumption of isolated nutrients or chemicals does not fare so well. The most striking example is that of supplementary β-carotene, which has been administered in several large, long-term clinical trials, with the effect of increasing disease *(32)*. Higher antioxidant nutrient intake was associated with more diabetic retinopathy in one study *(33)*. Other provocative examples from the author's observational work include that supplemental vitamin C in diabetics was associated with increased coronary heart disease *(34)*, and that supplemental iron in association with breakfast cereal intake (which is often fortified with supplemental iron) was associated with an increased rate of distal colon cancer *(35)*.

These findings are supportive of the concept that food synergies are important: the compounds in question are part of foods that appear to be healthy, but do not work outside their food matrix. The food matrix arises from a living organism consisting of thousands of compounds with checks and balances among those compounds to maintain homeostasis and life by preventing the action of any one compound from getting out of control. It is likely that some of this multiplicity of function is retained during human metabolism of the food. For example, whole grain breakfast cereals are associated with reduced risk of chronic disease *(14,36–38)*, as are fruits and vegetables *(32,39)*, which are high in β-carotene and vitamin C, among a wide variety of other phytochemicals.

In a very simple example of food synergy, vitamin E functions as an antioxidant by accepting electrons, after which it exists in an oxidized state, that is, as a pro-oxidant. To reduce the risk that it will cause damage, it must be reduced, which is done by vitamin C. The vitamin C is then oxidized and must be reduced, and so on until the cycle reaches an end. One important in vitro study was suggestive of the influence of balancing substances in food by showing that cell proliferation in a cancer cell line was much lower when incubated with apple or apple skin than it was when incubated with an amount of isolated vitamin C that had an equivalent total antioxidant capacity *(32)*.

A final aspect of diet that has been successfully studied is food patterns. Dietary patterns have been discovered using factor analysis. For example, Hu et al. *(40,41)* identified a "prudent" pattern associated with reduced incidence of cardiovascular disease and a "Western" pattern associated with increased incidence. Many other authors have followed a similar strategy, generally finding support for the general prudent pattern *(42)*. The association of a food pattern with incident disease is suggestive of a synergy between foods. There has been much advice about a diet that has potential to prevent chronic disease; the lower risk associated with the "prudent" pattern suggests that many people have apparently taken that advice and that the advised diets do have merit in risk reduction.

4. SUMMARY

Two particularly challenging issues in nutritional epidemiology were discussed in editorial fashion. Concerning how to find out what people eat, nutritional epidemiologists use variants of two basic methods. In the first, the participant records or recalls extensive detail about recent intake. The investigator then synthesizes this information into analytically usable variables. This method does not represent typical diet well unless multiple recalls/records are obtained. In the second method, the participant synthesizes his or her dietary information by responding to general questions about diet, such as how often a particular class of foods is eaten. This method does determine the typical diet, but fails to obtain details that are necessary for many types of analysis. It is hoped that advances in technology will enable simpler and more extensive collection and processing of dietary intake data.

Concerning how to think about the effect of diet on health, I suggest that simple nutrient pathways are inadequate for a full understanding of diet. It is proposed that considerable attention be paid to the foods and food patterns that people eat, as well as to the relations of these foods and food patterns to disease outcomes.

REFERENCES

1. Margetts BM, Nelson M, eds. Design Concepts in Nutritional Epidemiology. Second Edition. Oxford University Press, Oxford, 1997.
2. Willett W. Nutritional Epidemiology. Second Edition. Oxford University Press, New York, 1998.
3. Yang J, Meyers KJ, van der Heide J, Liu RH. Varietal differences in phenolic content and antioxidant and antiproliferative activities of onions. J Agric Food Chem 2004; 52:6787–6793.
4. McDonald A, Van Horn L, Slattery M, et al. The CARDIA dietary history: development, implementation, and evaluation. J Am Diet Assoc 1991; 91:1104–1112.
5. Liu K, Slattery M, Jacobs DR, Jr., et al. A study of the reliability and comparative validity of the CARDIA dietary history. Ethn Dis 1994; 4:15–27.
6. Liu K, Slattery M, Jacobs DR, Jr. Is the dietary recall the method of choice in black populations? Ethn Dis 1994; 4:12–14. (Letter to the editor)
7. Prewitt TE, Haynes SG, Graves K, Haines PS, Tyroler HA. Nutrient intake, lipids, and lipoprotein cholesterols in black and white children: the Lipid Research Clinics Prevalence Study. Prev Med 1988; 17:247–262.
8. Dennis BH, Zhukovsky GS, Shestov DB, et al. The association of education with coronary heart disease mortality in the USSR Lipid Research Clinics Study. Int J Epidemiol 1993; 22:420–427.
9. Dolecek TA, Johnson RL, Grandits GA, Farrand-Zukel M, Caggiula AW. Nutritional adequacy of diets reported at baseline and during trial years 1-6 by the special intervention and usual care groups in the Multiple Risk Factor Intervention Trial. Am J Clin Nutr 1997; 65(1 Suppl):305S–313S.
10. Dolecek TA, Stamler J, Caggiula AW, Tillotson JL, Buzzard IM. Methods of dietary and nutritional assessment and intervention and other methods in the Multiple Risk Factor Intervention Trial. Am J Clin Nutr 1997; 65(1 Suppl):196S–210S.

11. Graham S, Mettlin C, Marshall J, Priore R, Rzepka T, Shedd D. Dietary factors in the epidemiology of cancer of the larynx. Am J Epidemiol 1981; 113:675–680.
12. Singer MR, Moore LL, Garrahie EJ, Ellison RC. The tracking of nutrient intake in young children: the Framingham Children's Study. Am J Public Health 1995; 85:1673–1677.
13. Moore LL, Singer MR, Bradlee ML, et al. Intake of fruits, vegetables, and dairy products in early childhood and subsequent blood pressure change. Epidemiology 2005; 16:4–11.
14. Jacobs DR, Meyer KA, Kushi LH, Folsom AR. Whole grain intake may reduce risk of coronary heart disease death in postmenopausal women: the Iowa Women's Health Study. Am J Clin Nutr 1998; 68:248–257.
15. Willett WC, Stampfer MJ, Manson JE, et al. Intake of trans fatty acids and risk of coronary heart disease among women. Lancet 1993; 341:581–585.
16. Munger RG, Folsom AR, Kushi LH, Kaye SA, Sellers TA. Dietary assessment of older Iowa women with a food frequency questionnaire: nutrient intake, reproducibility, and comparison with 24-hour dietary recall interviews. Am J Epidemiol 1992; 136:192–200.
17. Willett WC, Sampson L, Browne ML, et al. The use of self-administered questionnaire to assess diet four years in the past. Am J Epidemiol 1988; 127:188–199.
18. Feskanich D, Rimm EB, Giovannucci EL, et al. Reproducibility and validity of food intake measurements from a semiquantitative food frequency questionnaire. J Am Diet Assoc 1993; 93:790–796.
19. Fraser GE. Diet, Life Expectancy, and Chronic Disease. Oxford University Press, New York, 2003, pp. 265–276.
20. Schatzkin A, Kipnis V. Could exposure assessment problems give us wrong answers to nutrition and cancer questions? J Natl Cancer Inst 2004; 96:1564–1565.
21. Pereira MA, O'Reilly E, Augustsson K, et al. Dietary fiber and risk of coronary heart disease: a pooled analysis of cohort studies. Arch Intern Med 2004; 164:370–376.
22. Knekt P, Ritz J, Pereira MA, et al. Antioxidant vitamins and coronary heart disease risk: a pooled analysis of 9 cohorts. Am J Clin Nutr 2004; 80:1508–1520.
23. University of Minnesota Nutrition Data System. http://www.ncc.umn.edu/. Last accessed January 2, 2005.
24. Svilaas, A., Sakhi, A. K., Andersen, L. F., et al. Intakes of antioxidants in coffee, wine, and vegetables are correlated with plasma carotenoids in humans. J Nutr 2004; 134,562–567.
25. Mertz W. The essential trace elements. Science 1981; 213:1332–1338.
26. Messina M, Lampe JW, Birt DF, et al. Reductionism and the narrowing nutrition perspective: time for reevaluation and emphasis on food synergy. J Am Diet Assoc 2001; 101:1416–1419.
27. Jacobs DR, Steffen LM. Nutrients, foods, and dietary patterns as exposures in research: a framework for food synergy. Am J Clin Nutr 2003; 78(Suppl 3):508S–513S.
28. Stover PJ. Physiology of folate and vitamin B12 in health and disease. Nutr Rev 2004; 62(6 Pt 2):S3–S12; discussion S13.
29. Rodriguez-Moran M, Guerrero-Romero F. Oral Magnesium supplementation improves insulin sensitivity and metabolic control in type 2 diabetic subjects: a randomized double blind controlled trial. Diabetes Care 2003; 26:1147–1152.
30. Halvorsen BL, Holte K, Myhrstad MC, et al. A systematic screening of total antioxidants in dietary plants. J Nutr 2002; 132:461–471.
31. Svilaas A, Sakhi AK, Andersen LF, et al. Intakes of antioxidants in coffee, wine, and vegetables are correlated with plasma carotenoids in humans. J Nutr 2004; 134:562–567.
32. Eberhardt MV, Lee CY, Liu RH. Antioxidant activity of fresh apples. Nature 2000; 405:903–904.
33. Clarke R, Armitage J. Antioxidant vitamins and risk of cardiovascular disease. Review of large-scale randomised trials. Cardiovasc Drugs Ther 2002; 16:411–415.
34. Mayer-Davis EJ, Bell RA, Reboussin BA, Rushing J, Marshall JA, Hamman RF. Antioxidant nutrient intake and diabetic retinopathy: the San Luis Valley Diabetes Study. Ophthalmology 1998; 105:2264–2270.
35. Lee DH, Aaron R, Folsom AR, Harnack L, Halliwell B, Jacobs DR. Does supplemental vitamin C increase cardiovascular disease risk in women with diabetes? Am J Clin Nutr 2004; 80:1194–1200.
36. Lee DH, Jacobs DR, Folsom AR. A hypothesis: interaction between supplemental iron intake and fermentation affecting the risk of colon cancer. The Iowa Women's Health Study. Nutr Cancer 2004; 48:1–5.

37. Jacobs DR, Gallaher DD. Whole grain intake and cardiovascular disease: a review. Curr Atheroscler Rep 2004; 6:415–423.

38. Liu S, Sesso HD, Manson JE, Willett WC, Buring JE. Is intake of breakfast cereals related to total and cause-specific mortality in men? Am J Clin Nutr 2003; 77:594–599.

39. Key TJ, Schatzkin A, Willett WC, Allen NE, Spencer EA, Travis RC. Diet, nutrition and the prevention of cancer. Public Health Nutr 2004; 7(1A):187–200.

40. Hu FB, Rimm E, Smith-Warner SA, et al. Reproducibility and validity of dietary patterns assessed with a food-frequency questionnaire. Am J Clin Nutr 1999; 69:243–249.

41. Hu FB, Rimm EB, Stampfer MJ, Ascherio A, Spiegelman D, Willett WC. Prospective study of major dietary patterns and risk of coronary heart disease in men. Am J Clin Nutr 2000; 72:912–921.

42. Newby PK, Tucker KL. Empirically derived eating patterns using factor or cluster analysis: a review. Nutr Rev 2004; 62:177–203.

3

The Nutrition Transition is Speeding Up

A Global Perspective

Barry M. Popkin

KEY POINTS

- The speed of increases in the prevalence of overweight and obesity in the developing world is greater than same changes in the prevalence rates among much higher-income developed countries. The major dietary changes are: increased intake of edible oil (an increase that is affordable by the world's poor in the majority of low-income countries); increased intake of caloric sweetener (particularly in sweetened beverages in some countries but also in many other processed food sources); and also a rapid increase in the total intake of animal source foods.
- A marked upward shift in the technologies available to the developing world for work, transportation, home production, and leisure are combining to rapidly increase sedentarianism.
- There is emerging research that indicates that there might be important biological differences between the populations found in Asia, Africa, and Latin America that might predispose many of them to higher risk of many nutrition-related noncommunicable diseases at lower body mass index levels than heretofore found in the United States and Europe. There are limited examples of national programs in Finland, South Korea, and other countries that offer some options for modifying these adverse shifts in diet and activity and obesity.

1. INTRODUCTION: WHAT IS THE NUTRITION TRANSITION?

The world is witnessing rapid shifts in diet and body composition, with resultant important changes in health profiles. In many ways, these shifts are a continuation of large-scale changes that have occurred repeatedly over time; the changes facing low- and moderate-income countries today, however, appear to be occurring very rapidly. Broad shifts in population size and age composition, disease patterns and dietary and physical-activity patterns are occurring worldwide. The former two sets of dynamic shifts are termed the

From: *Nutritional Health: Strategies for Disease Prevention, Second Edition*
Edited by: N. J. Temple, T. Wilson, and D. R. Jacobs © Humana Press Inc., Totowa, NJ

demographic and epidemiological transitions. Similarly, large shifts have occurred in dietary and physical activity and inactivity patterns. These changes are reflected in nutritional outcomes, such as changes in average stature and body composition. These dietary and physical activity changes, reflected in nutritional outcomes such as changes in average stature and body composition, are referred to as the nutrition transition.

Human diet and activity patterns and nutritional status have undergone a sequence of major shifts, defined as broad patterns of food use and corresponding to nutrition-related disease. Over the last three centuries, the pace of dietary and activity change appears to have accelerated to varying degrees in different regions of the world. In particular, changes have accelerated more in the past decade. These dietary and activity and body composition distribution changes are paralleled by major changes in health status, as well as by major demographic and socioeconomic changes. Obesity emerges early in the shift as does the level and age composition of morbidity and mortality. We can think of five broad nutrition patterns. They are not restricted to particular periods of human history. For convenience, the patterns are outlined as historical developments; however, "earlier" patterns are not restricted to the periods in which they first arose, but continue to characterize certain geographic and socioeconomic subpopulations.

1.1. Pattern 1: Collecting Food

This diet, which characterizes hunter–gatherer populations, is high in carbohydrates and fiber and low in fat, especially saturated fat (1,2). In meat from wild animals, the proportion of polyunsaturated fat is significantly higher than in meat from modern domesticated animals (3). Activity patterns are very high and little obesity is found among hunter–gatherer societies. It is important to note that much of the research on hunter–gatherers is based on modern and not prehistoric hunter–gatherer societies.

1.2. Pattern 2: Famine

The diet becomes much less varied and is subject to larger variations and periods of acute scarcity of food. These dietary changes are hypothesized to be associated with nutritional stress and a reduction in stature (estimated by some at about 4 in.) (4,5). During the later phases of this pattern, social stratification intensifies, and dietary variation according to gender and social status increases (6). The pattern of famine (as with each of the patterns) has varied over time and space. Some civilizations are more successful than others in alleviating famine and chronic hunger, at least for their more privileged citizens (7). The types of physical activities changed but there was little change in activity levels during this period of famine.

1.3. Pattern 3: Receding Famine

The consumption of fruits, vegetables, and animal protein increases, and starchy staples become less important in the diet. Many earlier civilizations made great progress in reducing chronic hunger and famine, but only in the last third of the last millennium have these changes become widespread, leading to marked shifts in diet. However, famines continued well into the 18th century in portions of Europe and remain common in some regions of the world. Activity patterns start to shift and inactivity and leisure become a part of the lives of more people.

1.4. Pattern 4: Nutrition-Related Noncommunicable Disease

A diet high in total fat, cholesterol, sugar, and other refined carbohydrates and low in polyunsaturated fatty acids and fiber, often accompanying an increasingly sedentary life, is characteristic of most high-income societies (and increasingly of portions of the population in low-income societies), resulting in increased prevalence of obesity and contributing to the degenerative diseases that characterize Omran's final epidemiological stage *(8)*. Omran's epidemiological transition moves from a pattern of high prevalence of infectious diseases and malnutrition to a pattern where chronic and degenerative diseases predominate.

1.5. Pattern 5: Behavioral Change

A new dietary pattern appears to be emerging as a result of changes in diet evidently associated with the desire to prevent or delay degenerative diseases and prolong health. Whether these changes, instituted in some countries by consumers and in others also prodded by government policy, will constitute a large-scale transition in dietary structure and body composition remains to be seen *(9–11)*. If such a new dietary pattern takes hold, it may be very important in enhancing "successful aging," that is, postponing infirmity and increasing the disability-free life expectancy *(12,13)*.

Our focus is increasingly on patterns three to five, in particular on the rapid shift in much of the world's low- and moderate-income countries from the stage of receding famine to nutrition-related noncommunicable disease (NR-NCD). Figure 1 presents this focus. The concern on this period is so great that the term "the nutrition transition" is synonymous for many with this shift from pattern 2 to 3.

2. WHAT ARE SOME CRITICAL DIMENSIONS?

2.1. The Speed of Change is Greater Today

Is there anything about the great rapidity of change in diet, activity, and body composition that matters? What does the high prevalence of the undernutrition and overweight combination in the same household mean in this context? Although there is no study that clearly explores these points, extant data from Europe and the United States would lead us to believe that the rates of change in diet, activity, and obesity today in the developing world are far beyond that experienced earlier by these countries. In a very short time many low- and middle-income countries have attained rates of overweight and obesity equal to or greater than that of the United States and Western Europe.

The pace of the rapid nutrition transition shifts in diet and activity patterns from the period, termed the "receding famine pattern," to one dominated by NR-NCDs seems to be accelerating in the lower- and middle-income transitional countries. We use nutrition rather than diet so that the term NR-NCD incorporates the effects of diet, physical activity, and body composition rather than solely focusing on dietary patterns and their effects. This is based partially on incomplete information that seems to indicate that the prevalence of obesity and a number of NR-NCDs are increasing far faster in the lower- and middle-income world than it has in the West. Another element is that the rapid changes in urban populations are much greater than those experienced a century or less ago in the West. Yet another is the shift in occupation structure and the rapid introduction of the

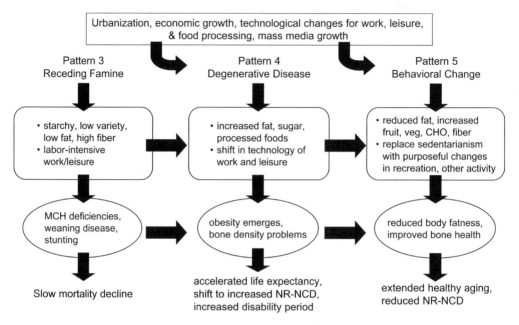

Fig. 1. Stages of the nutrition transition.

modern mass media. Underlying such changes is a general concern for rapid globalization as the root cause.

Clearly, there are quantitative and qualitative dimensions to these changes. On the one hand, changes toward a high-density diet, reduced complex carbohydrates and other important elements, and inactivity may be proceeding faster than in the past. The shift from labor-intensive occupations and leisure activities toward more capital-intensive, less strenuous work and leisure is also occurring faster. On the other hand, qualitative dimensions related to multidimensional aspects of the diet, activity, body composition, and disease shifts may exist. Social and economic stresses people face and feel as these changes occur might also be included.

At the start of the new millennium, scholars often feel as if the pace and complexity of life, reflected in all aspects of work and play, are increasing exponentially; there are also unanticipated developments, new technologies, and the impact of a very modern, high-powered communications system. It is this sense of rapid change that makes it so important to understand what is happening and anticipate the way changes in patterns of diet, activity, and body composition are occurring. Although the penetration and influence of modern communications, technology, and economic systems—related to what is termed globalization—have been a dominant theme of the last few decades, there seem to be some unique issues that have led to a rapid increase of "globalization and its impact."

Placing the blame on globalization is, on the one hand, focusing on broad and vaguely measured sets of forces; this ignores the need to be focused and specific, which would allow us to develop potentially viable policy options. It is difficult to measure each element of this globalization equation and its impact. These processes certainly have been expanded, as indicated by enhanced free trade, a push toward reduction of trade barriers in the developing world, and the increasing penetration of international corporations into

the commerce in each country (measured by share of gross national product or manufacturing). Similarly, other economic issues related to enhanced value given to market forces
and international capital markets are important. Equally, the increasing access to Western
media, the removal of communication barriers enhanced by the World Wide Web, cable
TV, mobile telephone systems, etc. is important. The accelerated introduction of Western
technology into manufacturing, basic sectors of agriculture, mining, and services is also
a key element.

Another way to consider the types of changes the developing world is facing is to
consider an urban squatter's life and a rural villager's life in China 20 yr ago, and today.
During the 1970s, food supply concerns still existed, there was no television, limited bus
and mass transportation, little food trade, minimal processed food existed, and most rural
and urban occupations were very labor intensive. Today, work and life activities have
changed: small gas-powered tractors are available, modern industrial techniques are
multiplying, offices are quite automated, soft drinks and many processed foods are found
everywhere, TVs are found in about 89% of households (at least one-fifth of whom are
linked to Hong Kong Star and Western advertising and programming), younger children
do not ride bicycles, and mass transit has become heavily used. Multiply such changes
by similar ones occurring in much of Asia, North Africa, the Middle East, Latin America,
and many areas (particularly cities) in sub-Saharan Africa and it is evident that the shift
from a subsistence economy to a modern, industrialized one occurred in a span of 10–20
yr, whereas, in Europe and other industrialized high-income societies, this occurred over
many decades or centuries.

To truly measure and examine these issues, we would need to compare changes in
the period between 1980 and 2000, for countries that are low and middle income, with
changes that occurred a half century earlier for the developing world. However, data on
diet and activity patterns are not available and there are only minimal data on NR-NCDs
and obesity.

The elements of the nutrition transition that we know to be negatively linked with NR-
NCDs are obesity, adverse dietary changes (e.g., shifts in the structure of diet toward a
greater role for higher fat and added sugar foods, reduced fruit and vegetable intake; shifts
in diets away from whole grain, nuts, and legumes with an overall reduction in fiber
intake, greater energy density, and greater saturated fat intake), and reduced physical
activity in work and leisure. We focus on these first, and then a few select underlying
factors. The causes of these elements of the nutrition transition are not as well understood
as the trends in each of them. In fact, there are few studies attempting to study the causes
of such changes, and there are only a few data sets that are equipped to allow such crucial
policy analyses to be undertaken.

2.2. Edible Oil

Prosperity has always been associated with the consumption of a fat-rich diet. Historians have long used meat consumption as an index of prosperity of an era or membership
in a higher social class (14). Fat-rich diets have long been regarded as richer and more
flavorful and often tend to be more varied (15). Until the decade following World War
II, the majority of fats available for human consumption were animal fats obtained from
milk, butter, and meat. Detailed information is provided on the revolution in the production and processing of oilseed-based fats in the past five decades (16).

2.3. Caloric Sweetener Revolution

Sugar is the world's predominant sweetener. It is not clear exactly when sugar became the world's principal sweetener—most likely in the 17th or 18th century, as the New World began producing large quantities of sugar at reduced prices *(17,18)*. Sugar use has since been linked with industrialization, and with the proliferation of processed foods and beverages that have sugar added to them (e.g., tea, coffee, and cocoa). We use the term "caloric sweetener" instead of added sugar as there is a range of nonsugar products in use today. High-fructose corn syrup is a prime example as it is the sweetener used in all US soft drinks. There are two major sugar crops: sugar beets and sugar cane. Sugar and syrups are also produced from the sap of certain species of maple trees, from sweet sorghum when cultivated explicitly for making syrup, and from sugar palm. Under the name sweeteners, the Food and Agriculture Organization (FAO) includes products used for sweetening that are either derived from sugar crops, cereals, fruits, milk, or produced by insects. This category includes a wide variety of monosaccharides (glucose and fructose) and disaccharides (sucrose and saccharose), which exist either in a crystallized state as sugar or in thick liquid form as syrups. Included in sweeteners are maple sugar and syrups, caramel, golden syrup, artificial and natural honey, maltose, glucose, isoglucose (also known as high-fructose corn syrup), other types of fructose, sugar confectionery, and lactose. In the last several decades, increasingly larger quantities of cereals (primarily maize) have been used to produce sweeteners derived from starch.

In separate study, we provide detailed information on the caloric sweetener revolution *(19)*. In 2000 there were 74 more kilocalories per capita of caloric sweetener consumed than in 1962. This represented an increase of 32% in the percentage of energy from caloric sweeteners and represents a 21% increase in the proportion of carbohydrates from refined caloric sweeteners.

We have also shown the profound changes that occurred between the 1960s and the past decade and also the large urbanization effect in the Drewnowski and Popkin paper *(16)*. This regression model predicts that rapid urbanization, usually associated with greater incomes and economic growth, can have independent effects on diet structure. In 1962 there was very little sweetener consumed by populations in lower-income countries. At lower income levels, according to the regression model, urbanization can more than double the amount of sweeteners in the diet. The model confirms previous observations that people living in urban areas consume diets distinct from those of their rural counterparts *(20,21)*. The potential impact of urbanization in flattening the income–sweetener relationship deserves further analysis; however, it is clear that the increased urbanization of lower-income nations is accelerating the shift to increased consumption of sweeteners and fats.

2.4. Animal Source Foods

The animal source foods (ASF) revolution refers to the increase in demand and production of meat, fish, and milk in low-income developing countries. Dr. Christopher Delgado from the International Food Policy Research Institute has studied this issue extensively in a number of seminal reports and papers *(22)*. Most of the world's growth in production and consumption in these foods is coming from the developing countries. Although cereal production is increasing, this is mainly a derived demand for additional

ASFs. The ASF revolution is driven by demand as ASFs are substituted into starch-based diets. Income elasticities of demand are high for red meat in China, South Korea, and Morocco *(23,24)*. Over time, we expect to see a larger share of household food expenditures on animal products. Price elasticities for cereals tend to be low; price changes will impact low-income groups faster than higher-income groups. Since 1970 relative prices of food have dropped considerably, most dramatically for beef. Owing to market saturation and technological changes that increase productivity, the *increase in demand for* ASF is projected to peak by 2020. As relative commodity prices decrease and income increases, people tend to both increase the diversity of their diet and to shift into higher priced foods that are more highly processed. While average income growth explains overall growth in total food expenditures, urbanization and population growth explain the greater increase in ASF demand in developing countries.

As Delgado has shown, 31% of food fish is from aquaculture, but 60% of world aquaculture is in China, as well as 40% of the world's pigs *(22)*. China is trying to promote beef consumption because beef requires less grain than pork. Projections to 2020 include huge increases in China's food fish consumption, as well as 31% of world beef production. India is the largest producer of milk, although 42% of the population still claim to not eat any ASF, and only the Muslim segment of the population consumes beef. India already has food safety systems in place, especially in urban areas. Large amounts of sweets containing mostly milk and sugar are processed and distributed in India.

Whether it is a curse or a blessing depends on policy and technology. The ASF revolution is driven by demand, substituting into starch-based diets. Developing countries will produce 63% of meat and 50% of milk in 2020. It is a global food activity, transforming the grain markets for animal feed. It also leads to resource degradation, rapid increases in feed grain imports, rapid concentration of production and consumption, and the promotion of social change.

3. INCREASED SEDENTARIANISM IS OCCURRING CONCURRENTLY

There are several linked changes in physical activity occurring jointly. One is a shift in the structure of the population away from the high-energy expenditure activities, such as farming, mining, and forestry, toward the service sector. Elsewhere, we have shown this large effect *(25)*.

A second change is the change in the level of energy expenditure in the same occupation. The proportion of urban adults (male and female) working in occupations where they participate in vigorous activity patterns has decreased, and increased where the activity pattern is light. In rural areas, however, there has been a shift toward increased physical activity linked to holding multiple jobs and more intensive effort. For rural women, there is a shift toward a larger proportion being engaged in more energy-intensive work, but there are also some for whom the shift is toward a lighter work effort. In contrast, for rural men there is a small decrease in the proportion engaged in light work effort. We have also shown how shifts in activity at an occupation represent a significant determinant of the increase in obesity in China *(26)*.

Other major changes relate to mode of transportation and activity patterns during leisure hours. In one study in China it has been demonstrated that the odds of being obese were 80% higher ($p < 0.05$) for men and women in households who owned a motorized vehicle compared with those who did not own such a vehicle (27). Fourteen percent of households acquired a motorized vehicle between 1989 and 1997. Compared with those whose vehicle ownership did not change, men who acquired a vehicle experienced a 1.8 kg greater weight gain ($p < 0.05$) and were twice as likely to become obese.

The final pattern is type of leisure activity. Television ownership has skyrocketed in China, leading to greater inactivity during leisure time (28). The consequences of this shift, not only in TV ownership but also in usage patterns for TV watching, remain to be fully studied.

4. IS THE BIOLOGY DIFFERENT?

There are a number of different ways in which this question could be answered in the affirmative. One is if the body composition and other unmeasured race–ethnic factors affect susceptibility to NR-NCDs. Another might be if previous disease patterns (e.g., the presence of malaria or other tropical diseases) led to disease patterns that predisposed the population to certain problems. There is limited but strong evidence that there are potentially important biological differences between those from the developing world and those from Western Europe or European genetic backgrounds. Do we need different body mass index (BMI) cut points for subpopulation groups and is this based on biological differences or just adiposity measurement that is missed with the use of BMI? That is, do we just have such imprecise measurement that this is the problem? Again, there is evidence from a range of body composition and BMI–disease studies that would lead us to believe that the answer is yes. That is, Asians, Africans, and Latin Americans are more likely than whites in the United States and Europe to have greater body fat and central fat for the same BMI and to have a higher likelihood of experiencing cardiovascular disease (CVD) outcomes of importance at lower BMI levels.

There is another pathway related to the role of previous health problems for which we have less understanding and no real documentation of its impact, e.g., malnutrition causing viral mutation, parasitic infections affecting long-term absorption patterns, or a parasite linked with an unknown genotype—comparable to sickle cell anemia and its evolutionary linkage with malaria. We have no basis for speculation about this potential pathway.

However, the final pathway—the effect of fetal and infant insults on subsequent metabolic function—is one that appears to be a critical area. If the rapid shifts toward positive energy imbalance are occurring concurrently with higher levels of low birthweight in a population, then this becomes a much more salient aspect of this argument. In the developing world, where intrauterine malnutrition rates are high and a high prevalence of nutrition insults during infancy exist, the work of Barker and many others portends important potential effects on the prevalence of NR-NCDs in the coming decades. Not only is there an emerging consensus that fetal insults, in particular with regard to thin, low-birth-weight infants who subsequently face a shift in the stage of the transition and become overweight, are linked with increased risk of the NR-NCDs, but infancy may equally be a period of high vulnerability. Termed "fetal origins" or "infant programming," this literature suggests that a rapid shift toward energy imbalance, preceded by high levels of thin babies and infant stunting, will have important long-term effects in increasing the probability that the subsequent energy imbalance leads to CVD and various conditions linked with CVD.

5. CAN WE TURN BACK THE CLOCK OR MODIFY THE ADVERSE DYNAMICS? PROGRAM AND POLICY ISSUES

A series of papers focused on the early efforts in low- and moderate-income countries to prevent many of the most adverse dimensions of the rapid shift to the NR-NCD pattern. The general message is that a combination of national and local efforts targeted on changes, not only in the economic and physical environment, but also use of the mass media and various settings (work, school, and community) are needed to create the wide-scale changes needed.

Puska et al. *(29)* provide a clear example of how an integrated approach to dietary change can affect the structure of the diet and considerably reduce NR-NCDs. They focused on the need for intersectoral collaboration with one responsible national agency as the focal point. Then they laid out how, in Finland, national price policy and food-labeling policies were combined with nutrition education programs and the enlistment of voluntary organizations, to tackle this effort. They also discussed the need to involve industry at the national and international level. Their paper shows how research and demonstration efforts also comprise important elements in the large-scale effort needed.

Matsudo et al. *(30)* presented some of the key elements used to launch a mass promotion of physical activity in São Paulo, Brazil. Termed the Agita São Paulo, it began as a multilevel, community-wide intervention designed to increase the knowledge about benefits and the level of physical activity in a megapopulation of 34 million of São Paulo State. It is slowly being expanded into a national effort. It begins with the main message that moderate intensity physical activity for 30 min/d (in one single or in multiple sessions) on most days of the week is important. The program encourages activity at home, leisure, and in transport between locations. It focuses all education materials and efforts on a "one step ahead" model. In order to reach all socioeconomic classes it has widely used mass activity Agita days where millions walk, as well as a wide range of messages and approaches. The Agita approach focuses on partnering with many different sectors to empower persons of all ages and classes. This Agita movement began after the reduction in obesity noted in the Monteiro et al. paper *(31)*. It promises to be an important dimension of the Brazilian effort to improve diet and reduce sedentarianism.

Zhai et al. *(32)* and Coitinho et al. *(33)* provide important overviews of China and Brazil, countries that have begun to address this topic. China began in the late 1980s to consider price policies and other food policies that might retard or arrest the rapid shift toward an energy-dense diet but did little else in the last decade. The Chinese Academies of Agricultural Sciences and Preventive Medicine (including as a key component the Institute of Nutrition and Food Safety) along with the State Council met in one international meeting to review evidence in 1990 regarding the shift in the structure of the Chinese diet and patterns of morbidity and mortality. They have now begun to consider a wide-ranging set of activities in the nutrition and other sectors to address the very rapid increase of NR-NCDs seen in China. In the health sector, efforts related to reducing hypertension and diabetes are becoming more widespread, but there is limited work in the nutrition sector aside from the creation of dietary guidelines. This paper points to some unique strengths from past Chinese efforts and to an agenda for the next several decades.

In Brazil, a more coordinated and systematic effort is underway. The effort began more recently, but has created a number of important legislative and regulatory policies, revised one very large school feeding program, and done much to focus on the national policy environment. At the same time efforts at mass communication directly via the mass media and through schools and food stores are underway. Furthermore, efforts at long-term capacity building have begun. The Matsudo et al. *(30)* effort noted above is a key component of this effort.

Earlier work in South Korea has also shown how that country used a variety of educational and other nutrition programs to promote the traditional high-vegetable and low-fat diet *(34,35)*.

6. SUMMARY

This chapter explores shifts in nutrition transition from the period termed the receding famine pattern to one dominated by NR-NCDs. It examines the speed of these changes, summarizes dietary and physical activity changes, and provides some sense of the health effects and economic costs. The focus is on the lower- and middle-income countries of Asia, Africa, the Middle East, and Latin America. The article shows that changes are occurring at great speed and at earlier stages of countries' economic and social development. The burden of disease from NR-NCDs is shifting towards the poor and the costs are also becoming greater than those for undernutrition. Policy options are identified.

REFERENCES

1. Truswell AS. Diet and Nutrition of Hunter-gathers. Health and Diseases in Tribal Societies. Ciba Foundation Symposium 149. Elsevier, Amsterdam, 1977.
2. Harris DR. The prehistory of human subsistence: a speculative outline, In: Food, Nutrition and Evolution: Food as an Environmental Factor in the Genesis of Human Variability, Walcher DN, Kretchmer N, eds., Masson, New York, 1981.
3. Eaton SB, Shostak M, Konner M. The Paleolithic Prescription: A Program of Diet and Exercise and a Design for Living. Harper & Row, New York, 1988.
4. Eaton SB, Konner M. Paleolithic nutrition: A consideration on its nature and current implications. N. Engl. J. Med. 1985; 312:283–289.
5. Vargas LA. Old and new transitions and nutrition in Mexico, In: Disease in Populations in Transition, Swedlund AC, Armelagos GJ, eds., Greenwood, Westport, CT, 1990.
6. Gordon KD. Evolutionary perspectives on human diet, In: Nutritional Anthropology, Johnson, FE, ed., Liss, New York, 1987, pp. 3–41.
7. Newman LF, Kates RW, Matthews R, Millman S. Hunger in History. Basil Blackwell, Cambridge, MA, 1990.
8. Omran AR. The epidemiologic transition: a theory of the epidemiology of population change. Milbank Mem. Fund Q. 1971; 49(4, pt. 1):509–538.
9. Milio N. Nutrition Policy for Food-rich Countries: a Strategic Analysis. The Johns Hopkins University Press, Baltimore, 1990.
10. Popkin BM, Haines PS, Reidy KC. Food consump¬≠tion of U.S. women: patterns and determinants between 1977 and 1985. Am. J. Clin. Nutr. 1989; 49:1307–1319.
11. Popkin BM, Haines PS, Patterson R. Dietary changes among older Americans, 1977–87. Am. J. Clin. Nutr. 1992; 55:823–830.
12. Manton KG, Soldo BJ. Dynamics of health changes in the oldest old: New perspective and evidence. Milbank Mem. Fund Q. Health Soc. 1985; 63:206–285.
13. Crimmins EM, Saito Y, Ingegneri D. Changes in life expectancy and disability-free life expectancy in the United States. Popul. Dev. Rev. 1989; 15:235–267.

14. Fischler C. L'Homnivore: le Gôvt, la Cuisine et le Corps. Odile Jacob, Paris, 1990.
15. Drewnowski A. Dietary fats: perceptions and preferences. J. Am. Coll. Nutr. 1990; 9:431–435.
16. Drewnowski A, Popkin BM. The nutrition transition: new trends in the global diet. Nutr. Rev. 1997; 55:31–43.
17. Galloway JH. Sugar, In: The Cambridge World History of Food. Vol I, Kiple KF, Ornelas KC, eds., Cambridge University Press, New York, 2000, pp. 437–449.
18. Mintz S. Time, sugar, and sweetness, In: Food and Culture: A Reader. Counihan C, Van Esterik P, eds., Routledge, New York, 1977, pp. 357–369.
19. Popkin BM, Nielsen SJ. The sweetening of the world's diet. Obesity Res. 2003; 11, 1325–1332.
20. Popkin BM, Bisgrove E. Urbanization and nutrition in low-income countries. Food Nutr. Bull. 1988; 10:3–23.
21. Solomons NW, Gross R. Urban nutrition in developing countries. Nutr. Rev. 1995; 53:90–95.
22. Delgado CL. Rising consumption of meat and milk in developing countries has created a new food revolution. J. Nutr. 2003; 133:3907S–3910S.
23. Popkin BM, Du S. Dynamics of the nutrition transition toward the animal foods sector in China and its implications: a worried perspective. J. Nutr. 2003; 33(1):3898S–3906S.
24. Guo X, Mroz TA, Popkin BM, Zhai F. Structural changes in the impact of income on food consumption in China, 1989–93. Econ. Devel. Cult. Change 2000; 48:737–760.
25. Popkin BM. Urbanization, lifestyle changes and the nutrition transition. World Devel. 1999; 27:1905–1916.
26. Bell C, Ge K, Popkin BM. Weight gain and its predictors in Chinese adults. Int. J. Obes. 2001; 25:1079–1086.
27. Bell AC, Ge K, Popkin BM. The road to obesity or the path to prevention? Motorized transportation and obesity in China. Obes. Res. 2002; 10:277–283.
28. Du S, Lu B, Zhai F, Popkin BM. The nutrition transition in China: a new stage of the Chinese diet, In: The Nutrition Transition: Diet and Disease in the Developing World. Caballero, B., Popkin, B. M., Academic Press, London, 2002, pp. 205–222.
29. Puska P, Pietinen P, Uusitalo U. Influencing public nutrition for noncommunicable disease prevention: from community intervention to national programme —experiences from Finland. Public Health Nutr. 2002; 5(1A):245–251.
30. Matsudo V, Matsudo S, Andrade D, et al. Promotion of physical activity in a developing country: The Agita São Paulo experience. Public Health Nutr. 2002; 5(1A):253 and 261.
31. Monteiro CA, Benicio MHD'A, Conde WL, Popkin BM. Shifting obesity trends in Brazil. Eur. J. Clin. Nutr. 2000; 54:342–346.
32. Zhai F, Fu D, Du S, Ge K, Chen C, Popkin BM. What is China doing in policy-making to push back the negative aspects of the nutrition transition? Public Health Nutr. 2002; 5(1A):269–273.
33. Coitinho D, Monteiro CA, Popkin BM. What Brazil is doing to promote healthy diets and active lifestyles? Public Health Nutr. 2002; 5(1A):263–267.
34. Kim S, Moon S, Popkin BM. The nutrition transition in South Korea. Am. J. Clin. Nutr. 2000; 71:44–53.
35. Lee M-J, Popkin BM, Kim S. The unique aspects of the nutrition transition in South Korea: the retention of healthful elements in their traditional diet. Public Health Nutr. 2002; 5(1A):197–203.e

4 Medical Nutrition Therapy for Diabetes

Prioritizing Recommendations Based on Evidence

Marion J. Franz

KEY POINTS

- Long-term clinical trials have documented the importance of metabolic control of glucose, lipids, and blood pressure in patients with diabetes. Although new medications and insulins are now available, medical nutrition therapy (MNT) is essential if medical goals are to be achieved. Successful MNT is an ongoing process.
- Recommendations for carbohydrate, protein, fat, micronutrients, and alcohol are graded according to the level of available evidence. The grading of recommendations can be used to prioritize nutrition care.
- For persons with type 1 diabetes, the first priority is to identify a food/meal plan that can be used to integrate an insulin regimen into the person's lifestyle. Physiological insulin regimens consisting of a basal or background insulin and bolus or mealtime insulin or insulin pumps provide flexibility in timing and frequency of meals, amounts of carbohydrate eaten at meals, and timing of physical activity. Insulin-to-carbohydrate ratios are used to adjust the mealtime rapid-acting insulin dose needed to cover the planned carbohydrate content of the meal.
- Type 2 diabetes results from a combination of insulin resistance and insulin deficiency (β-cell failure) and is a progressive disease. Just as medical management of type 2 diabetes progresses from nutrition therapy as monotherapy to nutrition therapy plus medications including insulin, the nutrition care process must also change. Nutrition therapy for type 2 diabetes progresses from prevention of obesity or weight gain to improving insulin resistance to contributing to improved metabolic control.
- Monitoring of glucose, lipids, and blood pressure is essential to assess the outcomes of lifestyle interventions and/or to determine if additional changes in lifestyle or medications are necessary.

From: *Nutritional Health: Strategies for Disease Prevention, Second Edition*
Edited by: N. J. Temple, T. Wilson, and D. R. Jacobs © Humana Press Inc., Totowa, NJ

1. INTRODUCTION

Diabetes mellitus is a group of diseases characterized by an elevated blood glucose concentration resulting from defects in insulin secretion, insulin action, or both. Insulin, a hormone produced by the β-cells of the pancreas, is necessary for the use or storage of body fuels. In diabetes abnormalities in the metabolism of carbohydrate, protein, and fat are present. Without effective insulin, hyperglycemia occurs causing both the short-term and long-term complications of diabetes mellitus.

Approximately 16.7 million US adults have diagnosed diabetes; an increase from 4.9% of the adult population in 1990 to 7.9% in 2001—a 61% increase *(1)*. If undiagnosed diabetes is also included, it is likely that almost 10% of US adults have the disease. Prevalence increases with age, affecting 18.4% of those 65 yr of age or older *(2)*. The disease is particularly prevalent in ethnic populations, such as African Americans, Hispanic populations (Latinos and Mexican Americans), Native Americans and Alaskan Natives, Asian Americans, and Pacific Islanders *(2)*. Much of the increase is because the prevalence of diabetes increased by 76% among people in their 30s *(2)*. The prevalence of newly diagnosed type 2 diabetes among children has also increased from less than 4% in the years before 1990 to nearly 45% in recent years in certain racial/ethnic groups *(2)*.

Of concern are the more than 20 million adults with impaired glucose tolerance (IGT), the 13–14 million with impaired fasting glucose (IFG), and the 40–50 million with metabolic syndrome *(2)*. These individuals are at high risk for conversion to type 2 diabetes and for cardiovascular disease (CVD) if lifestyle prevention strategies are not implemented.

2. DIAGNOSIS AND SCREENING FOR DIABETES MELLITUS

Three ways to diagnosis diabetes are available and in the absence of unequivocal hyperglycemia with acute metabolic decompensation, each must be confirmed on a subsequent day. Normal and diagnostic criteria are listed in Table 1 *(3)*.

Testing or screening for diabetes should be considered in all individuals aged 45 yr of age and older, particularly in those with a body mass index (BMI) of 25 kg/m² or more, and, if normal, the test should be repeated at 3-yr intervals *(3)*. Testing should be considered at a younger age, or be carried out more frequently, in individuals who are overweight (BMI ≥ 25 kg/m²) and have additional risk factors:

- Are habitually physically inactive.
- Have a first-degree relative with diabetes.
- Are members of a high-risk ethnic population cited in the Introduction.
- Have delivered a baby weighing more than 9 kg or have been diagnosed with gestational diabetes mellitus (GDM).
- Are hypertensive (blood pressure ≥140/90 mmHg).
- Have a high-density lipoprotein (HDL) cholesterol level 0.90 mmol/L or less (35 mg/dL) or a triglyceride level 2.82 mmol/L or higher (250 mg/dL).
- Have polycystic ovary syndrome (PCOS).
- Had IGT or IFG on previous testing.
- Have other clinical considerations associated with insulin resistance (e.g., PCOS or acanthosis nigricans—gray-brown skin pigmentations).
- Have a history of vascular disease.

Table 1
Criteria for the Diagnosis of Diabetes Using Fasting Plasma Glucose,
2-h Postprandial Glucose, or Casual Glucose

Normoglycemia	Impaired fasting glucose (IFG) or impaired glucose tolerance (IGT)	Diabetes[a]
• Fasting plasma glucose (FPG) < 5.6 mmol/L (<100 mg/dL) • 2-h postprandial glucose (PG)[b] <7.8 mmol/L (<140 mg/dL)	• IFG: FPG≥5.6 and <7.0 mmol/L (≥100 and < 126 mg/dL) • IGT: 2-h PG[b] ≥7.8 and <11.1 mmol/L (≥140 and <200 mg/dL)	• FPG≥7.0 mmol/L (≥126 mg/dL) • 2-h PG[b] ≥11.1 mmol/L (≥200 mg/dL) • Symptoms of diabetes and casual plasma glucose concentration ≥11.1 mmol/L (≥200 mg/dL)

[a]The FPG test is preferred because of ease of administration, convenience, acceptability in patients, and lower cost.

[b]This test requires the use of a glucose load containing the equivalent of 75 g anhydrous glucose dissolved in water. (Adapted from ref. 3.)

Consistent with screening recommendations for adults, children, and youth at increased risk for type 2 diabetes should be tested if they are both:
- Overweight (BMI > 85th percentile for age and sex, or weight for height > 85th percentile, or > 120% of ideal weight for height).
- Two of the following risk factors are present—family history of type 2 diabetes in first- or second-degree relative, member of high-risk ethnic populations, signs of insulin resistance or conditions associated with insulin resistance (acanthosis nigricans, hypertension, dyslipidemia, or PCOS) (3).

Screening should be initiated at 10 yr of age or at onset of puberty, if puberty occurs at a younger age, and, if normal, repeated every 2 yr. The preferred test is the fasting plasma glucose test.

2.1. Type 1 Diabetes

Type 1 diabetes accounts for 5–10% of all diagnosed cases of diabetes. The primary defect is pancreatic β-cell destruction, usually leading to absolute insulin deficiency and resulting in hyperglycemia, polyuria, polydipsia, weight loss, dehydration, electrolyte disturbance, and ketoacidosis. The capacity of a healthy pancreas to secrete insulin is far in excess of what is needed normally; therefore, the clinical onset of diabetes may be preceded by an extensive asymptomatic period of months to years, during which β-cells are undergoing gradual destruction. Persons with type 1 diabetes are dependent on exogenous insulin to prevent ketoacidosis and death. Although it can occur at any age, even in the eighth and ninth decades of life, most cases are diagnosed in people younger than 30 yr of age, with peak incidence at around ages 10–12 yr in girls and 12–14 yr in boys.

The etiology involves a genetic disposition and an autoimmune destruction of the islet β-cells that produce insulin. At diagnosis, 85–90% of persons with type 1 diabetes have one or more circulating autoantibodies. Antibodies identified as contributing to the destruction of β-cells are as follows:

1. Islet cell autoantibodies.
2. Insulin autoantibodies, which may occur in persons who have never received insulin therapy.
3. Autoantibodies to glutamic acid decarboxylase (GAD_{65}), a protein on the surface of β-cells that appears to provoke an attack by the T-cells (killer T-lymphocytes) and to destroy the β-cells.
4. Autoantibodies to the tyrosine phosphatases IA-2 and IA-2β.

The disease also has strong human leukocyte antigen *HLA* associations, with linkage to the *DQA* and *DQB* genes, and is influenced by the *DRB* genes. These *HLA-DR/DQ* alleles can be either predisposing or protective *(4)*.

Frequently, after diagnosis and the correction of hyperglycemia, metabolic acidosis, and ketoacidosis, there is a recovery of endogenous insulin secretion. During this "honeymoon phase," exogenous insulin requirements decrease dramatically. However, the need for exogenous insulin is inevitable, and within 8–10 yr after clinical onset, β-cell loss is complete and insulin deficiency is absolute.

Latent autoimmune diabetes of adults describes a minority of patients with adult-onset diabetes. Typically, patients are positive for glutamic acid decarboxylase antibodies, 35 yr of age or older, nonobese, and present without ketosis and weight loss. Although many maintain good glycemic control for several years with sulfonylureas, these persons become "insulin-dependent" more rapidly than antibody-negative persons with type 2 diabetes *(5)*.

2.2. Type 2 Diabetes

Lifestyle interventions for the prevention and control of type 2 diabetes is the subject of Chapter 5. This condition may account for 90–95% of all diagnosed cases of diabetes and is a progressive disease that is often present long before it is diagnosed. Persons may or may not experience the classic symptoms of uncontrolled diabetes and they are not prone to develop ketoacidosis. Although persons with type 2 diabetes do not require exogenous insulin for survival, approx 40% or more will eventually require exogenous insulin for adequate glycemic control *(6)*.

Risk factors include genetic and environmental factors. Although approx 50% of men and 70% of women are obese at the time of diagnosis, type 2 diabetes also occurs in nonobese individuals, especially in the elderly, whereas, conversely, many obese individuals never develop type 2 diabetes *(2)*.

Type 2 diabetes results from a combination of insulin resistance and insulin deficiency (β-cell failure). Endogenous insulin levels may be normal, depressed, or elevated, but they are inadequate to overcome concomitant insulin resistance (decreased tissue sensitivity or responsiveness to insulin). As a result of this, hyperglycemia ensues, which is first exhibited as an elevation of postprandial glucose owing to insulin resistance at the cellular (muscle and liver) level. As insulin secretion decreases, hepatic glucose production increases causing elevations in fasting glucose levels. Compounding the problem is the deleterious effect of hyperglycemia itself—glucotoxicity—on both insulin sensitivity and insulin secretion, hence the importance of achieving near-euglycemia in persons with type 2 diabetes *(7)*.

Insulin resistance is also demonstrated in adipocytes, leading to lipolysis and an elevation in circulating free fatty acids. Increased free fatty acids further cause a decrease in insulin sensitivity at the cellular level, impair insulin secretion by the pancreas, and augment hepatic glucose production (lipotoxicity) *(8)*. To slow the progressive nature of type 2 diabetes requires that both conditions (hyperglycemia and lipotoxicity) be corrected.

2.3. Gestational Diabetes Mellitus

GDM is defined as any degree of glucose intolerance with onset or first recognition during pregnancy. It occurs in approx 7% of all pregnancies, resulting in more than 200,000 cases annually *(9)*. It is usually diagnosed during the second or third trimester, at which point insulin-antagonist hormones increase and insulin resistance occurs. Risk assessment for GDM should be undertaken at the first prenatal visit. Women at high risk (marked obesity, personal history of GDM, glycosuria, or a strong family history of diabetes) should be tested as soon as feasible. Other women are tested between 24 and 28 wk of gestation.

2.4. Other Types of Diabetes

Diabetes associated with or secondary to other conditions may occur in about 2% of all disorders comprising the syndrome of diabetes. These conditions include pancreatic disease, hormonal disease, drug or chemical exposure, insulin receptor abnormalities, and certain genetic syndromes *(4)*.

2.5. Prediabetes

Prediabetes is the preferred term for the condition previously referred to as impaired glucose homeostasis and includes IGT and IFG *(4)*. Prediabetes refers to a stage intermediate between normal glucose homeostasis and diabetes. *See* Table 1 for diagnostic criteria. Individuals with prediabetes are at high risk for future diabetes and CVD, which are both associated with the metabolic syndrome. Central to the metabolic syndrome is insulin resistance and the constellation of associated cardiovascular risk factors—visceral (abdominal) obesity, dyslipidemia (characterized by small, dense low-density lipoprotein [LDL] cholesterol particles, hypertriglyceridemia, and low levels of HDL cholesterol), and elevated blood pressure.

3. IMPORTANCE OF METABOLIC CONTROL

3.1. Type 1 Diabetes

Evidence relating hyperglycemia and other metabolic consequences of insulin deficiency to the development of complications comes from a series of studies in Europe and North America. The Diabetes Control and Complications Trial (DCCT) demonstrated beyond a doubt the clear link between glycemic control and development of noncardiovascular and microvascular complications in persons with type 1 diabetes and that any improvement in glycemic control reduces the risk of developing complications *(10)*. The Diabetes Control and Complications Trial, sponsored by the US National Institutes of Health, was a long-term, prospective, randomized, controlled, multicenter trial that studied approx 1400 young adults (aged 13–39 yr) with type 1 diabetes who were treated with either intensive therapeutic regimens (multiple injections of insulin or use of insulin infusion pumps guided by blood glucose monitoring results) or conventional regimens (one or two insulin injections per day). Patients who achieved control similar to that of the intensively treated patients in the study could expect a 50–75% reduction in the risk of progression to retinopathy, nephropathy, and neuropathy after 8–9 yr.

3.2. Type 2 Diabetes

The United Kingdom Prospective Diabetes Study (UKPDS) demonstrated conclusively that elevated blood glucose levels cause long-term complications in type 2 diabetes just as in type 1 diabetes (11). The UKPDS recruited and followed 5102 newly diagnosed individuals with type 2 diabetes for an average of 10–11 yr. Subjects randomized into a group treated conventionally, primarily with nutrition therapy, had an average hemoglobin A1c (A1C) of 7.9% compared to subjects randomized into an intensively treated group, initially treated with sulfonylureas, who had an average A1C of 7.0%. In the intensive therapy group, the microvascular complications rate decreased significantly by 25% and the risk of macrovascular disease decreased by 16%. Combination therapy (combining insulin or metformin with sulfonylureas) was needed in both groups to meet glycemic goals as loss of glycemic control was noted during the 10-yr trial. Aggressive treatment of even mild-to-moderate hypertension was also beneficial in both groups (12).

This study documented the progressive nature of type 2 diabetes. Before randomization into intensive or conventional treatment, subjects received individualized intensive nutrition therapy for 3 mo. During this run-in period, the mean A1C decreased by 1.9% (from ~9 to ~7%) and patients lost an average of 3.5 kg (8 lb). UKPDS researchers concluded that a reduction of energy intake was at least as important, if not more important than, the actual weight lost in determining the fasting plasma glucose (13). An important lesson learned from the UKPDS is that therapy needs to be intensified over time and that as the disease progresses, medical nutrition therapy (MNT) alone is not enough to keep the majority of the patients' A1C levels at 7%. Medication(s), and for many individuals eventually insulin, needs to be added to the treatment regimen. It is not the "diet" failing, but instead it is the pancreas failing to secrete enough insulin to maintain adequate glucose control.

4. GLUCOSE, LIPID, AND BLOOD PRESSURE GOALS

It is important that persons with diabetes need to know their target blood glucose, lipid, and blood pressure goals. Self-monitoring of blood glucose (SMBG) is used on a day-to-day basis to adjust treatment regimens; however, laboratory measurement of glycated hemoglobin provides the best available index of overall diabetes control. The healthcare team, including the individual with diabetes, should work together to implement blood glucose monitoring and establish individual target blood glucose goals (see Table 2 for a listing of target goals). The frequency of monitoring depends on the type of diabetes and overall therapy.

4.1. Self-Monitoring of Blood Glucose

SMBG can be performed up to eight times per day—before breakfast, lunch, and dinner; at bedtime; 1–2 h after the start of meals; during the night; or when needed to determine causes of hypoglycemia or hyperglycemia. For most patients with type 1 diabetes, SMBG is recommended four or more times a day, namely before each meal and at bedtime. SMBG in persons with type 2 diabetes should be sufficient to facilitate

Table 2
Glucose, Lipids, and Blood Pressure Recommendations for Adults With Diabetes

Glycemic control	
A1C	<7.0%[a]
Preprandial plasma glucose	5.0–7.2 mmol/L (90–130 mg/dL)
Postprandial plasma glucose	<10.0 mmol/L (180 mg/dL)
Blood pressure	<130/80 mmHg
Lipids	
LDL cholesterol	<2.6 mmol/L (<100 mg/dL)
Triglycerides	<1.7 mmol/L (<150 mg/dL)
HDL cholesterol	>1.1 mmol/L (>40 mg/dL)[b]

[a]Referenced to a nondiabetic range of 4.0–6.0% using a Diabetes Control and Complications Trial -based assay.

[b]For women, it has been suggested that the high-density lipoprotein goal be increased by 10 mg/dL.
LDL, low-density lipoprotein; HDL, high-density lipoprotein; A1C, hemoglobin A1c.
(Adapted from ref. 3.)

reaching glucose goals and is often performed one to four times a day, often before breakfast and before and 2 h after the largest meal, but only 3 or 4 d/wk. When adding to or modifying therapy, patients with type 1 and type 2 diabetes should test more often than usual *(14)*.

Because the accuracy of SMBG is dependent on the instrument and user, it is important for health care providers to evaluate each individual's monitoring techniques, both initially and at regular intervals thereafter. Comparisons between results from patient self-testing in the clinic and simultaneous laboratory testing are useful to assess the accuracy of patient results. Most meters now automatically convert the capillary whole blood test to plasma glucose values so comparisons can readily be made with laboratory values.

It is important that the results of SMBG be written in a record book, and that individuals be taught how to adjust their management program based on the results. The first step in using such records is to learn how to identify patterns in blood glucose levels and how to adjust insulin and/or medication doses. For example, if blood glucose levels are consistently (generally 3 d in a row) elevated at a specific testing time, adjustments are made in the insulin or medication acting at that time. After pattern management is mastered, algorithms for insulin dose changes to compensate for an elevated or low glucose value can be added.

In using blood glucose monitoring records, it should be remembered that factors other than food affect blood glucose concentrations. An increase in blood glucose can be the result of insufficient insulin or insulin secretagogues, too much food, or increases in glucagon and other counterregulatory hormones as a result of stress, illness, or infection. Factors contributing to hypoglycemia include too much insulin or insulin secretagogues, not enough food, unusual amounts of exercise, and skipped or delayed meals.

It is now possible to do continuous ambulatory blood glucose monitoring to determine 24-h blood glucose patterns and to detect unrecognized hypoglycemia. One such system consists of a subcutaneous sensor that monitors interstitial glucose levels for up to 72 h. Data can be downloaded in the physician's office after completion of the prescribed cycle.

4.2. Glycated Hemoglobin

Glycated hemoglobin can be assayed by several methods and is expressed as the percentage of hemoglobin that has glucose attached to it. Hemoglobin A1 is an evaluation of a combination of all fractions of the hemoglobin molecule. A1C is a measurement of the glycation of the "c" fraction and the values are lower because only one fraction is measured.

4.3. Lipids and Blood Pressure

Other parameters besides glucose that must be regularly monitored are lipids and blood pressure (see Table 2 for lipid and blood pressure goals). In adults with diabetes, lipid tests should be done at least annually and more often if needed to achieve goals (3). Lifestyle interventions, including MNT and increased physical activity, may allow some persons to reach lipid goals. Glucose control can also beneficially modify plasma lipid levels while smoking cessation to decrease risk of CVD is important. Pharmacological treatment is indicated if lipid goals are not reached with lifestyle modifications and improved glycemia. However, in patients with clinical CVD and LDL cholesterol higher than 2.6 mmol/L (>100 mg/dL), pharmacological therapy is initiated at the same time that lifestyle interventions are started (3). The first priority of pharmacological therapy is to lower LDL cholesterol to less than 2.6 mmol/L (<100 mg/dL) using statins, the drugs of choice for this purpose (15). A lower LDL cholesterol goal of less than 1.8 mmol/L (<70 mg/dL), using a high dose of a statin, is an option in high-risk patients with diabetes and overt CVD (3).

Patients with diabetes should be treated to achieve a systolic blood pressure less than 130 mmHg and a diastolic blood pressure less than 80 mmHg (3). If lifestyle modifications—moderate weight loss, reduction of dietary sodium, increased consumption of fruits, vegetables, and low-fat diary products, avoidance of excessive alcohol consumption, and increased physical activity levels—do not achieve these goals, medication should be added until blood pressure goals are met. Multiple drug therapy (two or more agents at proper doses) is generally required to achieve blood pressure targets (3).

4.4. Ketone Tests

Urine or blood testing can be used to detect ketones. Testing for ketonuria or ketonemia should be performed regularly during periods of illness and when blood glucose levels consistently exceed 13.3 mmol/L (240 mg/dL). The presence of persistent, moderate, or large amounts of ketones, along with elevated blood glucose levels, requires insulin adjustments. Persons with type 2 diabetes rarely have ketosis. However, ketone testing should be done in the presence of a serious illness.

5. MEDICATIONS

5.1. Insulin

Persons with type 1 diabetes depend on insulin to survive. In individuals with type 2 diabetes, insulin may be needed to restore glycemia to normal. Circumstances that require the use of insulin in type 2 diabetes include failure to achieve adequate control with use of oral medications; periods of acute injury, infection, or surgery; pregnancy; and allergy or serious reactions to sulfonylurea agents.

Table 3
Insulin Therapy

Type of insulin	Onset of action	Peak action	Usual effective duration	Monitor effect in
Bolus insulin				
Rapid-acting				
Lispro (Humalog)	<15 min	0.5–1.5 h	2–4 h	2 h
Aspart (Novolog)				
Glulisine (Apidra)	0.5–1 h	2–3 h	3–6 h	4 h (next meal)
Short-acting				
Regular				
Basal insulin				
Long-acting				
Glargine (Lantus)	~1 h	—	24 h	10–12 h
Intermediate-acting				
NPH	2–4 h	6–10 h	10–16 h	8–12 h
Mixtures				
70/30 (70% NPH, 30% regular)	0.5–1 h	Dual	10–16 h	
Humalog Mix 75/25 (75% neutral protamine lispro [NPL] 25% lispro)	<15 min	Dual	10–16 h	
Novolog Mix 70/30 (70% neutral protamine aspart [NPA] 30% aspart)	<15 min	Dual	10–16 h	

NPH, neutral protamine hagedorn.

57

Insulin regimens are designed to mimic normal insulin action. After eating, plasma glucose and insulin concentrations increase rapidly, peak in 30–60 min, and return to basal concentrations within 2–3 h. To mimic this, rapid-acting (or short-acting) insulin is given before meals and is referred to as bolus or mealtime insulin. Mealtime insulin doses are adjusted based on the carbohydrate in the meal *(16)*. An insulin-to-carbohydrate ratio can be established for an individual that will determine the amount of bolus insulin to inject. (*See* Table 2 for types of insulin, onset, and approximate duration of action.)

The basal or background insulin dose is that amount of insulin required in the postabsorptive state to restrain endogenous glucose output primarily from the liver, and to limit lipolysis and excess flux of free fatty acids to the liver. Glargine is a frequently used 24-h peakless insulin and is given at bedtime (or at any consistent time during the day). To better mimic the physiological action of insulin, basal insulin, such as glargine, can be used with rapid-acting insulin given at mealtimes to control postprandial glucose levels and to reduce the risk of hypoglycemia. Determir is another peakless insulin and is used as a basal insulin. Historically, neutral protamine hagedorn insulin has also been used as basal insulin. It must be administered twice a day, usually before breakfast and the evening meal, but because of its peaking action, it often results in erratic glucose levels and overnight hypoglycemia.

Insulin pump therapy provides basal rapid-acting or short-acting insulin pumped continuously by a mechanical device in micro amounts through a subcutaneous catheter that is monitored 24 h a day. Boluses of the insulin are then given before meals.

The administration of basal insulin once or twice a day and often in combination with oral glucose-lowering medications, may suffice for individuals with type 2 diabetes who still have significant endogenous insulin. A commonly used regimen combines a short-acting or rapid-acting insulin and a basal insulin, such as neutral protamine hagedorn, given twice a day. However, many individuals with type 2 diabetes will eventually require an insulin regimen that better mimics the physiological actions of endogenous insulin.

5.2. Oral Glucose-Lowering Medications for Type 2 Diabetes

Pharmacological options before the mid-1990s were limited to sulfonylureas and insulin. However, since that time new classes of oral medications have been introduced to the market that target the mechanisms underlying insulin resistance and insulin deficiency. Administered as monotherapy, each of the classes of medications (except α-glucosidase inhibitors) result in an approx 1–2% reduction in A1C compared with placebo in controlled clinical trials *(17)*.

Sulfonylureas, such as glimepiride and glyburide, are known as insulin secretagogs and cause insulin release from β-cells. They depend on the concentration of intracellular calcium. Sulfonylureas bind to receptors on pancreatic β-cell surfaces to enhance the entry of calcium into β-cells with a resultant increase in insulin secretion.

Nonsulfonylurea insulin secretagogs, such as repaglinide and nateglinide, also bind to receptors on pancreatic β-cell surfaces to enhance the entry of calcium into the β-cells with a resultant increase in insulin secretion. The effect is glucose-dependent. Insulin secretion is rapidly stimulated when needed and then insulin concentrations are allowed to return to normal.

Biguanides, especially metformin, are categorized as insulin sensitizers because they reduce insulin-stimulated liver glucose production. This is manifested as an improvement in fasting glucose values.

The thiazolidinediones, such as rosiglitazone and pioglitazone, reduce insulin resistance by binding to a nuclear peroxisome-proliferation activated receptor γ in muscle and adipose cells. This changes transcription of genes mediating carbohydrate and lipid metabolism resulting in an increase in insulin stimulated uptake of glucose by skeletal muscle cells. They also reduce lipolysis with a resultant reduction in free fatty acid, increase HDL cholesterol, and decrease triglyceride levels.

α-Glucosidase inhibitors, such as acarbose and miglitol, unlike other classes of medications do not target the mechanisms underlying insulin resistance or deficient insulin secretion. Instead, they competitively inhibit the intestinal epithelial enzyme that catalyzes the conversion of polysaccharides and disaccharides to monosaccharides in the small intestine, thereby delaying carbohydrate absorption and reducing postprandial glucose levels.

Because of the multifactorial nature of type 2 diabetes, combination therapy in which medications with complementary mechanisms of action are used is effective. In a patient whose A1C is more than 2% above target, combination therapy with two or more classes is considered at the onset of therapy as it yields additive reductions in A1C. No particular combination has been shown to be more effective than any other.

Long-term studies demonstrate that oral medications, used first as monotherapy and later in combination therapy, often fail to control blood glucose levels (11). Accordingly, combination therapies of insulin and oral medications are often used. Inclusion of insulin has the additional merit that it may slow the reduction in β-cell function (18). Starting insulin earlier in the course of the disease is one approach that offers the possibility of preserving endogenous insulin secretion by providing the body with an outside source of insulin. Furthermore, this approach can lead to improvements in glycemic control at lower insulin doses than if insulin is used as monotherapy.

5.3. New Injectable Drugs

Two new injectable drugs have recently been approved. Exenatide (Byetta) is the first in a class of drugs called "incretin mimetics," and is derived from lizard saliva of the Gila monster. It mimics the action of a hormone called glucagon-like peptide-1, secreted by the small intestine, which promotes insulin secretion by the pancreas. It is approved for patients taking either metformin (a sulfonylurea) or both, and is injected in fixed doses of 5 or 10 μg less than 1 h before morning and evening meals. Aside from lowering A1C levels it appears to have a weight-loss effect (average weight loss of 3.5 lb), whereas most antidiabetic drugs tend to increase weight.

The second drug is an analog of human amylin, a hormone made in the β-cells of the pancreas. It is called symlin (pramlinitide) and is used as adjunctive therapy to insulin to help control postprandial blood glucose in patients with type 1 and type 2 diabetes who have failed to achieve desired glucose control despite optimal insulin therapy. Samall reduction in weight compared with persons on insulin alone are also reported.

6. MEDICAL NUTRITION THERAPY: EVIDENCE-BASED NUTRITION RECOMMENDATIONS

Evidence-based nutrition practice begins with evidence-based recommendations that translate research data and clinically applicable evidence into the nutrition care process. This requires using the best available evidence while still taking into account individual circumstances, preferences, cultural and ethnic concerns, and involving the person with diabetes in the decision-making process. By collecting and using outcome data, nutrition care and the health and well-being of the patient is improved.

Nutrition recommendations for diabetes illustrate the history of developing recommendations and the evidence-based process. Before 1994, nutrition recommendations for diabetes attempted to define an "ideal" nutrition prescription that would apply to all persons with the disease and one that identified ideal percentages of macronutrients. The nutrition prescription was based on a theoretical calculation of required calories and percentages of carbohydrate, protein, and fat. Individualization, although recommended, needed to be done within the confines of this prescription, which did not allow for much, if any, individualization. Not surprisingly, persons with diabetes often found it difficult, if not impossible, to adhere to these recommendations.

In 1994, the American Diabetes Association (ADA) recommended a different approach *(19,20)*. The nutrition prescription, instead of being rigid, was to be based on an assessment of lifestyle changes that would assist the individual in achieving and maintaining therapeutic goals and changes that he or she is willing and able to make. For example, if an individual with type 2 diabetes has been eating 3000 kcal with 40% of the calories from fat, it is unlikely that the individual would adhere for long to a 1500-kcal weight-reduction diet. A more realistic approach would be to negotiate manageable lifestyle changes that will lower energy and fat intake and that are of the individual's choosing.

This more realistic and flexible approach continues with the 2002 ADA nutrition principles and recommendations *(21,22)*. Historically, nutrition recommendations have been based on scientific knowledge, clinical experience, and expert consensus, but which of these factors are used to make recommendations and to define the quality of the evidence is often unclear. The 2002 nutrition principles and recommendations are classified based on the level of supporting evidence using the ADA system for grading clinical recommendations *(23)*. Recommendations have been assigned a level of evidence, A, B, or C, depending on the quality of the evidence, and E, expert consensus. A-level recommendations have multiple, well-designed and conducted, randomized controlled trials with similar outcomes. B-level recommendations have multiple studies but often with differing outcomes; however, the preponderance of the evidence suggests a particular recommendation. C-level recommendations may have one well-conducted randomized trial, studies with small numbers, or studies that were not as well designed and conducted.

6.1. Goals and Outcomes of Medical Nutrition Therapy for Diabetes

Improving health through food choices and physical activity is the basis of all nutrition recommendations for diabetes. However, a primary goal of MNT is to attain and maintain blood glucose levels in the normal range or as close to normal as is safely possible. MNT must also focus on the effect of lifestyle modifications on lipid and lipoprotein profiles and blood pressure so as to prevent and treat the cardiovascular complications associated with diabetes. However, because lifestyle modifications impact almost immediately on glycemia, glucose goals are often the first focus.

Research supports MNT as an effective therapy in reaching treatment goals. Results from randomized, controlled trials support observational studies of diabetes MNT provided by registered dietitians in demonstrating improved glycemic outcomes with

Table 4
Effectiveness of Medical Nutrition Therapy

End point	Expected outcome	When to evaluate
Glycemic control		6 wk to 3 mo
A1C	1–2% (15–22%) decrease	
Plasma fasting glucose	50 mg/dL (2.78 mmol/L) decrease	
Lipids		6 wk; if goals are
Total cholesterol	24–32 mg/dL (0.62–0.082 mmol/L) (10–16%) decrease	not achieved intensify MNT
LDL cholesterol	19–25 mg/dL (0.46–0.65 mmol/L) (12–16%) decrease	evaluate again in 6 wk
Triglycerides	15–17 mg/dL (0.17–0.19 mmol/L) (8%) decrease	
HDL cholesterol	3 mg/dL (0.08 mmol/L) (7% decrease)	
With no exercise	No decrease	
With exercise		
Blood pressure (in hypertensive patients)	Decrease of 5 mmHg in systolic and 2 mmHg in diastolic	Measured at every medical visit

A1C, hemoglobin A1c; MNT, medical nutrition therapy; HDL, high-density lipoprotein; LDL, low-density lipoprotein. (Reprinted from ref. *25* with permission.)

decreases in A1C of approx 1–2% (a 12–24% decrease in A1C) *(24,25)*. These outcomes are similar to those from oral glucose-lowering medications. Furthermore, the outcomes will be known by 6 wk–3 mo *(26)*. At this point, it is essential that the outcomes of nutrition interventions be evaluated. If the goals have not been met by lifestyle modifications, medications need to added or adjusted. Table 4 is a summary of the mean expected metabolic outcomes from MNT on glucose, lipids, and/or blood pressure.

6.2. Evidence-Based Nutrition Recommendations for Diabetes

The grading of nutrition recommendations also allows professionals to prioritize nutrition care. Nutrition interventions can implement A-level recommendations first, and B-, C-, and expert consensus recommendations would follow. Those based on expert consensus should be noted as not having enough research support to be graded A, B, or C.

6.2.1. CARBOHYDRATE

Because carbohydrate is the nutrient that most affects postprandial glycemia and is the major determinant of bolus insulin doses, it is addressed first. Foods containing carbohydrate—grains, fruits, vegetables, and low-fat milk—are important components of a healthful diet and should be included in the food/meal plan of persons with diabetes (Grade: A). This recommendation reflects the concern that low-carbohydrate diets eliminate many foods that are important for all persons to eat as part of a healthy lifestyle.

There is strong evidence to suggest that in regard to the effects of carbohydrate on glucose concentrations, the total amount of carbohydrate in meals (or snacks) is more important than the source (starch or sugar) or the type (low or high glycemic index [GI])

(Grade: A). Numerous studies have reported that when subjects are allowed to choose from a variety of starch and sugars, the glycemic response is similar, as long as the total amounts of carbohydrate is kept constant *(27)*. All persons with diabetes can benefit from basic information about carbohydrates—what foods contain carbohydrates (starches, fruit, starchy vegetables, milk, sweets), average 15-g portion sizes, and how many servings to select for meals (and snacks if desired) *(28)*. The first decision for food and meal planning is the total number of carbohydrate servings the person with diabetes chooses to eat at meals or for snacks. Individuals on physiological insulin therapy or insulin pumps can adjust their bolus insulin according to the amount of carbohydrate they plan to ingest (Grade: B) *(16)*. Individuals using fixed insulin regimens and who do not self-adjust their insulin doses need to be consistent in day-to-day carbohydrate intake (Grade: C) *(29)*.

Although different carbohydrates do have different glycemic responses (GI), there is limited evidence to show long-term glycemic benefit when low-GI diets vs high-GI diets are implemented *(27)*. In a meta-analysis, low-GI diets compared with high-GI diets reduced A1C by approx 0.43% (a 7.4% decrease) *(30)*. This is in contrast to the studies summarized in Subheading 6.1. that demonstrate a reduction by MNT in A1C of approx 1–2% (a 15–22% decrease). Therefore, for a primary nutrition therapy intervention, an approach documented to have the greatest impact on metabolic outcomes should be selected and information on the glycemic responses of foods can perhaps best be used for fine-tuning glycemic control *(31)*.

Fiber is an important component of a healthful diet, but there is no reason to recommend that people with diabetes eat a greater amount of fiber than other Americans (Grade: B). The effect of fiber on glucose is controversial. Well-controlled studies in individuals with type 1 diabetes *(32)* and with type 2 diabetes *(33)* have reported benefits from very large amounts of fiber (~50 g/d, usual intake is 15–20 g/d) on postprandial glucose, insulin, and lipid levels, whereas other studies using similar amounts have not shown benefit *(34,35)*. It is not known if the majority of persons with diabetes can regularly consume enough fiber long term to see benefit (Grade: Expert Consensus).

6.2.2. PROTEIN

There is minimal evidence to suggest that usual intake of protein (15–20% of energy intake) be changed in people who do not have renal disease (Grade: Expert Consensus). There is some evidence that lowering protein intake to 0.8–1.0 g/kg/d in patients with microalbuminuria or to 0.8 g/kg/d with overt nephropathy may slow the progression of renal disease (Grade: C). Furthermore, in persons with controlled diabetes, ingested protein does not increase plasma glucose concentrations, although protein is just as potent a stimulant of insulin secretion as carbohydrate (Grade: B).

Protein is probably the most misunderstood nutrient with inaccurate advice frequently given to persons with diabetes. Although patients are often told that 50–60% of protein becomes glucose and enters the bloodstream 3–4 h after it is eaten, research documents the inaccuracy of this statement. Although nonessential amino acids undergo gluconeogenesis, in subjects with controlled diabetes the glucose produced does not enter the general circulation *(36,37)*. It is often suggested to patients that adding protein to a meal or snack will slow the absorption of carbohydrate but several studies show that this is not the case. If differing amounts of protein are added to meals or snacks, the peak glucose response is not affected by the addition of protein *(36,38,39)*. There is also no evidence that adding protein to bedtime snacks is helpful or will assist in the immediate treatment of hypoglycemia or prevent blood glucose levels from dropping again after the initial treatment *(40)*.

The long-term effects of a diet high in protein and low in carbohydrate in persons with diabetes are unknown. Although initially blood glucose levels may improve and weight may be lost, it is unknown whether long-term weight loss is maintained any better with these diets than with other low-calorie diets (Grade: Expert Consensus). In a recent randomized trial comparing a low-carbohydrate, high-protein diet with a low-calorie, high-carbohydrate, low-fat (conventional) diet, the low-carbohydrate diet produced a greater weight loss than the conventional diet for the first 6 mo, but the difference was not significant at 1 yr *(41)*. The low-carbohydrate group experienced greater weight regain at 1 yr and an approx 40% attrition rate was reported in both groups.

6.2.3. DIETARY FAT

Limiting intake of saturated fats, trans-fatty acids, and dietary cholesterol is recommended, especially in individuals with LDL cholesterol 100 mg/dL or higher (Grade: A). Research data supporting these guidelines are from studies conducted in the general population. Unfortunately, studies have not been done in people with diabetes demonstrating the effects of specific percentages of saturated fatty acids (e.g., 10 vs 7% of energy) or specific levels of dietary cholesterol.

To lower LDL cholesterol, energy intake from saturated or trans fats can be reduced if weight loss is desirable, or replaced with either carbohydrate or mono- or polyunsaturated fat when weight loss is not a goal (Grade: B). Ethnic or cultural preferences may play a role in determining whether saturated fat is to be replaced with carbohydrate or unsaturated fats. There should be caution in recommending an increased intake of unsaturated or polyunsaturated fat: increasing any type of fat intake may result in increased caloric intake and weight gain (*see* Chapter 13). Careful attention must therefore be paid to total energy intake (Grade: Expert Consensus). In general, research suggests that low-fat diets are usually associated with modest weight loss, which can be maintained as long as the diet is continued *(42)*. With this modest weight loss, a decrease in total cholesterol and triglycerides and an increase in HDL cholesterol are observed.

6.2.4. MICRONUTRIENTS

There is no evidence of benefit from vitamin or mineral supplementation in individuals with diabetes who do not have underlying deficiencies (Grade: B). Exceptions are for folate in the prevention of birth defects and calcium in the prevention of bone disease.

Routine supplementation of the diet with antioxidants has not proven beneficial and therefore supplements are not recommended (Grade: A). The initial enthusiasm for the clinical use of antioxidant vitamins in the prevention of cardiovascular disease stemmed from positive results in the preclinical setting. Data suggested that antioxidants, particularly vitamin E, prevented initiation of disease progression in laboratory animals without known atherosclerosis. The early positive findings and the presumed safety of antioxidant supplementation led to large, prospective cohort studies, in which an association was found between antioxidant vitamin intake, serum vitamin concentrations, or both, and improved cardiovascular outcomes *(43)*. However, a recent meta-analysis reviewed seven large clinical trials of vitamin E (three studies had significant numbers of subjects with diabetes) involving more than 80,000 subjects taking anywhere from 50–800 IU of vitamin E and who were followed for as long as 6 yr *(44)*. No dose of vitamin E proved to be of benefit for reducing death from CVD (or any other cause). Of particular interest is the Heart Outcomes Prevention (HOPE) trial involving 9541 subjects that evaluated the effects of vitamin E and of ramipril in patients with a high risk of cardiovascular events and reported no effects of vitamin E on cardiovascular outcomes or nephropathy *(45)*. The MICRO-HOPE study involved a subgroup of the HOPE subjects of 3654 persons with diabetes and at high risk for cardiovascular events given 400 IU of α-tocopherol for an average of 4.5 yr *(46)*. Vitamin E had a neutral effect on cardiovascular outcomes, on microvascular complications, and on glycemic control. Of concern are the outcomes from the HDL-Atherosclerosis Treatment Study, in which antioxidant combinations including 800 IU of vitamin E blunted the HDL-raising effects of niacin and simvastatin and resulted in poor clinical outcomes (47).

None of the randomized trials indicated a favorable effect of β-carotene in preventing atherosclerotic disease *(44)*. Two studies reported an increased incidence of lung cancer, whereas in the meta-analysis *(44)* involving more than 130,000 people, β-carotene supplements (as opposed to food) led to a small but significant increase in all-cause mortality (7.4 vs 7.0%) and a slight increase in cardiovascular death (3.4 vs 3.1%) compared with control treatment.

6.2.5. ALCOHOL

Recommendations for alcohol intake are similar to those for the general public. Alcoholic drinks should be limited to less than two per day for men and less than one per day for women. One drink is defined as a 12 oz beer, 5 oz wine, or 1.5 oz of distilled spirits, each of which contains approx 15 g of alcohol. In persons with diabetes, moderate amounts of alcohol when ingested with food have minimal, if any, effect on blood glucose and insulin concentrations. For individuals using insulin or insulin secretagogs, if alcohol is consumed, it should be consumed with food to prevent hypoglycemia. Previous recommendations had suggested that alcoholic beverages should be substituted for fat servings. However, alcoholic beverages should be considered an addition to the regular food/meal plan for all patients with diabetes with no food being omitted (Grade: Expert Consensus).

Observational studies suggest a U- or J-shaped association with moderate consumption of alcohol (~15–30 g/d) and decreased risk of type 2 diabetes, coronary heart disease, and stroke *(48–50)*. In persons with type 2 diabetes, light to moderate amounts of alcohol are associated with a decreased risk of atherosclerosis and coronary heart disease *(51)*, perhaps owing to increases in HDL cholesterol. Furthermore, moderate amounts of alcohol are reported to improve insulin resistance *(52,53)*, to not increase triglyceride levels in hypertriglyceridemic individuals *(54)*, and to have a beneficial effect on triglyceride levels in postmenopausal women *(52)*. Some evidence suggests that heavy alcohol consumption (>3 drinks/d) may be associated with an increased risk of diabetes.

A recent systematic review *(55)* concluded that moderate alcohol consumption is associated with a decreased risk of diabetes and a decreased incidence of heart disease in persons with diabetes. However, because the available evidence is primarily observational, it does not support recommending alcohol consumption to persons who do not currently drink. The relationship between alcohol and various aspects of health is discussed in Chapter 12.

7. PRIORITIZING NUTRITION INTERVENTIONS FOR TYPE 1 AND TYPE 2 DIABETES

7.1. Type 1 Diabetes

Persons with this condition can lead normal lives, provided careful attention is given to appropriate treatment. Many individuals with type 1 diabetes have competed successfully in all levels of sports including collegiate and professional events. One example is Gary Hall, who won the gold medal in the 50-m freestyle swimming at the 2004 Athens Olympics.

The first priority for persons requiring insulin therapy is to integrate an insulin regimen into the patient's lifestyle. With the many insulin options now available, a regimen can usually be developed that will conform to the individual's preferred food choices and meal routine. The food/meal plan is developed first and is based on the individual's appetite, preferred foods, and usual schedule of meals and physical activity. After the dietitian, working with the individual with diabetes, develops a food plan, this information is shared with the professional determining the insulin regimen. Insulin therapy can then be integrated into food and physical activity schedules.

The preferred type of insulin regimen consists of a basal insulin, such as glargine, and a bolus insulin, such as a rapid-acting insulin (lispro or aspart) at mealtimes. This type of regimen is referred to as physiological or intensive insulin therapy and provides increased flexibility in timing and frequency of meals, amounts of carbohydrate eaten at meals, and timing of physical activity. After determining the amount of insulin required to cover the individual's usual meal carbohydrate, they can be taught how to adjust mealtime insulin doses based on the planned carbohydrate content of the meal (insulin-to-carbohydrate ratios). This was confirmed in the dose adjustment for normal eating (DAFNE) randomized, controlled trial (56). In this study individuals with type 1 diabetes using routinely prescribed insulin therapy, in which insulin is determined first and eating must then be consistent and matched to the time actions of insulin (conventional insulin therapy), were either immediately provided with the skills needed to determine their bolus insulin based on their desired carbohydrate intake on a meal-to-meal basis (DAFNE) or attended the training 6 mo later. In the group receiving the DAFNE training, A1C levels were significantly improved by approx 1%, with no significant increase in severe hypoglycemia, along with positive effects on quality of life, satisfaction with treatment, and psychological well-being, despite an increase in the number of insulin injections (but not in total amount of insulin) and in blood glucose monitoring compared with the controls who received the training later.

Conventional or fixed insulin therapy usually consists of rapid-acting (or short-acting) and intermediate-acting insulins given before breakfast and the evening meal. For this type of insulin therapy, consistency in the day-to-day carbohydrate content of meals, as well as the timing of meals, is important.

Table 5
Progressive Nutrition Therapy for the Prevention and Treatment of Type 2 Diabetes

Stage	Goal	Strategies
Overweight individuals (BMI ≥25)	• Prevent obesity • Stop weight gain	• Decrease calorie intake by 100 kcal/d • Inrease number of steps by 2000/d
Metabolic syndrome	• Improve insulin sensitivity	• Increase physical activity/exercise • Reduce energy intake, modest weight loss
Prediabetes	• Prevent/delay type 2 diabetes	• Reduce energy and fat intake to achieve a modest weight loss (5–7% of body weight) • Accumulate 150 min/wk of physical activity
Type 2 diabetes	• Attain and maintain normal/optimal metabolic profiles—glucose, lipids, and blood pressure • Prevent weight gain with use of medications	• Learn carbohydrate counting • Decrease energy intake • Increase physical activity • Use medications when needed

Although carbohydrate counting is emphasized, total energy intake cannot be ignored. Weight gain is common as treatment intensifies; therefore, individuals must also be knowledgeable about the protein, fat, and calorie content of foods.

7.2. Type 2 Diabetes

Just as medical management of type 2 diabetes progresses from nutrition therapy as monotherapy to nutrition therapy plus medications, the nutrition care process also changes. Table 5 reviews the stages of the condition, the goals of nutrition therapy, and strategies that can be implemented to facilitate goal achievement.

Although there are similarities, MNT recommendations for those with type 2 diabetes differ in several aspects from the recommendations for prevention. MNT progresses from prevention of obesity or weight gain to improving insulin resistance to contributing to improved metabolic control of glucose, lipids, and blood pressure.

7.2.1. OVERWEIGHT/OBESITY: HALTING THE EPIDEMIC

Although it may not be possible to decrease the numbers of overweight and obese persons in the United States, obesity researchers suggest focusing on preventing of the increase in obesity that has been occurring at an alarming rate (57). In this regard, America on the Move is a program designed to prevent weight gain. The strategy is to decrease energy intake by 100 kcal/d and to increase physical activity by increasing the number of steps a person takes during the day by about 2000 (57).

7.2.2. METABOLIC SYNDROME: IMPROVING INSULIN RESISTANCE

Persons with the metabolic syndrome are at increased risk of developing prediabetes, type 2 diabetes, and CVD. Central to the metabolic syndrome is insulin resistance and associated cardiovascular risk factors—visceral (abdominal) obesity, elevated blood pressure, and dyslipidemia (characterized by small, dense LDL cholesterol particles, hypertriglyceridemia, and low levels of HDL cholesterol). Genetic and environmental (obesity, sedentary lifestyle, and aging) factors contribute to insulin resistance.

There is no evidence to suggest that a high-carbohydrate diet contributes to insulin resistance. Instead, studies suggest that insulin sensitivity and the ability of insulin to lower blood glucose levels is improved as total dietary carbohydrate is increased *(59)*. Conversely, a lower intake of carbohydrate and higher intake of dietary fat, particularly saturated fat, are associated with a decline in insulin sensitivity *(60,61)*. An analysis of the National Health and Nutrition Examination Survey III data reported that carbohydrate intake was not associated with an elevation in A1C, plasma glucose, or serum insulin concentrations. However, a low carbohydrate intake was associated with elevated serum C-peptide concentrations (a measure of basal insulin secretion), which indicates an association between low-carbohydrate diets and increased basal insulin secretion *(62)*. Reduced energy intake and modest weight loss improve insulin sensitivity in the short term. Long-term effects of weight loss on insulin sensitivity have not been well studied. For instance, in a 48-wk supervised weight loss and maintenance program, insulin sensitivity was improved substantially with weight loss: a weight loss of 14 kg was associated with a 62% decrease in insulin levels *(63)*. However, even though subjects maintained a loss of approx 10% of initial weight, by week 96 insulin levels had returned to elevated baseline values—a marked increase in insulin levels with partial weight regain.

The lifestyle factor most consistently reported to improve insulin resistance and glucose tolerance is physical training *(64)*. Several long-term studies reported improved insulin action in exercise-trained obese individuals, independent of weight loss *(65,66)*. Exercise also decreases blood pressure and triglyceride levels. Although reported to increase HDL cholesterol in the general population, it is not clear if this is also the case in people with insulin resistance *(67)*. Physical activity in the absence of calorie restriction has only a modest, if any, effect on weight loss *(68)*, but is useful as an adjunct to other weight-loss strategies and is important in long-term maintenance of weight loss *(69–71)*. It is especially noteworthy that overweight, fit men are reported to have a lower risk of mortality from chronic disease than lean, unfit men *(72)*.

7.2.3. PREDIABETES: PREVENTING TYPE 2 DIABETES

For individuals who have progressed to prediabetes, the benefits of lifestyle modifications were conclusively documented in the Finnish Prevention Study *(73)* and the Diabetes Prevention Program *(74)*. The Finnish Diabetes Study used intensive lifestyle interventions, including weight reduction of 5% or more, reduction of total and saturated fat (<30% of energy and <10% of energy, respectively), increased fiber (>15 g/1000 kcal), and increased physical activity (>4 h/wk). On average, the percentage of individuals achieving the intervention goals ranged from 86% for exercise to 25% for fiber consumption. After 4 yr, the overall risk of diabetes was reduced by 58% in the intervention group, an outcome attributed specifically to changes in the lifestyles of participants.

The Diabetes Prevention Program was a 27-center clinical trial with 45% of participants from ethnic and racial minorities. The pharmacological intervention included either metformin (850 mg/d for 4 wk and 850 mg twice a day after 4 wk) or a placebo. The intensive lifestyle intervention involved a modest weight loss of approx 5–7% of body weight through reduced intake of energy and dietary fat, and increased physical activity of 150 min/wk. Structured programs that emphasized regular contact with study participants were necessary to accomplish the study objectives.

Diabetes risk was reduced by 31% in the metformin group but in the intensive lifestyle group it was reduced by 58%. Furthermore, lifestyle intervention was successful among all groups, whereas metformin was ineffective in some groups, including older individuals and those who were only slightly overweight. Based on these findings, the ADA and the National Institute of Diabetes, Digestive, and Kidney Disease recommend that lifestyle modifications—modest weight loss (5–10% of body weight) and modest physical activity (30 min/d)—should be the first line of defense to prevent or delay the onset of type 2 diabetes (75).

7.2.4. TYPE 2 DIABETES: ACHIEVING EUGLYCEMIA

As individuals move from being insulin resistant to insulin deficient, MNT shifts from weight loss to glucose, lipid, and blood pressure control. The goal of therapy is to achieve euglycemia to slow β-cell exhaustion. Although moderate weight loss may be beneficial for some individuals, primarily those who are still insulin resistant, for most it is too late for weight loss to improve hyperglycemia (76,77). At later stages of the disease when medications—including insulin—need to be combined with nutrition therapy, weight gain often occurs and preventing this weight gain becomes a factor. However, glycemic control must still take precedence over concern about weight.

Teaching individuals how to make appropriate food choices (usually by means of carbohydrate counting) and using data from blood glucose monitoring to evaluate short-term effectiveness are important components of successful MNT for type 2 diabetes. Furthermore, fitness, independent of BMI and body fatness, is related to a decrease in all-cause death rates in men with diabetes (78). This again highlights the importance of clinicians giving greater attention to counseling for increasing physical activity and improving fitness in persons with diabetes, primarily for the benefits associated with enhanced cardiorespiratory fitness that are independent of weight. The impact of nutrition interventions on glycemic control are evident by 6 wk–3 mo. At this point, it can be determined if MNT alone is to be continued or if medications need to be added (or adjusted) to MNT.

Many individuals with type 2 diabetes also have dyslipidemia and hypertension, so decreasing intakes of saturated fat, cholesterol, and sodium should also be a priority. Lifestyle strategies should be implemented as soon as diabetes is diagnosed to prevent the chronic complications of the disorder. When insulin is required, consistency in timing of meals and of their carbohydrate content becomes important.

8. APPLYING NUTRITION EVIDENCE TO CLINICAL PRACTICE

MNT begins by developing a rapport with the individual with diabetes. Whether provided individually or in groups, nutrition therapy involves a common process: nutri-

Table 6
Carbohydrate Servings[a]

Starch	Milk
1 slice of bread (1 oz)	1 cup skim/reduced-fat milk
1/3 cup cooked rice or pasta	2/3 cup fat-free fruited yogurt sweetened with
3/4 cup dry cereal	nonnutritive sweetener (6 oz)
4–6 crackers	
1/2 large baked potato with skin (3 oz)	
3/4 oz pretzels, potato, or tortilla chips	
Fruit	*Sweets and desserts*
1 small fresh fruit (4 oz)	2 small cookies
1/2 cup fruit juice	1 tablespoon jam, honey, syrup
1/4 cup dried fruit	1/2 cup ice cream, frozen yogurt, or sherbet

[a]One serving contains 15 g of carbohydrate.

tion assessment, nutrition diagnosis (problem identification), nutrition intervention (including self-management education), and nutrition monitoring and evaluation *(79)*.

Integrating nutrition recommendations into diabetes management requires professionals with a high level of clinical skills, not only in regard to nutrition recommendations for diabetes but also in the overall management of diabetes. The intervention is individualized based on the needs of the person with diabetes and whether the intervention is for initial, continuing, or intensive care. Providing nutrition therapy in groups is becoming increasingly important as reimbursement criteria for diabetes self-management education recommends that, when possible, group sessions are preferable. Group interventions for diabetes self-management education, including nutrition therapy, are as effective as individual interventions *(80)*.

The nutrition prescription and meal/food plan is a modification of the usual food intake that is individualized to meet treatment goals. Appropriate educational materials are selected. Traditionally, all persons with diabetes were taught the use of exchange lists for meal planning. The exchange lists are still of value in helping dietitians to assess the energy and macronutrient intake of both the usual and modified diet. However, many dietitians and persons with diabetes find that carbohydrate counting, either basic *(28)* or advanced *(81)*, is a more helpful method of meal planning.

Regardless of the methods and materials used for interventions, measurement, and documentation of outcomes is essential and requires a system of planned follow-up and ongoing education and support.

8.1. Carbohydrate Counting

Carbohydrate counting is useful in the management of all types of diabetes. Instead of grouping foods into six lists as in the exchange system, it groups foods into three groups: carbohydrate, meat and meat substitutes, and fat. The carbohydrate list is composed of starches, starchy vegetables, fruits, milk, and sweets; one serving is the amount of food that contains 15 g carbohydrate. Table 6 list some examples of a carbohydrate serving.

Table 7
The Old vs the New Nutrition Paradigm

Outdated nutrition advice	Updated nutrition recommendations
MNT is a calculated American Diabetes Association (ADA) diet (energy and percentage of macronutrients).	There no longer is an ADA diet that applies to all persons with diabetes. An ADA diet can only be defined as an individualized food/meal plan based on assessment, therapy goals, and use of approaches that meet the patient's needs. Diet sheets or a one time "diet instruction" is rarely sufficient to change eating habits. For people to make lifestyle changes that result in positive clinical outcomes requires education, counseling, and support over time.
Weight loss is essential.	Weight loss is typically helpful but not an essential treatment for improving blood glucose. Weight loss recommendations may be a barrier for those who have unsuccessfully tried multiple times to lose weight. It is often possible to improve glucose control by changing food habits without weight loss. For those who are already at or below an appropriate weight, weight loss is not a treatment goal.
Ideal body weight is the goal; this often requires a weight loss of 40–50 lb (18–23 kg).	Research has shown that even small amounts of weight loss can improve glucose, lipids, and insulin resistance in the short term. It is unknown if this can be maintained long term.
Sugars and sweets are forbidden as they are more rapidly digested and absorbed and cause blood glucose levels to go higher	Evidence from many clinical studies has demonstrated that sugars do not increase glycemia more than isocaloric amounts of starch. Therefore, the total amount of carbohydrate eaten is more important than the source of the carbohydrate.
Protein is recommended because it slows the absorption of carbohydrates and prevents hypoglycemia.	Ingested protein does not slow the absorption of carbohydrate nor does adding protein prevent or assist in the treatment of hypoglycemia. Protein is as potent a stimulant of insulin as is carbohydrate.
Chromium and vitamin E are often recommended because they improve blood glucose and/or lipid levels.	If individuals are not deficient in a micronutrient, supplements are unlikely to be beneficial. It is difficult to determine who is and who is not deficient in chromium. Supplementation with vitamin E has not been shown to be beneficial in intervention trials.
"When diet and exercise fail," add medications; at this point there is no need to pay attention to lifestyle.	Type 2 diabetes is a progressive disease and MNT should always be part of the diabetes care plan; beta cells fail, not diet and exercise.

MNT, medical nutrition therapy. (Reprinted from ref. *83* with permission.)

Carbohydrate counting does not mean that meat and fat portions can be ignored. Individuals with diabetes must also know the approximate number of meat and fat servings they should select for meals and snacks. Weight control is important, as is the maintenance of a healthy balance of food choices.

Women with type 2 diabetes often do well with three or four carbohydrate servings per meal and one to two for a snack. Men with type 2 diabetes may need four to five carbohydrate servings per meal and one to two for a snack. Food records along with blood glucose monitoring data can then be used to evaluate if treatment goals are being met, or if there is a need for additional lifestyle and/or medication changes *(82)*.

Learning how to use Nutrient Facts on food labels is also useful. First, individuals should take note of the serving size and the total amount (grams) of carbohydrate. The total grams of carbohydrate are then divided by 15 to determine the number of carbohydrate servings in the serving size.

8.2. Insulin-to-Carbohydrate Ratios

Insulin-to-carbohydrate ratios are used to determine the bolus (mealtime) insulin doses. Individuals must be consistent in their carbohydrate intake and the bolus insulin adjusted to cover that amount of carbohydrate. The servings or grams of carbohydrate per meal are then divided by the bolus insulin dose to determine how many units of insulin are needed to cover the servings or grams of carbohydrate. For example, if an individual usually eats 75 g (five servings) carbohydrate servings for dinner and the postmeal glucose is within target range by taking 5 U of rapid-acting insulin premeal, the insulin-to-carbohydrate ratio is 1:15 g (1 serving) (75 ÷ 5, which equals 1 U of insulin per 15 g of carbohydrate). Individuals can then adjust their bolus insulin based on the carbohydrate they plan to eat.

9. SUMMARY

There have been major changes in nutrition recommendations and therapy over the past decade. Table 7 illustrates the paradigm shift that has occurred in nutrition therapy for diabetes *(83)*. Monitoring of glucose, A1C, lipids, and blood pressure is essential in persons with diabetes to assess the outcomes of lifestyle interventions and/or to determine if changes in medication(s) are necessary. MNT is essential for effective diabetes management, but to be successful it involves an ongoing process. It is important that all health care providers understand nutrition issues and guide the individual's efforts by referring patients with prediabetes or diabetes for MNT as soon as the diagnosis is made, by promoting and reinforcing the importance of lifestyle modifications, and by providing support for the lifestyle intervention process.

REFERENCES

1. Mokad AH, Bowman BA, Ford ES, Vinicor F, Marks JS, Koplan JP. The continuing epidemics of obesity and diabetes in the United States. JAMA 2001; 286:1195–1200.
2. American Diabetes Association. Diabetes 2001 Vital Statistics. American Diabetes Association, Alexandria, VA, 2001.
3. American Diabetes Association. Standards of medical care in diabetes (Position Statement). Diabetes Care 2005; 28(Suppl 1):54–536.
4. American Diabetes Association. Diagnosis and classification of diabetes mellitus (Position Statement). Diabetes Care 2004; 27(Suppl 1):S5–S10.
5. Zimmet, P. Z. The pathogenesis and prevention of diabetes in adults: genes, autoimmunity, and demography. Diabetes Care 1994 18:1050–1064.
6. DeWitt DE, Hirsch IB. Outpatient insulin therapy in type 1 and type 2 diabetes mellitus. JAMA 2003; 289:2254–2264.
7. Yki-Jarvinen H. Acute and chronic effects of hyperglycemia on glucose metabolism: implications for the development of new therapies. Diabetes Med 1997; 14(S3):S32–S37.
8. Boden G, Chen X. Effects of fat on glucose uptake and utilization in patients with non-insulin dependent diabetes. J Clin Invest 1995; 3:1261–1268.

9. American Diabetes Association. Gestational diabetes mellitus (Position Statement). Diabetes Care 2004; 27(Suppl 1):S88–S90.

10. Diabetes Control and Complications Trial Research Group. The effect of intensive treatment of diabetes on the development and progression of long-term complications in insulin-dependent diabetes mellitus. N Eng J Med 1993; 339:977–986.

11. UK Prospective Diabetes Study Group. Intensive blood-glucose control with sulphonylureas or insulin compared with conventional treatment and risk of complications in patients with type 2 diabetes (UKPDS 34). Lancet 1998; 352:854–865.

12. UK Prospective Diabetes Study Group. Tight blood pressure control and risk of macrovascular complications in type 2 diabetes (UKPDS 38). BMJ 1998; 317:703–713.

13. UKPDS Group. UK Prospective Study 7: Response of fasting glucose to diet therapy in newly presenting type II diabetic patients. Metabolism 1990; 39:905–912.

14. American Diabetes Association. Tests of glycemia in diabetes (Position Statement). Diabetes Care 2004; 27(Suppl 1):S91–S93.

15. The National Cholesterol Education Program (NCEP) Expert Panel on Detection, Evaluation and Treatment of High Blood Cholesterol in Adults (Adult Treatment Panel III). Executive summary of the third report of the National Cholesterol Education Program (NCEP) Expert Panel on Detection, Evaluation and Treatment of High Blood Cholesterol in Adults (Adult Treatment Panel III). JAMA 2001; 285:2486–2497.

16. Rabasa-Lhoret R, Garon J, Langlier H, Poisson D, Chiasson J-L. Effects of meal carbohydrate on insulin requirements in type 1 diabetic patients treated intensively with the basal-bolus (ultralente-regular) insulin regimen. Diabetes Care 1999; 22:667–673.

17. Inzucchi SE. Oral antihyperglycemic therapy for type 2 diabetes. JAMA 2002; 287:360–372.

18. Buse JB. Overview of current therapeutic options in type 2 diabetes. Rationale for combining oral agents with insulin therapy. Diabetes Care 1999; 22(Suppl 3):C65–C70.

19. Franz MJ, Horton ES, Bantle JP, et al. Nutrition principles for the management of diabetes and related complications (Technical Review). Diabetes Care 1994; 17:490–518.

20. American Diabetes Association. Nutrition recommendations and principles for people with diabetes mellitus (Position Statement). Diabetes Care 1994; 17:519–522.

21. Franz MJ, Bantle JP, Beebe CA, et al. Evidence-based nutrition principles and recommendations for the treatment and prevention of diabetes and related complications (Technical Review). Diabetes Care 2002; 25:148–198.

22. American Diabetes Association. Evidence-based nutrition principles and recommendations for the treatment and prevention of diabetes and related complications (Position Statement). Diabetes Care 2004; 27(Suppl 1):S36–S46.

23. American Diabetes Association Clinical Practice Recommendations. Diabetes Care 2004; 27(Suppl 1): S1, S2.

24. Pastors JG, Warshaw H, Daly A, Franz M, Kulkarni K. The evidence for the effectiveness of medical nutrition therapy in diabetes management. Diabetes Care 2002; 25:608–613.

25. Pastors JG, Franz MJ, Warshaw H, Daly A, Arnold M. How effective is medical nutrition therapy in diabetes care? J Am Diet Assoc 2003; 103:827–831.

26. Franz MJ, Monk A, Barry B, et al. Effectiveness of medical nutrition therapy provided by dietitians in the management of non-insulin-dependent diabetes mellitus: a randomized controlled clinical trial. J Am Diet Assoc 1995; 95:1009–1017.

27. Franz MJ. Carbohydrate and diabetes: is the source or the amount of more importance? Curr Diab Rep 2001; 1:177–186.

28. American Dietetic Association, American Diabetes Association. Basic Carbohydrate Counting. American Dietetic Association, Chicago; American Diabetes Association, Alexandria, VA, 2003.

29. Wolever TMS, Hamad S, Chiasson J-L, et al. Day-to-day consistency in amount and source of carbohydrate intake associated with improved glucose control in type 1 diabetes. J. Am Coll Nutr 1999; 18:242–247.

30. Brand-Miller J, Hayne S, Petocz P, Colagiuri S. Low-glycemic index diets in the management of diabetes: a meta-analysis of randomized controlled trials. Diabetes Care 2003; 26:2261–2267.

31. Franz MJ. The glycemic index. Not the most effective nutrition therapy intervention (Editorial). Diabetes Care 2003; 26:2466–2468.

32. Giacco R, Parillo M, Rivellese AA, et al. Long-term dietary treatment with increased amounts of fiber-rich low-glycemic index natural food improves blood glucose control and reduces the number of hypoglycemic events in type 1 patients with diabetes. Diabetes Care 2000; 23:1461–1466.
33. Chandalia M, Garg A, Luthohann D, von Bergmann K, Grundy SM, Brinkley LJ. () Beneficial effects of a high dietary fiber intake in patients with type 2 diabetes. N Engl J Med 2000; 342:1392–1398.
34. Hollenbeck CB, Coulston AM, Reaven GM. To what extent does increased dietary fiber improve glucose and lipid metabolism in patients with noninsulin-dependent diabetes mellitus (NIDDM)? Am J Clin Nutr 1986; 43:16–24.
35. Lafrance L, Rabasa-Lhoret R, Poisson D, Ducros F, Chiasson J-L. The effects of different glycaemic index foods and dietary fiber intake on glycaemic control in type 1 patients with diabetes on intensive insulin therapy. Diabet Med 1998; 15:972–978.
36. Nuttall FQ, Mooradian AD, Gannon MC, Billington C, Krezowski P. Effect of protein ingestion on the glucose and insulin response to a standardized oral glucose load. Diabetes Care 1984; 7:465–470.
37. Gannon MC, Nuttall JA, Damberg G, Gupta V, Nuttall FQ. Effect of protein ingestion on the glucose appearance rate in people with type 2 diabetes. J Clin Endocrinol Metab 2001; 86:1040–1047.
38. Peters AL, Davidson MB. Protein and fat effects on glucose response and insulin requirements in subjects with insulin-dependent diabetes mellitus. Am J Clin Nutr 1993; 58:555–600.
39. Franz MJ. Protein and diabetes: much advice, little research. Curr Diab Rep 2002; 2:457–464.
40. Gray RO, Butler PC, Beers TR, Kryshak EJ, Rizza RA. Comparison of the ability of bread versus bread plus meat to treat and prevent subsequent hypoglycemia in patients with insulin-dependent diabetes mellitus. J Clin Endocrinol Metab 1996; 81:1508–1511.
41. Foster GD, Wyatt HR, Hill JO, et al. A randomized trial of a low-carbohydrate diet for obesity. N Engl J Med 2003; 348:2082–2090.
42. Lichtenstein AH, Ausman LM, Carrasco W, Jenner JL, Ordovas JM, Schaefer EJ. Short-term consumption of a low fat diet beneficially affects plasma lipid concentrations only when accompanied by weight loss. Arterioscler Thromb 1994; 14:1751–1760.
43. Hasanain B, Mooradian AD. Antioxidant vitamins and their influence in diabetes mellitus. Current Diabetes Reports 2002; 2:448–456.
44. Vivekananthan DP, Penn MS, Sapp SK, Hsu A, Topol EJ. Use of antioxidant vitamins for the prevention of cardiovascular disease: meta-analysis randomized trials. Lancet 2003; 361:2017–2023.
45. Yusuf S, Dagenais G, Pogue J, Bosch J, Sleight P. Vitamin E supplementation and cardiovascular events in high-risk patients. The Heart Outcomes Prevention Evaluation Study Investigators. N Engl J Med 2000; 342:154–160.
46. Lonn E, Yusuf S, Hoogwerf B, et al., on behalf of the Heart Outcomes Prevention Evaluation (HOPE) investigators. Effects of vitamin E on cardiovascular and microvascular outcomes in high-risk patients with diabetes. Diabetes Care 2002; 25:1919–1927.
47. Brown BG, Zhao XQ, Chait A, et al. Simvastin and niacin, antioxidant vitamins, or the combination for the prevention of coronary disease. N Eng J Med 2001; 345:1583–1592.
48. Reynolds K, Lewis LB, Nolen JDL, Kinney GL, Sthya B, He J. Alcohol consumption and risk of stroke. JAMA 2003; 289:579–588.
49. Wannamethee SG, Camargo CA, Manson JE, Willett WC, Rimm EB. Alcohol drinking patterns and risk of type 2 diabetes mellitus among younger women. Arch Intern Med 2003; 163:1329–1336.
50. Wei M, Gibbon LW, Mitchell TL, Kampert JB, Blair SN. Alcohol intake and incidence of type 2 diabetes in men. Diabetes Care 2000; 23:18–22.
51. Tanasescu M, Hu FB. Alcohol consumption and risk of coronary heart disease among individuals with type 2 diabetes. Current Diabetes Reports 2001; 1:187–191.
52. Davies MJ, Baer DJ, Judd JT, Brown ED, Campbell WS, Taylor PR. Effects of moderate alcohol intake on fasting insulin and glucose concentrations and insulin sensitivity in postmenopausal women. JAMA 2002; 287:2559–2562.
53. Bell RA, Mayer-Davis EJ, Artin MA, D'Agostino RB, and Haffner SM. Association between alcohol consumption and insulin sensitivity and cardiovascular disease risk factors: the Insulin Resistance and Atherosclerosis Study. Diabetes Care 2000; 23:1630–1636.
54. Pownall HJ, Ballantyne CH, Kimball KT, Simpson SL, Yeshurun D, Grotto AM. Effect of moderate alcohol consumption on hypertriglyceridemia. Arch Intern Med 1999; 159:981–987.

55. Howard AA, Arnsten JH, Gourevitch MN. Effect of alcohol consumption on diabetes mellitus. A systematic review. Ann Intern Med 2004; 140:211–219.
56. DAFNE Study Group. Training in flexible, intensive insulin management to enable dietary freedom in people with type 1 diabetes: dose adjustment for normal eating (DAFNE) randomized trial. BMJ 2002; 325:746–752.
57. Dausch JG. The obesity epidemic: what's being done? J Am Diet Assoc 2002; 102:638, 639.
58. America on the Move. Simple steps to better health. Available at: http://www.americaonthemove.org. Accessed January 12, 2004.
59. Bessesen DH. The role of carbohydrates in insulin resistance. J Nutr 2001; 131:2782S–2786S.
60. Swinburn BA, Boyce VL, Bergman RN, Howard BV, Bogardus C. Deterioration in carbohydrate metabolism and lipoprotein changes induced by modern, high fat diet in Pima Indians and Caucasians. J Clin Endo Metab 1991; 73:156–165.
61. Lovejoy JC. The influence of dietary fat on insulin resistance. Curr Diab Rep 2002; 2:435–440.
62. Yang EJ, Kerver JM, Park K, Kayitsinga J, Allison DB, Song WO. Carbohydrate intake and biomarkers of glycemic control among US adults: the third National Health and Nutrition Examination Survery (NHANES III). Am J Clin Nutr 2003; 77:1426–1433.
63. Weinstock RS, Dai H, Wadden TA. Diet and exercise in the treatment of obesity: effects of 3 interventions on insulin resistance. Arch Intern Med 1998; 158:2477–2483.
64. Kovisto VA, Yki-Jarvinen H, DeFronzo RA. Physical training and insulin resistance. Diabetes Metab Res 1996; 1:445–481.
65. Oshita Y, Yamagouchi K, Hayantzu G, Sato Y. Long-term jogging increases insulin action despite no influence on body mass index or VO2 max. J Appl Physiol 1990; 66:2206–2210.
66. Duncan GE, Perri MG, Theriaque DW, Hutson AD, Eckel RH, Stacpoole PW. Exercise training without weight loss, increases insulin sensitivity and postheparin plasma lipase activity in previously sedentary adults. Diabetes Care 2003; 26:557–562.
67. American Diabetes Association. Physical activity/exercise and diabetes mellitus (Position Statement). Diabetes Care 2004; 27(Suppl 1):S58–S62.
68. Bouchard C, Deprés JP, Tremblay A. Exercise and obesity. Obes Res 1993; 1:133–147.
69. Pronk NP, Wing RR. Physical activity and long-term maintenance of weight loss. Obes Res 1994; 2:587–599.
70. Wing RR. Physical activity in the treatment of adulthood overweight and obesity: current evidence and research issues. Med Sci Sports Exerc 1999; 31:547S–553S.
71. Anderson RE, Wadden TA, Bartlett SJ, Zemel BS, Verde TJ, Franckowiak SC. Effects of lifestyle activity vs. structured aerobic exercise n obese women: a randomized trial. JAMA 1999; 281:335–340.
72. Lee DC, Blair SN, Jackson AS. Cardiorespiratory fitness, body composition, and all-cause and cardiovascular disease mortality in men. Am J Clin Nutr 1999; 69:373–380.
73. Tuomilehto J, Lindstrom J, Eriksson JG, et al. for the Finnish Diabetes Prevention Study Group. Prevention of type 2 diabetes by changes in lifestyle among subjects with impaired glucose tolerance. N Engl J Med 2001; 344:1343–1350.
74. Diabetes Prevention Program Research Group. Reduction in the incidence of type 2 diabetes with lifestyle intervention or metformin. N Engl J Med 2003; 346:393–403.
75. American Diabetes Association and National Institute of Diabetes and Digestive and Kidney Diseases. The prevention or delay of type 2 diabetes. Diabetes Care 2003; 26(Suppl 1):S62–S69.
76. Watts NB, Spanheimer RG, DiGirolamo M, et al. Prediction of glucose response to weight loss in patients with non-insulin-dependent diabetes mellitus. Arch Intern Med 1990; 150:803–806.
77. Wolf AM, Conaway MR, Crowther JQ, et al. Translating lifestyle intervention to practice in obese patients with type 2 diabetes. Diabetes Care 2004;27:1570–1576.
78. Church TS, Cheng YJ, Earnest CP, et al. Exercise capacity and body composition as predictors of mortality among men with diabetes. Diabetes Care 2004; 27:83–88.
79. Lacey K, Pritchett E. Nutrition care process and model: ADA adopts road map to quality care and outcomes management. J Am Diet Assoc 2003;103:1061–1072.
80. Rickheim PL, Weaver TW, Flader JL, Kendall DM. Assessment of group versus individual diabetes education. Diabetes Care 2002; 25:269–274.

81. American Diabetes Association. Advanced Carbohydrate Counting. American Dietetic Association, Chicago; American Diabetes Association, Alexandria, VA, 2003.
82. Franz MJ, Reader D, Monk A. Implementing Group and Individual Medical Nutrition Therapy for Diabetes. American Diabetes Association, Alexandria, VA 2002.
83. Fran MJ, Warshaw H, Daly AE, Green-Pastors J. Arnold BJ. Evolution of diabetes medical nutrition therapy. Postgrad Med J 2003; 79:30–35.

5

Diet and the Prevention of Type 2 Diabetes

Norman J. Temple and Nelia P. Steyn

KEY POINTS

- The prevalence of type 2 diabetes is increasing rapidly in all parts of the world.
- Obesity and physical inactivity are major modifiable risk factors.
- Whereas cohort studies indicate that cereal fiber, a major source of insoluble fiber, is most potent for preventing diabetes, intervention studies indicate that soluble fiber is most effective for improving glycemic control.
- Evidence from cohort studies is inconsistent in establishing an association between the glycemic index or the glycemic load of the diet and the risk of diabetes. However, foods with a low glycemic index help improve glycemic control when given to persons with type 2 diabetes.
- Saturated fat appears to increase the risk of diabetes whereas polyunsaturated fat appears to be protective.
- Diets poor in magnesium and chromium may increase the risk of diabetes. Supplements of chromium, especially chromium picolinate, may improve glycemic control in diabetics and others, especially where the diet has been poor in the mineral.

1. INTRODUCTION

The focus of this chapter is the role of diet in the prevention of type 2 diabetes. Chapter 4 focuses on the therapy for diabetes.

1.1. Background

By far the most common type of diabetes is type 2. In the United States about 5% of people with diabetes have type 1 and the remainder have type 2. By 2000 there were approx 150 million people around the world with the disease, a number that is expected to double by 2025 (1). It is the fourth or fifth leading cause of death in most developed countries.

The lowest rates of type 2 diabetes are found in rural communities where people retain traditional lifestyles (2). But dramatic increases in the prevalence and incidence of type 2 diabetes have been observed in communities where the diet has shifted from a tradi-

From: *Nutritional Health: Strategies for Disease Prevention, Second Edition*
Edited by: N. J. Temple, T. Wilson, and D. R. Jacobs © Humana Press Inc., Totowa, NJ

tional indigenous diet to a typical "Western" diet. There is growing evidence that the disease has reached epidemic proportions in many developing and newly industrialized countries (2). We can confidently ascribe these changes in disease rates to changes in lifestyle, most notably diet and a reduction in physical activity.

1.2. Classification and Diagnosis

Type 2 diabetes was formerly known as noninsulin-dependent diabetes. As many as half of all people with the disease have not been diagnosed. For this reason, unless systematic testing of a population is carried out, estimates of the prevalence of the disease are likely to be serious underestimates. Furthermore, because of the differences in criteria, comparisons of rates from recent and earlier studies must be made with caution.

The fasting plasma glucose (FPG) concentration is now given greater importance as a criterion for diagnosis. The FPG concentration considered diagnostic of diabetes is 7.0 mmol/L or more ($\geq$126 mg/dL) (3,4). This value was introduced in the late 1990s and is a decrease from the former value of 7.8 mmol/L (140 mg/dL). Diagnosis can also be made based on an oral glucose tolerance test using 75 g of glucose. A 2-h postload glucose level of 11.1 mmol/L or more (200 mg/dL) indicates diabetes. If the oral glucose tolerance test reveals a level above normal (7.8 mmol/L or 140 mg/dL) but below the cut-off for diabetes, this is indicative of impaired glucose tolerance (IGT). An additional category, impaired fasting glycemia (IFG), has been introduced. This refers to a FPG level that is above normal but below the cut-off for diabetes, i.e., 6.1 mmol/L (110 mg/dL) to less than 7.0 mmol/L (125 mg/dL). Only a minority of individuals with IGT have IFG, and conversely, only a minority of those with IFG have IGT (5,6). The above values are World Health Organization criteria. The criteria used by the American Diabetes Association (ADA) are almost the same (see Table 1 in Chapter 4). The one notable difference is that the ADA uses a slightly lower cut-off for IFG: an FPG concentration of 5.6 mmol/L or more ($\geq$100 mg/dL).

2. EPIDEMIOLOGY

2.1. Prevalence and Incidence of Type 2 Diabetes

In the United States the most complete information on the prevalence of type 2 diabetes has come from the US National Health Examination Surveys (NHANES) (7,8). Data from the health examination surveys show that among persons age 40–74 yr the prevalence of diabetes (based on the fasting criteria) increased from 8.9% in 1976–1980 to 12.3% in 1988–1994—a 38% increase over the course of a decade (7). Data from the Behavioral Risk Factor Surveys, carried out on representative samples of American adults, reveal that the prevalence of diagnosed diabetes increased between 1991 and 1999 from 4.1 to 6.0% in men, and from 5.6 to 7.6% in women, an increase of approx 40% in less than a decade (9,10). Based on the National Health Interview Survey, the estimated lifetime risk of developing diabetes for an individual born in the United States in 2000 is 32.8% for men and 38.5% for women (11). However, the authors of this estimate note that the true risk may well be higher.

The prevalence of type 2 diabetes differs considerably between different ethnic groups living in the same country in apparently similar environments (8,12). For example, in the United Kingdom and other countries Asian Indians have high prevalence rates of diabetes compared with the indigenous populations *(13,14)*. Similarly, the prevalence in Hispanic Americans is slightly higher than in African Americans, whereas the white population has a much lower prevalence *(11)*. Native American populations have the highest prevalence rates *(15,16)*. The Pima Indians of Arizona have the unfortunate distinction of having the highest prevalence rates in the world; roughly 50% of all adults have the condition *(17)*. The one other population with a comparable prevalence (about 40%) are the Micronesians of the Pacific island of Nauru *(18)*.

Globally, there have been dramatic increases in recent decades in the frequency of type 2 diabetes, especially in developing countries *(18)*. In South Africa, for example, the disease was formerly rare in rural areas, whereas the prevalence in urban areas was only 1.1% *(19)*. However, in strong contrast, the disease is now more common in black Africans than in the white population *(20)*. Within the next decade India and China are expected to have more cases than any other countries in the world *(1)*.

2.2. Mortality

Age-adjusted mortality rates among persons with type 2 diabetes are 1.5–2.5 times higher than in the general population, and this translates to a reduction of life expectancy of approx 10 yr *(21)*. Other researchers estimated that for an individual diagnosed at age 40 yr with the condition, the number of years of life lost will be 11.6 in men and 14.3 in women; for quality-adjusted life years the loss will be 18.6 and 22.0 yr, respectively *(11)*. This is strongly related to the considerably higher risk of cardiovascular disease, especially coronary heart disease *(22)*, as well as of renal disease. This risk is greatest where other risk factors are also present—notably hyperlipidemia, hypertension, and smoking—and if the diabetes has been present for a long period of time.

3. METABOLIC CHANGES DURING DEVELOPMENT OF TYPE 2 DIABETES: INSULIN RESISTANCE AND IMPAIRED GLUCOSE HOMEOSTASIS

The underlying metabolic defect in type 2 diabetes is resistance to the action of insulin *(23,24)*. The β-cells of the pancreas respond to this by increasing output of insulin to maintain normal blood glucose levels. Therefore, insulin resistance is indicated by elevated insulin concentrations, either in the fasting state or after a glucose load.

In the early stages of the disease process glucose tolerance may be normal. However, hypersecretion of insulin is usually insufficient to maintain normal glucose levels indefinitely and, resultingly, there is progression to IGT and IFG. At this stage insulin secretion declines at a variable rate and the disease process advances from IGT and IFG to overt diabetes. The early abnormalities of glucose metabolism are steps on the road to type 2 diabetes *(23,24)*. This occurs either as a result of an inherent defect of the β-cell or because of glucotoxicity whereby the β-cell is damaged as blood glucose levels rise. As will be discussed under Heading 6, we have growing evidence that this sequence of events can be slowed or even reversed by appropriate intervention, especially lifestyle change.

IGT, IFG, and type 2 diabetes are often associated with a cluster of clinical and metabolic abnormalities including central obesity, hypertension, hyperuricemia, raised levels of plasminogen activator inhibitor-1, and an abnormal blood lipid pattern, namely raised levels of triglyceride and reduced levels of high-density lipoprotein cholesterol.

This constellation of features constitute the "syndrome" now known as the metabolic syndrome or insulin resistance syndrome *(25)*. These features all contribute to the increased risk of cardiovascular disease associated with IGT and type 2 diabetes and may coexist with hyperinsulinemia before abnormalities of blood glucose are detectable.

A wide range of lifestyle-related factors have been implicated, including physical inactivity, several aspects of the diet, and the subsequent development of overweight and obesity. These factors may be associated both with the development of insulin resistance, as well as with its progression to impaired glucose metabolism (IFG, IGT) and eventually to type 2 diabetes. The nutritional status of a person before birth, as well as in infancy and childhood, appears to be a significant factor as discussed in Chapter 15.

4. IRREVERSIBLE RISK FACTORS

4.1. Genetic Factors

As discussed in Subheading 4.1., the prevalence of type 2 diabetes varies considerably among different ethnic groups living in apparently similar environments. Although differences in lifestyle undoubtedly account for some of this, inherent genetic differences in susceptibility to the disease are also probably involved.

The importance of genetic factors is further strongly suggested by studies of family history as a risk factor. The risk of having type 2 diabetes is increased two- to sixfold if a parent or sibling has the disease *(26)*. At present it is impossible to quantify the relative contributions of genetic and environmental factors. The disease is believed to be polygenic; some relevant genes have been identified, but by no means all.

4.2. Age

Among Caucasians in the developed world the prevalence of type 2 diabetes increases with age, at least into the 70s. But in developing countries many cases occur in younger adults.

A newly emerging feature of type 2 diabetes is its occurrence in childhood and adolescence *(27)*. This has been observed in many ethnic groups in recent years. In Japan, for example, increasing numbers of cases are seen in school children so that the disease is now more common than type 1 diabetes *(28)*. Caucasians, however, have largely escaped this trend. As in adults, type 2 diabetes in children is frequently asymptomatic and is detected mainly by screening.

5. MODIFIABLE RISK FACTORS

5.1. Obesity

Many studies have documented that obesity is a major risk factor. For example, data from the Nurses' Health Study revealed that the risk of diabetes is 20-fold greater in obese women (body mass index [BMI] 30–35) as compared with slim women (BMI <23) *(29)*. Even being at the high end of normal may carry significant risk: the risk ratio was 2.7 when comparing those with a BMI of 23–25 with those with a BMI of less than 23 *(29)*. Obesity has increased rapidly in many populations in recent years and this is associated with a parallel rise in the prevalence of type 2 diabetes *(10)*.

The distribution of body fat may be a more reliable predictor than BMI of the risk of developing diabetes. Several studies indicate that a high-waist circumference or a high-waist-to-hip ratio (an apple shape) is an important risk factor *(30)*. For example, in a study of Japanese-American men, the anthropometric measure that best predicted the disease was the amount of intra-abdominal fat *(31)*. As there are relatively little data available concerning the waist circumference or waist-to-hip ratio in different populations, BMI is still the most common tool used to measure risk associated with excess adiposity and to provide guidelines. However, future studies may permit guidelines to be established that use waist circumference or waist-to-hip ratio. Waist circumference is generally considered a more useful parameter than waist-to-hip ratio as it is easier to measure and has good predictive ability *(32)*.

5.2. Physical Inactivity

Physical activity has repeatedly been shown to have a protective association with the risk of diabetes *(33–36)*. The relationship is most pronounced in subjects who also have other risk factors, such as obesity, hypertension, or parental diabetes.

Guidelines used today typically recommend moderate exercise on at least 5 d/wk but do not specify heart rate targets. However, more recent evidence suggests that vigorous exercise may be required to improve insulin sensitivity. This was shown in a study conducted by McAuley et al. *(37)* on normoglycemic, insulin-resistant adults. Insulin sensitivity improved in those who engaged in vigorous exercise but not in those who participated in moderate exercise. The vigorous exercise program required participants to train five times per week for at least 20 min/session at an intensity of 80–90% of predicted maximum heart rate *(37)*.

5.3. Carbohydrates and Dietary Fat

A debate that has been ongoing for decades is the question of whether high intakes of either carbohydrate or fat predispose to diabetes *(38)*. One important piece of indirect evidence is that a relatively high intake of dietary fat increases the risk of obesity, a subject that is reviewed in Chapter 13. By extension, this also implicates dietary fat in the causation of diabetes.

In experimental animals, diets rich in any type of fat (with the exception of ω-3 fatty acids) have been shown to result in insulin resistance relative to high-carbohydrate diets *(39–42)*. The data from epidemiological studies are less consistent. Although some studies have suggested that a high-fat or low-carbohydrate intake may hasten the progress of diabetes *(43–49)*, most studies, especially large cohort studies, have shown little association between the quantity of fat or carbohydrate in the diet and the risk of the disease *(50–53)*. Thus, a wide range of carbohydrate intakes may be acceptable in terms of achieving a low risk of type 2 diabetes. We now examine a more important question, namely the impact of the type of carbohydrate-containing foods, especially the fiber content, and also the type of fat.

5.4. Dietary Fiber

During the 1970s Trowell proposed that dietary fiber had an important role in the prevention and management of a range of diseases, including type 2 diabetes *(54,55)*.

Subsequent research studies have clearly shown that dietary fiber is one of the factors that influence postprandial glucose and insulin response.

Cross-sectional studies have revealed an inverse relationship between fiber intake and blood insulin levels *(46,48,56,57)*, implying that fiber improves insulin sensitivity. Four large cohort studies—the Health Professionals Follow-up Study carried out on men aged 40–75 yr *(50)*, the (original) Nurses' Health Study carried out on women aged 40–65 yr *(58)*, the Nurses' Health Study II carried out on women aged 24–44 yr *(59)*, and the Iowa Women's Health Study carried out on women aged 55–69 yr *(52)*—have studied the effects of fiber on the risk of developing diabetes. All four studies clearly showed that a relatively low intake of dietary fiber poses a significantly increased risk for the disease. The association was found to be strongest for cereal fiber: comparison of the extreme quintiles revealed a risk ratio of 0.64–0.72, after correcting for confounding variables, such as age, BMI, smoking, and physical activity. These findings suggest that insoluble fiber is strongly protective against diabetes. By contrast, a much weaker protective association was seen for sources of soluble fiber.

As the main dietary source of cereal fiber is whole grain products, these findings strongly imply that whole grains are protective against the development of diabetes. There are many substances contained in whole grains that may deserve the credit for this. We must be cautious, therefore, before bestowing the credit on dietary fiber. Other possibilities include vitamin E, antioxidants, phytochemicals, isoflavins, and lignans. Because many of these factors occur together in cereals, it is extremely difficult to determine the precise benefits of each.

Dietary intervention studies have been conducted in which supplements of dietary fiber have been given for several weeks. This has been shown to lower both postprandial glycemia and insulin levels *(60–62)* and to lead to an overall improvement in glycemic control as measured by HbA_{1C}. This is seen in both normal subjects and in those with type 2 diabetes. The effects were most pronounced when soluble fiber was given, regardless of whether it was taken as a supplement or in food. Lesser effects have been reported using insoluble fiber. We therefore see a clear contrast between what has been observed in the above cohort studies and in intervention studies: the former indicate that insoluble fiber from cereals is most potent for preventing diabetes, whereas the latter indicate that soluble fiber is most effective for improving glycemic control.

The studies discussed here leave little doubt that the great majority of people consume insufficient dietary fiber, especially cereal fiber; this is a significant factor in increasing the risk of diabetes while also worsening glycemic control in those with the disease. The required intake is likely to be at least as great as the median amount consumed by people in the highest quintile in the cohort studies discussed earlier. That amount was 24.1 g *(58)* and 26.5 g *(52)* in women and 29.7 g *(50)* in men. This is similar to the Dietary Reference Intakes for fiber published in the United States in 2002, which recommended an intake of 21–25 g in women and 30–38 g in men.

As there is still conjecture regarding both the ideal intake and most beneficial type of fiber, it makes most sense to emphasize appropriate carbohydrate sources rather than to specify quantities of fiber. In other words, people should be encouraged to eat generous amounts of whole grain cereals, legumes, vegetables, and fruit. Nuts are also a modest source of fiber. Interestingly, the Nurses' Health Study revealed a protective association between the consumption of nuts and risk of diabetes *(63)*.

5.5. Glycemic Index and Glycemic Load

Different forms of carbohydrate-rich foods cause very different postprandial glycemic responses. In recognition of this, the term glycemic index (GI) was coined in 1981 *(64)*. It is defined as the glycemic response elicited by a 50-g carbohydrate portion of a food expressed as a percentage of that elicited by a 50-g portion of a reference food (glucose or white bread). Low-GI foods have lower 2-h areas under the glucose curve than the reference food, whereas high-GI foods have higher areas.

GI is a valuable means for comparing different types of food. However, an important limitation of the term is that it ignores the quantity of carbohydrate in the food. For instance, carrots have a high GI but this is misleading as their content of carbohydrate is low. For that reason, the new concept of a glycemic load was developed. This is the mean GI of the diet multiplied by its carbohydrate content. Thus, a diet rich in foods that have both a high content of carbohydrate and a high GI will have a high glycemic load.

Three cohort studies reported that glycemic load or GI is associated with the risk of diabetes *(50,58,59)*. Two other cohort studies, however, failed to confirm this *(52,65)*. Numerous studies have demonstrated that foods with a low GI are beneficial when given to type 2 diabetics (i.e., glycemic control is improved) *(66)*. Furthermore, several studies have found that foods with a low GI are associated with improvements in blood lipids *(66)*.

Although the exact mechanisms by which a diet with a high glycemic load may accelerate the development of type 2 diabetes are not fully understood, there is evidence that the following is a reasonably accurate picture of the etiology of the disease *(66)*. A diet with a high glycemic load repeatedly causes hyperglycemia and thence hyperinsulinemia. The next step in the chain is insulin resistance (though other factors may also cause this). The cycle of hyperinsulinemia and insulin resistance places the β-cells of the pancreas under long-term increased demand. Eventually, the β-cells starts losing its ability to function properly and the body is now on the road from IGT to type 2 diabetes.

Even if the glycemic load concept is still to be firmly established, we can recommend that foods with a low glycemic load should be emphasized because, at worst, they will do no harm. Low glycemic-load foods include pasta, bran cereals, beans, nuts, apples, apple juice, milk, and yogurt. Intermediate foods include shredded wheat, muesli, banana, pineapple, orange juice, and ice cream. High glycemic-load foods include white bread, rye bread, instant rice, cornflakes, potatoes, and soft drinks. In brief, the diet should focus on fruit, vegetables, legumes, bran-rich cereals, and stone-ground bread, while limiting potatoes, white flour, and refined sugar. The recommended foods are more or less the same ones that were recommended above for achieving an ideal fiber intake.

5.6. Type of Dietary Fat

There is evidence that the type of dietary fat may modify glucose tolerance and insulin sensitivity *(67,68)*. In epidemiological studies, intake of saturated fat has been associated with poor glucose tolerance *(44)* and higher fasting levels of both glucose *(69,70)* and insulin *(46,71)*. Conversely, intake of polyunsaturated fat has been associated with lower fasting and 2-h glucose concentrations *(70,72)*, as well as lower risk of type 2 diabetes *(51,73,74)*. In two short-term intervention studies, substitution of saturated fat by unsaturated fat improved glucose tolerance in young, healthy women *(75)* and in middle-aged, glucose-intolerant hyperlipidemic subjects *(76)*. A longer-term study (3 mo) by Vessby et al. *(77)* showed that replacing saturated fat with monounsaturated fat significantly improved insulin sensitivity in healthy subjects.

These findings parallel the situation with heart disease: saturated fat appears to accelerate the metabolic process leading to diabetes whereas polyunsaturated fat is apparently protective.

5.7. Micronutrients

5.7.1. MAGNESIUM

Three large American cohort studies reported that intake of magnesium showed a strong inverse association with the risk of type 2 diabetes *(50,52,58)*. In each case the risk ratio was about 0.66 when comparing the extreme quintiles, after correcting for confounding variables such as age, BMI, smoking, and physical activity. Although the strength of the association was reduced after adjusting for cereal fiber, an important source of magnesium, it still remained strong and statistically significant. However, in the absence of any randomized trials it would be premature to make specific recommendations concerning magnesium intake.

5.7.2. CHROMIUM

The relationship between chromium and glucose metabolism has been under investigation since the late 1950s *(78–80)*. Anderson et al. *(81)* carried out a study in which they gave supplemental chromium to subjects who had been consuming a fairly low intake of the mineral. They reported that subjects with mildly impaired glucose tolerance showed an improvement in glucose tolerance and a lower level of blood insulin after receiving supplemental chromium. However, this was not seen in subjects with normal glucose tolerance. This suggests that when the intake of chromium is low, some people develop IGT, which can be corrected by chromium supplementation. The lowering in blood insulin level indicates that chromium improves tissue sensitivity to insulin. Comparable observations have been reported from studies in rats *(82–84)*.

Several clinical trials have been conducted on patients with type 2 diabetes. The study with the most rigorous design was done in Beijing, China *(85)*. In this double-blind study, 4 mo of supplemental chromium improved blood levels of both glucose and insulin, both fasting levels and after oral glucose. HbA$_{1C}$ also improved, consistent with the improved glucose tolerance. However, other clinical trials have given inconsistent results *(79)*. The most plausible explanation for this is as follows: first, the type of chromium that is most effective is chromium picolinate, the type used in the Beijing study. Some of the other studies used chromium chloride, which is poorly absorbed *(81)*. Second, chromium is only effective in persons who have been consuming a diet poor in the mineral *(79,80)*.

These studies support the view that a large fraction of many populations habitually consume a diet that is mildly deficient in chromium. Dietary sugar may aggravate this by increasing loss of chromium. The evidence is growing that a poor chromium status plays a significant role in the development of insulin resistance and IGT, and the progression of this state to type 2 diabetes.

5.8. Alcohol

Consumption of moderate amounts of alcohol has a protective association with the risk of diabetes. This is discussed further in Chapter 12.

6. LIFESTYLE MODIFICATIONS AND RISK REDUCTION

Studies have recently been conducted that examined the efficacy of lifestyle intervention to prevent or at least slow the progression of IGT to diabetes. Two randomized controlled trials on overweight subjects with IGT demonstrated that weight loss achieved by an increase in physical activity and dietary change, including a reduction in total and saturated fat and increased dietary fiber, can reduce the incidence of type 2 diabetes. The Finnish Diabetes Prevention Study (FDPS) assessed the efficacy of an intensive diet and exercise program in 522 adults *(86)*. The intervention group received individual counseling with respect to diet, weight loss, and physical activity. Weight loss was about 3 kg greater in the intervention group than in the control group. The cumulative incidence of diabetes after 4 yr was 23% in the control group and 11% in the intervention group. A similar intervention program, the Diabetes Prevention Program, was conducted in the United States on a larger sample of 3234 adults *(87)*. During the 3 yr of follow-up, about 29% of the control group developed diabetes as compared with only 14% of the diet and exercise group. (A second intervention group was treated with a drug.) In both studies the estimated risk reduction was about 58%.

The Da Qing Study, conducted in China, was undertaken over a longer intervention period (6 yr) than the above studies *(88)*. The 577 participants with IGT were randomized by clinic rather than as individuals, into a control group or into one of three lifestyle interventions: diet only (including weight loss if the BMI was >25), exercise only, or both diet and exercise. The cumulative incidence of diabetes after 6 yr was 68% in the control group, 44% in the diet group, 41% in the exercise group, and 46% in the diet plus exercise group. After adjusting for differences in baseline BMI and fasting glucose, reduction in risk was 31% with diet alone, 46% with exercise alone, and 42% with both diet and exercise.

These three studies provide strong evidence that for adults who are at high risk of developing type 2 diabetes, changes in lifestyle can be highly protective. This was achieved even though the average amount of weight lost was relatively small. This emphasizes the importance of even a small degree of weight loss in conjunction with an increase in physical activity in the prevention of diabetes. Although these lifestyle intervention studies show that quite modest changes can substantially reduce the progression from IGT to diabetes, it is not clear whether it will be possible to achieve this success in larger groups or to maintain these lifestyle changes for longer periods.

Although these trials are of enormous importance, it is nevertheless equally important to appreciate that even in the intensive intervention groups an appreciable proportion go on to develop diabetes, and this steadily worsens over the years. It is not clear whether this is caused by an inability to sustain the necessary intensive lifestyle interventions or whether there is an inevitable deterioration in β-cell function. It is well established that the increased insulin secretion has already started to decrease even during the phase of IGT and then declines progressively as the disease process continues, regardless of treatment. Thus the best hope of truly "preventing" type 2 diabetes probably lies not in identifying those with IGT but rather in implementing lifestyle intervention programs in individuals at the stage of insulin resistance or in the general population (especially in populations where the disease is common).

7. CONCLUSIONS

Type 2 diabetes was previously a disease of the middle-aged and elderly but in recent years has escalated in younger age groups and the condition is now seen in adolescence, especially in high-risk populations. The disease has a devastating health impact.

The fast growing epidemic of the disease has occurred in parallel with a dramatic rise in the frequency of overweight and obesity. There is convincing evidence that obesity, particularly when centrally distributed, increases insulin resistance and thence leads to IGT, and eventually to diabetes. The risk of diabetes is seen to increase with weight, even within the normal range of BMI. An optimum BMI is therefore at the lower end of the normal range (i.e., around 21). Weight loss in the overweight and obese has been convincingly shown to reduce insulin resistance and diabetes risk.

Lack of physical activity has a similar effect on diabetes risk as obesity, though the magnitude of its impact is much less. Ideally, people should engage in moderate or vigorous physical activity for at least 1 h every day. Vigorous activity appears to be more effective than moderate activity. Physical activity that results in weight loss is likely to prove especially effective.

Much research indicates that although both carbohydrates and fats are associated with diabetes, it is the type of carbohydrate-containing food and the type of fat that is probably critical, rather than the quantity. A generous intake of dietary fiber, especially the soluble type, appears to improve insulin sensitivity and glycemic control in type 2 diabetes. However, cohort studies have revealed that cereal fiber (i.e., insoluble fiber) is most closely associated with a reduced risk of the disease, consonant with a general benefit of whole grain foods. Other evidence indicates that replacement of foods with a high GI by foods with a lower GI, thereby lowering the glycemic load of the diet, is another beneficial step.

Saturated fat has been shown to be associated with higher fasting glucose and insulin levels, an increased risk of IGT, and increased rates of progression from IGT to diabetes. Replacing an appreciable proportion of dietary saturated fat with unsaturated fat, within the usual range of total fat intake, is associated with improved glucose tolerance and improved insulin sensitivity.

A dietary pattern that minimizes the risk of IGT and diabetes is therefore one that emphasizes foods with a low glycemic load and that are rich in fiber but low in saturated fat. However, the efficacy of this dietary strategy has not yet been conclusively established using intervention studies. Nevertheless, it should be noted that low rates of type 2 diabetes are seen in groups and populations consuming diets rich in whole grain cereals, legumes, fruit, and vegetables, and with low intakes of foods rich in saturated fat.

In view of the enormous and growing economic, social, and personal cost of the disease, it seems prudent that primary prevention should be a major priority. Accordingly, there is an urgent need to tackle the epidemic of overweight and obesity, and to encourage greater participation in physical activity. These are the two vital components of an antidiabetes strategy. Simultaneously, a healthy diet should be a central component of such a lifestyle approach.

The dietary factors and lifestyle changes that help prevent diabetes are also effective in therapy. In that regard diabetes resembles the conditions that are closely associated with it, namely obesity, hypertension, hyperlipidemia, and cardiovascular disease. Indeed, the similarity of these conditions goes much further: the lifestyle approach outlined earlier for the prevention of diabetes will, in general, help prevent all of them.

REFERENCES

1. King H, Aubert RE, Herman WH. Global burden of diabetes, 1995–2025: prevalence, numerical estimates, and projections. Diabetes Care 1998; 21:1414–1431.
2. Amos AF, McCarty DJ, Zimmet P. The rising global burden of diabetes and its complications: estimates and projections to the year 2010. Diabetic Medicine 1997; 14:S7–S85.
3. Gavin JR, III, Alberti KGMM, Davidson MB, et al. Report of the Expert Committee on the Diagnosis and Classification of Diabetes Mellitus. Diabetes Care 1997; 20:1183–1197.
4. WHO Consultation Group. Definition, Diagnosis and Classification of Diabetes Mellitus and its Complications. Part 1: Diagnosis and Classification of Diabetes Mellitus. World Health Organisation, Geneva, 1999.
5. Harris MI, Eastman RC, Cowie CC, et al. Comparison of diabetes diagnostic categories in the U.S. population according to the 1997 American Diabetes Association and 1980–1985 World Health Organization diagnostic criteria. Diabetes Care 1997; 20:1859–1862.
6. Bennett PH. Impact of the new WHO classification and diagnostic criteria. Diabetes Obes Metab 1999; 1(Suppl 2):S1–S6.
7. Harris MI, Flegal KM, Cowie CC, et al. Prevalence of diabetes, impaired fasting glucose, and impaired glucose tolerance in U.S. adults. The Third National Health and Nutrition Examination Survey, 1988–1994. Diabetes Care 1998; 21:518–524.
8. Harris MI, Hadden WC, Knowler WC, et al. Prevalence of diabetes and impaired glucose tolerance and plasma glucose levels in U.S. population aged 20–74 yr. Diabetes 1987; 36:523–534.
9. Mokdad AH, Bowman BA, Engelgau MM, et al. Diabetes trends among American Indians and Alaska natives: 1990–1998. Diabetes Care 2001; 24:1508, 1509.
10. Mokdad AH, Bowman BA, Ford ES, et al. The continuing epidemics of obesity and diabetes in the United States. JAMA 2001; 286:1195–1200.
11. Narayan KM, Boyle JP, Thompson TJ, Sorensen SW, Williamson DF. Lifetime risk for diabetes mellitus in the United States. JAMA 2003; 290:1884–1890.
12. Harris MI. Noninsulin-dependent diabetes mellitus in black and white Americans. Diabetes Metab Rev 1990; 6:71–90.
13. Mather HM, Chaturvedi N, Fuller JH. Mortality and morbidity from diabetes in South Asians and Europeans: 11- year follow-up of the Southall Diabetes Survey, London, UK. Diabet Med 1998; 15:53–59.
14. Omar MA, Seedat MA, Dyer RB, et al. South African Indians show a high prevalence of NIDDM and bimodality in plasma glucose distribution patterns. Diabetes Care 1994; 17:70–73.
15. Gohdes D. Diabetes in North American Indians and Alaska Natives. Diabetes in America. In: Harris MI, Cowie CC, Stern MP, et al., eds. National Institutes of Health, Bethesda, MD, 1995.
16. Knowler WC, Pettitt DJ, Saad MF, et al. Diabetes Mellitus in the Pima Indians: Incidence, Risk Factors and Pathogenesis. Diabetes/Metabolism Rev 1990; 6:1–27.
17. Bennett PH. Type 2 diabetes among the Pima Indians of Arizona: an epidemic attributable to environmental change? Nutr Rev 1999; 57(5 Pt 2):S51–S54.
18. King H, Rewers M. Global estimates for prevalence of diabetes mellitus and impaired glucose tolerance in adults. WHO Ad Hoc Diabetes Reporting Group. Diabetes Care 1993; 16:157–177.
19. Cosnett JE. Illness among Natal Indians: a survey of hospital admissions. S Afr Med J 1957; 31:1109–1115.

20. Omar MAK, Seedat MA, Motala AA, Dyer RB, Becker P. The prevalence of diabetes mellitus and impaired glucose tolerance in a group of urban South African blacks. S Afr Med J 1993; 83:641–643.
21. Gu K, Cowie CC, Harris MI. Mortality in adults with and without diabetes in a national cohort of the U.S. population, 1971–1993. Diabetes Care 1998; 21:1138–1145.
22. Stamler J, Vaccaro O, Neaton JD, et al. Diabetes, other risk factors, and 12-yr cardiovascular mortality for men screened in the Multiple Risk Factor Intervention Trial. Diabetes Care 1993; 16:434–444.
23. Edelstein SL, Knowler WC, Bain RP, et al. Predictors of progression from impaired glucose tolerance to NIDDM: an analysis of six prospective studies. Diabetes 1997; 46:701–710.
24. Weyer C, Bogardus C, Mott DM, et al. The natural history of insulin secretory dysfunction and insulin resistance in the pathogenesis of type 2 diabetes mellitus. J Clin Invest 1999; 104:787–794.
25. Klein BE, Klein R, Lee KE. Components of the metabolic syndrome and risk of cardiovascular disease and diabetes in Beaver Dam. Diabetes Care 2002; 25:1790–1794.
26. Everhart JE, Knowler WC, Bennett PH. Incidence and risk factors for noninsulin-dependent diabetes. Diabetes in America, Diabetes Data Compiled 1984. In: Harris MI, Hamman RF, eds. NIH Publication No. 85-1468, 1985.
27. Dabelea D, Hanson RL, Bennett PH, et al. Increasing prevalence of type II diabetes in American Indian children. Diabetologia 1998; 41:904–910.
28. Kitagawa T, Owada M, Urakami T, et al. Increased incidence of non-insulin dependent diabetes mellitus among Japanese schoolchildren correlates with an increased intake of animal protein and fat. Clin Pediatr (Phila) 1998; 37:111–115.
29. Hu FB, Manson JE, Stampfer MJ, et al. Diet, lifestyle, and the risk of type 2 diabetes mellitus in women. N Engl J Med 2001; 345:790–797.
30. Chan JM, Rimm EB, Colditz GA, et al. Obesity, fat distribution, and weight gain as risk factors for clinical diabetes in men. Diabetes Care 1994; 17:961–969.
31. Boyko EJ, Fujimoto WY, Leonetti DL, et al. Visceral adiposity and risk of type 2 diabetes: a prospective study among Japanese Americans. Diabetes Care 2000; 23:465–471.
32. Lean ME, Han TS, Seidell JC. Impairment of health and quality of life in people with large waist circumference. Lancet 1998; 351:853–856.
33. Manson JE, Rimm EB, Stampfer MJ, et al. Physical activity and incidence of non-insulin-dependent diabetes mellitus in women. Lancet 1991; 338:774–778.
34. Manson JE, Nathan DM, Krolewski AS, et al. A prospective study of exercise and incidence of diabetes among US male physicians. JAMA 1992; 268:63–67.
35. Kriska AM, LaPorte RE, Pettitt DJ, et al. The association of physical activity with obesity, fat distribution and glucose intolerance in Pima Indians. Diabetologia 1993; 36:863–869.
36. Helmrich SP, Ragland DR, Leung RW, et al. Physical activity and reduced occurrence of non-insulin-dependent diabetes mellitus. N Engl J Med 1991; 325:147–152.
37. McAuley KA, Williams SM, Mann JI, et al. Intensive lifestyle changes are necessary to improve insulin sensitivity: a randomized controlled trial. Diabetes Care 2002; 25:445–452.
38. Grundy SM. The optimal ratio of fat-to-carbohydrate in the diet. Ann Rev Nutr 1999; 19:325–341.
39. Storlien LH, Baur LA, Kriketos AD, et al. Dietary fats and insulin action. Diabetologia 1996; 39:621–631.
40. Hedeskov CJ, Capito K, Islin H, Hansen SE, Thams P. Long-term fat-feeding-induced insulin resistance in normal NMRI mice: postreceptor changes of liver, muscle and adipose tissue metabolism resembling those of type 2 diabetes. Acta Diabetol 1992; 29:14–19.
41. Storlien LH, Jenkins AB, Chisholm DJ, Pascoe WS, Khouri S, Kraegen EW. Influence of dietary fat composition on development of insulin resistance in rats. Relationship to muscle triglyceride and omega-3 fatty acids in muscle phospholipid. Diabetes 1991; 40:280–289.
42. Storlien LH, Kraegen EW, Chisholm DJ, Ford GL, Bruce DG, Pascoe WS. Fish oil prevents insulin resistance induced by high-fat feeding in rats. Science 1987; 237:885–888.
43. Marshall JA, Hamman RF, Baxter J. High-fat, low-carbohydrate diet and the etiology of non-insulin-dependent diabetes mellitus: the San Luis Valley Diabetes Study. Am J Epidemiol 1991; 134:590–603.
44. Feskens EJM, Virtanen SM, Räsänen L, et al. Dietary factors determining diabetes and impaired glucose tolerance. A 20-year follow-up of the Finnish and Dutch cohorts of the Seven Countries Study. Diabetes Care 1995; 18:1104–1112.

45. Marshall JA, Hoag S, Shetterly S, Hamman RF. Dietary fat predicts conversion from impaired glucose tolerance to NIDDM. The San Luis Valley Diabetes Study. Diabetes Care 1994; 17:50–56.

46. Marshall JA, Bessesen DH, Hamman RF. High saturated fat and low starch and fiber are associated with hyperinsulinemia in a non-diabetic population: The San Luis Valley Diabetes Study. Diabetologia 1997; 40:430–438.

47. Mayer EJ, Newman B, Quesenberry CP, Selby JV. Usual dietary fat intake and insulin concentrations in healthy women twins. Diabetes Care 1993; 16:1459–1469.

48. Lovejoy J, DiGirolamo M. Habitual dietary intake and insulin sensitivity in lean and obese adults. Am J Clin Nutr 1992; 55:1174–1179.

49. Tsunehara CH, Leonetti DL, Fujimoto WY. Diet of second-generation Japanese-American men with and without non-insulin-dependent diabetes. Am J Clin Nutr 1990; 52:731–738.

50. Salmeron J, Ascherio A, Rimm EB, et al. Dietary fiber, glycemic load and risk of NIDDM in men. Diabetes Care 1997; 20:545–550.

51. Salmeron J, Hu FB, Manson JE, et al. Dietary fat intake and risk of type 2 diabetes in women. Am J Clin Nutr 2001; 73:1019–1026.

52. Meyer KA, Kushi LH, Jacobs DR, Slavin J, Sellers TA, Folsom AR. Carbohydrates, dietary fiber, and incident type 2 diabetes in older women. Am J Clin Nutr 2000; 71:921–930.

53. Bessesen DH. The role of carbohydrates in insulin resistance. J Nutr 2001; 131:2782S–2786S.

54. Trowell HC. Dietary fiber, ischaemic heart disease and diabetes mellitus. Proc Nutr Soc 1973; 32:151–157.

55. Trowell HC. Dietary fiber hypothesis of the etiology of diabetes mellitus. Diabetes 1975; 24:762–765.

56. Feskens EJ, Loeber JG, Kromhout D. Diet and physical activity as determinants of hyperinsulinaemia: the Zutphen Elderly Study. Am J Epidemiol 1994; 140:350–360.

57. Ludwig DS, Pereira MA, Kroenke CH, et al. Dietary fiber, weight gain, and cardiovascular disease risk factors in young adults. JAMA 1999; 282:1539–1546.

58. Salmeron J, Manson JE, Stampfer MJ, Colditz GA, Wing AL, Willett WC. Dietary fiber, glycemic load, and risk of non-insulin-dependent diabetes mellitus in women. JAMA 1997; 277:472–477.

59. Schulze MB, Liu S, Rimm EB, Manson JE, Willett WC, Hu FB. Glycemic index, glycemic load, and dietary fiber intake and incidence of type 2 diabetes in younger and middle-aged women. Am J Clin Nutr 2004; 80:348–356.

60. McIntosh M, Miller C. A diet containing food rich in soluble and insoluble fiber improves glycemic control and reduces hyperlipidemia among patients with type 2 diabetes mellitus. Nutr Rev 2001; 59:52–55.

61. Jenkins DJ, Jenkins AL. Dietary fiber and the glycemic response. Proc Soc Exp Biol Med 1985; 180:422–431.

62. Anderson JW. Fiber and health: an overview. Am J Gastroenterol 1986; 81:892–897.

63. Jiang R, Manson JE, Stampfer MJ, Liu S, Willett WC, Hu FB. Nut and peanut butter consumption and risk of type 2 diabetes in women. JAMA 2002; 288:2554–2560.

64. Jenkins DJ, Wolever TM, Taylor RH, et al. Glycemic index of foods: a physiological basis for carbohydrate exchange. Am J Clin Nutr 1981; 34:362–366.

65. Stevens J, Ahn K, Juhaeri, Houston D, Steffan L, Couper D. Dietary fiber intake and glycemic index and incidence of diabetes in African-American and white adults: the ARIC study. Diabetes Care 2002; 25: 1715–1721.

66. Ludwig DS. The glycemic index: physiological mechanisms relating to obesity, diabetes, and cardiovascular disease. JAMA 2002; 287:2414–2423.

67. Lichtenstein AH, Schwab US. Relationship of dietary fat to glucose metabolism. Atherosclerosis 2000; 150:227–243.

68. Hu FB, van Dam RM, Liu S. Diet and risk of type II diabetes: the role of types of fat and carbohydrate. Diabetologia 2001; 44:805–817.

69. Feskens EJ, Kromhout D. Habitual dietary intake and glucose tolerance in euglycaemic men: the Zutphen Study. Int J Epidemiol 1990; 19:953–959.

70. Trevisan M, Krogh V, Freudenheim J, et al. Consumption of olive oil, butter and vegetable oils and coronary heart disease risk factors. The Research Group ATS-RF2 of the Italian National Research Council. JAMA 1990; 263:688–692.

71. Parker DR, Weiss ST, Troisi R, Cassano PA, Vokonas PS, Landsberg L. Relationship of dietary satu-rated fatty acids and body habitus to serum insulin concentrations: the Normative Aging Study. Am J Clin Nutr 1993; 58:129–136.
72. Mooy JM, Grootenhuis PA, de Vries H, et al. Prevalence and determinants of glucose intolerance in a Dutch caucasian population. The Hoorn Study. Diabetes Care 1995; 18:1270–1273.
73. Colditz GA, Manson JE, Stampfer MJ, Rosner B, Willett WC, Speizer FE. Diet and risk of clinical diabetes in women. Am J Clin Nutr 1992; 55:1018–1023.
74. Meyer KA, Kushi LH, Jacobs DR, Folsom AR. Dietary fat and incidence of type 2 diabetes in older Iowa women. Diabetes Care 2001; 24:1528–1535.
75. Uusitupa M, Schwab U, Mäkimattila S, et al. Effects of two high-fat diets with different fatty acid composi-tions on glucose and lipid metabolism in healthy young women. Am J Clin Nutr 1994; 59:1310–1316.
76. Vessby B, Gustafsson I-B, Boberg J, Karlström B, Lithell H, Werner I. Substituting polyunsaturated for saturated fat as a single change in a Swedish diet: effects on serum lipoprotein metabolism and glucose tolerance in patients with hyperlipoproteinaemia. Eur J Clin Invest 1980; 10:193–202.
77. Vessby B, Uusitupa M, Hermansen K, et al. Substituting dietary saturated for monounsaturated fat impairs insulin sensitivity in healthy men and women: the KANWU study. Diabetologia 2001; 44:312–319.
78. Schwarz K, Mertz W. Chromium (III) and the glucose tolerance factor. Arch Biochem Biophys 1959; 85:292–295.
79. Lukaski HC. Chromium as a supplement. Annu Rev Nutr 1999; 19:279–302.
80. Vincent JB. Quest for the molecular mechanism of chromium action and its relationship to diabetes. Nutr Rev 2000; 58(3 Pt 1):67–72.
81. Anderson RA, Polansky MM, Bryden NA, Canary JJ. Supplemental-chromium effects on glucose, insulin, glucagon, and urinary chromium losses in subjects consuming controlled low-chromium diets. Am J Clin Nutr 1991; 54:909–916.
82. Striffler JS, Polansky MM, Anderson RA. Dietary chromium decreases insulin resistance in rats fed a high-fat, mineral-imbalanced diet. Metabolism 1998; 47:396–400.
83. Striffler JS, Law JS, Polansky MM, Bhathena SJ, Anderson RA. Chromium improves insulin response to glucose in rats. Metabolism 1995; 44:1314–1320.
84. Anderson RA, Bryden NA, Polansky MM, Gautschi K. Dietary chromium effects on tissue chromium concentrations and chromium absorption in rats. J Trace Elem Exptl Med 1996; 9:11–25.
85. Anderson RA, Cheng N, Bryden NA, et al. Elevated intakes of supplemental chromium improve glucose and insulin variables in individuals with type 2 diabetes. Diabetes 1997; 46:1786–1791.
86. Tuomilehto J, Lindstrom J, Eriksson JG, et al. Prevention of type 2 diabetes mellitus by changes in lifestyle among subjects with impaired glucose tolerance. N Engl J Med 2001; 344:1343–1350.
87. Knowler WC, Barrett-Connor E, Fowler SE, et al. Reduction in the incidence of type 2 diabetes with lifestyle intervention or metformin. N Engl J Med 2002; 346:393–403.
88. Pan XR, Li GW, Hu YH, et al. Effects of diet and exercise in preventing NIDDM in people with impaired glucose tolerance. Diabetes Care 1997; 20:537–544.

6   Diet and the Control of Blood Lipids

Tricia L. Psota, Sarah K. Gebauer,
Gigi Meyer, and Penny M. Kris-Etherton

KEY POINTS

- Lipids and lipoproteins play a key role in modulating risk of coronary heart disease (CHD). Elevated levels of total cholesterol, low-density lipoprotein cholesterol (LDL-C), and triglyceride (TG) increase CHD risk, whereas high high-density lipoprotein cholesterol (HDL-C) levels exert a cardioprotective effect.
- The blood lipid profile is adversely affected by dietary saturated fatty acids, trans-fatty acids, and cholesterol, whereas unsaturated fatty acids and soluble fiber have favorable effects.
- Many clinical studies have demonstrated that designer diets low in saturated fatty acids, trans-fatty acids, and cholesterol and high in fiber lower total cholesterol and LDL-C levels, whereas the effects they have on TG and HDL-C levels are diet specific.
- New dietary interventions that can be implemented to control blood lipids provide a variety of options for individualizing diets to maximize CHD risk reduction and promote overall diet adherence.
- Current guidelines to achieve and maintain a healthy body weight, a desirable cholesterol profile, and a desirable blood pressure emphasize a diet including a variety of fruits, vegetables, grain products, including whole grains, low-fat or nonfat dairy products, fish, nuts, legumes, spices, poultry, and lean meats.

1. INTRODUCTION

Lipids and lipoproteins play a key role in modulating risk of coronary heart disease (CHD). It is well established that elevated levels of total cholesterol (TC), low-density lipoprotein-cholesterol (LDL-C), and triglyceride (TG) increase CHD risk. In contrast, an elevated high-density lipoprotein-cholesterol (HDL-C) level exerts a cardioprotective effect. Diet can increase or decrease CHD risk via changes in the lipid and lipoprotein profile. Many epidemiological and controlled clinical studies have demonstrated effects of single nutrients, specific foods, and total diets (with multiple changes in both nutrients and foods, resulting in different dietary patterns) on the lipid and lipoprotein profile. This research has culminated in dietary recommendations that can markedly lower risk of CHD. Consequently, a healthy diet is a cornerstone in CHD risk reduction.

From: *Nutritional Health: Strategies for Disease Prevention, Second Edition*
Edited by: N. J. Temple, T. Wilson, and D. R. Jacobs © Humana Press Inc., Totowa, NJ

This chapter will review both epidemiological and clinical studies, including regression and meta-analyses, which have evaluated single nutrients, specific foods, and different dietary patterns involving changes in both nutrients and foods on lipid and lipoprotein CHD risk factors. Identifying dietary factors that increase or decrease CHD lipid/lipoprotein risk factors is important to implementing diet strategies that maximally reduce CHD risk. The advent of new dietary interventions that can be implemented to control blood lipids provides a variety of options for individualizing diets to maximize CHD risk reduction and promote overall diet adherence.

2. INDIVIDUAL NUTRIENTS THAT MODIFY LIPIDS AND LIPOPROTEINS

The nutrients that modify plasma lipids and lipoproteins have been the most extensively studied diet components to date. The emphasis has been on examining the effects of different fatty acids, cholesterol, and fiber on lipids and lipoproteins. Saturated fatty acids (SFA), trans-fatty acids, and cholesterol adversely affect lipid and lipoprotein levels, whereas soluble fiber and unsaturated fatty acids (monounsaturated fatty acids [MUFA] and polyunsaturated fatty acids [PUFA]) have favorable effects (*see* Table 1).

2.1. Saturated Fatty Acids

The landmark Seven Countries Study reported a significant association between total SFA intake and TC among different populations *(1)*. Subsequent epidemiological studies also have found positive correlations between SFA intake and TC levels, as well as the incidence of CHD *(2,3)*. In a more recent analysis of the Seven Countries Study data, associations were reported between individual SFA and TC, as well as with SFA and CHD mortality. Intakes of lauric acid (12:0) and myristic acid (14:0) were most strongly associated with TC ($r = 0.84, 0.81$, respectively) *(4)*.

Results from earlier and subsequent clinical studies supported the epidemiological associations reported between SFA and TC. The early feeding studies by Keys et al. *(5)* and Hegsted et al. *(6)* in the 1950s and 1960s culminated in summary equations evaluating the effect of fatty acids on TC in humans, using regression analysis of data across their many clinical studies. The studies found that SFA raises TC levels compared with carbohydrates and MUFAs (which both had neutral effects) whereas PUFAs lowered TC levels.

Regression analyses demonstrate that for every 1% increase in energy from SFA, LDL-C levels increase approx 0.033–0.045 mmol/L *(7–9)*. In addition to raising TC and LDL-C, SFA has also been shown to increase HDL-C. Studies have shown that for every 1% increase in SFA, HDL-C levels increase by 0.011–0.013 mmol/L *(7–9)*.

Since the equations originally developed by Keys et al. *(5)* and Hegsted et al. *(6)* for TC, several equations have been published that predict the effects of SFA, MUFA, and PUFA on TC, LDL-C, and HDL-C levels *(7,10,11)*. In addition to equations that incorporate classes of fatty acids, equations have been generated to predict how changes in individual fatty acids, including trans-fatty acids, affect total and lipoprotein cholesterol levels. Recent regression analyses have demonstrated that stearic acid (18:0) has more of a neutral effect on TC, LDL-C, and HDL-C *(11)*, whereas myristic acid (14:0) is more hypercholesterolemic than lauric acid (12:0) and palmitic acid (16:0) *(10)*. A recent meta-analysis of 60 controlled trials determined the effects of different SFA relative to carbo-

Table 1
Summary of the Effects of Different Nutrients on Lipids and Lipoproteins

Nutrients	TC	LDL-C	HDL-C	TG
SFA	↑	↑	↑	—
Trans fat	↑	↑	↓[b]	—
MUFA[a]	—	—	↑	↓
n-6 PUFA	↓	↓	↑[c]	—
n-3 PUFA	—	—	—	↓
Cholesterol	↑	↑	—	—
Soluble fiber	↓	↓	—	↓

[a]When replacing carbohydrate.

[b]When replacing saturated fatty acids.

[c]At moderate levels.

SFA, saturated fatty acidsand legumes.; MUFA, monounsaturated fatty acids; PUFA, polyunsaturated fatty acids; TC, total cholesterol; LDL-C, low-density lipoprotein cholesterol; HDL-C, high-density lipoprotein cholesterol; TG, triglycerides.

hydrates using the TC/HDL-C ratio, a more specific marker of risk of coronary artery disease (CAD) *(12)*. Although lauric acid was found to have the greatest LDL-C raising effect, it decreased the ratio of TC/HDL-C as the result of an increase in HDL-C relative to carbohydrates. Myristic and palmitic acids had little effect on the ratio, whereas stearic acid reduced the ratio. As is evident in Fig. 1, individual fatty acids have remarkably different effects on lipids and lipoproteins *(13)*. In addition to showing the effects of SFA, the figure demonstrates the effects of elaidic acid (trans-18:1), oleic acid (*cis*-18:1, the most common MUFA), and linoleic acid (18:2 n-6, the most common PUFA).

2.2. Trans-Fatty Acids

In a follow up of the Seven Countries Study, elaidic acid, the predominant trans-fatty acid in hydrogenated vegetable oil, was significantly associated with TC ($r = 0.70$; $p < 0.01$) and 25-yr mortality rates from CHD ($r = 0.78$; $p < 0.001$) *(4)*. As seen in Fig. 1, trans-fat increases TC and LDL-C while slightly lowering HDL-C.

A recent clinical trial conducted by Judd et al. *(14)* assessed the change in LDL-C when replacing carbohydrates with trans-fatty acids. Subjects were fed experimental diets that provided approx 15% of energy from protein, 39% from total fat, and 46% from carbohydrate (CHO). TC and LDL-C were increased by 5.8% and 10.1%, respectively, when trans-fatty acids replaced 8% of the energy provided from CHO. When 8% of energy provided was replaced with a combination of 4% trans-fatty acids and 4% stearic acid, TC and LDL-C were increased by 5.6% and 8.7%, respectively. No significant differences were seen in HDL-C with either replacement compared to the CHO control diet.

Mensink and Katan *(15)* measured the effects of trans-fatty acids on HDL-C by placing subjects on three diets that were identical in nutrient composition except that 10% of total calories were either from oleic acid, trans-isomers of oleic acid, or SFA. The mean HDL-C level was the same on the SFA and oleic acid diets, but was 0.17 mmol/L lower on the trans-fatty acid diet ($p < 0.0001$).

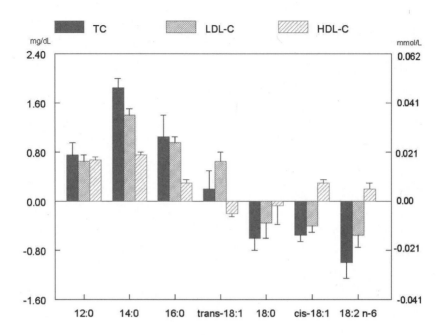

Fig. 1. Effects of individual fatty acids on changes in plasma cholesterol.

Lichtenstein et al. *(16)* conducted a clinical trial evaluating the effects of different hydrogenated fats on blood lipids and lipoproteins. The experimental diets provided 30% energy from total fat and were identical with the exception of the test fats fed. Two-thirds of the fat was provided by soybean oil (<0.5 g trans-fat/100 g of fat), semiliquid margarine (<0.5 g/100 g), stick margarine (20.1 g/100 g), or butter (1.25 g/100 g). Compared with the butter diet, the vegetable fat diets produced the following reductions in TC, LDL-C, and HDL-C:

1. Soybean-oil diet: 10, 12, and 3% respectively.
2. The semi-liquid margarine diet: 10, 11, and 4%, respectively.
3. The stick margarine diet: 3, 5, and 6%, respectively.

Although all of the vegetable fat diets resulted in decreases in TC, LDL-C, and HDL-C compared with the butter diet, stick margarine (containing the highest amount of trans-fatty acid) decreased LDL-C the least and decreased HDL-C the most compared with the other vegetable fats. This resulted in a 4% increase in the TC:HDL-C ratio, whereas the other vegetable fats slightly decreased the ratio. On balance, the soybean oil diet resulted in the most favorable effects on lipoproteins with the greatest reduction in TC and LDL-C and the smallest reduction in HDL-C, resulting in the greatest decrease in the TC:HDL-C ratio of 6%, whereas the semiliquid margarine diet resulted in a 5% reduction in the ratio.

This study demonstrates that increases in trans-fat result in a dose–response increase in LDL-C and decrease HDL-C at high levels (higher than typical consumption, which is about 2.6% of calories).

Through regression analysis, the effect of trans-fatty acids on TC, LDL-C, HDL-C, and TG levels have been compared with other fatty acids using predictive equations. Trans-fatty acids have been shown to increase TC and LDL-C, albeit somewhat less than

SFA; however, they lower HDL-C vs SFA. Furthermore, regression analysis has confirmed that myristic acid is the most hypercholesterolemic fatty acid; trans-fatty acids are less hypercholesterolemic then lauric and palmitic acids *(10)*. Recent data have demonstrated a linear dose-dependent relationship between trans-fatty acid intake and the raising effect on LDL-C:HDL-C ratio from intakes of 0.5 to 10% of total calories. The magnitude of this effect is greater for trans-fatty acids than it is for SFA *(17)*.

2.3. Monounsaturated Fatty Acids

Regression analyses and controlled feeding studies have shown that MUFA, and oleic acid in particular, have either a neutral or slight lowering effect on TC levels, particularly when SFA intake is low *(13)*. Figure 1 shows that oleic acid slightly decreases TC and LDL-C, and modestly increases HDL-C.

A meta-analysis of various studies conducted by Garg *(18)* evaluated the effects of high-MUFA diets (22–33% of total energy) vs high-CHO diets (49–60% of total energy). High-MUFA diets led to slight decreases in TC (3%), and decreases in very-low-density lipoprotein cholesterol (22%), and TG levels (19%), when compared with high-CHO diets. Effects of high-MUFA diets on HDL-C were inconsistent among studies with either slight increases or no changes reported. Overall, the studies conducted demonstrate a 4% increase in HDL-C in subjects on a high-MUFA diet, with no overall effect on LDL-C.

2.4. Polyunsaturated Fatty Acids

Some of the earliest clinical trials fed high levels of PUFAs (13–21% of energy) and evaluated effects on TC and CHD events *(19–22)*. Three of the studies reported a 13–15% decrease in TC that was accompanied by a 25–43% decrease in CHD events *(19–21)*. These studies established that feeding very high levels of PUFA led to a substantial decrease in TC. In parallel, many controlled clinical studies were conducted that provided data to develop predictive equations that demonstrated that PUFA lowered both TC and LDL-C. These equations predict that a 1% increase in PUFA reduces TC by 0.024 mmol/L and that this cholesterol-lowering effect is approximately half that of the cholesterol-raising effect of SFA *(5,6)*.

More recent predictive equations for individual fatty acids demonstrate that n-6 fatty acids, specifically linoleic acid (LA), is the most potent fatty acid in terms of lowering TC and LDL-C (*see* Fig. 1). In addition to these effects, LA raises HDL-C when compared with stearic acid (18:0) *(13)*. A study by Mattson and Grundy *(23)* reported an HDL-C lowering effect (-5.0 ± 1.7 mg/dL; $p < 0.02$) of PUFA at very high levels (28% of total calories) in normotriglyceridemic individuals; however, other studies have reported no significant change in HDL-C with a high PUFA intake *(24)*.

The marine long-chain n-3 fatty acids, eicosapentaenoic acid (EPA) and docosahexanoic acid (DHA), have been shown to significantly decrease TG levels. In a review of 36 human studies, consumption of 3–4 g/d of EPA and DHA resulted in a 25% and 34% decrease in TG levels in normolipemic (TG < 2.0 mmol/L) and hypertriglyceridemic patients (TG ≥ 2.0 mmol/L), respectively. However, LDL-C was increased by 4.5% and 10.8% in normolipemic and hypertriglyceridemic patients, respectively. EPA and DHA did not significantly affect TC or HDL-C levels *(25)*. The characteristic TG-lowering effect of marine n-3 fatty acids has generally not been found at physiologically relevant concentrations of plant sources of n-3 fatty acids. When reported, a TG-lowering effect was found only at very high levels (38 g) of α-linolenic intake *(25)*.

Numerous studies have shown a cardioprotective effect of marine n-3 fatty acids. This is discussed in Chapter 8. The exact mechanism by which these marine n-3 fatty acids protect against coronary disease still remains unclear. The mechanism does not appear to be the result of changes in blood lipids and lipoproteins, but rather is thought to be the result of stabilizing atherosclerotic plaques, decreased production of chemoattractants, growth factors, adhesion molecules, inflammatory eicosanoids and cytokines, and increased endothelial relaxation and vascular compliance (26).

In the Gruppo Italiano per lo Studio della Sopravvivenza nell'Infarto Miocardico (GISSI) Prevention Study (27), the largest prospective clinical trial to test the efficacy of n-3 fatty acids for secondary prevention of CHD, subjects randomized to the EPA + DHA supplement group (850 mg/d of n-3 fatty acid ethyl esters), with and without 300 mg/d of vitamin E, experienced a 15% reduction in the primary end point of death, nonfatal myocardial infarct, and nonfatal stroke ($p < 0.02$). In addition, all-cause mortality was reduced by 20% ($p = 0.01$) and sudden death by 45% ($p < 0.001$) compared with the control group. (Vitamin E provided no benefit.)

2.5. Dietary Cholesterol

Numerous studies have demonstrated that there is a positive linear relationship between dietary cholesterol intake and both TC and LDL-C. Based on a meta-analysis of 27 controlled feeding studies, for each 100 mg/d increase in dietary cholesterol (up to 400 mg/d) there is a corresponding increase of TC of 0.16 to 0.51 mmol/L, when baseline intake of dietary cholesterol is zero. But with a higher baseline cholesterol intake (300 mg/d), the increase in TC induced by an additional 100 mg/d of dietary cholesterol is now only 0.05–0.16 mmol/L (28). An increase in LDL-C accounts for 80% of the increases predicted in TC (28).

2.6. Dietary Fiber

Intervention studies have demonstrated that viscous fiber reduces both TC and LDL-C (28). A meta-analysis of 20 trials using viscous fiber from oat sources demonstrated that the reduction in TC per gram intake of viscous fiber ranged from 0.1–2.5% (29). Larger reductions were seen in studies conducted with subjects who had higher baseline blood cholesterol levels (≥5.9 mmol/L), specifically at viscous fiber intakes of at least 3 g/d. Studies have also found that adequate intake of soluble fiber prevents the increase in TG levels typically associated with diets low in fat and high in CHO (30). In a recent study by Obarzanek et al. (31), individuals with elevated cholesterol levels fed the Dietary Approaches to Stop Hypertension (DASH) diet (58% kcal from CHO, 27% from total fat) that provided 30 g/d of fiber had significantly lower TC and LDL-C ($p < 0.0001$) without any change in TG levels, compared with subjects fed a control diet (50% kcal from CHO, 37% from total fat) with intakes of only 11 g/d of fiber. Therefore, the lower-fat, high-fiber diet did not increase TG levels. A study conducted in subjects with type 2 diabetes who followed a diet that provided 55% of calories from CHO and 22 g of fiber per 1000 kcal, reported a 10.2% decrease ($p < 0.02$) in fasting serum TG levels compared with those consuming a diet that provided 55% CHO and only 10 g of fiber per 1000 kcal (32). Subjects consuming the high-fiber diet had additional benefits to the blood lipid profile, including a 6.7% reduction in TC and 12.5% reduction in LDL-C.

3. FOODS THAT MODIFY LIPIDS AND LIPOPROTEINS

Food-based dietary recommendations have been made by the American Heart Association (AHA) for healthy Americans to decrease risk for CHD. These guidelines recommend an overall healthy eating pattern to achieve and maintain a healthy body weight, a desirable cholesterol profile, and a desirable blood pressure. To achieve a healthy eating pattern, the diet should include a variety of fruits, vegetables, grain products (including whole grains), low-fat or nonfat dairy products, fish, legumes, poultry, and lean meats. To achieve a desirable cholesterol profile, the AHA Guidelines recommend limiting foods high in SFA, trans fat, and cholesterol that are provided by full-fat dairy products, fatty meats, partially hydrogenated vegetable oils, and egg yolks *(33)*. In addition, the AHA recommends that SFA be decreased and replaced with calories from either nutrient-dense carbohydrates (from grain products, fruits, vegetables, and fat-free dairy products) or unsaturated fat (from vegetables, fish, legumes, and nuts). The following is an overview of specific foods that beneficially affect blood lipids and can be incorporated in a diet to manage CHD risk.

3.1. Fruits and Vegetables

There is an impressive epidemiological database from 14 large studies that have found that increased intake of fruits and vegetables is associated with a significant reduction in at least one cardiovascular disease (CVD) outcome, including mortality *(34)*. The mechanisms of action are thought to be mediated, in part, through CVD risk factor reduction, including beneficial effects on lipids and lipoproteins. Using the National Health and Nutrition Examination Survey (NHANES) III data, Tande et al. *(35)* evaluated the relationship between the Food Guide Pyramid recommendations (i.e., food group) and serum lipids in 9111 participants. Fruit intake was inversely related to serum TC, LDL-C, and HDL-C ($p = 0.012, 0.014, 0.001$, respectively) and directly related to TG levels ($p = 0.003$). Part of the TC and LDL-C lowering associated with fruit consumption may result from a higher viscous fiber intake. Similar findings were reported in the National Heart, Lung, and Blood Institute Family Heart Study *(36)*. Based on a food frequency questionnaire, subjects consuming more fruits and vegetables (4 or more vs 1.9 or less servings/d) had lower LDL-C concentrations (3.17 vs 3.36 mmol/L for men, 3.11 vs 3.35 for women; $p < 0.0001$) *(36)*.

3.2. Whole Grain Breads and Cereals

Jacobs and Gallaher *(37)* reviewed 13 prospective epidemiological studies and found a 20–40% reduction in risk of atherosclerotic CVDs when comparisons were made between habitual consumers of whole grains vs those who seldom consumed these foods. In part, this likely is the result of beneficial effects on serum lipids and lipoproteins. Using NHANES III data, Tande et al. *(35)* found intake of grains to be inversely associated with both serum TC and HDL-C ($p = 0.020$ and 0.0001). In a cross-sectional analysis of data from the Framingham Offspring study, McKeown et al. *(38)* found that whole grain intake was associated with reduced body mass index, blood pressure, fasting insulin, and TG, and with increased HDL-C. The differences in the associations reported for HDL-C between the McKeown et al. *(38)* and Tande et al. *(35)* studies could be explained by differences in the types of grains evaluated. McKeown et al. evaluated whole grains, whereas Tande et al. simply evaluated grains. A high intake of refined grain would be associated with a high-carbohydrate, low-fat diet, which could explain the inverse association reported in their study.

Clinical studies have shown that viscous (soluble) fiber reduces TC and LDL-C levels, whereas insoluble fiber has no effect. A meta-analysis of 67 studies evaluating different sources of soluble fiber (oats, pectin, guar, and psyllium) reported that 2–10 g/d significantly reduced LDL-C *(39,40)*. The Adult Treatment Panel (ATP) III Report notes that an increase in viscous fiber of 5–10 g/d on average would be expected to lower LDL-C by approx 5% *(39)*.

3.3. Dairy Products

Based on an analysis of NHANES III data, Tande et al. *(35)* found that dairy consumption was directly related to LDL-C, which likely could be explained by the increase in SFA intake that is associated with dairy products that are not fat-free. A model community-based CHD intervention program, the North Karelia Project in eastern Finland, reported that a decrease in SFA intake (principally from dairy fat) from 20–21% of energy in 1972 to 14–15% of energy in 1997 was associated with a decrease in TC levels of 15–19% among men and women *(41)*. The main changes in diet were a decreased use of butter and increased use of low-fat and skim milk instead of whole milk. In the North Karelia Project, ischemic heart disease mortality declined 73% from 1971 to 1995 *(42)*. The reduced mortality was associated with a decrease in blood cholesterol levels and also beneficial changes in other CVD risk factors including blood pressure lowering and smoking cessation.

3.4. Lean Meat

Based on an analysis of NHANES III data, Tande et al. *(35)* found that meat consumption was associated with an increase in LDL-C, which, like dairy products, could be explained by the higher intake of SFA that is associated with higher-fat red meats. Controlled clinical studies have convincingly shown that incorporating lean red meat (beef, veal, and pork) into a National Cholesterol Education Program Step I diet in free-living individuals with hypercholesterolemia elicit similar reductions in LDL-C and increases in HDL-C levels as that seen in persons when given lean white meat (poultry and fish) *(43)*. Other clinical studies have reported similar results *(44,45)*. Thus, red meat can be included in a cholesterol-lowering diet provided that it is lean and the quantity is consistent with the daily amount recommended (5 oz/d for Therapeutic Lifestyle Changes [TLC]/step II diets; 6 oz/d for step I diets). Representative SFA and cholesterol values of selected cuts/species of red meat, poultry, and fish are shown in Table 2.

To put these values into perspective, a recommendation of less than 7% energy from SFA translates to 15 g/d and 21 g/d for diets with 1900 kcal and 2700 kcal, respectively. A meal containing 6 oz of lean beef will provide about 8 g of SFA. Dark meat from poultry is in saturated fat comparable to lean beef content as seen in Table 2. Lean red meats include bottom round and sirloin cuts, whereas lean poultry includes skinless white meat.

Table 2
Fatty Acid Composition, Cholesterol, and Caloric Value of Raw Meat, Fish, and Poultry in 100-g Portions

Source	Energy (kcal)	Total fat	SFA (g)	MUFA (g)	PUFA (g)	n-3 (g)	n-6 (g)	Cholesterol (mg)
Ground beef, 95% lean	137	5.0	2.2	2.1	0.2	0.035	0.224	62
Ham, lean	195	8.3	2.8	3.8	1.0	0.090	0.880	70
Chicken, light meat, no skin	114	1.7	0.4	0.4	0.4	0.050	0.280	58
Chicken, dark meat, no skin	178	8.75	2.4	3.3	2.0	0.07	1.9	75
Turkey, light meat, no skin	108	0.5	0.2	0.1	0.1	0.010	0.120	66
Salmon, farm-raised	183	10.9	2.2	3.9	3.9	2.162	1.738	59
Tuna, light, canned in water	116	0.8	0.2	0.2	0.3	0.292	0.043	30

SFA, saturated fatty acids; MUFA, monounsaturated fatty acids; PUFA, polyunsaturated acids. (Adapted from ref. 46.)

3.5. Fish

Epidemiological studies *(47–51)* and information from the evidence-based Agency for Healthcare Research and Quality Report, Effects of Omega-3 Fatty Acids on Cardiovascular Disease *(52)*, have reported the cardioprotective effects of fish consumption among healthy populations. Controlled clinical trials have shown that consumption of n-3 fatty acids from fish or from fish oil supplements reduces all-cause mortality and various CVD outcomes. The Diet and Reinfarction Trial (DART) reported that male myocardial infarct survivors who consumed 200–400 g/wk of fatty fish (which provided an additional 500–800 mg/d of n-3 fatty acids) had a 29% reduction in 2-yr all-cause mortality *(53)*.

The AHA and the Dietary Guidelines for Americans 2005 recommend two servings of fish per week, preferably fatty fish, to decrease CVD risk *(33,34)*. Fatty fish include salmon, tuna, mackerel, trout, herring, and sardines.

3.6. Nuts

Four large cohort studies have reported that frequent nut consumption is associated with a 30–50% decrease in risk of CHD *(54)*. In the Nurses' Health Study, women who ate more than 5 oz/wk had a significantly lower risk for total CHD (RR = 0.65; p = 0.0009) than women who ate less than 1 oz/mo after adjusting for age, smoking, and other risk factors for CHD *(55)*.

Nuts have a fatty acid profile that favorably affects blood lipids and lipoproteins *(56)*. They are low in SFA and high in unsaturated fatty acids *(see* Table 3), and are a rich sources of other nutrients. Furthermore, nuts contain plant sterols and dietary fiber, which would also be expected to contribute to their cholesterol-lowering effect. Numerous clinical studies have consistently reported a lowering effect on TC and LDL-C by diets low in SFA and cholesterol and high in unsaturated fat provided by a variety of nuts *(56)*. Based on the clinical studies conducted to date, an intake of 1–2 oz/d of nuts reduces LDL-C by 3–19%.

3.7. Vegetable Oils

Vegetable oils are rich sources of unsaturated fatty acids—MUFA and PUFA—depending on the seed oil *(see* Table 4). Beneficial effects of unsaturated fatty acids have been noted in both epidemiological and clinical trial literature. The Nurses' Health Study reported that, compared with equivalent energy from carbohydrates, a 5% increment in energy from MUFA was associated with a decreased risk of CHD (RR = 0.81; p = 0.05) *(3)*. Moreover, for a 5% increment in energy from PUFA (compared with CHO) the RR was 0.62 (p = 0.003).

The clinical trial literature convincingly affirms that the beneficial effect reported in the epidemiological literature of unsaturated fatty acids is owing, in part, to favorable effects on lipids and lipoproteins *(see* Subheadings 2.3 and 2.4). The varying fatty acid profile of different vegetable oils has enabled numerous clinical studies to be done that have manipulated dietary fatty acid composition in a myriad of ways. Consistently, these studies show that n-6 PUFAs lower TC and LDL-C and that MUFAs have a neutral to very slight cholesterol-lowering effect, when substituted isoenergetically for CHO *(7)*. The effect of different vegetable oils on cholesterol lowering will reflect the type and

Table 3
Fatty Acid Composition and Caloric Value in 1 oz of Nuts

	Amount, 1 oz (28.35 g)	Energy (kcal)	Total fat (g)	SFA (g)	MUFA (g)	PUFA (g)	n-3 (g)	n-6 (g)
Almonds	22 nuts	169	15.0	1.2	9.5	3.6	0.000	3.586
Brazil nuts	6–8 nuts	186	18.8	4.3	7.0	5.8	0.010	5.824
Cashews	12 nuts	163	13.1	2.6	7.7	2.2	0.046	2.172
Hazelnuts	12 nuts	183	17.7	1.3	13.2	2.4	0.017	2.382
Macadamia nuts	10–12 nuts	204	21.6	3.4	16.8	0.4	0.056	0.369
Peanuts	35 pieces	168	14.6	2.0	8.9	3.1	0.054	2.987
Pecans	15 halves	201	21.1	1.8	12.5	5.8	0.282	5.550
Pistachios	49 kernels	162	13.0	1.6	6.9	3.9	0.074	3.866
Walnuts	14 halves	175	16.7	1.0	4.3	9.9	0.569	9.376

All values given for dried or dry roasted nuts.
  SFA, saturated fatty acids; MUFA, monounsaturated fatty acids; PUFA, polyunsaturated acids. (Adapted from ref. 46.)

Table 4
Fatty Acid Composition and Caloric Value of Vegetable Oils in 1 Tbsp (14.2 g)

Oil	Kcal	Total fat (g)	SFA (g)	MUFA (g)	PUFA (g)	n-3 (g)	n-6 (g)
Canola	124	14.0	1.0	8.2	4.1	1.302	2.842
Corn	120	13.6	1.7	3.3	8.0	0.158	7.278
Cottonseed	120	13.6	3.5	2.4	7.1	0.027	7.004
Olive	119	13.5	1.8	10.0	1.4	0.107	1.243
Peanut	119	13.5	2.3	6.2	4.3	0.000	4.320
Safflower	120	13.6	0.8	10.2	2.0	0.000	10.149
Soybean	120	13.6	2.0	3.2	7.9	0.925	6.936
Sunflower	120	13.6	1.4	2.7	8.9	0.000	8.935

SFA, saturated fatty acids; MUFA, monounsaturated fatty acids; PUFA, polyunsaturated acids. (Adapted from ref. 46.)

amount of oil(s) used in the diet and the resulting fatty acid profile. Furthermore, the fatty acid profile of the total diet is the key determinant of the blood cholesterol response.

4. DESIGNER DIETS TO MODIFY LIPIDS AND LIPOPROTEINS

It is abundantly evident that many dietary patterns that are based on modifying certain nutrients and specific foods can be implemented to beneficially affect lipids and lipoproteins. The step I and II diets have been considered the "gold standard" dietary approaches for lipid management. A step I diet is defined as: total fat, less than 30% of calories; saturated fat, less than 10% of calories; and dietary cholesterol, less than 300 mg/d. A step II diet is defined as: total fat, less than 30% of calories; saturated fat, less than 7% of calories; and dietary cholesterol, less than 200 mg/d. The TLC diet is a contemporary derivative of a step II diet and provides 25–35% of calories from fat, less than 7% calories from saturated fat, and less than 200 mg/d of cholesterol, and is currently recommended to maximally lower LDL-C. Additional options for LDL-C lowering in the TLC diet include incorporation of 2 g/d of plant stanols/sterols and 10–25 g/d of viscous fiber *(39)*. There are other dietary patterns recommended for the management of lipids and lipoproteins, including vegetarian diets, very low-fat diets, and diets high in soy protein or ALA. Many clinical studies have evaluated the effects of these diets on blood lipids. Typically, these diets lower TC and LDL-C, whereas the effects they have on TG and HDL-C are diet specific. Availability of different dietary patterns for the management of lipids and lipoproteins provides options to target specific CHD risk factors, as well as to achieve maximal adherence.

4.1. National Cholesterol Education Program/AHA Recommendations

4.1.1. STEP I AND STEP II DIETS

Step I and step II diets favorably affect the lipid and lipoprotein profile, thereby reducing CHD risk. In a meta-analysis of 37 dietary intervention studies in free-living subjects conducted by Yu-Poth et al. *(57)*, a step I diet resulted in decreases in TC, LDL-C, and TG levels of 10, 12, and 10%, respectively, whereas a step II diet resulted in decreases of 13, 16, and 8%, respectively, and a 7% decrease in HDL-C (for step II: TC, LDL, TG: $p < 0.01$; for step II HDL-C: $p = 0.05$). In general, the studies summarized in this review reported a modest weight loss *(57)*, which could explain the decrease in TG reported despite a reduced-fat diet. It is important to appreciate that numerous studies have been conducted with step I and step II diets in many populations, including subjects of different ages with normal blood lipids, hypercholesterolemia, CAD, and combined hypercholesterolemia and hypertriglyceridemia. The lipid and lipoprotein responses among different populations to step I and II diets are comparable to the results summarized in the meta-analysis by Yu-Poth et al. with the exception that there is some variation in TG response. This seems to reflect whether subjects maintained or lost weight on a reduced-fat diet. In general, if there is no weight loss on these diets, there is an increase in TG *(58–61)*, whereas if weight loss occurs, there is either no change *(62)* or a decrease in TG *(57)*.

Table 5
Descriptions of Dietary Patterns That Beneficially Affect Blood Lipids

Diet	Featured food components
Step I	Fruits, vegetables, whole grains, low-fat and fat-free dairy, lean meats.
Step II	Fruits, vegetables, whole grains, low-fat and fat-free dairy, lean meats (while being lower in dietary cholesterol and saturated fat than step I).
TLC	Step II with food sources of plant stanol/sterols, such as margarine, orange juice, yogurt, etc., and of viscous fiber, such as fruits, vegetables, whole grains, and legumes.
Portfolio	Vegetarian. Oats, barley, psyllium, soy protein, almonds, eggplant, okra, and sterol-enriched margarine.
Mediterranean	Bread, root vegetables, green vegetables, fish, olive oil, canola oil, mustard oil, and/or soybean oil.
DASH	Fruits, vegetables, whole grains, low-fat dairy.
Lifestyle Heart	Vegetarian. Fruits, vegetables, grains, legumes, soy products.

TLC, Therapeutic Lifestyle Change; DASH, Dietary Approaches to Stop Hypertension.

4.1.2. THERAPEUTIC LIFESTYLE CHANGES

In addition to the inclusion of plant stanols/sterols and viscous fiber into a step II diet for maximal lowering of LDL-C levels, the TLC diet also emphasizes weight loss and physical activity. TLC is expected to decrease LDL-C by approx 20–30% (39). The decrease in LDL-C induced by each of these changes is as follows: approx 8–10% by the reduction in SFA to less than 7% of calories, 3–5% by the reduction in dietary cholesterol to less than 200 mg, up to 5% by the addition of 5–10 g/d of viscous fiber (39), about 5–8% by a weight loss of about 10 lbs, and 6–15% by the inclusion of 2 g/d of plant stanol/sterol esters.

4.2. Portfolio Diet

The Portfolio diet, a vegetarian diet including plant sterols and viscous fibers primarily from oat, barley, and psyllium, in addition to soy protein and almonds, meets the recommendations of the TLC diet (63,64). The goal of the Portfolio diet is to achieve the maximal LDL-C lowering effect possible by diet.

Jenkins et al. (63) investigated this diet in hypercholesterolemic subjects. The diet contained 22.4% of calories as protein (97% of which was vegetable protein), 50.6% CHO, 27.0% fat (4.3% SFA, 11.8% MUFA, and 9.9% PUFA), 10 mg cholesterol/1000 kcal, and 30.7 g fiber/1000 kcal. After 4 wk, there were marked reductions in TC and LDL-C of 22.4% and 29.0%, respectively ($p < 0.001$). HDL-C and TG were unaffected. In a follow-up study by Jenkins et al. (64) subjects consumed either a Portfolio diet (20.0% of calories as protein [99% of which was vegetable protein], 56.6% CHO, 23.2% fat [4.9% SFA, 9.5% MUFA, and 7.9% PUFA], 48 mg cholesterol/1000 kcal, 37.2 g fiber/1000 kcal) or a step II diet (19.6% of calories as protein [30% of which was vegetable protein], 58.8% CHO, 21.6% fat [4.4% SFA, 8.5% MUFA, and 7.5% PUFA], 34 mg cholesterol/1000 kcal, 26.6 g fiber/1000 kcal). After 4 wk, the Portfolio diet resulted in considerably greater cholesterol lowering than the step II diet. TC and LDL-C decreased by 26.6% and 35.0%, respectively, ($p < 0.001$) on the Portfolio diet but by only 9.9% and 12.1%, respectively, ($p < 0.001$) on the step II diet. Moreover, TG levels decreased 6.3% following the Portfolio diet but rose by 4.9% following the step II diet. Nonsignificant reductions in HDL-C occurred on both diets.

4.3. Mediterranean Diet

Given the broad geographical area that comprises the Mediterranean region there is no one common Mediterranean diet. However, there is a dietary pattern that is characteristic of Mediterranean-style diets. This pattern emphasizes a diet that is high in fruits, vegetables, bread, cereals, potatoes, beans, nuts, and seeds. It includes olive oil as an important fat source and also dairy products, fish, and poultry consumed in low to moderate amounts, eggs consumed zero to four times weekly, and little red meat. In addition, wine is consumed in low to moderate amounts. There is long-standing interest in the Mediterranean diet because populations that consume this dietary pattern have low rates of coronary disease. Epidemiological studies and clinical trials have evaluated blood lipids of populations living in this region.

The Seven Countries Study prompted interest in the Mediterranean diet when it reported that the 15-yr mortality rate from CHD in southern Europe was two to three times lower than that in northern Europe or the United States. However, measurements of TC levels for men (mean age 49) living in the Mediterranean region of southern Europe revealed a mean value of 5.19 mmol/L. These values are broadly similar to the levels in regions where CHD rates are high *(65)*. Findings from the Ustica Project and ATTICA Study confirmed that blood lipid levels in the Mediterranean population are not especially low. In the Ustica Project by Barbagallo et al. *(66)* the 576 participants living on the small island in the southern part of the Tyrrhenian sea, more than 18 yr of age, had mean TC and LDL-cholesterol levels of 5.39 and 3.68 mmol/L, respectively. Overall, 22.8% of the Ustica population was hypercholesterolemic and 22.5% had low HDL-C levels (<1.04 mmol/L). In the ATTICA Study, 43% of the 2282 participants more than 14 yr of age living in the Athens area had TC higher than 5.19 mmol/L, whereas 49% had LDL-C levels higher than 3.38 mmol/L. HDL-C levels were lower than 0.91 mmol/L in 14% of the participants *(67)*. These three studies suggest, therefore, that the cardiopro-tective effect of the Mediterranean diet may be mediated, in part, by factors other than lipids/lipoproteins.

One major secondary prevention clinical trial has demonstrated beneficial effects of a Mediterranean-style diet, rich in ALA, on recurrent coronary events *(68)*. In the Lyon Diet Heart Study there were no diet effects on blood lipids and lipoproteins.

The Lyon Diet Heart Study was a randomized, single-blind, secondary prevention trial that tested the effects of a Western diet vs a Mediterranean diet on the reoccurrence of myocardial infarction. Subjects consumed a control diet (32.7% of calories as fat [11.7% SFA, 10.3% 18:1, 5.3% 18:2, 0.27% 18:3], 318 mg/d cholesterol) or an experimental diet rich in ALA (30.5% fat [8.3% SFA, 12.9% 18:1, 3.6% 18:2, 0.81% 18:3], 217 mg/d cholesterol). After 104 wk on the experimental diet, TC, LDL-C, and TG levels were unchanged. Despite a similar coronary risk factor profile (plasma lipids and lipoproteins, blood pressure, and smoking status), subjects following the Mediterranean-style diet had a 50–70% lower risk of recurrent heart disease as measured by three different combinations of outcome measures including: (1) cardiac death and nonfatal heart attacks; (2) the preceding plus other measures (unstable angina, stroke, heart failure, and pulmonary or peripheral embolism); and (3) all of these measures plus events that required hospitalization.

Further studies are needed to identify the underlying mechanisms that account for the favorable effects of a Mediterranean-style diet rich in ALA on CVD risk. Although there is some evidence of a beneficial effect on lipids and lipoproteins, it is clear that other mechanisms also account for the effects observed.

4.4. DASH Diet

The DASH Trial was designed to compare the effects of three dietary patterns on blood pressure. In a secondary analysis, the responsiveness of blood lipids to diet was also assessed. A 3-wk run-in control diet was consumed by the 459 subjects, followed by 8 wk of one of three diets:

1. A control diet high in saturated fat (14% of calories) and low in dietary fiber (10.8 g/d).
2. A diet with increased amounts of fruit and vegetables but with a macronutrient profile similar to the control diet (52% of calories as CHO, 37% fat [13% SFA, 14% MUFA, and 7% PUFA], and 188 mg/d cholesterol) that is high in dietary fiber (29.9 g/d).
3. A DASH diet high in fruits (5.2 servings/d) and vegetables (4.4 servings/d), and low-fat dairy products (2 servings/d, and 0.7 servings/d of high-fat dairy). This diet was lower in fat and low in saturated fats but high in fiber (58% of calories as CHO, 27% fat [7% SFA, 10% MUFA, and 8% PUFA], 141 mg/d cholesterol, 29.7 g/d fiber).

Compared with the control group, TC, LDL-C, and HDL-C decreased by 1.9, 1.5, and 0.4%, respectively, in the fruit and vegetable group (not significant), but decreased significantly by 7.3, 9.0, and 7.5%, respectively, in the DASH group ($p < 0.0001$). Although TG levels decreased 8.4% in the fruit and vegetable group ($p = 0.076$), TG levels were not significantly affected by the DASH diet *(31)*. Thus, a high-fiber diet may prevent an increase in TG levels, which might be expected on a lower-fat diet, and results in a decrease in TG levels when following a moderate-fat diet.

4.5. Lifestyle Heart Program

In the Lifestyle Heart Trial, 48 patients with moderate to severe CHD were randomized to either a usual-care group or an intensive lifestyle change group. The intervention consisted of a very-low-fat vegetarian diet high in complex carbohydrates (15–20% of calories as protein, 70–75% CHO, 10% fat [PUFA:SFA >1], 5 mg/d cholesterol), moderate aerobic exercise, stress management training, smoking cessation, and group psychosocial support. After 1 yr on the program, TC and LDL-C significantly decreased by 27.6 and 39.8%, respectively ($p < 0.005$). Changes in HDL-C (decrease of 9.6%) and TG (increase of 13.4%) were not significant. Hand-in-hand with the change in lipid profile there was evidence of regression of atherosclerosis. After 5 yr the average percent diameter stenosis decreased in the experimental group by 3.1%, whereas in the control group it increased by 11.8% ($p = 0.001$). After 1 yr, the experimental group reported significantly less angina than the control group (91% reduction vs 186% increase; $p < 0.001$) *(69)*.

5. SUMMARY

CHD is the leading cause of death in the United States. Although much progress has been made in reducing CHD, it is apparent that major strategies are needed to prevent and treat coronary disease. As discussed in this chapter, diet plays a key role in modulating lipids and lipoproteins, important risk factors for CHD. Dietary patterns, which reflect a composite of foods, and nutrients consumed, can be modified in countless ways to reduce CHD risk. It is clear that saturated fat, trans fat, and dietary cholesterol increase LDL-C levels, whereas PUFA, viscous fiber, and stanol/sterol esters reduce LDL-C. Because LDL-C is the primary target for CHD intervention efforts, dietary strategies that lower LDL-C can consequently reduce CHD risk. In addition, there are dietary patterns that have major effects on CHD risk with little or no effect on LDL-C. It is evident that contemporary efforts to reduce CHD risk will entail those that target not only LDL-C, as well as other lipid/lipoprotein risk factors, but also will involve the use of dietary patterns that target the wide array of nonlipid/lipoprotein CHD risk factors. Clues from intervention studies have identified foods and dietary patterns that merit making recommendations for implementation in practice to reduce CHD. Cardioprotective foods include fruits and vegetables, whole grains, fish (preferably fatty), vegetable oils, nuts, legumes, spices, lean meats, and low-fat dairy products. The challenge we face, as always, is identifying effective population-based strategies for implementing healthy diets that reduce CHD risk.

REFERENCES

1. Keys A. Coronary heart disease in seven countries. Circulation 1970; 41:I1–211.
2. Posner BM, Cobb JL, Belanger AJ, Cupples LA, D'Agostino RB, Stokes J. Dietary lipid predictors of coronary heart disease in men. The Framingham Study. Arch Intern Med 1991; 151:1181–1187.
3. Hu FB, Stampfer MJ, Manson JE, et al. Dietary fat intake and the risk of coronary heart disease in women. N Engl J Med 1997; 337:1491–1499.
4. Kromhout D, Menotti A, Bloemberg B, et al. Dietary saturated and trans-fatty acids and cholesterol and 25-year mortality from coronary heart disease: The Seven Countries Study. Prev Med 1995; 24: 308–315.
5. Keys A, Anderson JT, Grande F. Serum cholesterol response to changes in the diet. IV. Particular saturated fatty acids in the diet. Metabolism 1965; 14:776–787.
6. Hegsted DM, McGandy RB, Myers ML, Stare EJ. Quantitative effects of dietary fat on serum cholesterol in man. Am J Clin Nutr 1965; 17:281–295.
7. Mensink RP, Katan MB. Effect of dietary fatty acids on serum lipids and lipoproteins. A meta-analysis of 27 trials. Arterioscler Thromb 1992; 12:911–919.
8. Clarke R, Frost C, Collins R, Appleby P, Peto R. Dietary lipids and blood cholesterol: Quantitative meta-analysis of metabolic ward studies. Br Med J 1997; 314:112–117.
9. Hegsted DM, Ausman LM, Johnson JA, Dallal GE. Dietary fat and serum lipids: an evaluation of the experimental data. Am J Clin Nutr 1993; 57:875–883.
10. Muller H, Kirkhus B, Pedersen JI. Serum cholesterol predictive equations with special emphasis on trans and saturated fatty acids. An analysis from designed controlled studies. Lipids 2001;36: 783–791.
11. Yu S, Derr J, Etherton TD, Kris-Etherton PM. Plasma cholesterol-predictive equations demonstrate that stearic acid is neutral and monounsaturated fatty acids are hypocholesterolemic. Am J Clin Nutr 1995; 61:1129–1139.

12. Mensink RP, Zock PL, Kester ADM, Katan MB. Effects of dietary fatty acids and carbohydrates on the ratio of serum total to HDL cholesterol and on serum lipids and apolipoproteins: a meta-analysis of 60 controlled trials. Am J Clin Nutr 2003; 77:1146–1155.

13. Kris-Etherton PM, Yu S. Individual fatty acid effects on plasma lipids and lipoproteins: human studies. Am J Clin Nutr 1997; 65(Suppl):1628–1644S.

14. Judd J, Baer D, Clevidence B, Kris-Etherton P, Muesing R. Dietary *cis* and trans monounsaturated and saturated fatty acids. Lipids 2002; 37:123–131.

15. Mensink RP, Katan MB. Effect of dietary trans fatty acids on high-density and low-density lipoprotein cholesterol levels in healthy subjects. N Engl J Med 1990; 323:439–445.

16. Lichtenstein AH, Ausman LM, Jalbert SM, Schaefer EJ. Effects of different forms of dietary hydrogenated fats on serum lipoprotein cholesterol levels. N Engl J Med 1999; 25:1933–1940.

17. Ascherio A, Willett WC. Health effects of trans-fatty acids. Am J Clin Nutr 1997; 66(Suppl):1006S–1010S.

18. Garg A. High-monounsaturated-fat diets for patients with diabetes mellitus: a meta-analysis. Am J Clin Nutr 1998; 67(Suppl):577S–582S.

19. Dayton S, Pearce ML, Goldman H, et al. Controlled trial of a diet high in unsaturated fat for prevention of atherosclerotic complications. Lancet 1968; 2:1060–1062.

20. Leren P. The Oslo-Diet Heart Study: eleven-year report. Circulation 1970; 42:935–942.

21. Turpeinen O, Karvonen MJ, Pekkarinen M, Miettinen M, Elosuo R, Paavilainen E. Dietary prevention of coronary heart disease: the Finnish Mental Hospital Study. Int J Epidemiol 1979; 8:99–118.

22. Frantz ID Jr, Dawson EA, Ashman PL, et al. Test of effect of lipid lowering by diet on cardiovascular risk: the Minnesota Coronary Survey. Arteriosclerosis 1989; 9:129–135.

23. Mattson FH, Grundy SM. Comparison of effects of dietary saturated, monounsaturated, and polyunsaturated fatty acids on plasma lipids and lipoproteins in man. J Lipid Res 1985; 26:194–202.

24. Gardner CD, Kraemer HC. Monounsaturated versus polyunsaturated dietary fat and serum lipids. A meta-analysis. Arterioscler Thromb Vasc Biol 1995; 15:1917–1927.

25. Harris WS. n-3 Fatty acids and serum lipoproteins: human studies. Am J Clin Nutr 1997; 65:1645S–1654S.

26. Calder PC. n-3 Fatty acids and cardiovascular disease: evidence explained and mechanisms explored. Clin Sci (Lond) 2004; 107:1–11.

27. GISSI-Prevenzione Investigators. Dietary supplementation with n-3 polyunsaturated fatty acids and vitamin E after myocardial infarction: results of the GISSI-Prevenzione Trial. Gruppo Italiano per lo Studio della Sopravvivenza nell'Infarto miocardio. Lancet 1999; 354:447–455.

28. National Academy of Sciences and the Institutes of Medicine. Dietary Reference Intakes: Energy, carbohydrate, fiber, fat, fatty acids, cholesterol, protein, and amino acids. The National Academies Press, Washington, DC, 2002.

29. Ripsin CM, Keenan JM, Jacobs DR, et al. Oat products and lipid lowering. A meta-analysis. J Am Med Assoc 1992; 267:3317–3325.

30. Anderson JW. Dietary fiber prevents carbohydrate-induced hypertriglyceridemia. Curr Atheroscler Rep 2000; 2:536–541.

31. Obarzanek E, Sacks F, Vollmer W, et al. DASH Research Group. Effects on blood lipids of a blood pressure-lowering diet: the Dietary Approaches to Stop Hypertension (DASH) Trial. Am J Clin Nutr 2001; 74:80–89.

32. Chandalia M, Garg A, Lutjohann D, von Bergmann K, Grundy SM, Brinkley J. Beneficial effects of high dietary fiber intake in patients with type 2 diabetes mellitus. N Engl J Med 2000; 342:1392–1398.

33. Krauss RM, Eckel RH, Howard B, et al. AHA Dietary Guidelines: revision 2000: A statement for healthcare professionals from the Nutrition Committee of the American Heart Association. Circulation 2000; 102:2284–2299.

34. Dietary Guidelines Advisory Committee, 2005 Report www.health.gov/dietaryguidelines/dga2005/report/. Accessed on August 5, 2005.

35. Tande DL, Hotchkiss L, Cotugna N. The associations between blood lipids and the Food Guide Pyramid: findings from the Third National Health and Nutrition Examination Survey. Prev Med 2004; 38:452–457.

36. Djousse L, Arnett DK, Coon H, Province MA, Moore LL, Ellison RC. Fruit and vegetable consumption and LDL cholesterol: the National Heart, Lung, and Blood Institute Family Heart Study. Am J Clin Nutr 2004; 79:213–217.

37. Jacobs DR, Gallaher DD. Whole grain intake and cardiovascular aisease: a review. Curr Atheroscl Rep 2004; 6: 415–423.

38. McKeown NM, Meigs JB, Liu S, Wilson PW, Jacques PF. Whole-grain intake is favorably associated with metabolic risk factors for type 2 diabetes and cardiovascular disease in the Framingham Offspring Study. Am J Clin Nutr 2002; 76:390–398.

39. Executive Summary of the Third Report of The National Cholesterol Education Program (NCEP) Expert Panel on Detection, Evaluation, and Treatment of High Blood Cholesterol in Adults (Adult Treatment Panel III). JAMA 2001; 285:2486–2497.

40. Brown L, Rosner B, Willett WW, Sacks FM. Cholesterol-lowering effects of dietary fiber: a meta-analysis. Am J Clin Nutr 1999; 69:30–42.

41. Vartiainen E, Jousilahti P, Alfthan G, Sundvall J, Pietinen P, Puska P. Cardiovascular risk factor changes in Finland, 1972-1997. Int J Epidemiol 2000; 29:49–56.

42. Pekka P, Pirjo P, Ulla U. Influencing public nutrition for non-communicable disease prevention: from community intervention to national programme—experiences from Finland. Public Health Nutr 2002; 5:245–251.

43. Davidson MH, Hunninghake D, Maki KC, Kwiterovich PO Jr, Kafonek S. Comparison of the effects of lean red meat vs lean white meat on serum lipid levels among free-living persons with hypercholesterolemia: a long-term, randomized clinical trial. Arch Intern Med 1999; 159:1331–1338.

44. Scott LW, Dunn JK, Pownall HJ, et al. Effects of beef and chicken consumption on plasma lipid levels in hypercholesterolemic men. Arch Intern Med 1994; 154:1261–1267.

45. Beauchesne-Rondeau E, Gascon A, Bergeron J, Jacques H. Plasma lipids and lipoproteins in hypercholesterolemic men fed a lipid-lowering diet containing lean beef, lean fish, or poultry. Am J Clin Nutr 2003; 77:587–593.

46. USDA Nutrient Data Lab, 2004 http://www.nal.usda.gov/fnic/foodcomp/search/. Accessed on August 15, 2005.

47. Dolecek TA. Epidemiological evidence of relationships between dietary polyunsaturated fatty acids and mortality in the Multiple Risk Factor Intervention Trial. Proc Soc Exp Biol Med 1992; 200:177–182.

48. Siscovick DS, Lemaitre RN, Mozaffarian D. The fish story: a diet-heart hypothesis with clinical implications: n-3 polyunsaturated fatty acids, myocardial vulnerability, and sudden death. Circulation 2003; 107:2632–2634.

49. Hu FB, Bronner L, Willett WC, et al. Fish and omega-3 fatty acid intake and risk of coronary heart disease in women. JAMA 2002; 287:1815–1821.

50. Mozaffarian D, Lemaitre RN, Kuller LH, Burke GL, Tracy RP, Siscovick DS. Cardiovascular Health Study. Cardiac benefits of fish consumption may depend on the type of fish meal consumed: the Cardiovascular Health Study. Circulation 2003; 107:1372–1377.

51. He K, Song Y, Daviglus ML, et al. Accumulated evidence on fish consumption and coronary heart disease mortality: a meta-analysis of cohort studies. Circulation 2004;109: 2705–2711.

52. Wang C, Chung M, Balk E, et al. Effects of omega-3 fatty acids on cardiovascular disease. In: Evidence Report/Technology Assessment No. 04-E009-2. (Prepared by Tufts-New England Medical Center Evidence-based Practice Center.) Agency for Healthcare Research and Quality, Rockville, MD, 2004.

53. Burr ML, Fehily AM, Gilbert JF, et al. Effects of changes in fat, fish, and fibre intakes on death and myocardial reinfarction: diet and reinfarction trial (DART). Lancet 1989; 30:757–761.

54. Fraser GE. Nut consumption, lipids, and risk of a coronary event. Clin Cardiol 1999;22(7 Suppl): 11–15.

55. Hu FB, Stampfer MJ, Manson JE, et al. Frequent nut consumption and risk of coronary heart disease in women: prospective cohort study. BMJ 1998; 317:1341–1345.

56. Kris-Etherton PM, Zhao G, Binkoski AE, Coval SM, Etherton TD. The effects of nuts on coronary heart disease risk. Nutr Rev 2001; 59:103–111.

57. Yu-Poth S, Zhao G, Etherton T, Naglak M, Jonnalagadda S, Kris-Etherton PM. Effects of the National Cholesterol Education Program's Step I and Step II dietary intervention programs on cardiovascular disease risk factors: a meta-analysis. Am J Clin Nutr 1999; 69:632–646.

58. Koh KK, Ahn JY, Choi YM, et al. Vascular effects of step I diet in hypercholesterolemic patients with coronary artery disease. Am J Cardiol 2003; 92:708–710.

59. Ginsberg HN, Karmally W, Barr SL, Johnson C, Holleran S, Ramakrishnan R. Effects of increasing dietary polyunsaturated fatty acids within the guidelines of the AHA step 1 diet on plasma lipid and lipoprotein levels in normal males. Arterioscler Thromb 1994; 14:892–901.

60. Lichtenstein AH, Ausman LM, Jalbert SM, et al. Efficacy of a therapeutic lifestyle change/Step 2 diet in moderately hypercholesterolemic middle-aged and elderly female and male subjects. J Lipid Res 2002; 43:264–273.

61. Ginsberg HN, Kris-Etherton P, Dennis B, et al. Effects of reducing dietary saturated fatty acids on plasma lipids and lipoproteins in healthy subjects: the DELTA Study, protocol 1. Arterioscler Thromb Vasc Biol 1998; 18:441–449.

62. Walden CE, Retzlaff BM, Buck BL, McCann BS, Knopp RH. Lipoprotein lipid response to the National Cholesterol Education Program step II diet by hypercholesterolemic and combined hyperlipidemic women and men. Arterioscler Thromb Vasc Biol 1997; 17:375–382.

63. Jenkins DJ, Kendall CW, Faulkner D, et al. A dietary portfolio approach to cholesterol reduction: combined effects of plant sterols, vegetable proteins, and viscous fibers in hypercholesterolemia. Metabolism 2002; 51:1596–1604.

64. Jenkins DJ, Kendall CW, Marchie A, et al. The effect of combining plant sterols, soy protein, viscous fibers, and almonds in treating hypercholesterolemia. Metabolism 2003; 52:1478–1483.

65. Keys A, Menotti A, Karvonen MJ, et al. The diet and 15-year death rate in the seven countries study. Am J Epidemiol 1986; 124:903–915.

66. Barbagallo CM, Polizzi F, Severino M, et al. Distribution of risk factors, plasma lipids, lipoproteins and dyslipidemias in a small Mediterranean island: the Ustica Project. Nutr Metab Cardiovasc Dis 2002; 12:267–274.

67. Panagiotakos DB, Pitsavos C, Chrysohoou C, Skoumas J, Stefanadis C. Status and management of blood lipids in Greek adults and their relation to socio-demographic, lifestyle and dietary factors: the ATTICA Study; blood lipids distribution in Greece. Atherosclerosis 2004; 173:351–359.

68. de Lorgeril M, Renaud S, Mamelle N, et al. Mediterranean alpha-linolenic acid-rich diet in secondary prevention of coronary heart disease. Lancet 1994; 343:1454–1459.

69. Ornish D, Scherwitz LW, Billings JH, et al. Intensive lifestyle changes for reversal of coronary heart disease. JAMA 1998; 280:2001–2007.

7

Diet and Blood Pressure

Moving Beyond Preoccupation With Salt to Composite Dietary Patterns

Karen E. Charlton

KEY POINTS

- Much evidence from epidemiological and intervention studies indicates that sodium (salt) is related to elevated blood pressure and that a reduced intake of sodium helps lower the blood pressure. However, there is uncertainty regarding the degree of compliance and effectiveness of low-sodium diets for long-term use.
- The average intake of sodium in the United States is around 3310 mg/d (8.3 g/d salt). This should be reduced to about 1600–2000 mg/d (4–5 g/d salt). This requires avoiding adding salt to food, avoiding eating salt-rich processed foods, and also a reduction in the salt content of processed foods, such as bread.
- Other minerals are also involved in hypertension. There is strong evidence that potassium is effective in treating hypertension and apparently counters the effects of a high intake of sodium, especially in black people. Calcium may also help lower blood pressure although the effect is quite small. This might also be true for magnesium but the evidence is not clear.
- A combination of nonpharmacological methods can reduce blood pressure as much as some antihypertensive drugs. The Dietary Approaches to Stop Hypertension diet (which is rich in fruit, vegetables, and low-fat dairy products, with a reduced saturated and total fat intake) combined with a low-sodium intake and weight loss can decrease blood pressure by about 9/4.5 mmHg.
- Other factors linked to hypertension are alcohol consumption beyond moderation, being overweight, and lack of exercise.

1. INTRODUCTION

Salt restriction as a form of treatment for hypertension was introduced at the beginning of the last century when chloride could first be measured. Interestingly, more than 100 yr later, the merits of the salt hypothesis and the utility of its application are still being debated. The medical community is seldom as bewildered and polarized about a public

From: *Nutritional Health: Strategies for Disease Prevention, Second Edition*
Edited by: N. J. Temple, T. Wilson, and D. R. Jacobs © Humana Press Inc., Totowa, NJ

health policy issue as it is regarding the role of salt in health and disease. In 2000, two opposing arguments—for *(1)* and against *(2)*— regarding the appropriateness of the current US dietary guideline for sodium which recommends less than 6 g sodium chloride (or <2.4 g sodium [Na]) per day, were published back-to-back in the *American Journal of Clinical Nutrition*. The salt–blood pressure (BP) hypothesis states that excessive salt intake (in physiological terms) leads to an increase in BP in genetically susceptible persons and, if the high intake is maintained over the long term, will ultimately lead to sustained hypertension. The hypothesis regards salt as the essential pathogenic factor; however, an excessive salt intake interacts with both genetic predisposition, as well as other environmental factors.

BP is a function of flow and resistance. The kidneys, which excrete almost all ingested electrolytes and much of the water consumed daily, are responsible for managing the electrolyte and water content in the body. Volume content is tightly controlled by the regulation of sodium (and thereby chloride) excretion. Almost all people living in westernized societies ingest a high-sodium diet, however not all individuals respond similarly to a high-salt intake. A relationship between renal salt and water excretion and blood pressure can be created for any level of BP and is termed the renal pressure–natriuresis or diuresis relationship. All forms of hypertension in animal models tested to date feature a shift in the pressure–natriuresis relationship to the right, so that a higher level of pressure is required to excrete any given amount of salt and water. In normotensive individuals the relationship between salt and water intake (and excretion) is very steep, so that little change in BP occurs when salt and water intake (and excretion) are modified over a large range. Conversely, a fairly flat pressure–natriuresis curve indicates a sensitivity to salt.

Because there is no quick and easy way to predict whether an individual is salt sensitive, the classification has remained in the research domain rather than being of practical or clinical importance. Even in the research arena, no standardized methodology for the determination of salt sensitivity exists. Discrepancies among investigators include the route of sodium administration (intravenous saline or oral dietary salt), the level of salt restriction and/or salt loading required to elicit a response, as well as the number of days on which subjects should be salt-loaded or -depleted.

The publication of the findings of the landmark Dietary Attempts to Stop Hypertension (DASH) clinical trial, which is discussed under Heading 6, signalled a move by health professionals away from a preoccupation with salt to the role of a holistic, composite diet in the prevention and management of hypertension. This chapter will first consider the influence of individual nutrients on BP, and then review the role of various dietary patterns, as well as other behavioral factors.

2. SODIUM

The INTERSALT ecological study *(3)*, which was conducted with more than 10,000 participants from 52 centers around the world, demonstrated that, across populations, level of BP, increment in BP with age, and the prevalence of hypertension are related to salt intake, measured using 24-h urinary sodium excretion. However, the within-population analyses indicated that wide variation in the BP–salt relationship occurs throughout a population. The main observations in the INTERSALT study are that: for individuals, a difference of 100 mmol/d of sodium (6 g NaCl) intake is associated with an average difference of between 3 and 6 mmHg in systolic BP, and for populations, a 100 mmol/d lower sodium intake is associated with attenuation of the age-associated rise in systolic BP by 10 mmHg in persons aged 25–55 yr. It is noteworthy that in four remote INTERSALT study sites, both sodium excretion and BP were low, there was little or no upward slope of BP with age, and little or no hypertension.

Several systematic reviews have reported that restricting sodium intake in people with hypertension reduces their BP *(4–8)*. Generally, in hypertensive subjects, a 100 mmol/d reduction in sodium intake is associated with an average reduction in systolic BP of between 2 and 5 mmHg, and a reduction in diastolic BP of about 1 mmHg. It has been argued that on a population level, this level of sodium restriction would lower diastolic BP by 1.4–2.5 mmHg, resulting in a 15% reduction in stroke risk *(9)*. However, most of the studies included in these reviews have been short in duration and have not followed subjects up over the long term to assess whether dietary changes are sustainable. A systematic review of the long-term effects of advice to restrict dietary sodium in adults, with and without hypertension, reported only small reductions in BP (average of 1.1/0.6 mmHg) at 13–60 mo of follow-up *(10)*.

The disappointing long-term results are undoubtedly owing to subjects' inability to comply with dietary advice to reduce salt intake. As follow-up in trials became longer, the difference in 24-h urinary sodium excretion among intervention and control subjects became progressively smaller (reduction of 49 mmol/d at 6–12 mo of follow-up, compared with 35 mmol/d at 13–60 mo, and 10 mmol/d in trials that reported follow-up of more than 60 mo). The results of the review reflect the best-case scenario because the cited trials all used intensive interventions, which are probably unsuited to primary care or population prevention programs. However, it was concluded that advice to reduce sodium intake may help people on antihypertensive medication to stop taking their drugs while maintaining good BP control. In this regard, moderate dietary sodium restriction (from 206 to 109 mmol urinary Na/24 h) has been shown to be as effective as the addition of a thiazide diuretic agent, as combination therapy, to the prescription of an angiotensin-converting enzyme (ACE) inhibitor *(11)*. The particular advantage of sodium restriction over diuretic therapy is that urinary potassium excretion is not increased in the former.

2.1. Dietary Sodium and End-Organ Damage

In addition to its influence on arterial pressure, there is some evidence that dietary sodium may exert some nonpressure-related effects on left ventricular mass in experimental models of hypertension *(12)*, as well as in human essential hypertension *(13–15)*. As long ago as 1972 it was observed that the addition of salt to food before tasting was associated with an increase in the prevalence of electrocardiographic evidence of left ventricular hypertrophy in hypertensive men *(16)*. Recently, it has been demonstrated that dietary sodium amplifies the effect of arterial pressure on target organ damage (microalbuminuria and left ventricular mass), even in normotensive humans; thus, an excessive sodium intake can be considered to be an independent risk factor for cardiovascular risk *(17)*. Further, moderate sodium restriction in patients with mild-to-moderate essential hypertension has been shown to decrease left ventricular hypertrophy *(18)*.

2.2. Dietary Sodium, Cardiovascular Disease Risk, and All-Cause Mortality

It has been argued for decades that a high-salt intake may not be detrimental in subjects who are not sensitive to the BP elevating effects of sodium. However, a prospective study of 1173 men and 1263 women in Finland found that coronary heart disease (CHD), cardiovascular disease (CVD), and all-cause mortality all rose significantly with increasing 24-h urinary sodium excretion, independently of other cardiovascular risk factors, including BP *(19)*. In another 19-yr cohort study, high reported dietary sodium intake at baseline was strongly and independently associated with an increased risk of cardiovascular disease and all-cause mortality in overweight persons *(20)*.

2.3. Dietary Sources of Salt and Recommended Levels of Salt Restriction

Sodium chloride is approx 40% sodium and 60% chloride. The mean daily sodium intake of Americans adults is 3290 mg (equivalent to a salt intake of a little more than 8 g) *(21)*, which greatly exceeds the estimated minimum requirements of healthy nonpregnant, nonlactating adults of about 500 mg *(22)*. It is estimated that about three-quarters of sodium intake comes from food processing, about 15% is discretionary (half of which is contributed by table salt and half by added salt in cooking), 10–11% is naturally occurring (inherent) in foods, whereas less than 1% is provided by water *(23–25)*. The largest single source of sodium in the American diet comes from grain products, including bread, which contributes about one-quarter of total intake *(26)*. In contrast, in South Africa, between one-third and one-half of total sodium intake is provided from discretionary sources, whereas the large amount of salt added by bakers to bread and the high reliance on a few staple foods, results in this food item alone providing 40% of total nondiscretionary sodium intake in the black population *(27)*. In both black and white South Africans, bread and cereal is the food group that contributes half of total nondiscretionary sodium intake. Population-specific dietary information, such as this, allows commonly consumed food items to be targeted for intervention purposes.

The Joint National Committee (JNC) VII guidelines of the US National Heart Lung and Blood Institute *(28)* recommends a maximum sodium intake of 100 mmol (2400 mg) per day, which equates to about 6 g salt (Table 3). If an individual is prepared to give up salt added to food and to avoid eating salt-rich processed foods, salt intake can be reduced from the average intake of around 8.3 g (approx 140 mmol or 3320 mg Na) to about 6 g/d. This is the level of sodium restriction that is usually referred to as "No added salt" regimen (i.e., 80–100 mmol/d). To reduce sodium intake further requires bread intake to be limited, as well as the moderation of portion sizes of foods with relatively high natural sodium, such as meat, milk, and eggs. This type of restriction generally results in poor compliance. The most recent dietary guidelines of the World Health Organization recommend more stringent restrictions of sodium for the prevention of CVD (CHD, hypertension, and stroke), namely 70 mmol/d (4 g/d sodium chloride) (*see* Table 2) *(29)*. In patients with hypertension, consideration of the degree or stage of the condition is required, together with an assessment of the presence of major risk factors, target organ damage, or clinical CVD, to decide on a first line of management (*see* Tables 3 and 4). Lifestyle modification (*see* Table 3) is recommended for all patients with hypertension, regardless of whether or not drug therapy is initiated. A new classification, "pre-hypertension" (120–139/80–89 mmHg), has been included in the most recent version of the

Table 1
Lifestyle Modifications for Hypertension Prevention and Management

Modification	Recommendation	Average systolic BP reduction range (mmHg)[a]
Weight reduction	Maintain normal body weight (BMI = 18.5–24.9 kg/m²)	5–20 per 10 kg
DASH eating plan	Adopt a diet rich in fruits, vegetables, and low-fat dairy products with reduced content of saturated and total fat.	8-14
Dietary sodium restriction	Reduce dietary sodium intake to ≤100 mmol/d (2.4 g sodium or 6 g NaCl).	2–8
Aerobic physical activity	Regular aerobic physical activity (e.g., brisk walking) at least 30 min/d most days of the week.	4–9
Moderation of alcohol consumption	Men: limit to ≤2 drinks/d Women and lighter weight persons: limit to ≤1 drink/d.	2–4

[a]Effects are dose and time-dependent.
[b]1 drink = 1/2 oz or 15 mL ethanol (e.g., 12 oz beer, 5 oz wine, or 1.5 oz 80-proof whiskey).
DASH, Dietary Approaches to Stop Hypertension; BMI, body mass index.
(Adapted from ref. 28.)

JNC VII guidelines, for which lifestyle modification is also recommended. This recognizes the need for increased education of health care professionals and the public to reduce blood pressure levels and thus prevent the development of hypertension in the general population.

A randomized, controlled trial in elderly British people aged 60–78 yr who were not receiving antihypertensive medication found that a modest salt restriction from 10 to 5 g/d resulted in a reduction of blood pressure of 7.2/3.2 mmHg over a 4-wk period (30). Importantly, unlike studies in younger subjects, similar drops in blood pressure were seen for both normotensive and hypertensive subjects. Low-salt bread was provided to subjects, which greatly improved compliance with the reduced sodium regimen. The findings are consistent with predictions that a reduction in sodium intake of 50 mmol/d (about 3 g salt) in older people would lower the population's systolic BP by an average of 5 mmHg (4). This magnitude of BP reduction is similar to trials of drug therapy with thiazide diuretics in this age group, in which a 36% reduction in the 5-yr incidence of stroke has been estimated (31). To prevent one vascular event (particularly stroke) over a given period of time, four times as many younger people need to be treated than those past the age of 60 yr. These studies provide convincing motivation for universal sodium restriction in all elderly people.

Table 2
Dietary Goals for the Prevention of Cardiovascular Disease,
Including the Prevention of Hypertension

- A reduction of total sodium intake to an optimal 70 mmol/d (1.7 g sodium or 4.2 g NaCl). A more realistic population goal of 5 g/d NaCl is advised. Minimal consumption of other forms of Na consumption, such as food additives and preservatives (e.g., monosodium glutamate).
- Maintain potassium intake at a level which will keep the Na:K ratio close to 1 (i.e., daily K intake of 70–80 mmol/d). Achieved through the adequate daily consumption (400–500 g/d) of fruit and vegetables (including berries, green leafy and cruciferous vegetables, and legumes), as well as the use of K-enriched, low-sodium salt substitutes.
- To prevent excess energy consumption and weight gain, total daily fat intake should range from 15% to a maximum of 30% energy, except in very active groups with stable healthy weight (up to 35% total energy).
- Low intake of saturated fatty acids (<7% total energy intake); foods rich in myristic and palmitic acids should be especially reduced.
- Very low intake of trans-fatty acids (<1% total energy intake).
- Adequate intake of polyunsaturated fatty acids (6–10% total energy intake).
- Monounsaturated fatty acids to make up the rest of daily energy intake from fats.
- Dietary cholesterol restricted to less than 300 mg/d, mainly through restriction of dairy fats.
- Dietary goals related to fat quantity and quality can be met by: limiting intake of fat from dairy and meat sources; avoiding the use of hydrogenated fats and oils in cooking and in processed foods; using appropriate edible vegetable oils in moderation; having a regular intake of fish (1–2 times/wk, providing >200 mg DHA and EPA) and/or plant sources of α-linolenic acid; and preferentially employing nonfrying methods of cooking.
- Fiber is protective against CHD and has also been used in blood pressure-lowering trials. Adequate intake may be achieved through intake of fruits, vegetables, and whole grain cereals.
- Although regular low-to-moderate alcohol consumption is protective against CHD, concerns about other cardiovascular and health risks (including stroke, hypertension, and some cancers) do not favor a general recommendation for its use.

DHA, docosahexanoic acid; EPA, eicosapentaenoic acid; CHD, coronary heart disease. (Adapted from ref. *29*.)

As long ago as 1984, it was suggested that a relatively easy way to lower habitual sodium intakes in Australians would be to encourage the food industry to use less sodium in bread *(32)*. A successful partnership in Australia between the food industry and professional bodies in lowering sodium content of foods has been reported *(33)*. In response to a 1982 government report in Australia, in which lower levels of sodium intake were recommended for the general population, together with national dietary guidelines in the country and the accreditation criterion of the National Heart Foundation's "Pick the Tick" program (i.e., <400 mg Na per 100 g food), Kellogg's reformulated 12 of their breakfast cereal products to comprise, on average, 40% less sodium. As a result, 235 tons of salt were removed annually from the Australian food supply. Regular consumers

Table 3
Classification and Management of Blood Pressure for Adults[a]

BP classification	Systolic BP[a] (mmHg)	Diastolic BP[b] (mmHg)	Lifestyle modification	Initial drug therapy	
				Without compelling indication	With compelling indications[b]
Normal	<120	<80	Encourage	No antihypertensive drug indicated.	Drug(s) for compelling indications
Prehypertension	120–139	Or 80–89	Yes		
Stage 1 hypertension	140–159	Or 90–99	Yes	Thiazide-type diuretics for most. May consider ACEI, ARB, BB, CCB or combination	Drug(s) for compelling indications. Other antihypertensive drugs (diuretics, ACEI, ARB, CCB) as needed.
Stage 2 hypertension	≥160	Or ≥100	Yes	Two-drug combination for most (usually thiazide-type diuretic and ACEI or ARB or BB or CCB.	

ACEI, angiotensin converting enzyme inhibitor; ARB, angiotensin receptor blocker; BB, beta-blocker; CCB, calcium channel blocker.
[a]Treatment determined by highest blood pressure (BP) category.
[b]Compelling indications include heart failure, postmyocardial infarction, high coronary heart disease risk, diabetes, chronic kidney disease, or recurrent stroke prevention.
[c]Initial combined therapy should be used cautiously in those at risk for orthostatic hypotension.
[d]Treat patients with chronic kidney disease or diabetes to BP goal of less than 130/80 mmHg.
(Adapted from ref. 28.)

Table 4
Cardiovascular Risk Factors

Major risk factors	Target organ damage
• Hypertension[a]	• Heart disease
• Cigarette smoking	- Left ventricular hypertrophy
• Obesity[a] (BMI ≥30 kg/m^2)	- Angina or prior myocardial infarction
• Physical inactivity	- Prior coronary revascularization
• Dyslipidemia[a]	- Heart failure
• Diabetes mellitus[a]	• Brain
• Microalbuminuria or estimated GFR <60 mL/min	- Stroke or transient ischemic attack
• Age (>55 for men, >65 for women)	• Chronic kidney disease
• Family history of premature cardiovascular disease:	• Peripheral arterial disease
- Women <65 yr	• Retinopathy
- Men <55 yr	

[a]Components of the metabolic syndrome. GFR, Glomerular filtration rate; BMI, body mass index. (Adapted from ref. 28.).

of breakfast cereals (40% of the population or 7.1 million people) would have a reduction in salt intake of 90 mg/d, based on this simple change in product formulation. Importantly, consumer food appeal was not affected.

2.4. Salt Intake Patterns: Does "Salt Appetite" Exist?

The following questions arise: Why do humans consume sodium in quantities that far exceed physiological requirements? And is there a "salt appetite" that manifests in certain individuals as a result of either genetic programming or learned taste through exposure to high-salt intakes? Cultural practices may contribute to salt intake patterns as the following example illustrates. A 10-fold difference in sodium intake has been reported between two populations of the Solomon Islands, which has been attributed to the practice by one group's of steaming foods with fresh water, whereas the other group cooks with sea water (34).

The transduction of the salty taste involves passage of sodium through a specific ion channel in the apical membrane of receptor cells. The channel can be blocked with the drug amiloride, a potassium-sparing diuretic, and is specific; lithium, which can pass through readily, tastes salty, whereas other cations, such as potassium, which do not fit, do not taste salty. This specificity explains the difficulty in finding an acceptable salt substitute. There is some evidence that long-term adherence to a diet low in sodium can lead to a hedonic shift whereby both normotensive (35) and hypertensive (36) persons develop an increased acceptance of foods with a reduced sodium content, presumably because the salt taste receptors become more sensitive, and a lower sodium concentration provides the same salty taste as previously.

3. POTASSIUM

Mechanisms of the BP-lowering effect of potassium include its vasodilator activity, an increased loss of water and sodium, suppression of secretion of renin and angiotensin, stimulation of the sodium–potassium pump, and reduction in adrenergic tone. Data from more than 60 reports of the BP-lowering effects of potassium supplementation, and from a meta-analysis of randomized clinical trials (37), suggest that potassium supplementation should be considered more widely in therapeutic and preventive strategies for hypertension, particularly in certain subgroups. A mean increase in urinary potassium excretion of 53 mmol/d resulted in a decrease in systolic and diastolic BP of 3.1 and 2.0 mmHg, respectively. In almost all the trials, potassium was given as a chloride salt supplement, but both the JNC VII and the World Health Organization dietary guidelines recommend an increased intake of *foods* rich in potassium.

Experimental studies have shown that in most normotensive black men, but not white men, sensitivity to sodium occurs when dietary potassium is even marginally deficient, and is dose-dependently suppressed when dietary potassium is increased within the normal range, to 70 mmol/d (38). Such suppression of salt sensitivity may prevent or delay the occurrence of hypertension in many black people, in whom dietary potassium intake is often deficient. In studies in which dietary potassium was controlled at normal intakes ranging from 60 to 100 mmol/d throughout a dietary salt loading period, salt intakes as high as 400–600 mmol/d failed to induce a mean pressor effect in groups of either black or white normotensive men (39–42). Presumably, the potassium intake was sufficient to block the pressor effect of the high salt intake. Similarly, a marginally deficient potassium intake has been shown to result in an enhanced vasopressor responsiveness to sympathetic stress, induced either by experimental cold or mental stress *(43)*.

The earlier (1997) version of the JNC guidelines (VI) recommends an intake of 90 mmol of potassium per day (*see* Table 1), although the 2003 World Health Organization report recommends a potassium intake that will keep the sodium:potassium ratio close to one (i.e., a potassium intake of 70–80 mmol/d, if their guidelines on sodium restriction are achieved; Table 2).

4. CALCIUM

An inverse association between dietary calcium and BP has been shown in many observational epidemiological studies. However, this relationship is more convincing at low levels of calcium consumption (i.e., in groups that habitually consume calcium intakes of 300–600 mg/d). It has been suggested that there may be a threshold of dietary calcium intake (700–800 mg/d) above which any further potential BP-lowering effect of calcium may not be seen. In at least three animal models of hypertension, calcium supplementation has produced a significant decrease in BP, although in human studies the most consistent pressure-lowering effect of calcium has been seen in subjects during a high-sodium intake *(44–46)*. Studies performed in normotensive offspring of hypertensive subjects demonstrated altered calcium metabolism when they were given a high-salt diet *(47)*.

Two meta-analyses of controlled trials have shown that calcium supplementation (mostly with 1 or 1.5 g/d calcium) results in small reductions in systolic BP (0.9–1.7 mmHg) *(48,49)*. These reductions are not considered to be relevant at a public health level. Among hypertensives, calcium supplementation is more likely to reduce BP in older or black subjects *(50–54)*. Another subgroup of individuals for whom an increased calcium intake may be beneficial includes those with moderate-to-high chronic alcohol consumption *(55)*. Hypertensives have been shown to have an increase in urinary calcium excretion despite a lower calcium intake *(56)*, which has been referred to as a renal calcium "leak." A high intake of dietary salt, as well as of protein and caffeine, further aggravates obligatory urinary calcium loss. It has been estimated that one teaspoon of salt per day (100 mmol Na) raises urinary calcium by 40 mg/d.

5. MAGNESIUM

There is evidence, albeit indirect, from both experimental and metabolic studies, to suggest that an increased level of magnesium may be beneficial in lowering BP in otherwise healthy free-living individuals. In vitro studies have shown that magnesium influences cell membrane sodium pump activity, which in turn affects sodium–potassium transport across cell membranes, and subsequently vascular tone and reactivity *(57)*. Clinical studies have demonstrated significant BP reductions with parenteral high-dose magnesium in patients with eclampsia and glomerulonephritis *(58,59)*.

In addition, observational epidemiological studies have reported an inverse association between dietary magnesium intake and BP *(60)*. However, the imprecision of dietary intake reporting, together with the colinearity of magnesium intake with other dietary components that affect BP, limit the interpretation of epidemiological data. Since 1983, many magnesium supplementation trials have been conducted in humans but the results have been inconsistent, owing in part to small sample sizes or other design limitations.

A meta-analysis of 20 randomized clinical trials was performed to determine whether magnesium supplementation reduces BP, to identify the dose–response relationship, and to determine trial characteristics associated with the greatest reduction in BP *(61)*. The pooled estimate of the effect of magnesium supplementation was a small reduction of 0.6 mmHg in systolic BP and 0.8 mmHg for diastolic BP, but neither change was significant. A dose-dependent effect of magnesium was found, with reductions of 4.3/2.3 mmHg for each 10 mmol/d increase in magnesium dose. However, few of the studies included the higher dose range of magnesium (20–40 mmol/d) and the authors of the meta-analysis recommended that properly designed and adequately powered trials at higher dose ranges be performed to confirm the dose–response relationship. The median amount of magnesium administered in the trials included in the meta-analysis was 15 mmol/d (range: 10–40 mmol/d), which results in about a doubling of usual magnesium intake, at least in the American public. This dosage may not, however, be sufficiently large to produce a clinically significant effect.

A South African study published in 1987 reported on the relationship between serum and erythrocyte electrolytes, specifically magnesium and calcium, and BP in 296 urbanized black male laborers in Johannesburg *(62)*. A significant, inverse association was found between both serum and erythrocyte magnesium and BP, as well as between both serum calcium and potassium and BP. Of all the electrolytes assessed, magnesium (either serum or erythrocyte) correlated most strongly with BP. The authors concluded that body magnesium status, and its interactions with calcium, sodium, and potassium, may play an important role in the development and maintenance of elevated BP in the South African black population. As with calcium, further work on the association between magnesium and BP control in populations who habitually consume very low intakes of magnesium appears warranted.

6. COMPOSITE DIETARY INTERVENTIONS TO PREVENT AND MANAGE HYPERTENSION

The DASH randomized, controlled trial provided unequivocal evidence that nonpharmacological methods can reduce BP as much as some antihypertensive drugs *(63)*. Subjects fed a diet rich in fruit and vegetables for 8 wk achieved a significantly reduced systolic and diastolic BP of 2.8 and 1.1 mmHg, respectively, as compared with control subjects on a typical American diet. Subjects randomized to the DASH diet, rich in fruit, vegetables, and low-fat dairy products, and with a reduced saturated and total fat intake (*see* Table 5), had an even greater reduction in BP (5.5/3.0 mmHg). It was estimated that a population-wide reduction in BP of the magnitude observed with the DASH diet would reduce incident CHD by approx 15% and stroke by about 27%. It is noteworthy that the effects of the 8-wk DASH diet were greatest in hypertensive African Americans, in which a BP reduction of 13.2/6.1 mmHg was recorded *(64)*. Increased efficacy of the DASH diet among African Americans supports other data suggesting ethnic differences in BP response to diet. For example, African Americans tend to consume less potassium than their white counterparts, and this may explain some of the increased efficacy in this segment of the population.

Table 5
The Dietary Attempts to Stop Hypertension Diet

Food group	Daily servings	Serving sizes	Examples and notes	Significance to the DASH diet pattern
Grains and grain products	7–8	1 slice bread 1/2 cup dry cereal 1/2 cup cooked rice, pasta, or cereal	Whole wheat bread, muffin, pita bread, bagel, cereals, oatmeal	Major sources of energy and fiber
Vegetables	4–5	1 cup raw, leafy vegetables 1/2 cup cooked vegetables, 200 mL vegetable juice	Tomatoes, potatoes, carrots, peas, squash, broccoli, turnip greens, kale, spinach, artichokes, green beans, sweet potatoes	Rich sources of potassium, magnesium, and fiber
Fruits	4–5	1 medium fruit, 1/4 cup dried fruit, 200 mL fruit juice, 1/2 cup fresh, frozen, or canned fruit	Apricots, bananas, dates, oranges, orange juice, grapefruit, grapefruit juice, mangoes, melons, peaches, pineapples, prunes, raisins strawberries, tangerines	Important sources of potassium, magnesium, and fiber
Low-fat or nonfat diary foods	2–3	8 oz mL milk, 1 cup yogurt, 1.5 oz cheese	Skim or low-fat (2%) milk or buttermilk; nonfat or low-fat yogurt cheese	Major sources of calcium and protein
Meats, poultry, and fish	≤2	3 oz cooked meats, poultry, or fish	Select only lean meats; trim away visible fats; broil, roast, or boil, instead of frying; remove skin from poultry	Rich sources of protein and magnesium
Nuts, seeds and legumes	4–5/wk	1.5 oz or 1/3 cup nuts, 1/2 oz or 2 tbsp seeds, 1/2 cup cooked legumes	Almonds, mixed nuts, peanuts, walnuts, sunflower seeds, kidney beans, lentils, split peas	Rich sources of energy, magnesium, potassium, protein, and fiber

The Dietary Attempts to Stop Hypertension (DASH) eating plan shown above is based on 2000 kcal/d (8400 kJ/d). Depending on energy needs, the number of daily servings in a food group may vary from those listed. (Adapted from ref. 28.).

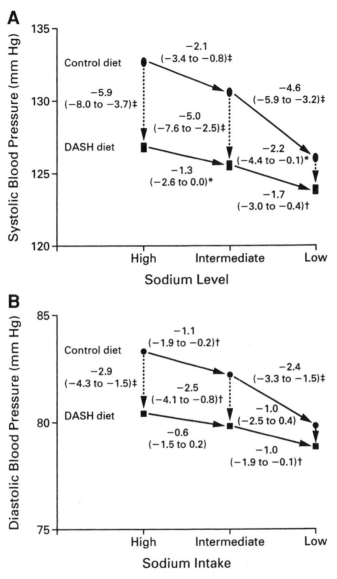

Fig. 1. The effect on systolic blood pressure (**A**) and diastolic blood pressure (**B**) of reduced sodium intake and the Dietary Attempts to Stop Hypertension diet. (From ref. *65*. Reprinted with permission of the Massachusetts Medical Society.)

The follow-up DASH Sodium study investigated the additional benefits of salt restriction as compared with the DASH diet alone (*65*). Reducing sodium intake from a high (150 mmol/d) to either an intermediate (100 mmol/d) or low (65 mmol/d) intake resulted in a stepwise reduction in BP (*see* Fig. 1). This was approximately twice as great in subjects on the control diet (6.7/3.5 mmHg) than on the DASH diet (3.0/1.6 mmHg); all differences were highly significant ($p < 0.001$). This indicates that the greatest benefits of sodium restriction are seen in those with a poor diet (i.e., a typical "American" high-fat diet with a low nutrient density), and that subjects who eat a large amount of fruit and vegetables, together with low-fat diary products, may be able to tolerate higher amounts of salt. Comparing the high-sodium phase of the control diet with the low-sodium phase of the DASH diet indicates that the combined effect of the two dietary changes was a decrease in BP of 8.9/4.5 mmHg.

In a subsequent study, the Diet, Exercise and Weight loss Intervention Trial (DEW-IT) *(66)*, overweight hypertensives demonstrated a net change of 9.5/5.3 mmHg in ambulatory BP, using a low-calorie version of the DASH diet, in combination with weight loss. In a fourth dietary intervention trial (PREMIER), the effects of combining the DASH diet with "established" lifestyle modification recommendations (weight loss, exercise, and restriction of salt and alcohol) were investigated *(67)*. Surprisingly, the addition of the DASH diet to lifestyle modification resulted in an incremental decrease of BP of only 0.6/0.9 mmHg (1.7/1.6 mmHg in hypertensive individuals).

Possible explanations regarding why the effects of combined interventions on blood pressure do not appear to be additive were recently suggested by Pickering *(68)*. Patients in the PREMIER study were not following the DASH diet as closely as in the three earlier DASH studies. PREMIER is the first study to investigate the effects of the DASH diet when patients are required to purchase their own food, rather than being provided with prepared meals. In the original DASH study, patients were provided with 9.6 daily servings of fruits and vegetables, whereas in the PREMIER study, the intake increased from 4.8 servings per day at baseline to 7.8 servings. This was evident in the difference in urinary potassium excretion in the two studies: there was a 105% increase in the original DASH study but only a 28% increase in the PREMIER study. Similarly, the effects of sodium restriction in the DASH Sodium follow-up study greatly exceeded the changes observed in almost all other studies in which participants prepared their own low-salt meals, presumably owing to greater compliance with a low-sodium regimen.

The authors of the PREMIER study suggest a "subadditivity of intervention effects." In other words, the combination of two or more interventions has a smaller effect on BP than the sum of the effects of the individual interventions. In the DEW-IT study, in which obese hypertensives were given a hypocaloric version of the DASH diet and a mean weight loss of 5.5 kg was achieved, the net reduction in BP was comparable to the effects of the DASH diet alone. In the Trials of Hypertension (TOHP) II study, the effect of adding sodium restriction to weight loss produced no further decrease in BP, even though moderate sodium restriction alone produced a modest, but significant, decrease *(69)*. Similarly, the DASH Sodium trial demonstrated a lower combined effect of the DASH diet and sodium restriction than the effects of either intervention on its own *(65)*.

It is often assumed that most individuals are not capable of changing more than one lifestyle factor at a time. However, it is probable that participants in the DASH Sodium trial were diligently consuming the prescribed diet because all food was provided. Similarly, in the TOHP II trial, which comprised three intervention groups (weight loss, sodium restriction, and combination), the magnitude of weight loss and reductions in urinary Na excretion were only marginally less in the combined group than the other two single intervention groups. This indicates that subjects were able to simultaneously achieve both lifestyle changes. An alternative explanation for a lack of additive effects is that different lifestyle interventions may act through the same physiological interventions, thus resulting in a nonlinear dose–response relationship. Much the same way as doubling the dose of antihypertensive drugs produces only a small further decline in BP *(70)*, a combination of lifestyle modifications—such as weight loss, increase in physical activity patterns, and altering the cation composition of the diet—may all be operating through the same physiological pathway. However, much remains to be learned regarding the mechanisms by which obesity and other lifestyle factors affect BP *(71)*. It has consistently been shown in intervention studies conducted in the United States that African Americans with raised BP benefit the most from nonpharmacological interventions, such as dietary changes and weight loss. Evidence of the impact of such interventions on BP is awaited from other ethnic populations. It is likely that the DASH diet cannot be applied to ethnically diverse populations in a "one size fits all" manner. As with all food-based dietary guidelines, recommendations for dietary change need to take into account affordability, accessibility, and sustainability, as well as cultural acceptability of the dietary patterns being promoted.

The evidence relating to the BP-lowering effects of composite dietary intervention supports the shifting paradigm in the provision of nutrition messages to the (often confused) public, in that a holistic approach needs to be taken, rather than the targeting of individual messages.

7. ALCOHOL

Epidemiological studies over the past two decades have firmly established a relationship between regular, excessive alcohol consumption and hypertension. This association has been found in both sexes and in those of differing ethnicity, and is independent of the type of alcoholic beverage, adiposity, education, smoking, salt intake, and several other factors *(72)*. It has been shown that a habitual intake of alcohol greater than 30–60 g/d (i.e., about 2.5–5 alcoholic drinks) results in BP elevation in both men and women. A rule of thumb can be derived: for subjects who consume an habitual intake of 30 g (about 2.5 drinks) or more of alcohol per day, an increment of 10 g alcohol per day increases systolic BP by an average of 1–2 mmHg and diastolic BP by 1 mmHg. As well as its direct effect on BP, alcohol can cause resistance to antihypertensive therapy *(73)* and is a risk factor for stroke *(74)*. The US National High Blood Pressure Education Program (NHBPEP) recommends that in those who drink alcohol, an intake of no more than 25 g of alcohol (two drinks) be consumed a day for men and no more than 15 g of alcohol per day for women and lighter weight people (*see* Table 1). The topic of alcohol is discussed further in Chapter 12.

8. WEIGHT REDUCTION AND BP

Weight reduction has been the single most effective component used in large-scale lifestyle approaches to the reduction of blood pressure, such as in the TOHP Phase I and II studies *(75,76)* and the Trial of Antihypertensive Interventions and Management (TAIM) study *(77)*. A systematic review of all randomized trials of nonpharmacological interventions that included at least 6 mo of follow-up revealed that net BP reductions were greatest for trials of the effects of weight loss, averaging a 5.2-mmHg reduction in systolic BP *(78)*. It has been estimated that for every 1 kg decrease in body weight, obese hypertensive patients can expect a decrease in BP of 2.4/1.5 mmHg *(79)*. A subsequent meta-analysis reported that a loss of 3–9% of body weight in overweight hypertensive subjects is associated with BP reductions of approx 3 mmHg in both systolic and diastolic BP *(80)*. Clearly, when inches come off the waist, millimeters come off the BP.

Weight reduction may decrease dosage requirements for antihypertensive medications. It is not yet clearly established whether weight reduction is superior to sodium restriction and/or potassium supplementation and/or exercise in reducing BP. It is unlikely that weight loss alone will achieve BP control in patients with stage 2 hypertension or in those who are not sufficiently motivated to lose weight.

Various explanations have been proposed to describe the mechanisms by which obesity leads to increased sensitivity to dietary sodium and increased BP levels. Obesity has been linked with suppressed kallikrein levels, an enzymatic precursor of bradykinin, and nitric oxide formation *(81,82)*, as well as with increased serum ACE or kinase II activity. Compared with their nonobese counterparts, obese Jamaicans (body mass index >31) have been shown to have higher serum ACE activity and angiotensinogen levels *(83)*. (The latter is expressed in adipose tissue.) It is hypothesized that obese persons have more renin substrate (i.e., angiotensinogen) and perhaps greater conversion of angiotensin I to angiotensin II, along with an increased leptin production, as well as accelerated breakdown of bradykinin to inactive metabolites, leading to impaired nitric oxide production. The sympathetic nervous system would thus be stimulated, resulting in vasoconstriction and increased plasma volume, leading to hypertension. There is some promising work that suggests that genetic determinants of hypertension may be located at the adipocyte level and influence local renin–angiotensin production. However, the complex, multifactorial nature of hypertension probably involves many gene polymorphisms, interacting at different levels.

Another emerging body of evidence relates to the low birth-weight hypothesis, whereby an adverse intrauterine environment programs the fetus to an increased susceptibility in later life to components of the metabolic syndrome (*see* Table 4), such as hypertension. An inverse association between birth-weight and BP has been found in studies of children, adolescents, and adults. In developing countries, one possible method of primordial prevention of hypertension may be to ensure adequate weight gain and appropriate nutrient intake in women during pregnancy.

9. PHYSICAL ACTIVITY

It is outside the scope of this chapter to review the effect of physical activity on BP; however, mention of it needs to be made because exercise is often recommended to help lower BP, especially in the context of a weight-reducing strategy (*see* Table 1). It is well established that increased levels of physical activity are associated with a decreased risk of CHD and stroke. A meta-analysis, which included only trials in which the exercise intervention had lasted 4 wk or longer, concluded that exercise reduced systolic BP by 4.7 mmHg and diastolic BP by 3.1 mmHg *(84)*.

Recommendations for the prescription of the optimal intensity, duration, and type of exercise for a hypertensive patient remain imprecise. For previously sedentary individuals, a prudent approach would be to commence exercise cautiously and at low intensity (40–50% of maximal oxygen uptake). In high-risk individuals, an initial, thorough medical evaluation, including an electrocardiogram, is advised before beginning an exercise program. There is little or no evidence for extra benefit from higher intensity exercise (>70% maximal oxygen uptake) or from more than three bouts of exercise per week. The challenge for most individuals is to maintain long-term compliance with exercise programs. In this regard, the encouragement of low-intensity activities, which can be incorporated into everyday lifestyle (such as walking instead of using the car), rather than structured high-intensity aerobic exercise programs, shows more promise and appears to result in comparable reductions in BP *(85)*. For both the prevention and management of hypertension, the current JNC VII guidelines recommend an increase in moderately intense physical activity (50–65% maximal oxygen uptake), such as 30 min of brisk walking on most days of the week.

10. CONCLUSIONS

Undoubtedly, nonpharmacological lifestyle changes represent a safe and effective approach to BP reduction, and offer broad advantages for lowering cardiovascular risk. Furthermore, using this approach, the need for antihypertensive medications can be decreased in subjects with established hypertension. Dietary advice for the prevention and management of hypertension needs to address changes in dietary patterns as a whole, rather than focusing on one or more nutrients. It appears that the most beneficial dietary pattern is a DASH-type diet that is low in total and saturated fat and alcohol (and reduced in total energy, if the subject is obese), and high in fiber, potassium, calcium, and magnesium, and moderately high in protein. In terms of foods, this translates into a diet rich in fruit and vegetables and low-fat dairy foods. Regarding sodium restriction, the greatest benefits are seen in those with a diet of poor quality (high in fat and low in nutrient density), However various subgroups, such as elderly hypertensives, obese individuals, and subjects of African descent, may particularly benefit from reducing dietary sodium intake.

To empower and encourage individuals to make sustainable, lifestyle changes, a systematic team approach is required, using health care professionals and community resources wherever possible, so as to provide necessary education, support, and follow-up. Nutrition professionals and legislators involved in food policy development need to work closely with the food industry to develop and market products that are reduced in sodium, or contain an optimal combination of cations known to be beneficial to BP reduction, namely potassium, magnesium, and calcium.

REFERENCES

1. Kaplan NM. The dietary guideline for sodium: should we shake it up? No! Am J Clin Nutr 2000; 71: 1020–1026.
2. McCarron DA. The dietary guideline for sodium: should we shake it up? Yes! Am J Clin Nutr 2000;71: 1013–1019.
3. INTERSALT Cooperative Research Group. INTERSALT: an international study of electrolyte excretion and blood pressure. Results for 24 hour urinary sodium and potassium excretion. BMJ 1988; 297:319–328.
4. Law MR, Frost CD, Wald NJ. By how much does dietary salt reduction lower blood pressure? III. Analysis of data from trials of salt reduction. BMJ 1991; 302:819–824.
5. Midgely JP, Matthew AG, Greenwoood CMT, Logan AG. Effect of reduced dietary sodium on blood pressure. JAMA 1996; 275:1590–1597.
6. Cutler JA, Follmann D, Allender PS. Randomized trials of sodium reduction: an overview. Am J Clin Nutr 1997; 65(Suppl 2):643–651S.
7. Graudal NA, Galloe AM, Garred P. Effects of sodium restriction on blood pressure, renin, aldosterone, caecholamines, cholesterols, and triglycerides: a meta-analysis. JAMA 1998; 279:1383–1391.

8. Alam S, Johnson AG. A meta-analysis of randomised controlled trials (RCT) among healthy normotensive and essential hypertensive elderly patients to determine the effect of high salt (NaCl) diet on blood pressure. J Hum Hypertens 1999; 13:367–374.

9. Cook NR, Cohen J, Hebert P, Taylor JO, Hennekens CH. Implications of small reductions in diastolic blood pressure for primary prevention. Arch Intern Med 1995; 155:701–709.

10. Hooper L, Bartlett C, Smith GD, Ebrahim S. Systematic review of long term effects of advice to reduce dietary salt intake in adults. BMJ 2002; 325:628–637.

11. Singer DRJ, Markandu ND, Cappuccio FP, Miller MA, Sagnella GA, MacGregor GA. Reduction of salt intake during converting enzyme inhibitor treatment compared with addition of a thiazide. Hypertension 1995; 25:1042–1044.

12. Pasquie JL, Jover B, du Cailar G, Mimran A. Sodium but not chloride ion modulates left ventricular hypertrophy in two-kidney one-clip hypertension. J Hypertens 1994; 12:1013–1018.

13. Schmeider RE, Messerli FH, Garavaglia GE, Nunez BS. Salt intake as a determinant of cardiac involvement in essential hypertension. Circulation 1998; 78:951–956.

14. Du Cailar G, Ribstein J, Daures JP, Mimran A. Sodium and left ventricular mass in untreated hypertensive and normotensive subjects. Am J Physiol 1992; 263:H177–H181.

15. Liebson PR, Grandits GA, Prineas RJ, Grimm RH Jr, Neaton JD, Stamler J. Echocardiographic correlates of left ventricular structure among 844 mildly hypertensive men and women in the treatment of mild hypertension study (TOMHS). Circulation 1993; 87:476–486.

16. Swaye PS, Gifford RW, Berretoni JN. Dietary salt and hypertension. Am J Cardiology 1972; 72:95–102.

17. Du Cailar G, Ribstein J, Mimran A. Dietary sodium and target organ damage in essential hypertension. Am J Hypertension 2002; 15:222–229.

18. Jula AM, Karanko HM. Effects on left ventricular hypertrophy of long-term nonpharmacological treatment with sodium restriction in mild-to-moderate essential hypertension. Circulation 1994; 89:1023–1031.

19. Tuomilehto J, Jousilahti P, Rastenyte D, Moltchanov V, Tanskanen A, Pietinen P. Urinary sodium excretion and cardiovascular mortality in Finland: a prospective study. Lancet 2001; 357:848–851.

20. Jiang H, Ogden LG, Vupputuri S, Bazzano LA, Loria C, Whelton PK. Dietary sodium intake and subsequent risk of cardiovascular disease in overweight adults. JAMA 1999; 282:2027–2034.

21. Briefel R, Alaimo K, Wright J, McDowell M. Dietary sources of salt and sodium. Presented at the NHLBI Workshop on Implementing Recommendations for Dietary Salt Reduction, Aug. 25-26, 1994.

22. National Research Council. Diet and health: implications for reducing chronic disease. National Academy Press, Washington, DC, 1989.

23. Sanchez-Castillo CP, Warrender S, Whitehead TP, James WP. An assessment of the sources of dietary salt in a British population. Clin Sci 1987; 72: 95-102.

24. Sanchez-Castillo CP, Branch WJ, James WP. A test of the validity of the lithium -marker technique for monitoring dietary sources of salt in men. Clin Sci 1987; 72:87-94.

25. James WPT, Ralph A, Sanchez-Castillo CP. The dominance of salt in manufactured food in the sodium intake of affluent societies. Lancet 1987; I:426-429.

26. Block G, Dresser CM, Hartman AM, Carroll MD. Nutrient sources in the American diet: quantitative data from the NHANES II survey. I. Vitamins and minerals. Am J Epidemiol 1985; 12:13-26.

27. Charlton KE, Steyn K, Levitt NS, et al. Diet and blood pressure in South Africa: the intake of foods containing sodium, potassium, calcium and magnesium in three ethnic groups. Nutrition 2005;21:39–50.

28. National High Blood Pressure Education Program. The seventh report of the Joint National Committee on Prevention, Detection, Evaluation, and Treatment of High Blood Pressure. US Department of Health and Human Services: NIH Publication No. 03-5231, May 2003.

29. Diet, nutrition and the prevention of chronic diseases. WHO Technical Report Series, 916. World Health Organization, Geneva, 2003, pp. i-viii, 1–149.

30. Cappuccio FP, Markandu ND, Carney C, Sagnella GA, MacGregor GA. Double-blind randomised trial of modest salt restriction in older people. Lancet 1997; 350:850-854.

31. Mulrow CD, Cornell JA, Herrera CR, Kadri A, Farnett L, Aguilar C. Hypertension in the elderly: implications and generalizability of randomised trials. JAMA 1994; 272:1932-1938.

32. Greenfield H, Smith AM, Maples J, Wills RBH. Contributions of foods to sodium in the Australian food supply. Hum Nutr Appl Nutr 1984; 38:203-210.

33. Williams P, McMahon A, Boustead R. A case study of sodium reduction in breakfast cereals and the impact of the Pick the Tick food information program in Australia. Health Promot Int 2003; 18:51-56.
34. Mattes RD. The taste for salt in humans. Am J Clin Nutr 1997; 65(Suppl):692S-697S.
35. Beauchamp GK, Bertino M, Engelman K. Failure to compensate decreased sodium intake with increased table salt usage. JAMA 1987; 258:3275-3278.
36. Thaler BI, Paulin JM, Phelan EL, Simpson FO. A pilot study to test the feasibility of salt restriction in a community. NZ Med J 1982; 95:839-842.
37. Whelton PK, He J, Cutler JA, et al. Effects of oral potassium on blood pressure. Meta-analysis of randomized controlled clinical trials. JAMA 1997;277: 1624–1632.
38. Morris RC, Sebastian A, Forman A, Tanaka M, Schmidlin O. Normotensive salt sensitivity. Effects of race and dietary potassium. Hypertension 1998; 33:18–23.
39. Brier ME, Luft FC. Sodium kinetics in white and black normotensive subjects: possible relevance to salt-sensitive hypertension. Am J Med Sci 1994; 307:S38–S42.
40. Dimsdale JE, Ziegler M, Mills P, Berry C. Prediction of salt sensitivity. Am J Hypertens 1990; 3:429–435.
41. Luft RC, Rankin LI, Bloch R, Weyman AE, Willis LR, Murray RH, Grim CE, Weinberger MH. Cardiovascular and humoral responses to extremes of sodium intake in normal black and white men. Circulation 1979; 60:697–706.
42. Kirkendall WM, Connor WE, Abboud F, Rastogi SP, Anderson TA, Fry M. The effect of dietary sodium chloride on blood pressure, body fluids, electrolytes, renal function, and serum lipids of normotensive men. J Lab Clin Med 1976; 87:418–434.
43. Sudhir K, Forman A, Yi S-L, Sorof J, Schmidlin O, Sebastian A, Morris RC Jr. Reduced dietary potassium reversibly enhances vasopressor response to stress in African-Americans. Hypertension 1997; 29:1083–1090.
44. Castenmiller JJM, Mensink RP, van der Heijden L, et al. The effect of dietary sodium on urinary calcium and potassium excretion in normotensive men with different calcium intakes. Am J Clin Nutr 1985;41:52–60.
45. Rich GM, McCullogh M, Olmedo A, et al. Blood pressure and renal blood flow responses to dietary calcium and sodium intake in humans. Am J Hypertens 1991;4:642S–645S.
46. Saito K, Sano H, Furuta Y, Yamanishi J, et al. Calcium supplementation in salt-dependent hypertension. Contrib Nephrol 1991; 90:25–35.
47. Yamawaka H, Suzuki H, Nakamura M, et al. Disturbed calcium metabolism in offspring of hypertensive parents. Hypertension 1992; 19:528–534.
48. Bucher HC, Cook RJ, Guyatt GH, Lang JD, Cook DJ, Hatala R, Hunt KD. Effects of dietary calcium supplementation on blood pressure: a meta-analysis of randomised controlled trials. JAMA 1996; 275:1016–1022.
49. Allender PS, Cutler JA, Follmann D, Cappuccio FP, Pryer J, Elliott P. Dietary calcium and blood pressure: a meta-analysis of randomised clinical trials. Ann Intern Med 1996; 124:825–831.
50. Tabuchi Y, Ogihara T, Hashizuma K, et al. Hypotensive effect of long-term oral calcium supplementation in elderly patients with essential hypertension. J Clin Hypertens 1986 ;2:254–262.
51. Takagi Y, Fukase M, Takata S, et al. Calcium treatment of essential hypertension in elderly patients evaluated by 24 h monitoring. Am J Hypertens 1991; 4:836–839.
52. Morris CD, McCarron DA. Effect of calcium supplementation in an older population with mildly increased blood pressure. Am J Hypertens 1992; 5:230–237.
53. Lyle RM, Melby CL, Hyner GC. Metabolic differences between subjects whose blood pressure did or did not respond to oral calcium supplementation. Am J Clin Nutr 1988; 47:1030–1035.
54. Zemel MB, Gualdoni SM, Walsh MF, et al. Effects of sodium and calcium on calcium metabolism and blood pressure regulation in hypertensive black adults. J Hypertens 1986; 4(Suppl 5):S364–S366.
55. Dwyer JH, Li L, Dwyer KM, Curtin LR, Feinleib M. Dietary calcium, alcohol, and incidence of treated hypertension in the NHANES I epidemiologic follow-up study. Am J Epidemiol 1996; 144:828–838.
56. Strazullo P, Nunziata V, Cirillo M, et al. Abnormalities of calcium metabolism in essential hypertension. Clin Sci 1983; 65:137–141.
57. Motoyama T, Sano H, Fukuzaki H. Oral magnesium supplementation in patients with essential hypertension. Hypertension 1989; 13:227–232.

58. Winkler AW, Smith PK, Hoff HE. Intravenous magnesium sulfate in the treatment of nephritic convulsions in adults. J Clin Invest 1942; 21:207–216.

59. Albert DG, Morita Y, Iseri LT. Serum magnesium and plasma sodium levels in essential vascular hypertension. Circulation 1958; 17:761–764.

60. Ma J, Folsom AR, Melnick SL, et al. Associations of serum and dietary magnesium with cardiovascular disease, hypertension, diabetes, insulin, and carotid wall thickness: the ARIC Study. J Clin Epidemiol 1995; 48:927–940.

61. Jee SH, Miller ER, Guallar E, Singh VK, Appel LJ, Klag MJ. The effect of magnesium supplementation on blood pressure: a meta-analysis of randomised clinical trials. Am J Hypertension 2002; 15:691–696.

62. Touyz RM, Milne FJ, Seftel HC, Reinach SG. Magnesium, calcium, sodium and potassium status in normotensive and hypertensive Johannesburg residents. S Afr Med J 1987; 72:377–381.

63. Appel L, Moore T, Obarzanek, et al. A clinical trial of the effects of dietary patterns on blood pressure. N Engl J Med 1997; 336:1117-1124.

64. Svetky LP, Simons-Morton D, Vollmer WM, et al. Effects of dietary patterns on blood pressure: Subgroup analysis of the Dietary Approaches to Stop Hypertension (DASH) randomised controlled trial. Arch Intern Med 1999; 159:285–293.

65. Sacks FM, Svetky LP, Vollmer WM, et al. for the DASH-Sodium collaborative research group. Effects on blood pressure of reduced dietary sodium and the dietary approaches to stop hypertension (DASH) diet. N Engl J Med 2001; 344:3–10.

66. Miller ER III, Erlinger TP, Young RD, et al. Results of the Diet, Exercise and Weight Loss intervention trial (DEW-IT). Hypertension 2002; 40:612–618.

67. Writing Group of the PREMIER Collaborative Research Group. Effects of comprehensive lifestyle modification on blood pressure control: main results of the PREMIER clinical trial. JAMA 2003; 289:2083–2093.

68. Pickering TG. Lifestyle modification and blood pressure control: Is the glass half full or half empty? JAMA 2003; 289:2131, 2132.

69. The Trials of Hypertension Prevention Collaborative Group. Effects of weight loss and sodium reduction intervention on blood pressure and hypertension incidence in overweight people with high-normal blood pressure: the Trials of Hypertension prevention, Phase II. Arch Intern Med 1997; 157:657–667.

70. Flack JM, Gushman WC. Evidence for the efficacy of low-dose diuretic monotherapy. Am J Med 1996; 101(3A):53S–60S.

71. Hall JE. The kidney, hypertension, and obesity. Hypertension 2003; 41:625–633.

72. Klatsky AL. Alcohol and hypertension. Clin Chim Acta 1996; 246:91-105.

73. Puddey IB, Parker M, Beilen LJ, Vandongen R, Masarei JRL. Effects of alcohol and caloric restrictions on blood pressure and serum lipids in overweight men. Hypertension 1992; 20:533-541.

74. Gill JS, Shipley MJ, Tsementzis SA, et al. Alcohol consumption—a risk factor for haemorrhagic stroke. Am J Med 1991; 90:489-497.

75. The Trials of Hypertension Prevention Collaborative Research Group. The effects of nonpharmacologic interventions on blood pressure of persons with high normal levels. Results of the Trials of Hypertension Prevention, Phase I. JAMA 1992; 267:1213-1220.

76. The Trials of Hypertension Prevention Collaborative Research Group. Effects of weight loss and sodium reduction intervention on blood pressure and hypertension incidence in overweight people with high-normal blood pressure. The Trials of Hypertension Prevention, phase II. Arch Intern Med 1997; 157:657-667.

77. Langford HG, Davis BR, Blaufox D, et al. Effect of drug and diet treatment of mild hypertension on diastolic blood pressure. The TAIM Research Group. Hypertension 1991; 17:210-217.

78. Ebrahim S, Smith GD. Lowering blood pressure: a systematic review of sustained effects of non-pharmacological interventions. J Public Health Med 1998; 20:441-448.

79. Staessen J, Fagard R, Amry A. The relationship between body weight and blood pressure. J Hum Hypertens 1988; 2:207–217.

80. Mulrow CD, Chiquette E, Angel L, et al. Dieting to reduce body weight for controlling hypertension in adults (Cochrane review). In: The Cochrane Database of Systematic Reviews 1998, Issue 4. Art. No: CD000484. DOI:10.2002/14651858. CD 000484.

81. Bellini C, Ferri C, Carlomagno A, et al. Impaired inactive to active kallikrein conversion in human sat-sensitive hypertension. J Am Soc Nephrol 1996; 7:2565–2577.

82. Higashi Y, Oshima T, Watanabe M, Matsuura H, Kajiyama G. Renal response to L-arginine in salt-sensitive patients with essential hypertension. Hypertension 1996; 27:643–648.

83. Forrester T, McFarlane-Anderson N, Bennett FI, et al. The angiotensin converting enzyme and blood pressure in Jamaicans. Am J Hypertens 1997; 10:519–524.

84. Halbert JA, Silagy CA, Finucane P, Withers RT, Hamdorf PA, Andrews GR. The effectiveness of exercise training in lowering blood pressure: a meta-analysis of randomised controlled trials of 4 weeks or longer. J Hum Hypertens 1997; 11:641–649.

85. Dunn AL, Marcus BH, Kampert JB, Garcia ME, Kohl HW, Blair SN. Comparison of lifestyle and structured interventions to increase physical activity and cardiorespiratory fitness. A randomized trial. JAMA 1999; 281:327–334.

8

Fish, n-3 Polyunsaturated Fatty Acids, and Cardiovascular Disease

Jayne V. Woodside and Ian S. Young

KEY POINTS

- n-3 Fatty acids are long-chain polyunsaturated fatty acid (PUFAs). The fish-based and fish oil-based n-3 PUFAs consist of eicosapentaenioc acid (C20:5 n-3) and docosahexaenoic acid (C22:6 n-3).
- Studies suggest that n-3 fatty acids protect against coronary heart disease and sudden cardiac death. The results of clinical trials are awaited.
- Both US and UK health agencies recommend an increase in consumption of fish and n-3 PUFAs.
- In the general population, the benefits of fish consumption within recommended amounts outweigh the risk posed by environmental contaminants.
- Evidence indicates that n-3 PUFAs may also protect against the development of a number of other diseases.

1. INTRODUCTION

Cardiovascular disease (CVD) is a major cause of morbidity and mortality in the Western world *(1)*. There are a number of well-established risk factors for CVD including smoking, hypertension, and family history *(2)*. In terms of nutrition, a diet high in fat, particularly saturated fat, has been shown to be associated with CVD incidence *(3)*. The observation that Greenland Eskimos (Inuit) have a low incidence of CVD despite a high saturated fat intake *(4)* has led to much scientific and public interest in the role of n-3 fatty acids found in fish and fish oils in the prevention and treatment of disease, and particularly CVD. In this chapter, the biochemistry and normal dietary intake of these compounds will be discussed, and the evidence linking them and their food sources with CVD reviewed. The safety of both fish-oil supplements and fish will be assessed, and the potential effect of fish and fish-oil consumption on other diseases will be considered.

2. BIOCHEMISTRY OF n-3 FATTY ACIDS

n-3 Fatty acids are long-chain polyunsaturated fatty acids (PUFAs) (18–22 carbon atoms) with the first of two or more double bonds beginning with the third carbon atom

From: *Nutritional Health: Strategies for Disease Prevention, Second Edition*
Edited by: N. J. Temple, T. Wilson, and D. R. Jacobs © Humana Press Inc., Totowa, NJ

(when counting from the methyl end). The fish-based and fish-oil-based n-3 PUFAs consist of eicosapentaenioc acid (EPA, C20:5 n-3) and docosahexaenoic acid (DHA, C22:6 n-3). Dietary α-linolenic acid (C18:3 n-3) can also be converted into EPA and DHA (e.g., in the brain, liver, and testes). However, the extent of this conversion is likely to be modest, and remains under debate. For example, Emken et al. *(5)* reported a 15% conversion, whereas more recently Pawlosky et al. *(6)* reported only a 0.2% conversion. Both reported that conversion to DHA was much lower than to EPA. The metabolism of the n-3 PUFAs is shown schematically in Fig. 1.

3. FOOD SOURCES OF n-3 PUFAS

The major food sources of α-linolenic acid are vegetable oils, principally canola and soybean oils *(7)*. Other rich sources include flaxseed and walnuts *(7)*. Fish are the main source of EPA and DHA *(7)*. All fish contain EPA and DHA; however, content can differ dramatically by species, and also within species, with factors such as the diet of the fish and wild vs farm-raised, influencing EPA and DHA content. Fatty fish, such as mackerel, salmon, herring, and trout, store fat in muscle and contain more EPA and DHA than white fish, such as cod, hake, and haddock, which store fat in the liver. Examples of food sources of α-linolenic acid and of EPA and DHA are shown in Table 1.

4. EVIDENCE LINKING CONSUMPTION OF FISH AND n-3 PUFAS TO CVD

4.1. Coronary Heart Disease

Epidemiological studies have consistently shown that consumption of at least one portion of fish weekly may decrease the risk of fatal coronary heart disease (CHD) by approx 40% compared with consumption of no fish *(8–11)*. More recently, in a 30-yr follow-up of the Chicago Western Electric Study, men who consumed 35 g/d or more of fish compared with those who consumed none had a relative risk of death from CHD of 0.62 *(12)*. The association was also shown for fatal CHD, although the association was not demonstrated for nonfatal myocardial infarction (MI) in a prospective study in the elderly *(13)*. A meta-analysis of prospective studies has confirmed the association, but only in high-risk groups *(14)*, although a more recent meta-analysis also found a protective effect of fish consumption on CHD (RR = 0.86; $p < 0.005$) *(15)*. The inverse association between fish consumption and mortality from CHD has been shown to be consistent across countries in an ecological study of 36 countries *(16)*.

Fewer studies have examined the effect of tissue n-3 PUFA levels rather than dietary intake on CHD risk. In the EURAMIC (European Multicentre Case–Control Study on Antioxidants, Myocardial Infarction and Breast Cancer) study, a large international case–control study, no association between adipose tissue DHA and MI risk was demonstrated *(17)*. However, in the EUROASPIRE study, which examined the fatty acid composition of serum cholesteryl esters in relation to secondary prevention of CHD, the relative risk of death, adjusted for CVD risk factors, for subjects in the highest tertile of fatty acids compared with those in the lowest tertile was 0.33 for α-linolenic acid, 0.33 for EPA, and 0.31 for DHA (p for trend = 0.063, 0.056, and 0.026, respectively) *(18)*.

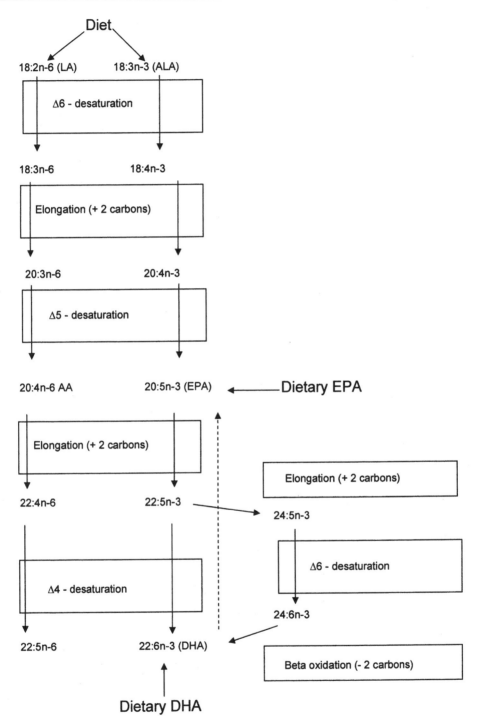

Fig. 1. Metabolism of n-3 polyunsaturated fatty acid. LA, linoleic acid; ALA, α-linolenic acid; AA, arachidonic acid.

Table 1
Food Sources of α-Linolenic Acid, EPA, and DHA

Food	α-Linolenic acid content (g/100 g)
Walnut oil	11.5
Canola oil	9.6
Walnuts, English	7.47
Soybean oil	7.30
Corn oil	0.9
Olive oil	0.7
	EPA + DHA content (g/100 g)
Mackerel	1.81
Sardines	1.71
Salmon	1.41
Trout, rainbow	0.97
Crab	0.92
Mussels	0.57
Plaice	0.26
Cod	0.24
Tuna (light, canned in water, drained)	0.16
Haddock	0.15

Data based on ref. 7.
EPA, eicosapentaenioc acid; DHA, docosahexaenoic acid.

Some notable studies have not reported a significant association between fish consumption and CHD risk. In the Health Professionals Follow-up Study, there was no significant association between fish intake (and n-3 PUFA intake), and risk of CHD (19). Similarly, the Physicians Health Study also failed to show an association between fish consumption or n-3 PUFA intake and risk of MI, nonsudden cardiac death, or total CVD mortality, although there was a reduced risk of total mortality (20). The Seven Countries data also showed a lack of association between fish consumption and both CHD incidence and mortality (21). The Alpha-Tocopherol, Beta-Carotene Cancer Prevention Study in fact found that estimated n-3 PUFA intake from fish was associated with a trend towards increased risk of coronary death (after adjustment for trans, saturated, and cis-monounsaturated fatty acids) (22).

The authors of the AHA scientific statement on fish consumption, fish oil, n-3 fatty acids, and CVD have summarized the possible reasons for the conflicting data from the epidemiological studies (23). There have been suggestions that the conflicting data reflect differences in the definition of sudden death and the residual confounding of reference groups that had a less healthy lifestyle (24), variability in end points studied, experimental design or dietary assessment of fish intake, different study populations (25), and the possible confounding effect of an increase in hemorrhagic stroke. Albert et al. (20) attempted to explain the lack of association in their study by pointing out that only a small fraction of their population reported little or no fish consumption, whereas the studies reporting an inverse association between fish consumption and coronary mortality have been on populations with relatively large numbers of noneaters of fish. The EURAMIC study only examined MI survivors, and it is possible that those who did not survive ate less fish. Another explanation, based on a summary of 11 prospective studies, is that fish is only protective in populations at high risk of CHD (RR = 0.4–0.6), but not in populations at low risk *(14)*. Another consideration is the type of fish consumed and how it is prepared: Oomen et al. *(26)* report a lower CHD mortality (RR = 0.66) only in those eating fatty fish, and not in those eating lean fish. Another emerging explanation relates to levels of methylmercury in fish (*see* Heading 7) with several, although not all, studies showing an association between methylmercury exposure and CHD risk *(27,28)*. Thus, methylmercury in fish may mask the beneficial effects of n-3 PUFAs on CHD risk. This is an area that clearly requires further study.

4.2. Intervention Studies

The first randomized, controlled trial (RCT) using n-3 PUFAs was the Diet and Reinfarction Trial (DART) study, which examined the effects of increased fatty fish intake on secondary prevention of CHD *(29)*. There was a 29% reduction in all-cause mortality over a 2-yr period in male MI survivors advised to increase intake of fatty fish by 200–400 g/wk (providing an extra 500–800 mg/d of n-3 PUFAs). Analysis of a subset of patients that received fish-oil capsules (900 mg/d EPA + DHA) suggested the effect was caused by these fatty acids *(30)*.

A number of more recent trials have also been carried out. Singh et al. *(31)*, in the Indian Experiment of Infarct Survival, randomized patients with suspected acute MI to either fish-oil capsules (1.8 g/d EPA + DHA), mustard oil (20 g/d providing 2.9 g/d α-linolenic acid), or placebo. Follow-up at 1 yr showed that total cardiac events occurred in 25 and 28% of the fish oil and mustard oil groups, respectively, compared with 35% of the placebo group, and this was statistically significant ($p < 0.01$).

The largest RCT so far carried out using n-3 PUFAs is the Italian Gruppo Italiano per lo Studio della Sopravvivenza nell'Infarto Miocardico Prevention Study (GISSI-P) *(32)*. In this secondary prevention study, 11,324 patients with pre-existing CHD were randomized to either 300 mg of vitamin E, fish oil (850 mg of EPA + DHA), both, or neither. After a 3.5-yr follow-up, those given n-3 PUFAs alone had a 15% reduction in the primary end point of death, nonfatal MI, and nonfatal stroke ($p < 0.02$), a 20% reduction in all-cause mortality ($p = 0.01$), and a 45% reduction in sudden death ($p < 0.001$) compared with the control group. Vitamin E had no apparent effect on the primary end point, whether given alone or when added to the n-3 PUFAs, although *p*-values approached significance. This trial was large and carried out in a relatively usual care setting (in that subjects were receiving conventional cardiac therapy). However, it was not placebo controlled (the control group received no intervention) and therefore is methodologically weaker than if a placebo control had been used. Dropout rates were also high (>25%).

The final intervention study with a clinical end point compared corn oil with 3.5 g/d of fish oil that was concentrated in DHA + EPA. No effect was seen on cardiac events in post-MI patients ($n = 300$) after 1.5 yr of intervention *(33)*. The authors speculated that this may be caused by the high habitual fish intake in western Norway.

No intervention trials have so far been carried out examining the effect of n-3 PUFA supplementation on primary prevention of CHD, although such trials are underway.

However, several studies have examined the effect of supplementation on intermediate CHD end points.

The first study of n-3 PUFAs on angiographic progression rates showed no effect of 6 g/d of n-3 PUFAs or olive oil over 2 yr *(34)*. However, a larger trial in patients presenting for coronary angiography (*n* = 223) randomized to either placebo or 3 g/d for 3 mo followed by 1.5 g/d for 21 mo, showed the n-3 PUFA supplementation was associated with less progression, more regression, and a trend towards fewer clinical events (7 vs 2; *p* = 0.1) *(35)*.Supplementation with n-3 PUFAs (3.4 g/d) has also been shown to lower vein graft occlusion rates from 33 (control) to 27% (*p* = 0.03) *(36)*.

Several trials examined the effect of n-3 fish oils on restenosis (the closing or narrowing of an artery that was previously opened by a cardiac procedure, such as angioplasty) after coronary angioplasty. Although an early meta-analysis (of 7 studies) showed a beneficial effect of supplementation *(37)*, more recent trials have not supported a benefit *(38,39)*. These later trials were large studies using 5–7 g/d n-3 fatty acids, and therefore, further studies are not considered necessary.

4.3. Sudden Death

A number of studies have been consistent in showing an association between fish consumption and a reduced risk of sudden cardiac death. In the Physicians' Health Study, men who consumed fish once per week or more had a relative risk of sudden death of 0.48 (*p* = 0.04) compared with men who consumed fish less than once per month *(20)*. A similar effect was reported when blood levels of n-3 PUFAs were examined, with the relative risk of sudden death being significantly lower in men in the third and fourth quartiles compared with those in the first quartile *(40)*. In another nested case–control study, fish intake was also associated with a reduced risk of sudden death. Intake of 5.5 g/mo of n-3 fatty acids were associated with a 50% reduced risk of primary cardiac arrest *(41)*.

The GISSI-P trial, which was mentioned earlier, tested the effect of fish-oil supplementation on CVD. Although not a stated primary end point, there was a 45% reduction in sudden cardiac death *(32)*. The results from this study were reanalyzed and it was determined that the reduction in risk of sudden cardiac death approached significance after 3 mo of consumption, accounting for 57% of the overall mortality benefit. The reduction became significant at 4 mo, and was highly significant (*p* = 0.0006) at 3.5 yr, the end of the study, when it accounted for 59% of the n-3 PUFA advantage in mortality *(42)*.

The evidence linking n-3 fatty acids with sudden cardiac death has recently been reviewed by Leaf et al. *(43)*. Overall, evidence relating n-3 PUFAs to disease is greater for sudden death than CHD events, and it would also appear that the effect is stronger for fatal CHD than for nonfatal MI. A meta-analysis of all RCTs examining n-3 PUFAs (including α-linolenic acid) has confirmed this, with the risk ratios for nonfatal MI, fatal CHD, and sudden death being 0.8, 0.7, and 0.7, respectively *(44)*.

4.4. Stroke

Compared with those focusing on CHD, relatively few studies have examined the effects of n-3 PUFAs on stroke. Ecological, cross-sectional, and case–control studies generally show an inverse association between consumption of fish and fish oils and stroke risk *(45)*. Results from the six prospective studies so far carried out have been less consistent, with two showing no association *(46,47)*, one showing a possible inverse association *(48)*, and three demonstrating a significant inverse association *(49–51)*. In the largest of these, the Nurses' Health Study, the relative risk of total stroke was lower, although this was not statistically significant, among women who regularly ate fish than among those who did not. A significant decrease in the risk of thrombotic stroke (RR = 0.49) was observed among women who ate fish at least two times per week compared with women who ate fish less than once per month, after adjustment for age, smoking, and other cardiovascular risk factors. The results also showed a nonsignificant decrease among women in the highest quintile of n-3 PUFA intake. No association was observed between fish or fish-oil consumption and hemorrhagic stroke *(48)*.

In the most recent prospective study, the Health Professionals Follow-up Study, a protective effect of eating fish at least once per month or more on ischemic stroke after 12-yr follow-up was demonstrated, but no effect on hemorrhagic stroke *(51)*. In a recent review, Skerrett and Hennekens *(45)* concluded that the data currently support the hypothesis that consumption of fish several times per week reduces the risk of thrombotic stroke, but does not increase the risk of hemorrhagic stroke. However, in both the Lyon Diet Heart Study *(52)* and the GISSI-P study *(32)*, there was no significant effect of n-3 PUFA supplementation on total stroke. More intervention studies must be carried out examining type-specific stroke risk rather than total stroke in high-risk populations.

Studies have also been carried out examining CVD risk factors as an end point. In a study of Japanese living in Japan or Brazil, Mizushima et al. *(53)* reported a dose–response relationship between the frequency of weekly fish intake and reduced CVD risk factors (e.g., obesity, hypertension, glycohemoglobin, and ST-T segment change on the echocardiogram).

The evidence detailed here suggests that regular consumption of fish (and n-3 PUFAs) is associated with reduced risk of the major forms of CVD: CHD, sudden death, and stroke. The potential mechanisms by which this reduction in risk occurs are explored in Subheading 4.5.

4.5. Mechanisms

There are a number of possible mechanisms of action for n-3 PUFAs.

4.5.1. DECREASED RISK OF ARRHYTHMIAS

Sudden cardiac death is a major cause of death in industrialized countries. Mortality statistics from the United States indicate that up to 80% of sudden cardiac deaths are caused by ventricular fibrillation, which is the most common arrhythmia *(54)*. Studies in cell cultures and animal models, observational studies, and human intervention trials all suggest that n-3 PUFAs may protect against fatal arrhythmia *(54,55)*. The proposed mechanism appears to involve a stabilizing effect on the myocardium itself *(55,23,56)*. This mechanism may well be the most important as indicated by the strong protective association observed between n-3 PUFAs and sudden death and the fact that n-3 PUFAs appear to exert their protective effect early in an intervention *(42)*.

4.5.2. REDUCED TRIGLYCERIDES

The reduction of triglycerides with n-3 PUFA supplementation is well established *(23)*. In a review of human studies, Harris *(57)* reported that around 4 g/d of n-3 PUFAs from fish oil decreases serum triglycerides by 25–30%, with an accompanying increase in low-density lipoprotein (LDL) cholesterol (*see* Heading 6) and high-density lipopro-tein-cholesterol of 1–3%. The lowering effect increases as the supplement dose increases *(57)*. Therefore, fish oil can have a therapeutic role in hypertriglyceridemia at doses of 3–5 g/d, levels only consistently obtainable by supplementation *(23)*. Both EPA and DHA appear to be able to reduce triglycerides *(58)*.

4.5.3. LOWERED BLOOD PRESSURE

n-3 PUFAs seem to have a small, dose-dependent, hypotensive effect *(59)*. The extent of blood pressure lowering appears to be dependent on the initial degree of hypertension *(59)*. A meta-analysis indicated a significant reduction in blood pressure of 3.4/2.0 mmHg in hypertensive subjects consuming 5.6 g/d of n-3 PUFAs *(60)*. As this is a relatively high dose, these fats probably have a limited role to play in the management of hypertension. Indeed, no relation in epidemiological studies has been detected between fish intake and blood pressure *(61)*.

4.5.4. REDUCED THROMBOSIS AND HEMOSTASIS

n-3 PUFAs have been shown to reduce platelet aggregation *(62,63)*, thereby reducing hemostasis. Their effect on thrombosis has yet to be clearly determined. A negative association between n-3 PUFA intake and levels of fibrinogen, Factor VIII, and von Willebrand factor has been demonstrated *(64)*, but the more recent CARDIA study found no such association between either fish or n-3 PUFA intake and these coagulation factors *(65)*. There have been both positive *(66)* and negative *(67)* studies of n-3 PUFA supple-mentation and coagulation factors. Therefore, although it seems clear that n-3 PUFAs beneficially influence platelet aggregation, thereby affecting hemostasis, their effects on thrombosis remains unclear and further well-designed intervention studies are required.

4.5.5. REDUCED ATHEROSCLEROTIC PLAQUE GROWTH

n-3 PUFAs appear to have an anti-atherogenic action in that they can inhibit new plaque development *(36)*. For example, EPA and DHA may alter expression of adhesion molecules. Abe et al. *(68)* reported a 9% reduction in intercellular adhesion molecule-1 and a 16% reduction in E-selectin but no change in vascular cell adhesion molecule-1 in hypertriglyceridemic subjects receiving n-3 PUFA supplementation for 7–12 mo. How-ever, other studies have failed to confirm these results *(66,69)*.

4.5.6. IMPROVED ENDOTHELIAL FUNCTION

Several studies have shown that n-3 PUFAs improve endothelial function, and this has been reviewed by Chin and Dart *(70)*. They have also been shown to favorably influence arterial compliance *(71)*.

4.5.7. REDUCED INFLAMMATORY RESPONSE

In vitro data exist suggesting that DHA reduces the expression of interleukin (IL)-6 and IL-8 in stimulated cells (and endothelial expression of adhesion molecules) *(72,73)*. Fish oil also affects other inflammatory mediators, such as tumor necrosis factor-α, and these molecules may affect atherogenesis and plaque stability *(74)*. A recent study by Trebble et al. *(75)* has shown that dietary fish-oil supplementation is associated with decreases in prostaglandin E_2 production and simultaneous increases in lymphocyte proliferation and interferon-γ production, and a trend towards increased IL-4 production by peripheral blood mononuclear cells (75). n-3 PUFAs have been proposed to play a role in rheumatoid arthritis, inflammatory bowel disease, and psoriasis, perhaps through a suppression of immune and inflammation responses, although few controlled human studies have been carried out (76).

4.5.8. Increased Plaque Stability

A recent study has shown that n-3 PUFAs are readily incorporated from dietary fish-oil supplements into advanced atherosclerotic plaques and that this incorporation is associated with structural changes consistent with increased plaque stability (77).

4.6. Effects on CVD of Plant-Derived vs Marine-Derived n-3 Fatty Acids

α-Linolenic acid, in contrast to EPA and DHA, is found in plant foods and not marine sources (Table 1). Evidence from epidemiological studies of α-linolenic acid and CVD indicates that α-linolenic acid is associated with a lower risk of both MI and fatal CHD in both women and men (23). In addition, in a recent observational study, higher consumption of linolenic acid was associated with a lower prevalence of carotid plaques, and with lesser thickness of segment-specific carotid intima-media thickness (78).

The effect of α-linolenic acid supplementation in CHD prevention has been examined in four trials. The Indian Experiment of Infarct Survival discussed above reported a significant decrease in total cardiac events in the group assigned to mustard seed oil (31). In the Lyon Diet Heart Study, a randomized, controlled trial of an α-linolenic acid-rich Mediterranean diet with free-living subjects, those in the intervention group had a 50–70% reduction of cardiac end points (52). In the final report of this study, de Lorgeril et al. (52) reported significant reductions in three composite outcomes (CO): CO1 (cardiac death and nonfatal MI), CO2 (CO1 plus unstable angina, stroke, heart failure, pulmonary or peripheral embolism), and CO3 (CO2 plus minor events requiring hospital admission), with adjusted risk ratios ranging from 0.28 to 0.53.

In terms of dietary change, subjects in the control group averaged 34% of calories from fat, 12% from saturated fat, 11% from monounsaturated fat, 6% from polyunsaturated fat, and 312 mg/d of cholesterol. In contrast, subjects on the Mediterranean-style diet averaged 30% of calories from fat, 8% from saturated fat, 13% from monounsaturated fat, 5% from PUFA, and 203 mg/d of cholesterol. Those on the Mediterranean diet consumed less linoleic acid (3.6 vs 5.3% kcal), but more oleic acid (12.9 vs 10.8% kcal), α-linolenic acid (0.84 vs 0.29% kcal), and dietary fiber. Plasma fatty acid analysis conducted after 52 wk of follow-up confirmed the dietary fatty acid data (79). Although the plasma levels of α-linolenic acid were significantly associated with CO1, it is impossible to ascribe the benefit unambiguously to α-linolenic acid because of the many other dietary variables present.

These two positive studies of α-linolenic acid are balanced by two negative studies. In the Norwegian Vegetable Oil Experiment, 13,000 men aged 50–59 yr with no history of MI were randomly assigned to consume either 5.5 g/d of α-linolenic acid (from 10 mL linseed oil) or 10 mL sunflower oil for 1 yr. There were no differences in sudden death, death from CHD, or all deaths within the groups (80). Similarly, the Mediterranean Alpha-Linolenic Enriched Groningen Dietary Intervention (MARGARIN) examined 282 subjects with multiple CVD risk factors and randomized them to receive margarines rich in either α-linolenic acid or linoleic acid. Follow-up was for 2 yr. There was no difference among groups in CHD risk, although there was a trend toward reduced CVD events in the α-linolenic acid group (p = 0.20) (81).

These contradictory studies indicate that further well-designed trials must be carried out to determine the role of α-linolenic acid in CVD etiology. Currently, the effects of plant vs marine n-3 PUFAs is difficult to determine as few, if any, studies have set out to test this. For example, a meta-analysis of the available RCTs examined all intervention trials whether they used marine or plant sources of n-3 PUFAs and found significant reductions in risk of nonfatal MI, fatal MI, and sudden death, but did not distinguish between the two sources of n-3 PUFAs (44).

5. FISH AND FISH-OIL INTAKE: RECOMMENDATIONS FOR HEALTH

The mean current daily intake of EPA and DHA combined in a typical North American diet (which includes about one fish serving every 10 d) approaches 130 mg/d, which is about 0.15% of total dietary fat intake. This is markedly lower than Japanese intakes and only a small fraction of the EPA and DHA consumed by the Greenland Inuit. Fish consumed 2.5–3 times per week would provide an EPA + DHA intake of about 500 mg/d, an intake about four times that currently consumed in North America. Epidemiological data from the MRFIT study in the United States have indicated that progressively higher intakes of fish-derived n-3 PUFAs (up to about 665 mg/d) during 10.5 yr were associated with a reduction in CHD mortality, as well as total mortality. A National Institutes of Health workshop in 1999 resulted in the recommendation of a combined average EPA + DHA intake of 650 mg/d for healthy adults. The American Heart Association (AHA) guidelines include the following recommendations with respect to n-3 PUFAs in patients with CHD (23):

> Consumption of one fatty fish meal per day (or alternatively, a fish-oil supplement) could result in an n-3 PUFA intake of around 900 mg/d, an amount shown to beneficially affect CHD mortality rates in patients with coronary disease.

Current mean intake in adults of EPA + DHA are far below these targets (i.e., about 20% of 650 mg/d or 14% of 900 mg/d). For healthy adults, the AHA recommends eating fish, particularly fatty fish, at least twice a week (23). Furthermore, in hypertriglyceridemic patients, the AHA suggests that an EPA + DHA supplement may be useful. These recommendations are summarized in Table 2.

In the United Kingdom, the 1991 COMA report made recommendations for essential fatty acid intake (linoleic and α-linolenic acids), but only on the basis of prevention of EFA deficiency, and did not divide the recommendations into n-6 and n-3 subgroups (82). Since then, however, COMA has published recommendations on nutritional aspects of CVD (83). In this publication they recommended no further increase in average intakes of n-6 PUFA, but an increase in the population average consumption of n-3 PUFA from about 100 mg/d to about 200 mg/d (1.5 g/wk) (83).

6. SAFETY AND SIDE-EFFECTS OF n-3 PUFA SUPPLEMENTS

Although the ratio of n-6 to n-3 fatty acid intake of early humans is estimated to have been about 1:1 (84), the ratio in the United States is now around 10:1 owing to both the reduction in n-3 fatty acid intake and the increase in use of vegetable oils rich in linoleic-acid (23). The Food and Drug Administration (FDA) has ruled that intakes of up to 3 g/d

Table 2
Summary of AHA Recommendations for n-3 PUFA Intake
in Different Population and Patient Groups

Population	Recommendation
Patients without documented CHD	Eat a variety of (preferably oily) fish at least twice a week. Include oils and foods rich in α-linolenic acid (flaxseed, canola, and soybean oils; flaxseed and walnuts).
Patients with documented CHD	Consume ~1 g/d of EPA + DHA, preferably from oily fish. EPA + DHA supplements could be considered in consultation with the physician.
Hypertriglyceridemic patients	2–4 g/d of EPA + DHA provided as capsules under a physician's care.

AHA, American Heart Association; PUFA, polyunsaturated fatty acid; CHD, coronary heart disease; EPA, eicosapentaenoic acid; DHA, docosahexaenoic acid.

of marine n-3 PUFAs are generally recognized as safe *(23)*. The FDA has also approved a qualified health claim for EPA and DHA in dietary supplements *(23)*.

Some side effects of n-3 fatty acid supplementation can occur *(85)*, with the most common complaint being reports of a fishy aftertaste. In the GISSI-P intervention study, which provided 0.85 g of n-3 PUFAs daily for 3.5 yr, 3.8% of subjects in the n-3 PUFA arm reported discontinuing their supplements because of side effects, compared with 2.1% in the vitamin E group. The most commonly reported side effects were gastrointestinal upset and nausea *(32)*.

High doses of n-3 PUFAs seem to modestly prolong skin bleeding time, and may also increase the tendency for nosebleeds *(61)*. However, a daily intake of 3 g/d or less of EPA + DHA does not appear to appreciably increase bleeding time. Similarly, in the clinical trials using more than 3 g/d, no clinically significant bleeding has been reported.

Although n-3 PUFAs are known to reduce triglycerides, they can also increase LDL cholesterol. Harris reported that around 4 g/d of n-3 PUFAs from fish oil increases LDL cholesterol by 5–10% *(87)*. There is also a suggestion that consumption of n-3 PUFAs may be associated with a higher susceptibility to in vitro oxidation of LDL *(88,89)*, although this remains to be confirmed *(90–92)*. However, it is likely that the established beneficial effects of n-3 PUFAs on other cardiovascular risk factors far outweigh their effects on either LDL-cholesterol or its oxidizability.

7. FISH: SAFETY ISSUES

There have been recent safety concerns about the levels of environmental contaminants in fish. Some species of fish may contain significant levels of methylmercury, polychlorinated biphenyls, dioxins, and other potentially toxic chemicals. Although these compounds are present at low levels in both fresh and sea water, they bioconcentrate in the aquatic food chain such that levels may be significant in larger predatory fish and marine mammals.

Fish and seafood are a major source of human exposure to these environmental contaminants. Polychlorinated biphenyls and methylmercury have long half-lives and can accumulate in people who regularly consume contaminated fish.

In the United States, the Environmental Protection Agency regulates sport-caught fish, whereas the FDA regulates all commercial fish. The Environmental Protection Agency recommends that women who are pregnant or may become pregnant, and nursing mothers should limit their consumption of fish to one 6-oz (170 g) meal per week *(23)*. They also recommend that young children consume 2 oz or less (60 g) of fish per week. The FDA recommends that pregnant women, nursing mothers, and young children eliminate shark, swordfish, king mackerel, and tilefish (also known as golden bass or golden snapper) from their diet completely and limit other fish consumption to 12 oz/wk (340 g or three to four servings/wk) to minimize methylmercury exposure *(23)*. The FDA also recommends that for adults other than pregnant women or those who may become pregnant, the maximum intake should be less than 7 oz/wk (200 g) of fish with very high (around 1 ppm) methylmercury levels (as listed previously) and less than 14 oz/wk (400 g) of fish with high (around 0.5 ppm) methylmercury levels (fresh tuna, marlin, red snapper).

In the United Kingdom, the Food Standards Agency has advised pregnant and breastfeeding women, and women who intend to become pregnant, to limit their consumption of tuna to no more than two medium-size cans or one fresh tuna steak per week. These women were also advised to avoid eating shark, swordfish, and marlin. For children, the Food Standards Agency advises that children under 16 should avoid shark, marlin, and swordfish, but they can still eat tuna *(93)*.

In summary, for adults excluding pregnant women or those who may become pregnant, the benefits of fish consumption within the amounts recommended far outweigh the risks imposed by environmental contaminants. Consumption of a wide variety of species within the guidelines of the particular country is the best approach to minimizing mercury exposure and increasing n-3 PUFA intake.

8. OTHER DISEASES

8.1. Cancer

Recent reviews of the evidence have concluded that an increase in the consumption of fish may contribute to lower risk of colorectal, prostate, and breast cancer *(94,95)*. EPA and DHA have consistently been shown to inhibit the proliferation of breast and prostate cancer cell lines in vitro and to reduce both the risk and progression of these tumors in animal models *(94)*. A series of case–control studies in Italy and Switzerland also appear to support a role for n-3 PUFAs in the reduction of cancer risk *(96)*. However, further well-designed epidemiological studies are required before definitive conclusions can be reached. Multiple mechanisms would appear to be involved in any chemopreventive activity of n-3 fatty acids, including suppression of neoplastic transformation, cell growth inhibition, enhanced apoptosis, and anti-angiogenesis *(95)*.

8.2. Alzheimer's Disease

Epidemiological investigation of dietary n-3 PUFAs and Alzheimer's disease is limited *(97)*. One case–control study reported that n-3 PUFA levels in plasma phospholipids of Alzheimer's patients were 60–70% of those found in age-matched control subjects

(98). Two prospective studies have found that fish consumption is inversely associated with risk of incident Alzheimer's disease *(99,100)*. A recent study adds to this evidence of an association. In a prospective study of Alzheimer's disease in a biracial community in Chicago, it was found that subjects who ate fish once a week or more had a 60% lower risk of developing Alzheimer's disease compared with those who never or rarely ate fish in a model adjusted for age and other risk factors *(101)*. Total intake of n-3 PUFAs was also associated with reduced risk of Alzheimer's disease *(101)*.

8.3. Rheumatoid Arthritis

Rheumatoid arthritis (RA) is a debilitating disease and is associated with increased risk of CVD and osteoporosis. Poor nutrient status in RA patients has been reported, and some drug therapies, such as nonsteroidal anti-inflammatory drugs, prescribed to alleviate RA symptoms, may increase the requirement for nutrients because of reduced absorption*(102)*. Supplementation with n-3 PUFAs has consistently been shown to improve RA symptoms and to lead to a reduction in nonsteroidal anti-inflammatory drug usage *(102,103)*.

8.4. Diabetes

One study has suggested an adverse effect of n-3 PUFAs on glycemic control in diabetes *(104)*. However, a Cochrane review has examined the effect of fish-oil supplementation in people with type 2 diabetes mellitus *(105)*. Eighteen randomized, placebo-controlled trials, including 823 participants followed for a mean of 12 wk, were included. The reviewers concluded that fish-oil supplementation in type 2 diabetes lowers triglycerides, may raise LDL cholesterol (especially in hypertriglyceridemic patients on higher doses of fish oil), and has no statistically significant effect on glycemic control *(105)*. The reviewers also stated that trials with vascular events or mortality-defined end points are needed before definite conclusions can be made. A meta-analysis of 26 trials of subjects with type 1 or type 2 diabetes confirmed that fish oil has no effect on hemoglobin A_{1C}, although fasting glucose levels rose slightly in the type 2 diabetics *(106)*. A high consumption of fish and fish oils has been associated with a lower CHD incidence and total mortality among diabetic women *(107)*. Based on these data, the FDA has concluded that an intake of 3 g/d or less is safe with respect to glycemic control.

9. CONCLUSIONS

Evidence from epidemiological studies and clinical trials suggests that n-3 fatty acids protect against CHD and sudden cardiac death. Primary prevention trials are currently underway, and although the outcome of these is awaited, it would seem safe to follow the recommendations of the AHA regarding intake. Clinical trials are still required in high risk groups, such as patients with type 2 diabetes, dyslipidemia, and hypertension, and those with congestive heart failure, who are at high risk of sudden death, to ascertain the benefits of n-3 fatty acids in these patients. Fish-oil supplements would appear to be safe, whereas the benefits of fish consumption within recommended amounts outweigh the risk owing to environmental contaminants (excluding children and pregnant women for whom special recommendations apply). Fish and fish-oil consumption may also protect against a variety of other diseases including cancer and Alzheimer's disease.

REFERENCES

1. Ross R. The pathogenesis of atherosclerosis in a perspective for the 1990s. Nature 1993; 362:801–809.
2. Heller RF, Chinn S, Tunstall-Pedoe H, Rose G. How well can we predict coronary heart disease? Findings in the United Kingdom Heart Disease Prevention Project. Br Med J 1984; 288:1409–1411.
3. Mann JI. Diet and risk of coronary heart disease and type 2 diabetes. Lancet 2002; 360:783–789.
4. Dyerberg J, Bang HO. Haemostatic function and platelet polyunsaturated fatty acids in Eskimos. Lancet 1979; 2:433–435.
5. Emken EA, Adlof RO, Gulley RM. Dietary linoleic acid influences desaturation and acylation of deuterium-labelled linoleic and linolenic acids in young adult males. Biochim Biophys Acta 1994; 1213:277–288.
6. Pawlosky RJ, Hibbeln JR, Novotny JA, Salem N Jr. Physiological compartmental analysis of alpha-linolenic acid metabolism in adult humans. J Lipid Res 2001; 42:1257–1265.
7. Ministry of Agriculture, Fisheries and Food. Fatty acids. Seventh supplement to the Fifth Edition of McCance and Widdowson's The Composition of Foods. HMSO, London, 1998.
8. Kromhout D, Bosschieter EB, de Lezenne Coulander C. The inverse relation between fish consumption and 20-year mortality from coronary heart disease. N Engl J Med 1985; 312:1205–1209.
9. Kromhout D, Feskens EJ, Bowles CH. The protective effect of a small amount of fish on coronary heart disease mortality in an elderly population. Int J Epidemiol 1995; 24:340–345.
10. Shekelle RB, Missell L, Paul O, Shryock AM, Stamler J. Fish consumption and mortality from coronary heart disease. N Engl J Med 1985; 313: 820.
11. Dolecek TA, Granditis G. Dietary polyunsaturated fatty acids and mortality in the Multiple Risk Factor Intervention Trial (MRFIT). World Rev Nutr Diet 1991; 66:205–216.
12. Daviglus ML, Stamler J, Orencia AJ, et al. Fish consumption and the 30-year risk of fatal myocardial infarction. N Engl J Med 1997; 336:1046–1053.
13. Lemaitre RN, King IB, Mozaffarian D, Kuller LH, Tracy RP, Siscovick DS. N-3 polyunsaturated fatty acids, fatal ischemic disease, and nonfatal myocardial infarction in older adults: the Cardiovascular Health Study. Am J Clin Nutr 2003; 77:319–325.
14. Marckmann P, Gronbaek M. Fish consumption and coronary heart disease mortality: a systematic review of prospective cohort studies. Eur J Clin Nutr 1999; 53:585–590.
15. Whelton SP, He J, Whelton PK, Muntner P. Meta-analysis of observational studies on fish intake and coronary heart disease. Am J Cardiol 2004; 93:1119–1123.
16. Zhang J, Sasaki S, Amano K, Kestelot H. Fish consumption and mortality from all causes, ischemic heart disease, and stroke: an ecological study. Prev Med 1999; 28:520–529.
17. Guallar E, Aro A, Jimenez FJ, et al. Omega-3 fatty acids in adipose tissue and risk of myocardial infarction: the EURAMIC study. Arterioscler Thromb Vasc Biol 1999; 19:1111–1118.
18. Erkkila AT, Lehto S, Pyorala K, Uusitupa MI. n-3 Fatty acids and 5-y risks of death and cardiovascular disease events in patients with coronary artery disease. Am J Clin Nutr 2003; 78:65–71.
19. Ascherio A, Rimm EB, Stampfer MJ, Giovannucci EL, Willett WC. Dietary intake of marine n-3 fatty acids, fish intake, and the risk of coronary heart disease among men. N Engl J Med 1995; 332:977–982.
20. Albert CM, Hennekens CH, O'Donnell CJ, et al. Fish consumption and risk of sudden cardiac death. JAMA 1998; 279:23–28.
21. Kromhout D, Bloemberg BP, Feskens EJ, Hertog MG, Menotti A, Blackburn H. Alcohol, fish, fibre and antioxidant vitamin intake do not explain population differences in coronary heart disease mortality. Int J Epidemiol 1996; 25:753–759.
22. Pietinen P, Ascherio A, Korhonen P, et al. Intake of fatty acids and risk of coronary heart disease in a cohort of Finnish men: the Alpha-Tocopherol, Beta-Carotene Cancer Prevention Study. Am J Epidemiol 1997; 145:876–887.
23. Kris-Etherton PM, Harris WS, Appel LJ, for the Nutrition Committee. Fish consumption, fish oil, omega-3 fatty acids, and cardiovascular disease. Circulation 2002; 106:2747–2757.
24. Kromhout D. Fish consumption and sudden cardiac death. JAMA 1998;279:65-66.
25. Sheard NF. Fish consumption and risk of sudden cardiac death. Nutr Rev 1998; 56:177–179.
26. Oomen CM, Feskens EJ, Rasanen L, et al. Fish consumption and coronary heart disease mortality in Finland, Italy and the Netherlands. Am J Epidemiol 2000; 151:999–1006.

27. Salonen JT, Seppanen K, Lakka TA, Salonen R, Kaplan GA. Mercury accumulation and accelerated progression of carotid atherosclerosis: a population-based prospective 4-year follow-up study in men in eastern Finland. Atherosclerosis 2000; 148:265–273.

28. Ahlqwist M, Bengtsson C, Lapidus L, Gergdahl IA, Schutz A. Serum mercury concentration in relation to survival, symptoms, and diseases: results from the prospective population study of women in Gothenburg, Sweden. Acta Odontol Scand 1999; 57:168–174.

29. Burr ML, Fehily AM, Gilbert JF, et al. Effects of changes in fat, fish, and fibre intakes on death and myocardial reinfarction: diet and reinfarction trial (DART). Lancet 1989; 2:757–761.

30. Burr ML, Sweetnam PM, Fehily AM. Diet and reinfarction. Eur Heart J 1994; 15:1152, 1153.

31. Singh RB, Niaz MA, Sharma JP, Kumar R, Rastogi V, Moshiri M. Randomised, double-blind, placebo-controlled trial of fish oil and mustard oil in patients with suspected acute myocardial infarction: the Indian experiment of infarct survival-4. Cardiovasc Drugs Ther 1997; 11:485–491.

32. GISSI-Prevenzione Investigators. Dietary supplementation with n-3 polyunsaturated fatty acids and vitamin E after myocardial infarction: results of the GISSI-Prevenzione trial. Gruppo Italiano per lo Studio della Sopravvivenza nell'Infarcto miocardico. Lancet 1999; 354:447–455.

33. Nilsen DW, Albrektsen G, Landmark K, Moen S, Aarsland T, Woie L. Effects of a high dose concentrate of n-3 fatty acids or corn oil introduced early after an acute myocardial infarction on serum triacylglycerol and HDL cholesterol. Am J Clin Nutr 2001; 74:50–56.

34. Sacks FM, Stone PH, Gibson CM, Silverman DI, Rosner B, Pasternak RC. Controlled trial of fish oil for regression of human coronary atherosclerosis. HARP Research Group. J Am Coll Cardiol 1995; 25:1492–1498.

35. von Schacky C, Angerer P, Kothny W, Theisen K, Mudra H. The effect of dietary omega-3 fatty acids on coronary atherosclerosis: a randomised, double-blind, placebo-controlled trial. Ann Intern Med 1999; 130:554–562.

36. Eritsland J, Arnesen H, Gronseth K, Fjeld NB, Abdelnoor M. Effect of dietary supplementation with n-3 fatty acids on coronary artery bypass graft patency. Am J Cardiol 1996; 77:31–36.

37. Gapinski JP, VanRuiswyk JV, Heudebert GR, Schectman GS. Preventing restenosis with fish oils following coronary angioplasty: a meta-analysis. Arch Intern Med 1993; 153:1595–1601.

38. Cairns JA, Gill J, Morton B, et al. Fish oils and low-molecular weight heparin for the reduction of restenosis after percutaneous transluminal coronary angioplasty. The EMPAR Study. Circulation 1996; 94:1553–1560.

39. Johansen O, Seljeflot I, Hostmark AT, Arnesen H. The effect of supplementation with omega-3 fatty acids on soluble markers of endothelial function in patients with coronary heart disease. Arterioscler Thromb Vasc Biol 1999; 19:1681–1686.

40. Albert CM, Campos H, Stampfer MJ, et al. Blood levels of long-chain n-3 fatty acids and the risk of sudden death. N Engl J Med 2002; 346:1113–1118.

41. Siscovick DS, Raghunathan TE, King I, et al. Dietary intake and cell membrane levels of long-chain n-3 polyunsaturated fatty acids and the risk of primary cardiac arrest. JAMA 1995; 274:1363–1367.

42. Marchioli R, Barzi F, Bomba E, et al. Early protection against sudden death by n-3 polyunsaturated fatty acids after myocardial infarction: time course analysis of the results of the GISSI-Prevenzione. Circulation 2002; 105:1897–1903.

43. Leaf A, Kang JX, Xiao Y-F, Billman GE. Clinical prevention of sudden cardiac death by n-3 polyunsaturated fatty acids and mechanism of prevention of arrhythmias by n-3 fish oils. Circulation 2003; 107:2646–2652.

44. Bucher HC, Hengstler P, Schindler C, Meier G. n-3 polyunsaturated fatty acids in coronary heart disease: a meta-analysis of randomised controlled trials. Am J Med 2002; 112:298–304.

45. Skerrett PJ, Hennekens CH. Consumption of fish and fish oils and decreased risk of stroke. Prev Cardiol 2003; 6:38–41.

46. Orencia AJ, Daviglus ML, Dyer AR, Shekelle RB, Stamler J. Fish consumption and stroke in men: 30-year findings of the Chicago Western Electric Study. Stroke 1996; 27:204–209.

47. Morris MC, Manson JE, Rosner B, Buring JE, Willett WC, Hennekens CH. Fish consumption and cardiovascular disease in the Physicians' Health Study: a prospective study. Am J Epidemiol 1995; 142:166–175.

48. Iso H, Rexrode KM, Stampfer MJ, et al. Intake of fish and omega-3 fatty acids and risk of stroke in women. JAMA 2001; 285:304–312.

49. Keli SO, Feskens EJ, Kromhout D. Fish consumption and risk of stroke: the Zutphen Study. Stroke 1994; 25:328–332.

50. Gillum RF, Mussolino ME, Madans JH. The relationship between fish consumption and stroke incidence: the NHANES I Epidemiologic Follow-up Study. Arch Intern Med 1996; 156:537–542.

51. He K, Rimm EB, Merchant A, et al. Fish consumption and risk of stroke in men. JAMA 2002; 288:3130–3136.

52. de Lorgeril M, Salen P, Martin JL, Monjaud I, Delaye J, Mamelle N. Mediterranean diet, traditional risk factors, and the rate of cardiovascular complications after myocardial infarction. Final report of the Lyon Diet Heart Study. Circulation 1999; 99:779–785.

53. Mizushima S, Moriguchi EH, Ishikawa P, et al. Fish intake and cardiovascular risk among middle-aged Japanese in Japan and Brazil. J Cardiovasc Risk 1997; 4:191–199.

54. Charnock JS. Lipids and cardiac arrhythmia. Prog Lipid Res 1994; 33:355–385.

55. Nair SSD, Leitch JW, Falconer J, Garg ML. Prevention of cardiac arrhythmia by dietary (n-3) polyunsaturated fatty acids and their mechanism of action. J Nutr 1997; 127:383–393.

56. Lee KW, Lip GYH. The role of omega-3 fatty acids in the secondary prevention of cardiovascular disease. Q J Med 2003; 96:465–480.

57. Harris WS, Connor WE, Alam N, Illingworth DR. Reduction of postprandial triglyceridaemia in humans by dietary n-3 fatty acids. J Lipid Res 1988; 29:1451–1460.

58. Grimsgaard S, Bonaa KH, Hansen JB, Nordoy A. Highly purified eicosapentaenoic acid and docosahexaenoic acid in humans have similar triacylglycerol-lowering effects but divergent effects on serum fatty acids. Am J Clin Nutr 1997; 66:649–659.

59. Howe PR. Dietary fats and hypertension: focus on fish oil. Ann NY Acad Sci 1997; 827:339–352.

60. Morris MC, Sacks F, Rosner B. Does fish oil lower blood pressure? A meta-analysis of controlled trials. Circulation 1993; 88:523–533.

61. De Deckere EAM. Health effects of fish and n-3 polyunsaturated fatty acids from plant and marine origin. In: Wilson T, Temple NJ, eds. Nutritional Health: Strategies for Disease Prevention. Humana Press, Totowa, NJ, 2001, pp. 195–206.

62. Agren JJ, Vaisanen S, Hanninen O, Muller AD, Hornstra G. Hemostatic factors and platelet aggregation after a fish-enriched diet or fish oil or docosahexaenoic acid supplementation. Prostaglandins Leukot Essent Fatty Acids 1997; 57:419–421.

63. Mori TA, Beilin LJ, Burke V, Morris J, Ritchie J. Interactions between dietary fat, fish and fish oils and their effects on platelet function in men at risk of cardiovascular disease. Arterioscler Thromb Vasc Biol 1997; 17:279–286.

64. Shahar E, Folsom AR, Wu KK, et al. Associations of fish intake and dietary n-3 polyunsaturated fatty acids with a hypocoagulable profile. The Atherosclerosis Risk in Communities (ARIC) Study. Arterioscler Thromb 1993; 13:1205–1212.

65. Archer SL, Green D, Chamberlain M, Dyer AR, Liu K. Association of dietary fish and n-3 fatty acid intake with hemostatic factors in the coronary artery risk development in young adults (CARDIA) Study. Arterioscler Thromb Vasc Biol 1998; 18:1119–1123.

66. Johansen O, Brekke M, Seljeflot I, Abdelnoor M, Arnesen H. N-3 fatty acids do not prevent restenosis after coronary angioplasty: results from the CART study. Coronary Angioplasty Restenosis Trial. J Am Coll Cardiol 1999; 33:1619–1626.

67. Marckmann P, Bladbjerg EM, Jespersen J. Dietary fish oil (4 g daily) and cardiovascular risk markers in healthy men. Arterioscler Thromb Vasc Biol 1997; 17:3384–3391.

68. Abe Y, El-Masri B, Kimball KT, et al. Soluble cell adhesion molecules in hypertriglyceridaemia and potential significance on monocyte adhesion. Arterioscler Thromb Vasc Biol 1998; 18:723–731.

69. Seljeflot I, Arnesen H, Brude IR, Nenseter MS, Drevon CA, Hjermann I. Effects of omega-3 fatty acids and/or antioxidants on endothelial cell markers. Eur J Clin Invest 1998; 28:629–635.

70. Chin JP, Dart AM. How do fish oils affect vascular function? Clin Exp Pharmacol Physiol 1995; 22:71–81.

71. McVeigh GE, Brennan GM, Cohn JN, Finkelstein SM, Hayes RJ, Johnston GD. Fish oil improves arterial compliance in non-insulin-dependent diabetes mellitus. Arterioscler Thromb 1994; 14:1425–1429.

72. De Caterina R, Libby P. Control of endothelial leukocyte adhesion molecules by fatty acids. Lipids 1996; 31:S57–S63.

73. De Caterina R, Liao JK, Libby P. Fatty acid modulation of endothelial activation. Am J Clin Nutr 2000; 71:213S–223S.

74. Endres S, von Schacky C. n-3 Polyunsaturated fatty acids and human cytokine synthesis. Curr Opin Lipidol 1996; 7:48–52.

75. Trebble TM, Wootton SA, Miles EA, et al. Prostaglandin E_2 production and T cell function after fish-oil supplementation: response to antioxidant cosupplementation. Am J Clin Nutr 2003; 78:376–382.

76. Simopoulos AP. Omega-3 fatty acids in inflammation and autoimmune disease. J Am Coll Nutr 2002; 21:495–505.

77. Thies F, Garry JMC, Yaqoob P, et al. Association of n-3 polyunsaturated fatty acids with stability of atherosclerotic plaques: a randomized controlled trial. Lancet 2003; 361:477–485.

78. Djousse L, Folsom AR, Province MA, Hunt SC, Ellison RC. Dietary linolenic acid and carotid athero-sclerosis: the National Heart, Lung and Blood Institute Family Heart Study. Am J Clin Nutr 2003; 77:819–825.

79. de Lorgeril M, Renaud S, Mamelle N, et al. Mediterranean alpha-linolenic acid-rich diet in secondary prevention of coronary heart disease. Lancet 1994; 343:1454–1459.

80. Natvig H, Borchgrevink CF, Dedichen J, Owren PA, Schiotz EH, Westlund K. A controlled trial of the effect of linolenic acid on the incidence of coronary heart disease. Scand J Clin Lab Med 1968; 105:S1–S20.

81. Bemelmans WJ, Broer J, Feskens EJ, et al. Effect of an increased intake of alpha-linolenic acid and group nutritional education on cardiovascular risk factors: the Mediterranean Alpha-linolenic Enriched Groningen Dietary Intervention (MARGARIN) study. Am J Clin Nutr 2002; 75:221–227.

82. Committee on Medical Aspects of Food Policy. Dietary reference values for food energy and nutrients for the United Kingdom. Report of the Panel on Dietary Reference Values. Report on Health and Social Subjects No 41. HMSO, London, 1991.

83. Committee on Medical Aspects of Food Policy. Nutritional aspects of cardiovascular disease. Report on Health and Social Subjects No 46. HMSO, London, 1994.

84. Simopoulos AP. Evolutionary aspects of omega-3 fatty acids in the food supply. Prostaglandins Leukot Essent Fatty Acids 1999; 60:421–429.

85. Harris WS, Ginsberg HN, Arunakul N, et al. Safety and efficacy of Omacor in severe hyper-triglyceridaemia. J Cardiovasc Risk 1997; 4:385–391.

86. Lox CD. The effects of dietary marine oils (omega-3 fatty acids) on coagulation profiles in men. Gen Pharmacol 1990; 21:241–246.

87. Harris WS. N-3 fatty acids and serum lipoproteins: human studies. Am J Clin Nutr 1997; 65:1645S–1654S.

88. Hau MF, Smelt AH, Bindels AJ, et al. Effects of fish oil on oxidation resistance of VLDL in hyper-triglyceridemic patients. Arterioscler Thromb Vasc Biol 1996; 16:1197–1202.

89. Sorensen NS, Marckmann P, Hoy CE, van Duyvenvoorde W, Princen HM. Effect of fish-oil-enriched margarine on plasma lipids, low-density-lipoprotein particle composition, size, and susceptibility to oxidation. Am J Clin Nutr 1998; 68:235–241.

90. Brude IR, Drevon CA, Hjermann I, et al. Peroxidation of LDL from combined-hyperlipidemic male smokers supplied with omega-3 fatty acids and antioxidants. Arterioscler Thromb Vasc Biol 1997; 17:2576–2588.

91. Bonanome A, Biasia F, De Luca M, et al. n-3 Fatty acids do not enhance LDL susceptibility to oxidation in hypertriacylglycerolemic hemodialyzed subjects. Am J Clin Nutr 1996; 63:261–266.

92. Higdon JV, Du SH, Lee YS, Wu T, Wander RC. Supplementation of postmenopausal women with fish oil does not increase overall oxidation of LDL ex vivo compared to dietary oils rich in oleate and linoleate. J Lipid Res 2001; 42:407–418.

93. Food Standards Agency, Dietary recommendations for fish and shellfish. Available at: http://www.food standards.gov.uk/news/newsarchive/2004/jun/fishreport2004. Accessed July 2, 2004.

94. Terry PD, Rohan TE, Wolk A. Intakes of fish and marine fatty acids and the risks of cancers of the breast and prostate and of other hormone-related cancers: a review of the epidemiologic evidence. Am J Clin Nutr 2003; 77:532–543.

 95. Rose DP, Connolly JM. Omega-3 fatty acids as cancer chemopreventive agents. Pharmacol Therapeut 1999; 83:217–244.

 96. Tavani A, Pelucchi C, Parpinel M, Negri, et al. n-3 Polyunsaturated fatty acid intake and cancer risk in Italy and Switzerland. Int J Cancer 2003; 105:113–116.

 97. Friedland RP. Fish consumption and the risk of Alzheimer disease. Is it time to make dietary recommendations? Arch Neurol 2003; 60:923, 924.

 98. Conquer JA, Tierney MC, Zecevic J, Bettger WJ, Fisher RH. Fatty acid analysis of blood plasma of patients with Alzheimer's disease, other types of dementia, and cognitive impairment. Lipids 2000; 35:1305–1312.

 99. Barberger-Gateau P, Letenneur L, Deschamps V, Peres K, Dartigues JF, Renaud S. Fish, meat, and risk of dementia: cohort study. BMJ 2002; 325:932, 933.

100. Kalmijn S, Launer LJ, Ott A, Witteman JC, Hofman A, Breteler MM. Dietary fat intake and the risk of incident dementia in the Rotterdam Study. Ann Neurol 1997; 42:776–782.

101. Morris MC, Evans DA, Bienias J, et al. Consumption of fish and n-3 fatty acids and risk of incident Alzheimer disease. Arch Neurol 2003; 60:940–946.

102. Rennie KL, Hughes J, Lang R, Jebb SA. Nutritional management of rheumatoid arthritis: a review of the evidence. J Hum Nutr Diet 2003; 16:97–109.

103. Cleland LG, James MJ, Proudman SM. The role of fish oils in the treatment of rheumatoid arthritis. Drugs 2003; 63:845–853.

104. Vessby B, Karlsrom B, Boberg M, Lithell H, Berne C. Polyunsaturated fatty acids may impair blood glucose control in type 2 diabetic patients. Diabet Med 1992; 9:126–133.

105. Farmer A, Montori V, Dinneen S, Clar C. Fish oil in people with type 2 diabetes mellitus. Cochrane Database Syst Rev 2001; 3:CD003205.

106. Friedberg CE, Janssen MJ, Heine RJ, Grobbee DE. Fish oil and glycemic control in diabetes. A meta-analysis. Diabetes Care 1998; 21:494–500.

107. Hu FB, Cho E, Rexrode KM, Albert CM, Manson JE. Fish and long-chain omega-3 fatty acid intake and risk of coronary heart disease and total mortality in diabetic women. Circulation 2003; 107:1852–1857.

9   Diet and Cancer Prevention

Cindy D. Davis and John A. Milner

KEY POINTS

- Overweight (body mass index [BMI] >25 kg/m^2) and obesity (BMI >30 kg/m^2) are associated with increased risk for many of the most common cancers.
- Epidemiological and preclinical (animal and cell culture) studies indicate that increased consumption of fruits, vegetables, and whole grains is associated with reduced cancer risk.
- Alcohol consumption has been associated with an increased risk of some cancers.
- Many bioactive food components can simultaneously influence multiple sites involved in the cancer process.
- Not all individuals should be expected to respond identically to bioactive food components because of genetic and environmental factors.
- Variation in the response to foods likely depends on the "omics" of nutrition.

1. INTRODUCTION

"Cancer" is a general term that represents many diseases, each with their own etiology; it arises from both genetic and environmental factors including dietary habits. The process starts as multiple genetic changes within a cell, which, unless controlled or reversed, ultimately evolve into "cancer." The importance of this uncontrolled cellular division is illustrated by the fact that cancer is the second leading cause of death in the United States and is expected to become the leading cause of death within the next decade (1). The cancer process, which can occur over decades, includes wide ranging cellular events that can be influenced by diet, such as carcinogen bioactivation, cellular differentiation, DNA repair, cellular proliferation/signaling, and apoptosis. Recently, Hanahan and Weinberg (2) identified six critical elements for cancer: self-sufficiency in growth signals, insensitivity to antigrowth signals, tissue invasion and metastasis, limitless replication potential, sustained angiogenesis, and evading apoptosis. Each of these "elements" can be modified by dietary components (see Fig. 1).

Guidance aimed at promoting and encouraging diet-related behaviors for reducing cancer risk has been formulated by various organizations. The National Cancer Institute is continually sharing knowledge about risk factors associated with cancer, including

From: *Nutritional Health: Strategies for Disease Prevention, Second Edition*
Edited by: N. J. Temple, T. Wilson, and D. R. Jacobs © Humana Press Inc., Totowa, NJ

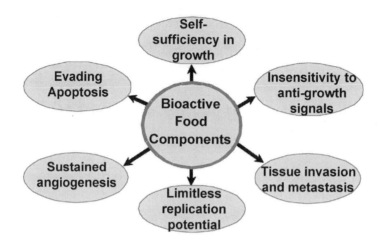

Fig. 1. Bioactive food components can modify the six critical elements for cancer. Targets are those identified as critical for cancer development by Hanahan and Weinberg. (From ref. *2.*)

diet, as it emerges (http://www.nci.nih.gov). Modifying dietary behaviors and nutritional habits based on current guidelines represents a proactive, practical, and cost-effective approach to cancer prevention that is also likely to promote overall good health. This chapter provides a synopsis of several areas that are germane to dietary components and cancer prevention.

2. DIETARY FAT

The epidemiological evidence suggesting a relationship between fat intake and cancer risk remains equivocal. Although geographic correlation studies and migrant studies, as well as some preclinical (animal and cell culture) studies, have demonstrated an association between per capita fat intake and breast, colon, and prostate cancers *(3,4)*, case–control and cohort studies have not always supported this relationship. Such variation in observations suggests that several factors may be intertwined, including absolute quantity and types of specific fatty acids consumed, and interactions among various dietary components and genetics.

Migrant studies generally support an increased risk for breast cancer as eating patterns shift from a low-fat, high-fiber diet to a high-fat, low-fiber "Western" diet *(5)*. Although these observations point to environmental or lifestyle factors, attribution of differences in breast cancer rates to dietary fat intake is tenuous based on these data alone *(4)*. The potential of known or suspected breast cancer risk factors to confound dietary associations is well recognized. For example, compared with countries with lower per capita fat intake, countries that tend to have higher per capita fat intake also tend to have lower age at menarche, later age at first birth, lower parity, and higher postmenopausal body weight. Some have suggested that much of the international variation in breast cancer risk and the proportion that is mediated by diet may be explained by nondietary risk factors *(4)*.

Case–control and cohort studies have not provided compelling evidence for an association between fat intake and breast cancer incidence. One meta-analysis of case-control studies found a relative risk of 1.21 for breast cancer, based on fat intake *(6)*. However, two separate meta-analyses of cohort studies reported relative risks of only 1.01 *(6)* and 1.05 *(7)*. More recently, a prospective analysis among premenopausal women enrolled in the Nurses' Health Study II demonstrated that relative to women in the lowest quintile of fat intake, women in the highest quintile had a slightly increased risk of breast cancer (RR = 1.25) *(8)*. The Women's Intervention Nutrition Study (WINS) also suggests that a low-fat diet protects against breast cancer recurrence *(8a)*.

As with studies involving breast cancer, human migration and animal studies provide some of the strongest evidence for a positive association between dietary fat and colorectal cancer risk *(3,4)*. However, analytic epidemiological studies generally fail to detect a positive association of total fat intake with risk of colorectal cancer *(4)*. A meta-analysis of 13 case–control studies indicated there was essentially no association with intake of total, saturated, monounsaturated, or polyunsaturated fat intakes with risk of colorectal cancer *(9)*. The preponderance of epidemiological evidence suggests that if an association exists, it may be attributable to an association with red meat intake *(4)*.

Similar to breast and colorectal cancer, there is a wide geographic variation in prostate cancer rates *(3,10)*. This likely reflects environmental and/or lifestyle factors. Of the 23 case–control studies that examined the association between total fat and prostate cancer, 13 revealed either a statistically significant relationship (6 studies) or a trend (7 studies) toward significance *(11)*. There have been six cohort studies that specifically analyzed the association between fat intake and the risk of prostate cancer *(11)*. In four of these, total fat intake was positively associated with risk of prostate cancer and the other two studies showed a trend toward significance *(11)*. Thus, case–control and cohort studies generally point to elevated fat intake as a risk factor for prostate cancer.

Overall, research findings suggest that the link between fat and cancer risk depends not only on the quantity, but also on the composition of specific fatty acids. The cancer-related effects of n-6 polyunsaturated fatty acids (PUFAs) (e.g., linoleic acid) vs those of n-3 PUFAs (e.g., α-linolenic acid [ALA], eicosapentanoic acid, and docosahexanoic acid) are of particular interest. Generally, n-6 PUFAs, found in common seed oils, tend to enhance the promotional phase of carcinogenesis in preclinical models for breast, colon, and prostate cancers, whereas n-3 PUFAs, particularly the longer-chain n-3 PUFAs, such as eicosapentanoic acid A and docosahexanoic acid found in fish oil, seem to exert inhibitory effects *(12–16)*. International evidence suggests that diets high in n-6 PUFAs are associated with increased breast cancer risk, whereas consumption of n-3 PUFAs do not increase and may reduce breast cancer risk *(17)*.

In a European multicenter breast cancer study, the ratio of long-chain n-3 PUFAs in adipose tissue to total n-6 PUFAs was inversely related to breast cancer risk, indicating that the balance between n-3 PUFAs and n-6 PUFAs may be important *(18)*. These findings are in agreement with ecological mortality data for breast cancer for 24 European countries that revealed an inverse correlation with fish and fish-oil consumption, when expressed as a proportion of animal fat, and that a high ratio of n-6 to n-3 PUFA in the diet is a risk factor for colon cancer *(12)*. A ratio of 1:1-2:1 (n-6:n-3) seems to be the most protective effect against the development and growth of mammary and colon tumors *(19)*. Recent preclinical studies have also demonstrated that n-3 PUFAs may be able to prevent colon cancer development *(19)*. n-3 PUFAs have been shown to act at different stages of cancer development and through several different mechanisms, including decreasing tumor cell proliferation, enhancing apoptosis, promoting cell differentiation, and limiting angiogenesis *(19,20)*. Nevertheless, a meta-analysis of 10 cohort and case-control studies that reported on the association between ALA and incidence or prevalence of prostate cancer showed an increased risk of prostate cancer in men with a high intake or blood level of ALA (RR = 1.6) *(13)*.

Other types of fatty acids may also influence cancer risk. Naturally occurring fatty acids are present in foods mainly as *cis* isomers; trans-fatty acids occur largely as a result of partial hydrogenation of vegetable oils, a process used to make oils more solid. Trans-fatty acids have been hypothesized to be carcinogenic *(21)*, although there are limited data in humans testing this hypothesis. The European Community Multicenter Study on Antioxidants, Myocardial Infarction, and Breast Cancer (Euramic) demonstrated a positive association between trans-fatty acids in adipose tissue and the incidence of cancers of the breast and colon, but not of the prostate *(21)*. However, a negative association between trans-fatty acids in adipose tissue and the incidence of metastasis in lymph nodes as a measure of the prognosis of breast cancer was observed *(22)*. Likewise, the impact of trans-fatty acids on colon cancer risk in humans are also inconsistent *(23,24)*. Overall, the effect of trans-fatty acids on cancer is still equivocal, though there are suggestions of a modestly increased risk.

Dairy products and meat from ruminants provide specific types of trans-fatty acids, namely conjugated linoleic acids (CLA). CLA is a collective term describing a mixture of conjugated diene isomers formed as intermediates in the biohydrogenation of linoleic acid by anaerobic bacteria in the rumen of ruminants *(25)*. Experiments have usually shown that CLA inhibits the formation of breast tumors in rats and inhibits the growth of transplantable breast and prostate cancer tumor cells in nude mice *(26)*. In contrast, in the Netherlands Cohort Study on Diet and Cancer, CLA intake showed a weak, positive relation with breast cancer incidence (RR = 1.24 for highest compared with lowest quintile) *(27)*. Further research is needed in humans to determine the relationship between consumption of trans-fatty acids and CLA and cancer susceptibility. Regardless, it is clear that not all trans-fatty acids are equivalent in their ability to modify cancer risk.

Butyrate is a short-chain fatty acid that may originate in foods or arise from the fermentation of dietary carbohydrates. Evidence exists that increased concentrations of it may protect against colorectal cancer *(20)*. Butyrate promotes growth arrest, differentiation, and apoptosis in colon *(28)* and breast cancer cell lines *(29)*. Animal studies have demonstrated that increased colonic butyrate concentrations correlate with a decreased incidence of colon cancer *(30)*, and dietary butyrate inhibits chemically induced mammary cancer in rats *(29)*. The chemopreventive benefits of butyrate depend, in part, on amount, time of exposure with respect to the tumorigenic process, and the type of fat in the diet *(31)*.

3. OBESITY, BODY WEIGHT, AND PHYSICAL ACTIVITY

Almost two-thirds of the US population is now considered either overweight or obese based on the 1999–2000 information from the National Health and Nutrition Examination Survey *(32)*. Both diet and exercise studies are beginning to document the power of lifestyle interventions in this area, as well as the extraordinary challenges in producing behavioral change. Undeniably, the social, behavioral, and biochemical complexities associated with obesity makes it an extremely complicated condition to prevent and/or treat. Nevertheless, recent advances are elucidating the points of intervention in the elaborate network of brain, gut, and fat cell-derived hormones that control appetite and the integrated regulation of metabolism *(33)*.

A comprehensive review by the International Agency on Research on Cancer *(34)* summarized the evidence linking obesity with cancer. Overall, 20–30% of some of the most common cancers in the United States, including prostate, colon, kidney, uterine, and postmenopausal breast, appear to be related to being overweight and/or physical inactivity. Increased mortality from cancers of the esophagus, liver, gallbladder, pancreas, and kidney, non-Hodgkin's lymphoma, and multiple myeloma are also positively related to increased body weight *(35)*. In addition, trends for increasing risk were observed for cancers of the stomach for both sexes and prostate in men, and for breast, uterus, cervix, and ovary in women. Calle et al. *(35)* estimated that overweight and obesity in the United States account for 14% of all cancer deaths in men and 20% in women.

Early in the 20th century, research began to emerge that caloric restriction was an effective strategy for increasing longevity and decreasing the risk of cancer *(36)*. Caloric restriction has several favorable effects on cancer processes including decreased mitogenic response, increased rates of apoptosis, reduced inflammatory response, induction of DNA repair enzymes, altered drug-metabolizing enzyme expression, and modified cell-mediated immune function *(37)*. At least part of these anticancer properties associated with caloric restriction likely involve the insulin-like growth factor (IGF)-1 pathway *(38)*.

The mechanisms by which excess weight may influence cancer risk are unresolved but may relate to homeostasis in the steroid hormones, IGFs, insulin resistance and lipid metabolism, and immune function and inflammatory factors, including cytokines and prostaglandins *(39)*. The identification of which lead to a change in cancer risk and adverse health outcomes in specific populations is fundamental to the development of public health initiatives and to personalized strategies for diet and exercise interventions. The interplay of dietary components with genetic susceptibility can modify the relationship between energy balance and cancer risk (*see* Fig. 2). Technological advances in genomics and posttranslational events (proteomics and metabolomics) hold promise to assist in deciphering the molecular basis by which energy balance influences cancer and identifying appropriate intervention strategies that incorporate personalized risk.

Despite considerable epidemiological evidence linking cancer with obesity and with lack of physical activity, the appropriate level and type of physical activity required to bring about protection remains unclear *(34)*. Although the 2002 Institute of Medicine report suggests that up to 60 min/d may be needed to prevent weight gain, others suggest that 150 min/d or more may be needed for cardiovascular benefit and weight control *(40)*. Additional controlled studies are needed to determine if the amount and duration of exercise needed to prevent obesity and to treat obesity are similar and to clarify the importance of the type of physical activity—moderate intensity or vigorous—that is needed to prevent weight gain and improve health *(41)*.

4. FRUITS, VEGETABLES, AND WHOLE GRAINS

Recommendations to consume larger quantities of fruit, vegetables, and whole grains for protection from chronic diseases, including cancer, come principally from epidemiological investigations and from a variety of animal and cell culture studies. Collectively, epidemiological studies suggest that increased consumption of fruits, vegetables, and

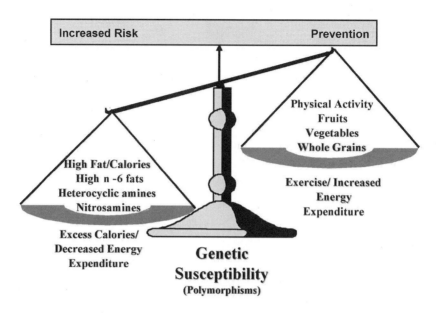

Fig. 2. Dietary components and genetic susceptibility (polymorphisms) can modify the relationship between energy balance and cancer risk.

whole grains may reduce cancer risk, yet it is evident that considerable inconsistencies exist in the literature *(42–44)*.

In 1997 the American Institute for Cancer Research and the World Cancer Research Fund summarized information arising from several hundred case–control and cohort studies *(3)*. They concluded that there is an inverse association between fruit and vegetable intake and numerous cancers. This is clear for cancer of the lung, stomach, colon/ rectum, esophagus, mouth, and pharynx; probable for cancers of the breast, larynx, pancreas, and bladder; and possible for cancers of the cervix, ovary, endometrium, prostate, thyroid, liver, and kidney. Similarly, a 2004 review by Key et al. *(45)* concluded the evidence that fruit and vegetable intake is associated with a reduced risk for several cancer sites, including the oral cavity, esophagus, stomach, and colorectum. Not all cancer sites appear equally influenced by fruit and vegetable intake. Michaud et al. *(46)* reported that consumption of these foods is not associated with risk of bladder cancer (RR = 1.28 for highest vs lowest quintile) among male smokers in a prospective cohort study. Likewise, no associations were observed for groups of fruits or vegetables (berries and cruciferous vegetables), or for specific fruits and vegetables and cancer at this site.

Some of the strongest evidence for the anticarcinogenic potency of fruit and vegetables emerges when consumers of at least five servings of fruit and vegetables per day are compared to those consuming only one or two offerings. In several case–control studies a high vs a low intake, particularly of vegetables, was associated with a marked reduction in cancer risk *(47)*. Key et al. *(45)* suggested that diets should include at least 400 g/d of fruit and vegetables. Unfortunately, relatively few studies have adequately examined the influence of the range of intakes of fruits and vegetables globally and thus the true impact across populations is difficult to quantify. Nevertheless, intakes higher than 350 or 400 g/d typically are not associated with added benefits in population-based studies *(44,48)*.

In a recent study with National Heart, Lung, and Blood Institute Family Heart Study subjects, Djousse et al. *(49)* found that the average daily servings of fruit and vegetables were 3.2 and 3.5 for adult men and women, respectively. It appears, therefore, that the majority of Americans consume insufficient amounts of these foods for optimal protection against cancer. Such findings point to the need for additional research to help define the most effective approaches for leading to a sustained change in dietary habits.

It seems logical to assume that all fruits and vegetables are not equivalent in their ability to influence health. Thus it is not that surprising that some types of vegetables surface more frequently as protective against cancer, including carrots and green, cruciferous, and allium vegetables *(46,48)*. A host of bioactive food components occurring within these and other foods may provide protection against cancer, including several nonessential components, such as isothiocyanates, allyl sulfides, flavonoids/isoflavones, and saponins, various essential minerals (e.g., selenium, zinc, iodine, and calcium), and several vitamins (e.g., C, D, E, and folic acid) *(46,50)*. Not all individuals should be expected to respond in exactly the same way to these dietary components because their attributions likely reflect their ability to influence specific molecular targets that can potentially be influenced by a host of genetic and environmental factors. Similarly, the magnitude of the response to fruit and vegetables is probably influenced by many factors, including the consumer's genetic background and a host of environmental factors, as well as the type, quantity, and duration of consumption of these foods *(48,51)*.

Enhanced whole grain intake has also been linked to a reduction in cancer risk. Jacobs et al. *(52)* concluded, based on a meta-analysis of 40 case–control studies, that whole-grain intake is associated with decreased risk for various cancers, particularly those of the colon/rectum (pooled OR = 0.79) and stomach (pooled OR = 0.57). Benefits attributed to whole grain consumption are observed at relatively low intakes (between 2 and 3 servings/d). However, typical consumption of whole grain foods in some Western countries is less than one serving per day. The main sources are wholemeal and rye breads and whole grain breakfast cereals. Unraveling the effects of grains is complicated by the fact that those consuming enhanced quantities in the United States tend to be older, from a high socioeconomic group, are less likely to smoke, and are more likely to exercise than those consuming low quantities *(53)*. Several compounds present in whole grains, including phytate, phytoestrogens (such as lignan, plant stanols, and sterols), and several vitamins and minerals, may contribute to the observed lower risk of cancer. Another feature of whole grains, and also of fruit and vegetables, that may help explain their anticarcinogenic action is that the high fiber content is satiating and therefore helps prevent over consumption of energy.

Overall, the quantitative influence of diet on cancer risk and tumor behavior remains a topic of considerable discussion and debate. Because the overall degree of protection is likely dependent on a number of factors, it may be unwise to focus attention on the average number of servings of fruits, vegetables, and whole grains consumed. Rather, it seems more prudent to focus future research on the identification of those individuals who will benefit most from specific foods or dietary patterns, and then develop appropriate preemption approaches to assist them in making wise food choices that are based on their own behaviors, genetic characteristics, and other factors, such as age and gender. Until this occurs it remains prudent to maintain or limit caloric intake to achieve a healthy weight by consuming more fruits, vegetables, and whole grains and less fat and refined carbohydrates.

5. DIETARY FIBER

Similar to high consumption of fruit and vegetables, numerous observational studies have reported an association between a high intake of fiber and a decreased risk of colorectal and breast cancer *(3)*. The term dietary fiber encompasses a complex mix of predominately nondigestible plant cell compounds with variable effects on gut physiology. Dietary fiber from different sources varies in composition, and it is unlikely that all will be equally protective against cancer. Fiber is thought to reduce the risk of colon cancer by decreasing gastrointestinal transit time, increasing stool bulk, and producing volatile short-chain fatty acids by fermentation. Dietary fiber, particularly from grains, cereals, and fruits, was associated with decreased risk of distal colon adenoma in the Prostate, Lung, Colorectal and Ovarian screening trial, a randomized, controlled trial designed to investigate methods for early detection of cancer *(54)*. Similarly, in a case–control study in California, relative to low fiber intake, high intake reduced the risk of rectal cancer *(55)*, and in a case–control study in Maryland increased intake of dietary fiber was associated with decreased risk of colon adenomas *(51)*. In the Cancer Prevention Study II Nutrition Cohort, men with very low intakes of vegetables and dietary fiber were at increased risk of colon cancer compared to those in the highest four quintiles *(56)*. In the European Prospective Investigation into Cancer and Nutrition cohort, the adjusted relative risk for the highest vs lowest quintile of fiber from food intake was 0.58 *(57)*. No food source of fiber was significantly more protective than others, and nonfood supplement sources of fiber were not investigated *(57)*. In contrast, the protective effect of dietary fiber against colon cancer has not been observed in randomized intervention trials, all of which used colon polyps as the outcome variable. Adopting a diet that is low in fat and high in fiber, fruits, and vegetables did not affect the risk of recurrence of colorectal adenomas *(58)* and did not alter rectal mucosal cell proliferation rates *(59)*. A Cochrane meta-analysis of five randomized controlled trials of increased dietary fiber found no difference between intervention and control groups for the development of adenomas *(60)*. The different results obtained between the observational and intervention studies may reflect the fact that the intervention studies used high-risk individuals. Nevertheless, study results linking dietary fiber and colon cancer remain inconclusive.

The effect of dietary fiber on mammary and prostate cancer risk has also been inconsistent. Whereas a high intake of fiber was protective against breast cancer in the Malmö Diet and Cancer Cohort *(61)*, dietary fiber and fiber fractions did not affect breast cancer risk in the Nurses' Health Study *(62)*. A large case–control study conducted in Italy found a moderate but significant inverse association between selected types of dietary fiber and prostate cancer risk *(63)*. The association was strongest for cellulose and for soluble and vegetable fibers *(63)*. The assessment of a cancer-protective effect for dietary fiber can be complicated by correlations among dietary fiber, dietary fat, and caloric intakes (i.e., high-fiber diets may be relatively low in fat and calories). A further confounding factor in examining the association between cancer risk and high-fiber diets is the possible effect on risk caused by micronutrients and phytochemicals in high-fiber foods.

6. MICRONUTRIENTS AND PHYTOCHEMICALS

A variety of micronutrients and phytochemicals occurring in fruits, vegetables, and whole grains have been proposed to be protective against cancer (64). Micronutrients, which include vitamins and minerals, are dietary components that are provided in small amounts. In contrast, phytochemicals are any plant chemicals. Phytochemicals are discussed in Chapter 10. Both micronutrients and phytochemicals can bring about a multitude of biological responses that may be important in the cancer process. An incomplete list of phytochemicals and some of their sources are listed in Table 1 and include thioethers (from allium foods including garlic and onions), terpenes (from citrus fruits), plant phenols (from grapes, strawberries, and apples), polyphenols (from green tea and chocolate), indoles and isothiocyanates (from cruciferous vegetables), and phytoestrogens (from soy and soy products). Because a comprehensive review of the interactions between micronutrients, phytochemicals, and cancer is beyond the scope of this chapter and has been published elsewhere (65,66), only some examples are provided to illustrate the principle that these food components are capable of modifying a variety of cancer processes. These examples show the magnitude and complexity of the potential interactions. Regardless, it is clear that several factors influence the response to these dietary components including the time of introduction, the quantity and duration of consumption, interactions among food components, and the genetic background of the consumer.

Epidemiological studies reveal that diets rich in fruits and vegetables containing vitamin C are linked to a decreased risk for stomach cancer and possibly also for cancers of the mouth, pharynx, esophagus, lung, pancreas, and cervix (3). Recent case–control data indicate a risk reduction of 40–60% for gastric cancer (67) and 66% for oral/pharyngeal cancer (68), and cohort data indicate a risk reduction of 23% for lung cancer in men (69) for the highest vs lowest intake of vitamin C (70).

Colorectal and prostate cancer rates are higher in the northern United States where sun exposure is lower (71). This has led to the hypothesis that sunlight-mediated dermal vitamin D synthesis provides protection (71). Several epidemiological studies support this hypothesis because decreased risk of colon and prostate tumors with higher serum levels of vitamin D has been observed (72,73). Although studies that include vitamin D from all sources or serum concentrations of $25(OH)D_3$ usually are associated with reduced incidence of colorectal cancer, analyses with only dietary vitamin D are mixed (74). This inconsistency may reflect that dietary sources provide only a portion of total vitamin D (74). Limited data also support a potential role of the vitamin in the prevention of breast cancer (75). Vitamin D is a steroid hormone that binds to the vitamin D receptor (76). Several genetic polymorphisms occur in the vitamin D receptor, which may influence the relationship between vitamin D, calcium, and colon cancer (77), but not prostate cancer (78), illustrating that the functional consequences of these polymorphisms are tissue specific.

Vitamin E is another fat-soluble nutrient that may influence cancer. Vitamin E is a collective term used to refer to a number of structurally and functionally different compounds that function, as least in part, as lipid-soluble antioxidants that can protect against the adverse effects of free radicals (79). Unfortunately, few epidemiological studies have investigated the association of cancer risk with diets providing large amounts of vitamin

Table 1
Examples of Dietary Phytochemicals That May Be Protective Against Cancer

Phytochemical	Dietary sources
Allyl sulfur compounds	Onions, garlic
β-Carotene[a]	Citrus fruit, carrots, squash, pumpkin
Catechins	Tea, berries
Ellagic acid	Grapes, strawberries, raspberries, walnuts
Indoles	Cruciferous vegetables
Isoflavones	Soybeans and other legumes
Isothiocyanates	Cruciferous vegetables
Lycopene	Tomatoes and tomato products
Quercetin	Onion, red grapes, citrus fruit, broccoli
Resveratrol	Grapes (skin), red wine
Terpenes	Citrus fruits
Thioethers	Garlic, onions

[a]In some cases, supplemental β-carotene may increase cancer risk in humans (*see* refs. *100–102*).

E. A recent review concluded that the vitamin possibly decreases the risk for lung and cervical cancers, but that evidence is insufficient for an effect on colon/rectum cancer, and that no relationship exists between vitamin E and breast or stomach cancer *(3)*. The vitamin has been reported to decrease the incidence of symptomatic oral radiation-induced mucositis in patients with cancer of the oropharynx and oral cavity *(80)*. A more recent review of the epidemiological data suggests that vitamin E from food offers some protection against breast cancer, whereas vitamin E supplements do not *(79)*; this again raises the issue that other food components in the food matrix may be important in determining the response. In the Alpha-Tocopherol, Beta-Carotene Prevention Study (ATBC), 34% fewer cases of prostate cancer and 16% fewer of colorectal cancer were diagnosed among male cigarette smokers who received daily vitamin E supplements compared to those given a placebo *(81)*. Although these results suggest a protective effect of vitamin E against prostate and colon cancers, these sites were not primary study end points and therefore additional studies are needed. In contrast, in the Cancer Prevention Study II Nutrition Cohort, the intake of vitamin E supplements was not associated with overall risk of prostate cancer or with risk of advanced prostate cancer *(82)*. Well designed randomized control trials, such as the Selenium and Vitamin E Cancer Prevention Trial (SELECT) (http://www.cancer.gov/clinicaltrials/select), which will investigate the independent and interactive roles of vitamin E and selenium in prostate cancer prevention, will assist in helping to understand the importance of these nutrients in cancer prevention.

International evidence points to an inverse association between selenium status and mortality from cancer of the large intestine, rectum, prostate, breast, ovary, lung, and leukemia *(83)*. Data from most case–control and cohort studies show a possible protective relationship of the mineral for lung and prostate cancer, but have not been overly convincing for other cancer sites, including breast and colon/rectum *(3)*. A meta-analysis suggests that selenium may afford some protection against lung cancer in populations where average selenium levels are low *(84)*. The evidence for these findings is greatest in studies using toenail selenium as an indicator of status *(84)*. Cohort studies also have identified low baseline serum or toenail selenium concentrations as a risk factor for prostate cancer *(85,86)*. Interestingly, an intervention study supports the protective effects of selenium against cancer. This randomized, controlled trial was designed to test selenium as a deterrent to the development of basal or squamous carcinomas. Secondary end point analyses showed that the mineral resulted in a significant reduction in total cancer mortality (RR = 0.5), total cancer incidence (RR = 0.63), and incidence of lung (RR = 0.54), colorectal (RR = 0.42), and prostate (RR = 0.37) cancer *(87)*. Participants with baseline plasma selenium concentration in the lowest two tertiles (<121.6 ng/mL) experienced reductions in total cancer incidence, whereas those in the highest tertile showed an elevated incidence (HR = 1.20; 95% CI = 0.77–1.86) *(88)*. Re-analysis of incidence data through the end of the blinded clinical trial indicated that supplementation significantly reduced lung *(89)* and prostate *(90)* cancer only in individuals with the lowest baseline selenium concentrations. Although these findings are intriguing, they need to be confirmed. The ongoing SELECT trial, which is the largest-ever prostate cancer study, should provide insights into the efficacy and possible mechanisms by which selenium might function as a dietary anticancer component.

Studies of folate and cancer are of particular interest as they show not only that this vitamin may exert an anticarcinogenic action but also demonstrate the importance of molecular nutrition studies. A large number of epidemiological and intervention studies support the role of folate in reducing the risk of colorectal cancer *(91)*. However, a common polymorphism in methylenetetrahydrolate reductase can potentially modify this relationship. Substituting C to T at nucleotide 677 results in reduced conversion of 5,10-methylenetetrahydrofolate to 5-methlenetetrahydrofolate, the form of folate that circulates in plasma. Individuals with this polymorphism appear to have an increased dietary folate requirement *(92–94)*. As compared with subjects with the CC or CT genotype having low plasma folate levels (<5.5 ng/mL), those with the TT genotype showed a decreased risk of colorectal adenomas when they had high levels of folate (adjusted OR = 0.58), and an increased risk when they had low levels (adjusted OR = 2.13) *(95)*. Because there was no clear relationship between plasma folate and colorectal adenomas among those with the CC or CT genotype, only a subset of the population may benefit from increased folate intakes *(95)*.

Common green, yellow/red, and yellow/orange vegetables and fruits contain a host of carotenoids. These include lutein, zeaxanthin, cryptoxanthin, lycopene, β-carotene, and α-carotene. Several dietary carotenoids and their byproducts have been identified in human serum, milk, and tissues. Despite much evidence that suggests that these compounds are anticarcinogenic, a 1998 comprehensive monograph concluded that the cancer preventative effects of carotenoids are largely unsubstantiated *(96)*.

Epidemiological studies have reported that high intakes of β-carotene-rich fruit and vegetables or high plasma concentrations of the nutrient usually have a significant inverse association with lung cancer risk *(97–99)*. The epidemiological data linking high intakes of β-carotene-rich fruit and vegetables to reduced lung cancer risk, along with animal data demonstrating that β-carotene inhibits cancer-related events, such as the induction of stimulation of intercellular communication via gap junctions, which can have a role in the regulation of cell growth, differentiation, and apoptosis, provides strong support for testing the effect of β-carotene supplements on lung cancer in randomized intervention trials, as was done in the ATBC Study *(81)*, the Physician's Health Study (PHS) *(100)*, and the Beta Carotene and Retinol Efficacy Trial (CARET) *(101)*. Unexpectedly, results from the ATBC and CARET studies showed adverse treatment effects in terms of increased lung cancer incidence in high-risk subjects *(102)*.

The different results obtained in supplementation trials compared to cohort studies may reflect that fruit and vegetables contain, in addition to β-carotene, numerous other compounds that may be protective against cancer. In fact, β-carotene may simply be a marker for the actual protective substances in fruit and vegetables. Alternately, β-carotene may have different effects when consumed as a supplement rather than in the food supply. The ATBC, CARET, and PHS studies illustrate that definitive evidence of both safety and efficacy is required for individual fruit and vegetable constituents before dietary guidelines beyond simply greater consumption can be proposed. Because β-carotene is the major source of vitamin A for much of the world's population, it is critical to define its safe intake from foods and supplements *(103)*. The CARET study also demonstrates the importance of large-scale primary prevention trials because the differences observed (lung cancer incidence of 4.6 and 5.9 per 1000 in the placebo and treatment groups, respectively) would not be detected in smaller studies *(101)*.

Lycopene is another carotenoid that has been proposed to have anticancer properties *(104)*. It is found most abundantly in tomatoes. However, to date this hypothesis has not been adequately investigated, using either foods or supplements. Like other carotenoids, lycopene can serve as a potent antioxidant and thereby influence exposures to reactive oxygen species *(105)*. Interestingly, at physiological concentrations it can also retard the growth of human cancer cells, possibly by influencing growth factor receptor signals and altering cell cycle progression. The gene, *connexin 43*, whose expression is sometimes upregulated by lycopene, may account for changes in intercellular gap junctional communications *(106)*. However, evidence also exists that lycopene may upregulate the expression of the urokinase plasminogen activator receptor and facilitate invasion *(107)*. As with many bioactive food components, a better understanding of molecular targets should assist in identification of those who might benefit and those who might be placed at risk as a result of dietary intervention *(108)*.

Although vitamin A activity is not required for carotenoids to be beneficial, at least experimentally, there is evidence that retinoids (vitamin A and its derivatives) can influence cancer biology, especially because they influence growth and differentiation *(109)*. Retinoids are thought to exert their biological functions through nuclear receptors, retinoic acid receptor, and retinoid X receptor. Experimental and clinical studies with retinoids reveal that they can inhibit or reverse the carcinogenic process in some organs, including hematological malignancy, as well as premalignant and malignant lesions in the oral cavity, head and neck, breast, skin, and liver *(109)*.

Epidemiological data suggest that some beverages may also influence cancer risk. Most notable is that tea consumption, both black (oxidized) and green (unoxidized), may reduce overall cancer mortality *(110)*. The protection associated with tea consumption has been highly variable and tumor site specific. Unfortunately, in many cases there may be significant error, partly because the measurement of intake is based on a single question, and also because of inconsistent adjustment for confounders, such as physical activity and consumption of coffee and alcohol *(111)*. Many animal and cell culture studies, although more consistent in producing a response, have focused on extracts of either black or green tea or have used isolated polyphenols *(111)*. Catechins predominate in green tea although black tea contains high amounts of theaflavins *(112)*. Because both classes of compounds can serve as antioxidants, shifts in free radicals may account for the observed biological responses *(112)*. However, a suppression in the activity of various growth factors, including platelet-derived growth factor, IGF, epidermal growth factor, fibroblast growth factor, and vascular endothelial growth factor, which transduce their mitogenic signals through the activation of tyrosine kinase receptors, may also account for the response to tea and its bioactive components *(113)*. Cell culture and animal studies provide ample evidence that individual catechins are potent natural inhibitors of several tyrosine kinase receptors.

The complexity of the relationship between dietary components and cancer is exemplified in a recent review that summarized the impact of diet on prostate cancer in 37 prospective cohort and 4 intervention studies *(114)*. Overall, these analyses support a protective role against prostate cancer for selenium, and possibly for vitamin E, tomatoes/lycopene, and pulses. However, the intake of meat, eggs, fruit, vegetables, coffee, tea, carotenoids, and vitamins A, C, and D were not consistently related to prostate cancer risk *(114)*. Intervention studies also indicate that supplementation with β-carotene does not lower prostate cancer risk, except possibly in men with low β-carotene status at the time that baseline measurements were made *(114)*.

7. ALCOHOL

Chronic ethanol abuse is accompanied by liver injury, neurotoxicity, hypertension, cardiomyopathy, immune incompetence, and increased risk for some cancers. When combined with cigarette smoking, alcohol is considered a primary factor associated with head and neck cancer; although the mechanism by which this effect occurs remains unclear *(115)*. Increased risks have also been noted for liver, breast, colon/rectum, and lung cancers following excessive alcohol consumption, although as with fruit and vegetable data, the findings are not always consistent *(3,116–118)*. Moderate alcohol intakes have been associated with an increased breast cancer risk of about 7% per alcoholic drink per day, perhaps as a result of altering estrogen concentrations *(119)*. A dose–response relationship has been observed, especially as intakes are markedly increased. In lifelong nonsmokers the risk for esophageal cancer was found to increase with daily consumption of four to eight drinks (RR = 2.7) and eight or more drinks (RR = 5.4), compared with more modest intakes (<4 drinks/d; RR = 1.0) *(117)*. Smoking combined with alcohol consumption increased the risk of oral cancer in Spanish men by two- to fourfold compared with alcohol only *(120)*.

Alcohol may alter several processes including shifts in sex hormone homeostasis, DNA damage, and nutrient balance *(121)*. Recent studies by Laufer et al. *(122)* suggest that vitamin B_{12} status in particular is influenced by moderate amounts of alcohol (30 g/d) in healthy women. Evidence also points to the central role for the mitogen-activated protein kinase family and the cascade in signaling caused by mitogen-activated protein kinase in the initiation of several cellular processes including proliferation, differentiation, apoptosis, and inflammatory responses *(123)*.

Although many factors likely contribute to cancer risk, at least some evidence suggests that interactions between alcohol intake and genetic polymorphisms may be involved.

Such an interrelationship has been reported between methylenetetrahydrofolate reductase and colon cancer risk *(124)*. High dietary intake of methionine (OR = 0.27) and low consumption of alcohol (OR = 0.11) has been associated with reduced incidence of colorectal cancer *(86)*.

8. FOOD PREPARATION AND PRESERVATION AND DIETARY CARCINOGENS

Although various carcinogens have been identified in foods and beverages, these appear to contribute only slightly to the overall impact of diet on cancer risk. Carcinogens present in food or as a result of cooking practices include aflatoxins, *N*-nitroso compounds, polycyclic aromatic hydrocarbons (PAHs), and heterocyclic amines (HCAs). Aflatoxin is a generic term for a group of fungal metabolites produced by *Aspergillus flavus* and *Aspergillus parasiticus (125)*. The most widely studied of the aflatoxins is aflatoxin B1, which can be found in moldy foods, particularly peanuts and corn *(125)*. Consumption of aflatoxin B1 has been associated with an increased risk of liver cancer in humans *(126)*.

Nitrites and nitrates are often used as preservatives in meats and other "cured" products. These additives are not carcinogenic in experimental animals; however, nitrate can interact with dietary substances, such as amines or amides to produce *N*-nitroso compounds, which are potent carcinogens in animals and probably humans *(127)*. Epidemiological studies have demonstrated a direct relationship between nitrosamine exposure and cancer of the stomach, esophagus, nasopharynx, urinary bladder, liver, and brain *(128)*. Several naturally occurring foods and their constituents, including tea, garlic, and cruciferous vegetables, may inhibit the formation of endogenous nitrosamines *(129–131)*. This reduction in carcinogen formation may contribute to the generally protective effect of fruit and vegetables on cancer risk.

Two classes of carcinogens derived from cooked meat have been shown to induce cancer in animal models. The first class is the PAHs associated with barbecued meats. These compounds are formed from the pyrolysis of fats that occurs when fat drips from meat onto hot coal, forming smoke that is redeposited on the meat surface. Eleven PAH compounds have been classified as carcinogenic to laboratory animals and as suspect carcinogens in humans *(132)*. The second class of compounds found in cooked meats are the HCAs. These are formed during high-temperature cooking by pyrolysis of proteins, amino acids, or creatinine. The amount in the diet can be substantial and is influenced by cooking habits such that prolonged high-temperature cooking of meats results in the greatest content *(132)*. Epidemiological studies have linked HCAs with cancers of the colorectum, breast, prostate, lung, and pancreas *(133)*. Polymorphisms in specific genes associated with metabolism or detoxification of HCAs (e.g., *CYP1A1, CYP1A2, GSTM1*, and *NAT2*) may explain variations in genetic susceptibility among individuals *(134)*. In view of the possible role of HCAs in human carcinogenesis, minimizing exposure seems prudent, i.e., avoiding overheating and overcooking.

9. CONCLUSIONS

The evidence linking diet to cancer prevention is impressive; nevertheless, much more personalized information is needed. The research highlighted here is only a small part of

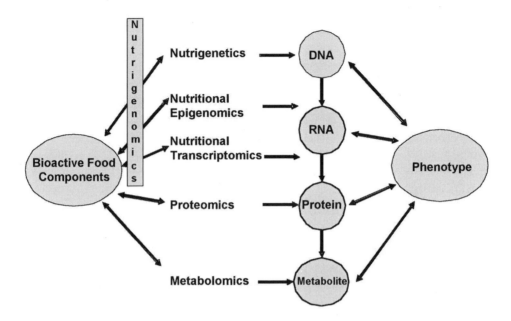

Fig. 3. Variation in the "omics" of nutrition (nutrigenetics, nutritional epigenomics, nutritional transcriptomics, proteomics, and metabolomics) likely contributes to the different phenotypic expression among individuals in response to bioactive food components.

the large body of evidence linking dietary habits with cancer risk and tumor behavior. Although a wealth of epidemiological and preclinical (animal and cell culture) investigations exist, more randomized prevention trials are needed. Overall, multiple cancer processes appear to be influenced by many dietary components, although the response is often variable. Variation in the "omics" of nutrition likely accounts for these inconsistencies (*see* Fig. 3). As discussed in this chapter, the response to these food components depends on a host of genomic and epigenomic events that ultimately influence cellular proteins and small molecular weight compounds. It will be increasingly important to define the amount of the specific bioactive component that needs to be consumed by an individual to achieve concentrations in target tissues that will lead to a phenotypic change. To achieve this change while minimizing harm, three elements are needed: (1) the discovery of relevant mechanisms; (2) the development of interventions for better diagnosis, treatment, and prevention; and (3) the delivery of effective approaches to those in need. Fundamental will be the elucidation of the specific molecular sites of action (targets) for specific dietary components and carefully designed randomized intervention trials to validate the diet and cancer hypothesis. Until more information surfaces, it is prudent to eat a variety of foods, maintain an appropriate body weight, and exercise.

REFERENCES

1. Stewart SL, King JB, Thompson TD, Friedman C, Wingo PA. Cancer mortality surveillance—United States, 1990-2000. MMWR Surveill Summ 2004; 53:1–108.

2. Hanahan D, Weinberg RA. The hallmarks of cancer. Cell 2000; 100:57–70.

3. World Cancer Research Fund/American Institute for Cancer Research. Food, Nutrition and the Prevention of Cancer: A Global Perspective. American Institute for Cancer Research, Washington, DC, 1997.

4. Kushi L, Giovannucci E. Dietary fat and cancer. Am J Med 2002; 113:63s–70s.

5. Ziegler RG, Hoover RN, Hildesheim A, et al. Migration patterns and breast cancer risk in Asian-American women. J Natl Cancer Inst 1993; 85:1819–1827.

6. Boyd NF, Martin LJ, Noffel M, Lockwood GA, Tritchler DL. A meta-analysis of studies of dietary fat and breast cancer risk. Br J Cancer 1993; 68:627–636.

7. Hunter DJ, Spiegelman D, Adarni H-O, et al. Cohort studies of fat intake and the risk of breast cancer-a pooled analysis. N Engl J Med 1996; 334:356–361.

8. Cho E, Spiegelman D, Hunter DJ, et al. Premenopausal fat intake and risk of breast cancer. J Natl Cancer Inst 2003; 95:1079–1085.

8a. Chlebowski RT, Blackburn GL, Elashoff RE, et al. Dietary fat reduction in postmenopausal women with primary breast cancer: phase III Women's Intervention Nutrition Study (WINS). Proc Amer Soc Clin Oncol 2005 24:10 (abstract).

9. Howe GR, Aronson, KJ, Benito E, et al. The relationship between dietary fat intake and risk of colorectal cancer-evidence from the combined analysis of 13 case–control studies. Cancer Causes Control 1997; 8:215–228.

10. Parker SL, Tong T, Bolden S, Wingo PA. Cancer statistics, 1997. CA Cancer J Clin 1997; 47:5–27.

11. Fleshner N, Bagnell PS, Klotz L, Venkateswaran V. Dietary fat and prostate cancer. J Urology 2004; 171:S19–S24.

12. Caygill CPJ, Charlett A, Hill MJ. Fat, fish, fish oil and cancer. Br J Cancer 1996; 74:159–164.

13. Brouwer IA, Katan MB, Zock PL. Dietary Œ±-linolenic acid is associated with reduced risk of fatal coronary heart disease, but increased prostate cancer risk: a meta-analysis. J Nutr 2004; 134:919–922.

14. Dwyer JT. Human studies on the effects of fatty acids on cancer: summary, gaps, and future research. Am J Clin Nutr 1997; 66:1581S–1586S.

15. Rose DP. Dietary fatty acids and cancer. Am J Clin Nutr 1997; 66:998–1003.

16. Deckere EAM. Possible beneficial effect of fish and fish n-3 polyunsaturated fatty acids in breast and colorectal cancer. Eur J Cancer Prev 1999; 8:213–221.

17. Chajes V, Bougnoux P. Omega-6/omega-3 polyunsaturated fatty acid ratio and cancer. In: Simopoulos AP, Cleland LG, eds. Omega-6/omega-3 essential fatty acid ratio: the scientific evidence. World Rev Nutr Diet: Karger, Basel, 2003; 92:133–151.

18. Simonsen N, van't Veer P, Strain JJ, et al. Adipose tissue omega-3 and omega-6 fatty acid content and breast cancer in the EURAMIC Study. Am J Epidemiol 1998; 147:342–352.

19. Roynette CE, Calder PC, Dupertuis YM, Pichard C. n-3 polyunsaturated fatty acids and colon cancer prevention. Clinical Nutr 2004; 23:139–151.

20. Nkondjock A, Shatenstein B, Maisonneuve P, Ghadirian P. Specific fatty acids and human colorectal cancer: an overview. Cancer Detect Prev 2003; 27:55–66.

21. Bakker N, van't Beer P, Zock PL. The Euramic Study group: adipose fatty acids and cancers of the breast, prostate and colon: an ecological study. Int J Cancer 1997; 72:587–597.

22. Petrek JA, Hudgins LC, Ho M, Bajorumas DR, Hirsch J. Fatty acid composition of adipose tissue and indication of dietary fatty acids and breast cancer prognosis. J Clin Oncol 1997; 15:1377–1384.

23. Slattery ML, Benson J, Ma K-N, Schaffer D, Potter JD. Trans-fatty acids and colon cancer. Nutr Cancer 2001; 39:170–175.

24. McKelevey W, Greenland S, Chem M-J, et al. A case–control study of colorectal adenomatous polyps and consumption of foods containing partially hydrogenated oils. Cancer Epidemiol 1999; 8:519–524.

25. Belury MA. Dietary conjugated linoleic acid in health: physiological effects and mechanisms of action. Ann Rev Nutr 2002; 22:505–531.

26. Masso-Welsch PA, Zangani D, Ip C, et al. Isomers of conjugated linoleic acid differ in their effects on angiogenesis and survival of mouse mammary adipose vasculature. J Nutr 2004; 134:299–307.

27. Voorrips LE, Brants HAM, Kardinaal AFM, Hiddink GJ, van den Brandt PA, Goldbohm RA. Intake of conjugated linoleic acid, fat, and other fatty acids in relation to postmenopausal breast cancer: the Netherlands Cohort Study on Diet and Cancer. Am J Clin Nutr 2002; 76:873–882.

28. Bordonaro M, Mariadason JM, Aslam F, Heerdt BG, Augenlicht LH. Butyrate-induced apoptotic cascade in colonic carcinoma cells: modulation of the beta-catenin pathway and concordance with effects of sulindac and trichostatin A but not curcumin. Cell Growth Differ 1999; 10:713–720.

29. Belobrajdic DP, McIntosh GH. Dietary butyrate inhibits NMU-induced mammary cancer in rats. Nutr Cancer 2000; 36:217–223.

30. Andoh A, Tsujikawa T, Fujiyama Y. Role of dietary fiber and short-chain fatty acids in the colon. Curr Pharm Des 2003; 9:347–358.

31. Lupton JR. Microbial degradation products influence colon cancer risk: the butyrate controversy. J Nutr 2004; 134:479–482.

32. Healthy United States, 2002. Healthy weight, overweight, and obesity among persons 20 years of age and over, according to sex, age, race, and Hispanic origin: United States, 1960–62, 1971–74, 1976–80, 1988–94, and 1999–2000.

33. Leibel RL. The role of leptin in the control of body weight. Nutr Rev 2002; 60:S15–S19.

34. IARC Working Group. Vanio H, Bianchini F, eds. IARC Working Group on the Evaluation of Cancer-Preventive Strategies. IARC Handbooks of Cancer Prevention, vol. 6. Weight control and physical activity. 1-315. IARC Press, Lyon, France, 2002.

35. Calle EE, Rodriguez C, Walker-Thurmond K, Thun MJ. Overweight, obesity and mortality from cancer in a prospectively studied cohort of U.S. adults. N Engl J Med 2003; 348:1625–1638.

36. Kritchevsky D. Caloric restriction and cancer. J Nutr Sci Vitaminol (Tokyo) 2001; 47:13–19.

37. Frame LT, Hart RW, Leakey JE. Caloric restriction as a mechanism mediating resistance to environmental disease. Environ Health Perspect 1998; 106:313–324.

38. Hursting SD, Lavigne JA, Berrigan D, Perkins SN, Barrett JC. Calorie restriction, aging, and cancer prevention: mechanisms of action and applicability to humans. Annu Rev Med 2003; 54:131–152.

39. Bray GA. Medical consequences of obesity. J Clin Endocrinol Metab 2004; 89:2583–2589.

40. Jakicic JM. Exercise in the treatment of obesity. Endocrinol Metab Clin North Am 2003; 32:967–980.

41. Hill, JO, Wyatt, HR, Reed, GW, Peters, JC. Obesity and the environment: Where do we go from here? Science 2003; 299:853–855.

42. Kris-Etherton PM, Hecker KD, Bonanome A, Coval SM, Binkoski AE, Hilpert KF, Griel AE, Etherton TD. Bioactive compounds in foods: their role in the prevention of cardiovascular disease and cancer. Am J Med 2002; 113:71S–88S.

43. Keck AS, Finley JW. Cruciferous vegetables: cancer protective mechanisms of glucosinolate hydrolysis products and selenium. Integr Cancer Ther 2004; 3:5–12.

44. Demark-Wahnefried W, Rock CL. Nutrition-related issues for the breast cancer survivor. Semin Oncol 2003; 30:789–798.

45. Key TJ, Schatzkin A, Willett WC, Allen NE, Spencer EA, Travis RC. Diet, nutrition and the prevention of cancer. Public Health Nutr 2004; 7:187–200.

46. Michaud DS, Pietinen P, Taylor PR, Virtanen M, Virtamo J, Albanes D. Intakes of fruits and vegetables, carotenoids and vitamins A, E, C in relation to the risk of bladder cancer in the ATBC cohort study. Br J Cancer 2002; 87:960–965.

47. Steinmetz KA, Potter JD. Vegetables, fruit, and cancer. I. Epidemiology. Cancer Causes Control 1991; 2:325–357.

48. Steinmetz KA, Potter JD. Vegetables, fruit, and cancer prevention: a review. J Am Diet Assoc 1996; 96:1027–1039.

49. Djousse L, Arnett DK, Coon H, Province MA, Moore LL, Ellison RC. Fruit and vegetable consumption and LDL cholesterol: the National Heart, Lung, and Blood Institute Family Heart Study. Am J Clin Nutr 2004; 79:213–217.

50. Milner JA. Incorporating basic nutrition science into health interventions for cancer prevention. J Nutr 2003; 133:3820S–3826S.

51. Mathew A, Peters U, Chatterjee N, Kulldorff M, Sinha R. Fat, fiber, fruits, vegetables and risk of colorectal cancer. Int J Cancer 2004; 108:287–292.

52. Jacobs DR, Jr, Marquart L, Slavin J, Kushi LH. Whole-grain intake and cancer: an expanded review and meta-analysis. Nutr Cancer 1998; 30:85–96.

53. Lang R, Jebb SA. Who consumes whole grains, and how much? Proc Nutr Soc 2003; 62:123–127.

54. Peters U, Sinha R, Chatterjee N, et al. Dietary fibre and colorectal adenoma in a colorectal cancer early detection programme. Lancet 2003; 361:1491–1495.

55. Slattery ML, Curtin KP, Edwards SL, Schaffer DM. Plant foods, fiber and rectal cancer. Am J Clin Nutr 2004; 79:274–281.

56. McCullough ML, Robertson AS, Chao A, et al. A prospective study of whole grains, fruits, vegetables and colon cancer risk. Cancer Causes Control 2003; 14:959–970.

57. Bingham SA, Day NE, Luben R, et al. Dietary fibre in food and protection against colorectal cancer in the European Prospective Investigation into Cancer and Nutrition (EPIC): an observational study. Lancet 2003; 361:1496–1501.

58. Schatzkin A, Lanza E, Corle D, et al. Lack of effect of a low-fat, high-fiber diet on the recurrence of colorectal adenomas. N Eng J Med 2000; 342:1149–1155.

59. Pfeiffer R, McShane L, Wargovich M, et al. The effect of a low-fat, high fiber, fruit and vegetable intervention on rectal mucosal proliferation. Cancer 2003; 98:1161–1168.

60. Asano TK, McLeod RS. Dietary fibre for the prevention of colorectal adenomas and carcinomas Cochrane Database Syst Rev 2002; 2:CD003430.

61. Mattison I, Wirfalt E, Johansson U, Bullberg B, Olsson H, Berglund G. Intakes of plant foods, fibre and fat and risk of breast cancer- a prospective study in the Malmo Diet and Cancer cohort. Br J Cancer 2004; 90:122–127.

62. Holmes MD, Liu S, Hankinson SE, Coldizt GA, Hunter DJ, Willett WC. Dietary carbohydrates, fiber and breast cancer risk. Am J Epidemiol 2004; 159:732–739.

63. Pelucchi C, Talamini R, Galeone C, et al. Fibre intake and prostate cancer risk. Int J Cancer 2004; 109:278–280.

64. Milner JA. Functional foods and health: a US perspective. Br J Nutr 2002; 88:S151–S158.

65. Bendich A, Deckelbaum RJ, eds. Preventive Nutrition: The Comprehensive Guide for the Health Professionals. Humana Press, Totowa, NJ, 1997.

66. Wildman REC, ed. Handbook of Nutraceuticals and Functional Foods. CRC Press LLC, Boca Raton, FL, 2004.

67. Estrom AM, Serafini M, Nyren O, Hansson LE, Ye W, Wolk A. Dietary antioxidant intake and the risk of cardia cancer and noncardia cancer of the intestinal and diffuse types: a population-based case-control study in Sweden. Int J Cancer 2000; 87:133–140.

68. Negri E, Franceschi S, Bosetti C, et al. Selected micronutrients and oral and pharyngeal cancer. Int J Cancer 2000; 86:122–127.

69. Voorrips LE, Goldbohm RA, Brants HA. A prospective cohort study on antioxidant and folate intake and male lung cancer risk. Cancer Epidemiol Biomarkers Prev 2000; 9:357–365.

70. Greenwald P, Clifford CK, Milner JA. Diet and cancer prevention. Eur J Cancer 2001; 37:948–965.

71. Holick MF. Vitamin D: importance in the prevention of cancers, type 1 diabetes, heart disease and osteoporosis. Am J Clin Nutr 2004; 79:362–371.

72. Peters U, Hayes RB, Chatterjee N, et al. Circulating vitamin D metabolites, polymorphism in the vitamin D receptor and colorectal adenoma risk. Cancer Epidemiol Biomarkers Prev 2004; 13:546–552.

73. Stewart LV, Weigel NL. Vitamin D and prostate cancer. Exp Biol Med 2004; 229:277–284.

74. Grant WB, Garland CF. A critical review of studies on vitamin D in relation to colorectal cancer. Nutr Canc 2004; 48:115–123.

75. Zhang SM. Role of vitamins in the risk, prevention, and treatment of breast cancer. Curr Opin Obstet Gynecol 2004; 16:19–25.

76. Cheteri MB, Stanford JL, Friedrichsen DM, et al. Vitamin D receptor gene polymorphisms and prostate cancer risk. Prostate 2004; 59:409–418.

77. Slattery ML, Yakuma K, Hoffman M, Neuhausen S. Variants of the VDR gene and the risk of colon cancer (United States). Cancer Causes Control 2001; 12:359–364.

78. Ntais C, Polycarpou A, Ionnidis JP. Vitamin D receptor gene polymorphisms and risk of prostate cancer: a meta-analysis. Cancer Epidemiol Biomarkers Prev 2003; 12:1395–1402.

79. Kline K, Lawson KA, Yu W, Sanders BG. Vitamin E and breast cancer prevention: current status and future potential. J. Mammary Gland Biol Neoplasia 2003; 8:91–102.

80. Ferreira PA, Fleck JF, Diehl A, et al. Protective effect of alpha-tocopherol in head and neck cancer radiation-induced mucositis: a double-blind randomized trial. Head Neck 2004; 26:313–321.

81. Heinonen OP, Huttunen IK, Albanes D et al. for the Alpha- Tocopherol Beta-Carotene Cancer Prevention Study Group. The effect of vitamin E and beta carotene on the incidence of lung cancer and other cancers in male smokers. N Engl J Med 1994; 330:1029–1035.

82. Rodriguez C, Jacobs EJ, Mondul AM, Calle EE, McCullough ML, Thun MJ. Vitamin E supplements and risk of prostate cancer in U.S. men. Cancer Epidemiol Biomarkers Prev 2004; 13:378–382.

83. Schrauzer GN, White DA, Schneider CI. Cancer mortality correlations studies III: statistical associations with dietary selenium intakes. Bioinorg Chem 1997; 7:23–34.

84. Zhuo H, Smith AH, Steinmaus C. Selenium and lung cancer: a quantitative analysis of heterogeneity in the current epidemiological literature. Cancer Epidemiol Biomarkers Prev 2004; 13:771–778.

85. Klein EA. Selenium: epidemiology and basic science. J Urol 2004; 171:S50–S53.

86. Li H, Stampfer MJ, Giovannucci EL, et al. A prospective study of plasma selenium levels and prostate cancer risk. J Natl Cancer Inst 2004; 96:696–703.

87. Clark LC, Combs GF, Turnbull BW, et al. Effects of selenium supplementation for cancer prevention in patients with carcinoma of the skin. A randomized controlled trial. JAMA 1996; 276:1957–1963.

88. Duffield-Lillico AJ, Reid ME, Turnbull BW, et al. Baseline characteristics and the effect of selenium supplementation on cancer incidence in a randomized clinical trial: a summary report of the Nutritional Prevention of Cancer Trial. Cancer Epidemiol Biomarkers Prev 2002; 11:630–639.

89. Reid ME, Duffield-Lillico AJ, Garland L, Turnbull BW, Clark LC, Marshall JR. Selenium supplementation and lung cancer incidence: an update of the nutritional prevention of cancer trial. Cancer Epidemiol Biomarkers Prev 2002; 11:1285–1291.

90. Duffield-Lillico AJ, Balkin BL, Reid ME, et al. Selenium supplementation, baseline plasma selenium status and incidence of prostate cancer: an analysis of the complete treatment period of the Nutritional Prevention of Cancer Trial. BJU Int 2003; 91:608–612.

91. Kim YI. Role of folate in colon cancer development and progression. J. Nutr 2003; 133:3731S–3739S.

92. Bailey LB, Gregory JF. Polymorphism of metheletetrahydrofolate reductase and other enzymes: metabolic significance, risks and impact on folate requirement. J Nutr 1999; 129:919–922.

93. Chen J, Giovannucci EL, Hunter DJ. MTHFR polymorphism, methyl-replete diets and the risk of colorectal carcinoma and adenoma among US men and women: an example of gene-environment interactions in colorectal tumorigenesis. J Nutr Suppl 1999; 129:560s–564s.

94. Frost P, Blom HJ, Milos R, et al. A candidate genetic risk factor for vascular disease: a common mutation in methylenetetrahydrofolate reductase. Nat Genet 1995; 10:111–113.

95. Marugame T, Tsuji E, Kiyohara C, et al. Relation of plasma folate and methyltetrahydrofolate reductase C677T polymorphism to colorectal adenomas. Int J Epidemiol 2003; 32:64–66.

96. IARC Working Group. IARC Handbooks of Cancer Prevention: Carotenoids, vol. 2. International Agency for Research on Cancer, Lyon, France, 1998.

97. Tapiero H, Townsend DM, Tew KD. The role of carotenoids in the prevention of human pathologies. Biomed Pharmacother 2004; 58:100–110.

98. Ziegler RA, Mayne ST, Swanson CA. Nutrition and lung cancer. Cancer Causes Control 1996; 7:157–177.

99. Cooper DA, Eldridge AL, Peters IC. Dietary carotenoids and lung cancer: a review of recent research. Nutr Rev 1999; 57:133–145..

100. Hennekens CH, Buring IE, Manson IE, et al. Lack of effect of long-term supplementation with beta carotene on the incidence of malignant neoplasms and cardiovascular disease. N Engl J Med 1996; 334:1145–1149.

101. Omenn OS, Goodman GE, Thomquist MD, et al. Effects of a combination of beta carotene and vitamin A on lung cancer and cardiovascular disease. N Eng J Med 1996; 334:1150–1155.

102. Mannisto S, Smith-Warner SA, Spiegelman D, et al. Dietary carotenoids and risk of lung cancer in a pooled analysis of seven cohort studies. Canc Epidemiol Biomarkers Prev 2004; 13:40–48.

103. Bendich A. From 1989 to 2001: what have we learned about the "biological actions of beta-carotene"? J Nutr 2004; 134:225S–230S.

104. Wu K, Erdman JW Jr, Schwartz SJ, Platz EA, Leitzmann M, Clinton SK, DeGroff V, Willett WC, Giovannucci E. Plasma and dietary carotenoids, and the risk of prostate cancer: a nested case-control study. Cancer Epidemiol Biomarkers Prev 2004; 13:260–269.

105. Heber D, Lu QY. Overview of mechanisms of action of lycopene. Exp Biol Med (Maywood). 2002; 227:920–923.
106. Livny O, Kaplan I, Reifen R, Polak-Charcon S, Madar Z, Schwartz B. Lycopene inhibits proliferation and enhances gap-junction communication of KB-1 human oral tumor cells. J Nutr 2002; 132:3754–3759.
107. Forbes K, Gillette K, Sehgal I. Lycopene increases urokinase receptor and fails to inhibit growth or connexin expression in a metastatically passaged prostate cancer cell line: a brief communication. Exp Biol Med (Maywood) 2003; 228:967–971.
108. Davis CD, Milner JA. Frontiers in nutrigenomics, proteomics, metabolomics and cancer prevention. Mut Res 2004; 551:51–64.
109. Okuno M, Kojima S, Matsushima-Nishiwaki R, Tsurumi H, Muto Y, Friedman SL, Moriwaki H. Retinoids in cancer chemoprevention. Curr Cancer Drug Targets 2004; 4:285–298.
110. Chung FL, Schwartz J, Herzog CR, Yang YM. Tea and cancer prevention: studies in animals and humans. J Nutr 2003; 133:3268S–3274S.
111. Gouni-Berthold I, Sachinidis A. Molecular mechanisms explaining the preventive effects of catechins on the development of proliferative diseases. Curr Pharm Des 2004; 10:1261–1271.
112. Arab L, Il'yasova D. The epidemiology of tea consumption and colorectal cancer incidence. J Nutr 2003; 133:3310S–3318S.
113. Frei B, Higdon JV. Antioxidant activity of tea polyphenols in vivo: evidence from animal studies. J Nutr 2003; 133:3275S–3284S.
114. Dagnelie PC, Schuurman AG, Goldbohm RA, Van den Brandt PA. Diet, anthropometric measures and prostate cancer risk: a review of prospective cohort and intervention studies. BJU Int 2004; 93:1139–1150.
115. Brennan P, Boffetta P. Mechanistic considerations in the molecular epidemiology of head and neck cancer. IARC Sci Publ 2004; 157:393–414.
116. Longnecker MP. Alcohol consumption and risk of cancer in humans: an overview. Alcohol 1995; 12:87–96.
117. Tavani A, Negri E, Franceschi S, La Vecchia C. Risk factors for esophageal cancer in lifelong non-smokers. Cancer Epidemiol Biomark Prev 1994; 3:387–392.
118. Potter JD. Methyl supply, methyl metabolizing enzymes and colorectal neoplasia. J Nutr 2002; 132:2410S–2412S.
119. Key TJ, Allen NE, Spencer EA, Travis RC. Nutrition and breast cancer. Breast 2003; 12:412–416.
120. Castellsague X, Quintana MJ, Martinez MC, et al. The role of type of tobacco and type of alcoholic beverage in oral carcinogenesis. Int J Cancer 2004; 108:741–749.
121. Singletary KW, Gapstur SM. Alcohol and breast cancer: review of epidemiologic and experimental evidence and potential mechanisms. JAMA 2001; 286:2143–2151.
122. Laufer EM, Hartman TJ, Baer DJ, et al. Effects of moderate alcohol consumption on folate and vitamin B12 status in postmenopausal women. Eur J Clin Nutr 2004, May 12 (electronic).
123. Aroor AR, Shukla SD. MAP kinase signaling in diverse effects of ethanol. Life Sci 2004; 74:2339–2364.
124. Sharp L, Little J. Polymorphisms in genes involved in folate metabolism and colorectal neoplasia: A HuGE review. Am J Epidemiol 2004; 159:423–443.
125. Paustenbach DJ. The practice of exposure assessment: a state of the art review. J Toxicol Environ Health B Crit Rev 2000; 3:179–291.
126. Nayak NC. Hepatocellular carcinoma-a model of human cancer: clinico-pathological features, etiology and pathogenesis. Indian J Pathol Microbiol 2003; 46:1–16.
127. Mirvish SS. Effects of vitamins C and E on N-nitroso compound formation, carcinogenesis and cancer. Cancer 1986; 58:1842–1850.
128. Ferguson LR. Natural and human-made mutagens and carcinogens in the human diet. Toxicology 2002; 181–182:79–82.
129. Milner JA. Mechanisms by which garlic and allyl sulfur compounds suppress carcinogen bioactivation. Garlic and carcinogenesis. Adv Exp Med Biol 2001; 492:69–81.
130. Weisburger JH, Chung FL. Mechanisms of chronic disease causation by nutritional factors and tobacco products and their prevention by tea polyphenols. Food Chem Toxicol 2002; 40:1145–1154.

131. Solt DB, Chang K, Helenowski I, Rademaker AW. Phenethyl isothiocyanate inhibits nitrosamine carcinogenesis in a model for study of oral cancer chemoprevention. Cancer Lett 2003; 202:147–152.

132. Goldamn R, Shields PG. Food Mutagens. J Nutr 2003; 133:965S–973S.

133. Snyderwine EG, Sinha R, Felton JS, Ferguson LR. Highlights of the eighth international conference on carcinogenic/mutagenic N-substituted aryl compounds. Mutation Res 2002; 506–507:1–8.

134. Murtaugh MA, Ma K, Sweeney C, Caan BJ, Slattery ML. Meat consumption patterns and preparation, genetic variants of metabolic enzymes, and their association with rectal cancer in men and women. J Nutr 2004; 134:776–784.

10 Health Benefits of Phytochemicals in Whole Foods

Rui Hai Liu

KEY POINTS

- Regular consumption of fruit and vegetables, as well as whole grains, is strongly associated with reduced risk of developing chronic diseases, such as cardiovascular disease (CVD), cancer, diabetes, Alzheimer's disease, cataracts, and age-related functional decline.
- Phytochemicals are defined as bioactive nonnutrient plant compounds in fruit, vegetables, grains, and other plant foods, which have been linked to reducing the risk of major chronic diseases. Phytochemicals are classified into carotenoids, phenolics, alkaloids, nitrogen-containing compounds, and organosulfur compounds.
- Oxidative stress can cause oxidative damage to large biomolecules such as proteins, DNA, and lipids, resulting in an increased risk for cancer and CVD. To prevent or slow down the oxidative stress induced by free radicals, sufficient amounts of antioxidants need to be consumed.
- The additive and synergistic effects of phytochemicals in fruit and vegetables are responsible for their potent antioxidant and anticancer activities. The benefit of a diet rich in fruit, vegetables, and whole grains is attributed to the complex mixture of phytochemicals present in these and other whole foods.
- Dietary modification by increasing the consumption of a wide variety of fruit, vegetables, and whole grains daily is a practical strategy for consumers to optimize their health and reduce the risk of chronic diseases. Antioxidants are best acquired through whole food consumption, not from expensive dietary supplements.

1. INTRODUCTION

Cardiovascular disease (CVD) and cancer are the top two leading causes of death in the United States and in most industrialized countries. Epidemiological studies have consistently shown that regular consumption of fruit and vegetables, as well as whole grains, is strongly associated with reduced risk of developing chronic diseases, such as CVD, cancer, diabetes, Alzheimer's disease, cataracts, and age-related functional decline (1–3). It is estimated that one-third of all cancer deaths in the United States could be avoided through appropriate dietary modification (3–5). This suggests that change in dietary

From: *Nutritional Health: Strategies for Disease Prevention, Second Edition*
Edited by: N. J. Temple, T. Wilson, and D. R. Jacobs © Humana Press Inc., Totowa, NJ

behavior, such as increasing consumption of fruit, vegetables, and whole grains, is a practical strategy for significantly reducing the incidence of chronic diseases. In addition, primary prevention of chronic diseases through dietary modification may be as effective, and less costly, than the secondary treatments commonly employed.

In 1982, the National Academy of Sciences of the United States, in their report on diet and cancer, included guidelines emphasizing the importance of fruit and vegetables (6). The value of adding citrus fruit, carotene-rich fruit and vegetables, and cruciferous vegetables to the diet for reducing the risk of cancer was specifically highlighted. In 1989, a report from the National Academy of Sciences on diet and health recommended consuming five or more servings of fruit and vegetables daily for reducing the risk of both cancer and heart disease (7). The Five-a-Day program was developed as a tool to increase public awareness of the health benefits of fruit and vegetable consumption and promote adequate intakes of known vitamins. Plant-based foods, such as fruit, vegetables, and whole grains, which contain significant amounts of bioactive phytochemicals, may provide desirable health benefits beyond basic nutrition to reduce the risk of chronic diseases (8).

2. PHYTOCHEMICALS

The "phyto-" of the word phytochemicals is the Greek word for plant. Therefore, phytochemicals are plant chemicals. Phytochemicals are defined as bioactive nonnutrient plant compounds in fruit, vegetables, grains, and other plant foods, some of which have been linked to reducing the risk of major chronic diseases. It is estimated that more than 5000 phytochemicals have been identified, but a large percentage still remain unknown and need to be identified before we can fully understand the health benefits of phytochemicals in whole foods (8). However, more and more convincing evidence suggests that the benefits of phytochemicals in fruit and vegetables may be even greater than is currently understood; for example, recent thinking supports defense by phytochemicals against oxidative stress induced by free radicals that are involved in the etiology of a wide range of chronic diseases (9).

Phytochemicals can be classified into carotenoids, phenolics, alkaloids, nitrogen-containing compounds, and organosulfur compounds (see Fig. 1). The most studied of the phytochemicals are phenolics and carotenoids.

2.1. Phenolics

Phenolics are compounds possessing one or more aromatic ring with one or more hydroxyl groups, and generally are categorized as phenolic acids, flavonoids, stilbenes, coumarins, and tannins (see Fig. 1). Phenolics are the products of secondary metabolism in plants, providing essential functions in the production and growth of the plants, acting as defense mechanisms against pathogens, parasites, and predators, as well as contributing to the color of plants. In addition to their roles in plants, phenolic compounds in our diet may provide health benefits associated with reduced risk of chronic diseases. Among the 11 most common fruits consumed in the United States, cranberry has the highest total phenolic content, followed by apple, red grape, strawberry, pineapple, banana, peach, lemon, orange, pear, and grapefruit (10). Among the 10 most common vegetables consumed in the United States, broccoli possesses the highest total phenolic content, follow by spinach, yellow onion, red pepper, carrot, cabbage, potato, lettuce, celery, and cucum-

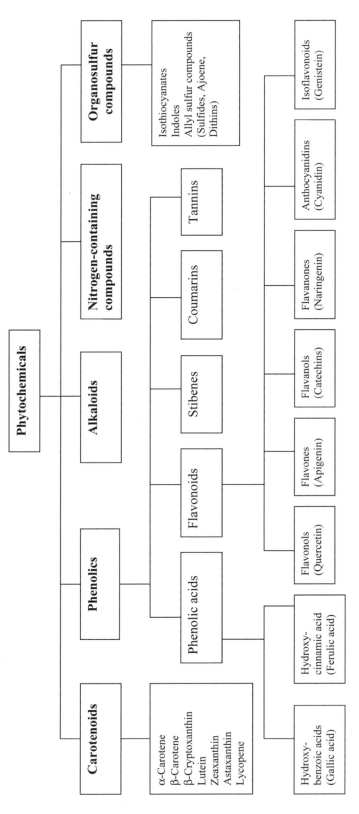

Fig. 1. Classification of dietary phytochemicals.

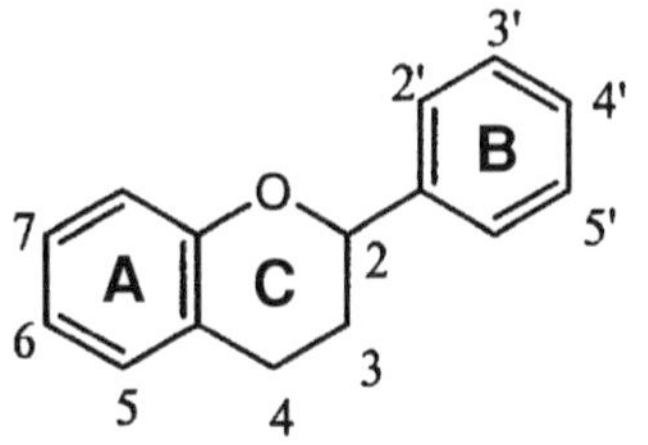

Fig. 2. The generic structure of flavonoids.

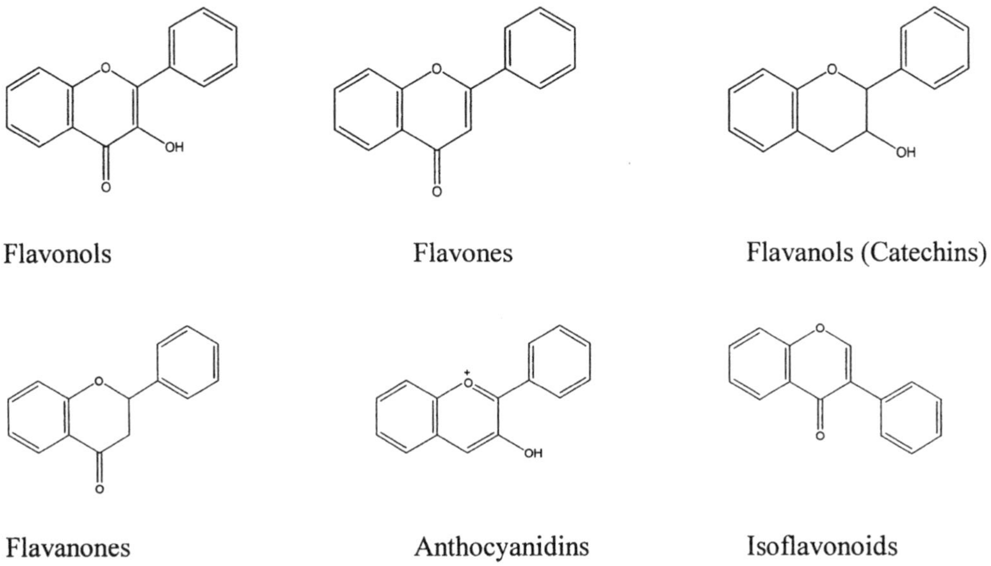

Flavonols   Flavones   Flavanols (Catechins)

Flavanones   Anthocyanidins   Isoflavonoids

Fig. 3. Structures of main classes of dietary flavonoids

ber *(11)*. It is estimated that flavonoids account for approximately two-thirds of the phenolics in our diet, and the remaining one-third are from phenolic acids.

2.1.1. FLAVONOIDS

Flavonoids are a group of phenolic compounds with antioxidant activity that have been identified in fruit, vegetables, and other plant foods, and have been linked to reducing the risk of major chronic diseases. More than 4000 distinct flavonoids have been identified. They commonly have a generic structure consisting of two aromatic rings (A and B rings) linked by three carbons that are usually in an oxygenated heterocycle ring, or C ring (*see* Fig. 2). Differences in the generic structure of the heterocycle C ring classify them as flavonols, flavones, flavanols (catechins), flavanones, anthocyanidins, and isoflavonoids (*see* Fig. 3). Flavonols (quercetin, kaempferol, and myricetin), flavones (luteolin and apigenin), flavanols (catechin, epicatechin, epigallocatechin, epicatechin gallate, and epigallocatechin gallate), flavanones (naringenin), and isoflavonoids (genistein) are common flavonoids in the diet (*see* Fig. 4). Flavonoids are most frequently found in nature as conjugates in glycosylated or esterified forms, but can occur as aglycones, especially because of the effects of food processing. Many different glycosides can be

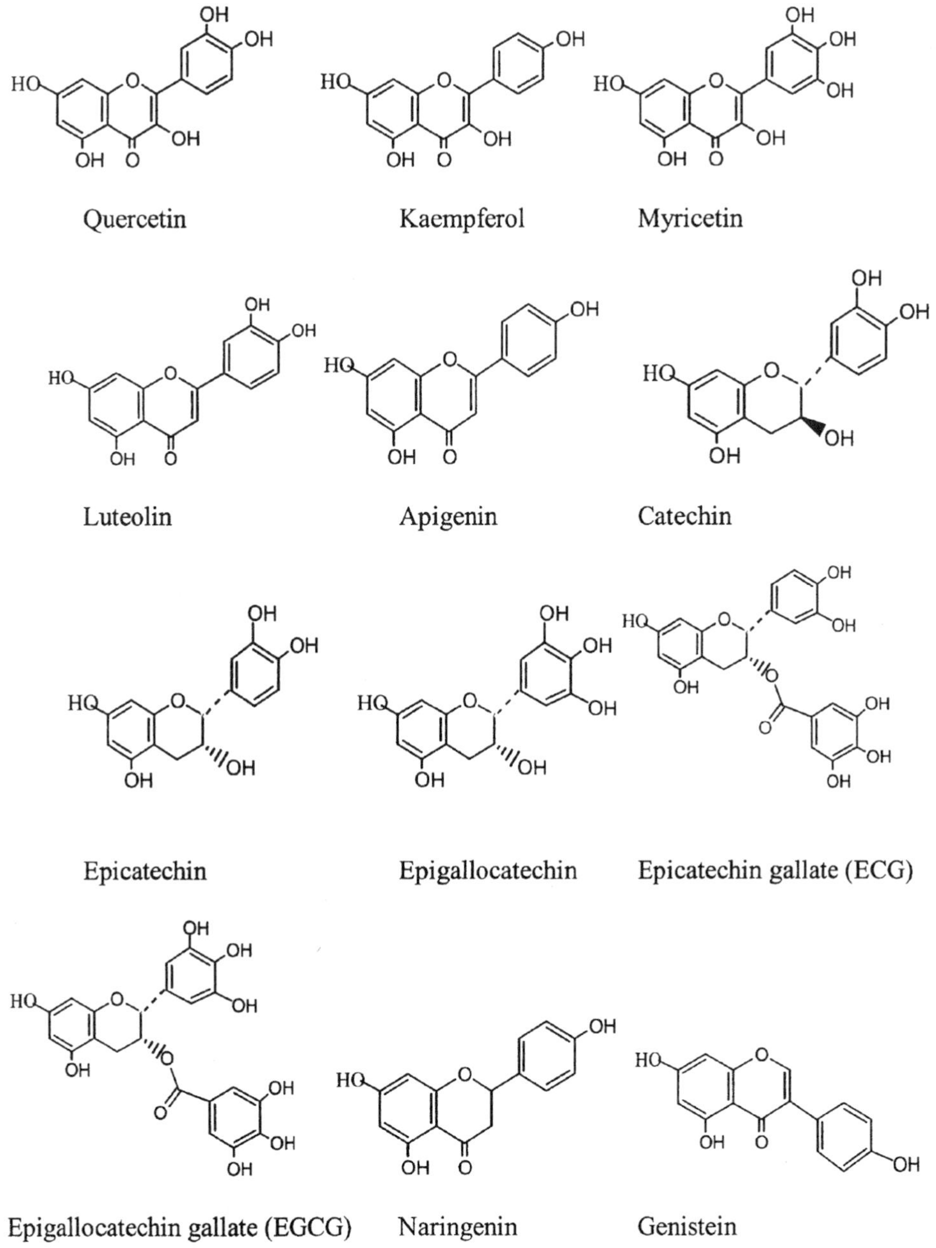

Fig. 4. Chemical structures of common dietary flavonoids.

found in nature as more than 80 different sugars have been discovered bound to flavonoids *(12)*. The red and blue colors in fruit and vegetables are caused by anthocyanins.

Human intake of all flavonoids is estimated to be between a few hundred milligrams *(13)* to 650 mg/d *(14)*. The total average intake of flavonols (quercetin, myricetin, and kaempferol) and flavones (luteolin and apigenin) was estimated as 23 mg/d, of which quercetin contributed about 70%; kaempferol, 17%; myricetin, 6%; luteolin, 4%; and apigenin, 3% *(15)*.

A Benzoic acid

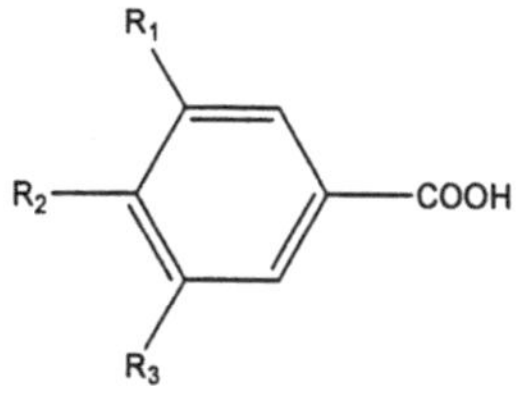

B Cinnamic acid

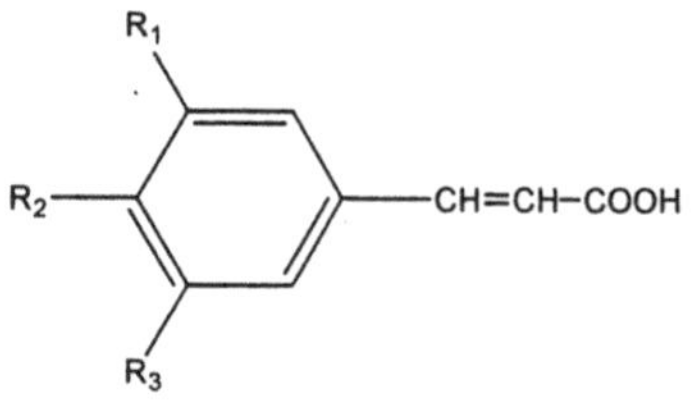

Benzoic acid Derivatives	Substitutions		
	R_1	R_2	R_3
p-Hydroxybenzoic	H	OH	H
Protocatechuic	H	OH	OH
Vannilic	CH_3O	OH	H
Syringic	CH_3O	OH	CH_3O
Gallic	OH	OH	OH

Cinnamic acid Derivatives	Substitutions		
	R_1	R_2	R_3
p-Coumaric	H	OH	H
Caffeic	OH	OH	H
Ferulic	CH_3O	OH	H
Sinapic	CH_3O	OH	CH_3O

Fig. 5. Structures of common phenolic acids: (**A**) benzoic acid and derivatives; (**B**) cinnamic acid and derivatives.

2.1.2. PHENOLIC ACIDS

Phenolic acids can be subdivided into two major groups, hydroxybenzoic acids and hydroxycinnamic acids (*see* Fig. 5). Hydroxybenzoic acid derivatives include *p*-hydroxybenzoic, protocatechuic, vannilic, syringic, and gallic acids. They are commonly present in the bound form and are typically a component of a complex structure like lignins and hydrolyzable tannins. They can also be found in the form of sugar derivatives and organic acids in plant foods.

Hydroxycinnamic acid derivatives include *p*-coumaric, caffeic, ferulic, and sinapic acids (*see* Fig. 5). They are mainly present in the bound form, linked to cell wall structural components such as cellulose, lignin, and proteins through ester bonds. Ferulic acids occur primarily in the seeds and leaves of plants, mainly covalently conjugated to mono- and disaccharides, plant cell-wall polysaccharides, glycoproteins, polyamines, lignin, and insoluble carbohydrate biopolymers. Wheat bran is a good source of ferulic acids, which are esterified to hemicellulose of the cell walls. Free, soluble-conjugated, and bound ferulic acids in grains are present in the ratio of 0.1:1:100 *(16)*. Food processing, such as thermal processing, pasteurization, fermentation, and freezing contributes to the release of these bound phenolic acids *(17)*.

Caffeic, ferulic, *p*-coumaric, protocatechuic, and vannilic acids are present in almost all plants. Chlorogenic acids and curcumin are also major derivatives of hydroxycinnamic acids present in plants. Chlorogenic acids are the ester of caffeic acid and are the substrate for enzymatic oxidation leading to browning, particularly in apples and potatoes. Curcumin is made of two ferulic acids linked by a methylene in a diketone structure, and is the major yellow pigment of mustard.

2.2. Carotenoids

Carotenoids are nature's most widespread pigments and have also received substantial attention caused by both their provitamin and antioxidant roles. There are more than 600 different carotenoids identified in nature. They occur widely in plants, micro-organisms, and animals. Carotenoids have a 40-carbon skeleton of isoprene units (see Fig. 6). The structure may be cyclized at one or both ends, have various hydrogenation levels, or possess oxygen-containing functional groups. Lycopene and β-carotene are examples of acyclized and cyclized carotenoids, respectively. Carotenoid compounds most commonly occur in nature in the all-trans form. The most characteristic feature of carotenoids is the long series of conjugated double bonds forming the central part of the molecule. This gives them their shape, chemical reactivity, and light-absorbing properties. β-Carotene, α-carotene, and β-cryptoxanthin are able to function as provitamin A. Zeaxanthin and lutein are the major carotenoids in the macular region (yellow spot) of the retina in humans.

Carotenoid pigments play important functions in photosynthesis and photoprotection in plant tissues. The photoprotection role of carotenoids originates from their ability to quench and inactivate reactive oxygen species, such as singlet oxygen formed from exposure of light and air. This photoprotection role is also associated with its antioxidant activity in human health. Carotenoids can react with free radicals and become radicals themselves. Their reactivity depends on the length of the chain of conjugated double bonds and the characteristics of the end groups. Carotenoid radicals are stable by virtue of the delocalization of the unpaired electron over the conjugated polyene chain of the molecules. This delocalization also allows addition reactions to occur at many sites on the radical (18). Astaxanthin, zeaxanthin, and lutein are excellent lipid soluble antioxidants that scavenge free radicals, especially in a lipid soluble enviroment. Carotenoids at sufficient concentrations can prevent lipid oxidation and related oxidative stress.

3. HEALTH BENEFITS OF PHYTOCHEMICALS

Cells in humans and other organisms are constantly exposed to a variety of oxidizing agents, some of which are necessary for life. These agents may be present in air, food, and water or they may be produced by metabolic activity within cells. The key factor is to maintain a balance between oxidants and antioxidants to sustain optimal physiological conditions in the body. Overproduction of oxidants can cause an imbalance, leading to oxidative stress, especially in chronic bacterial, viral, and parasitic infections (19). Oxidative stress can cause oxidative damage to large biomolecules, such as proteins, DNA, and lipids, resulting in an increased risk for cancer and CVD (9,20). To prevent or slow down the oxidative stress induced by free radicals, sufficient amounts and variety of antioxidants need to be consumed. Variety is believed to be important because antioxidant action is highly specific to the physiological situation that requires protection against oxidative stress. Fruit, vegetables, and grains contain a wide variety of antioxidant compounds (phytochemicals), such as phenolics and carotenoids, and may help protect cellular systems from oxidative damage and also lower the risk of chronic diseases (10,11,16,21–23).

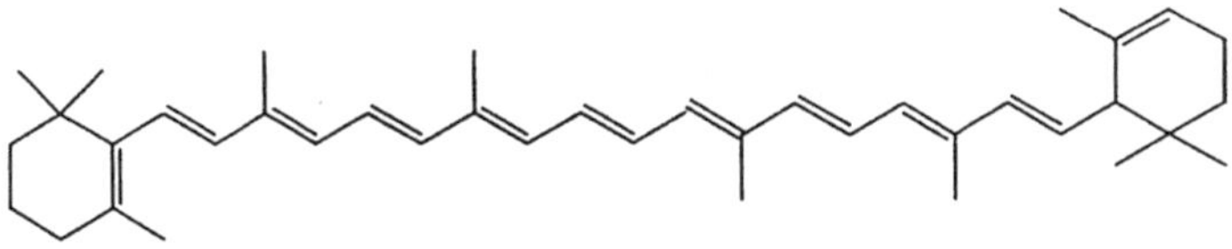

α-Carotene

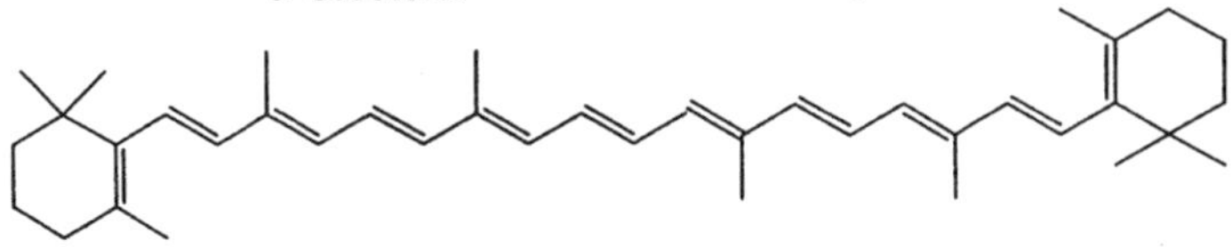

β-Carotene

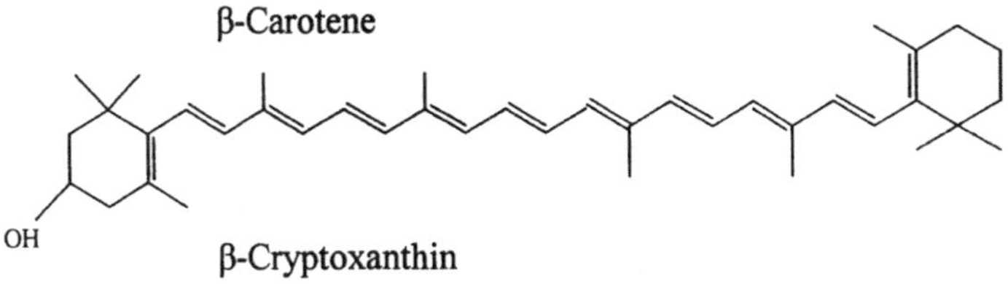

β-Cryptoxanthin

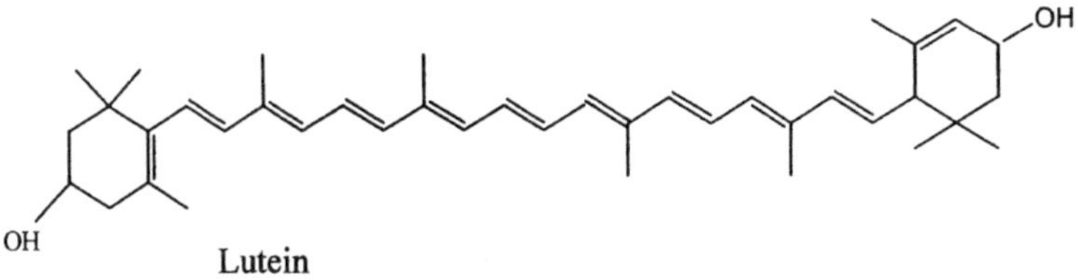

Lutein

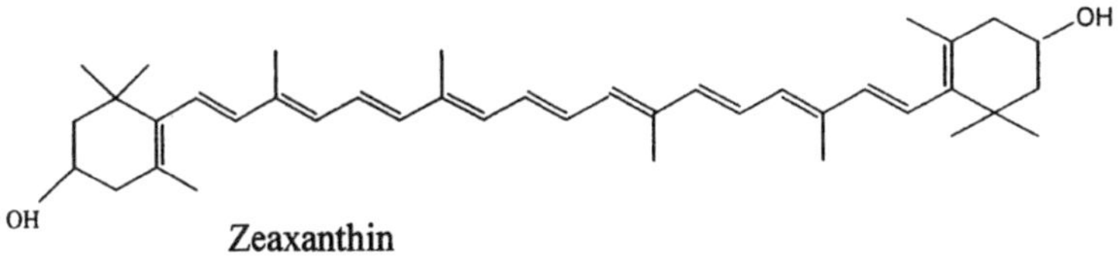

Zeaxanthin

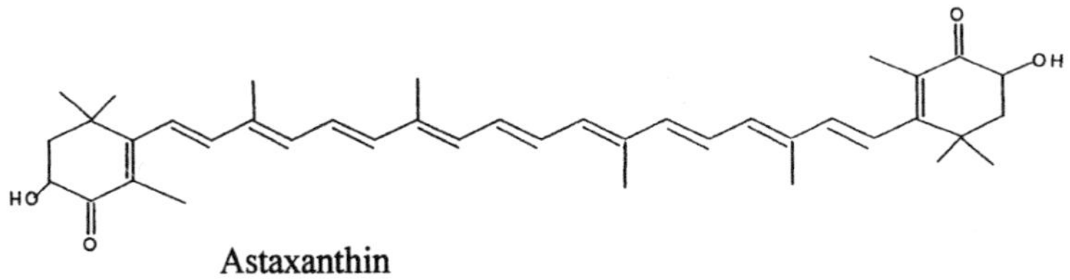

Astaxanthin

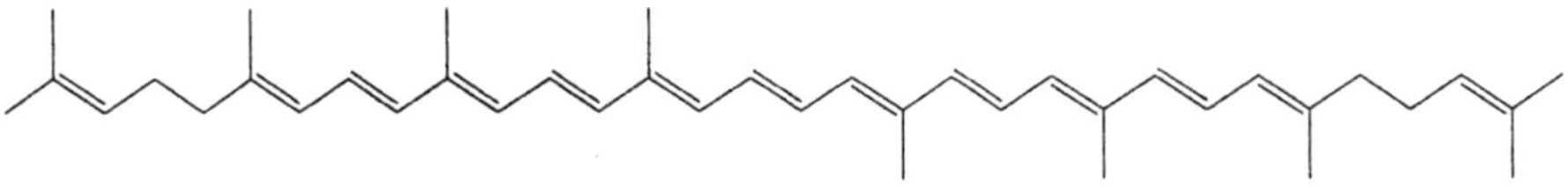

Lycopene

Fig. 6. Chemical structures of common dietary carotenoids.

3.1. Role of Phytochemicals in the Prevention of Cancer

Evidence suggests that regular consumption of fruit and vegetables can reduce cancer risk. Block et al. *(24)* established this in an epidemiological review of approx 200 studies that examined the relationship between intake of fruit and vegetables and cancer of the lung, colon, breast, cervix, esophagus, oral cavity, stomach, bladder, pancreas, and ovaries. In 128 of 156 dietary studies, the consumption of fruit and vegetables was found to have a significant protective effect. The risk of cancer was twofold higher in persons whose intake of fruit and vegetables was low compared with those with a high intake. Significant protection was found in 24 of 25 studies for lung cancer. Fruit was significantly protective in cancer of the esophagus, oral cavity, and larynx. In 26 of 30 studies, there was a protective effect of fruit and vegetable intake for cancer of the pancreas and stomach, and in 23 of 38 studies for colorectal and bladder cancer. A prospective study involving 9959 men and women in Finland showed an inverse association between the intake of flavonoids and incidence of cancer at all sites combined *(25)*. After a 24-yr follow-up, the risk of lung cancer was reduced by 50% in the highest quartile of flavonol intake. Consumption of quercetin from onions and apples was found to be inversely associated with lung cancer risk *(26)*. The effect of onions was particularly strong against squamous cell carcinoma.

Boyle et al. *(27)* showed that increased plasma levels of quercetin following a meal of onions was accompanied by increased resistance to strand breakage by lymphocyte DNA and decreased levels of some oxidative metabolites in the urine.

Carcinogenesis is a multistep process, and oxidative damage is linked to the formation of tumors through several mechanisms *(19,20)*. Oxidative stress induced by free radicals causes DNA damage, which, when left unrepaired, can lead to base mutation, single- and double-strand breaks, DNA cross-linking, and chromosomal breakage and rearrangement *(20)*. This potentially cancer-inducing oxidative damage might be prevented or limited by dietary antioxidants found in fruit and vegetables. Studies to date have demonstrated that phytochemicals in common fruit and vegetables can have complementary and overlapping mechanisms of action (*see* Table 1), including scavenging free radicals, regulation of gene expression in cell proliferation and apoptosis, modulation of detoxification enzymes, stimulation of the immune system, regulation of hormone metabolism, and antibacterial and antiviral effects *(28,29)*. It is logical to believe that antioxidant phytochemicals from other plant foods, such as whole grains, nuts, legumes, and spices act similarly.

3.2. Role of Phytochemicals in the Prevention of Cardiovascular Disease

Several epidemiological studies have examined the role of phytochemicals in CVD prevention. Dietary flavonoid intake was significantly inversely associated with mortality from coronary heart disease (CHD), and an inverse relation (weaker but significant) with incidence of myocardial infarction (MI) *(30,31)*. Intake of apples and onions, both high in quercetin, was inversely correlated with total and CHD mortality *(32)*. In a recent Japanese study, the total intake of flavonoids (quercetin, myricetin, kaempferol, luteolin, and ficetin) was inversely correlated with the plasma total cholesterol and low-density lipoprotein (LDL) cholesterol concentrations *(33)*. As a single phytochemical, quercetin intake was inversely related to total cholesterol and LDL plasma levels. Joshipura et al. *(34)* reported that total intake of both fruit and vegetables were each associated with

Table 1
Proposed Mechanisms by Which Dietary Phytochemicals May Prevent Cancer

- Antioxidant activity.
  - Scavenge free radicals and reduce oxidative stress.
  - Inhibit nitrosation and nitration.
  - Prevent DNA binding.
- Inhibition of cell proliferation.
- Induction of cell differentiation.
- Inhibition of oncogene expression and induction
    of tumor suppress gene expression.
- Induction of cell cycle arrest and apoptosis.
- Inhibition of signal transduction pathways.
- Enzyme induction and enhancing detoxification.
  - Phase II enzyme.
  - Glutathione peroxidase (GPX).
  - Catalase.
  - Superoxide dismutase (SOD).
- Enzyme inhibition.
  - Cyclooxygenase-2 (COX-2).
  - Inducible nitric oxide synthase (iNOS).
  - Xanthine oxide.
  - Phase I enzyme (block activation of carcinogens).
- Enhancement of immune functions and surveillance.
- Anti-angiogenesis.
- Inhibition of cell adhesion and invasion.
- Regulation of steroid hormone metabolism.
- Regulation of estrogen metabolism.
- Antibacterial and antiviral effects.

decreased risk for CHD. The inverse associations between total consumption of fruit and vegetables and CHD was observed with an intake of more than four servings per day. The Women's Health Study subjects had a relative risk of 0.68 for CVD when comparing the highest vs the lowest quintiles of fruit and vegetable intake, and the relative risk for MI was only 0.47. It was estimated that there was a 20–30% reduction in risk of CVD associated with high fruit and vegetable intake *(35)*. Most recently, in a study involving subjects from the National Health and Nutrition Examination Survey Epidemiologic Follow-up Study, there was a 27% lower CVD mortality with consumption of fruit and vegetables at least three times per day compared with only once per day. Fruit and vegetable intake was inversely associated with incidence of stroke, stroke mortality, CHD mortality, CVD mortality, and all-cause mortality *(36)*.

Mechanisms for the prevention of atherosclerosis by dietary antioxidants in fruit and vegetables have been proposed. In the LDL oxidation hypothesis, oxidized LDL cholesterol has been suggested as the atherogenic factor that contributes to CVD *(37,38)*. When circulating LDLs are present at high levels, they infiltrate the artery wall and increase intimal LDL, which can then be oxidized by free radicals. This oxidized LDL in the intima is more atherogenic than native LDL and serves as a chemotactic factor in the recruitment of circulating monocytes and macrophages. Oxidized LDL is typically taken up by macrophage scavenger receptors, thus inducing the formation of inflammatory cytokines and promoting cell proliferation, cholesterol ester accumulation, and foam cell formation. Gruel-like, lipid-laden foam cell accumulation in the blood vessel, forming fatty streak, would cause further endothelial injury and lead to atherosclerotic disease. Because oxidized LDL plays a key role in the initiation and progression of atherosclerosis, giving dietary supplements of antioxidants capable of preventing LDL oxidation has been an important therapeutic approach. Dietary antioxidants that are incorporated into LDL are themselves oxidized when the LDL is exposed to pro-oxidative conditions; this occurs before any extensive oxidation of the sterol or polyunsaturated fatty acids can occur *(39)*. Therefore, dietary antioxidants might retard the progression of atherosclerotic lesions. In addition, phytochemicals have been shown to have roles in the reduction of platelet aggregation, modulation of cholesterol synthesis and absorption, and reduction of blood pressure. Recently, C-reactive protein, a marker of systemic inflammation, has been reported to be a stronger predictor of CVD than is LDL cholesterol *(40)*, suggesting that inflammation is a critical factor in CVD. Inflammation not only promotes initiation and progression of atherosclerosis, but also causes acute thrombotic complications of atherosclerosis *(41)*. Dietary phytochemicals can lower C-reactive protein dramatically. Therefore, the anti-inflammatory activity of phytochemicals may play an important role in prevention of CVD.

4. HEALTH BENEFITS OF PHYTOCHEMICALS IN WHOLE FOODS: FOOD SYNERGY

The hypothesis that dietary antioxidants lower the risk of chronic disease has been developed from epidemiological studies. These have consistently shown that consumption of whole foods, such as fruit and vegetables, is strongly associated with reduced risk of chronic diseases. Therefore, it is reasonable for scientists to identify the bioactive compounds responsible, and hope to find the "magic bullet" to prevent those chronic diseases. The key question here is whether a purified phytochemical has the same health benefit as the compound does when its source is a food or a mixture of foods. It is now widely believed that the actions of the dietary supplements alone do not explain the observed health benefits of diets rich in fruit and vegetables, because, taken alone, the individual antioxidants studied in clinical trials do not appear to have consistent preventive effects *(42–44)*. The isolated pure compound either loses its bioactivity or may not behave the same way as the compound in whole foods. For example, numerous investigations have shown that the risk of cancer is inversely related to the consumption of green and yellow vegetables and fruit. Because β-carotene is present in abundance in these vegetables and fruit, it has been extensively investigated as a possible cancer-preventive agent. However, the role of carotenoids as anticancer supplements has recently been questioned as a result of several clinical studies *(42,45–47)*. In one study, the incidence of nonmelanoma skin cancer was unchanged in patients receiving a β-carotene supplement *(45)*. In other studies, smokers gained no benefit from supplemental β-carotene with respect to lung cancer incidence and may even have suffered a significant increase in lung cancer and total mortality *(42,47)*. In The Heart Outcomes Prevention Evaluation (HOPE)

Study, patients at high risk for cardiovascular events were given 400 IU of vitamin E per day or a placebo for 4.5 yr. No difference was found in deaths from cardiovascular causes, MIs, or deaths from CHD or strokes between the two groups *(48)*. In the Cambridge Heart Antioxidant Study (CHAOS), patients with CHD were given 400 or 800 IU of α-tocopherol or a placebo for a median of 510 d. α-Tocopherol intake was associated with a significantly reduced risk of MI; however, it insignificantly increased risk of cardiovascular death *(43)*. Vitamin E supplementation had no effect on the end points of death, MI, or stroke for the patients who had recently suffered an MI *(49,50)*. Vitamin C supplements also failed to lower the incidence of cancer or CHD *(51,52)*.

Phytochemical extracts from fruit and vegetables have recently been shown to have potent antioxidant and antiproliferative effects, and the combination of phytochemicals from fruit and vegetables has been proposed to be responsible for the potent antioxidant and anticancer activity of these foods *(10,11,53)*. The total antioxidant activity of phytochemicals in 1 g of apples with peel is equivalent to 83.3 μmol of vitamin C equivalents, or, to put it another way, the antioxidant value of 100 g apples is equivalent to 1500 mg of vitamin C *(53)*. This is far higher than the total antioxidant activity of 0.057 mg of vitamin C (the amount of vitamin C in 1 g of apples with peel) that is equivalent to 0.32 total oxyradical scavenging capacity (μmol vitamin C equivalent). In other words, vitamin C in apples contributes less than 0.4% of its total antioxidant activity. Thus, the vast majority of the antioxidant activity comes from phytochemicals, not vitamin C. The natural combination of phytochemicals in fruit and vegetables is responsible for its potent antioxidant activity. Apple extracts also contain bioactive compounds that inhibit tumor cell growth in vitro. Phytochemicals in apples with peel (50 mg/mL on a wet basis) inhibit colon cancer cell proliferation by 43%. However, this was reduced to 29% when apple without peel was tested *(53)*.

Different species and varieties of fruit, vegetables, and grains have different phytochemical profiles *(10,11,16)*. Therefore, consumers should obtain their phytochemicals from a wide variety of fruit, vegetables, and whole grains for optimal health benefits. In 2003, Temple and Gladwin reviewed more than 200 cohort and case–control studies that provided risk ratios concerning intake of fruit and vegetables and risk of cancer. They concluded that cancer prevention is best achieved by consumption of a wide variety of fruit and vegetables, although one group of fruit and vegetables may dominate a particular cancer *(54)*. To improve their nutrition and health, consumers should be obtaining antioxidants from their diet and not from expensive nutritional supplements, which do not contain the balanced combination of phytochemicals found in fruit and vegetables and other whole foods. More importantly, obtaining antioxidants from dietary intake by consuming a wide variety of foods is unlikely to result in consumption of toxic quantities because foods originating from plants contain many diverse types of phytochemicals in varying quantities. Fruit and vegetables eaten in the recommended amounts (5–10 servings per day of fruit and vegetables) are safe. Furthermore, health benefits from the consumption of fruit and vegetables extend beyond lowering the risk of developing cancers and CVD: it also has preventive effects on other chronic diseases, such as cataracts, age-related macular degeneration, central neurodegenerative diseases, and diabetes.

The additive and synergistic effects of phytochemicals in fruit and vegetables have been proposed to be responsible for their potent antioxidant and anticancer activities. The benefit of a diet rich in fruit and vegetables is attributed to the complex mixture of phytochemicals present in these and other whole foods (10,11,53). This partially explains why no single antioxidant can replace the combination of natural phytochemicals in fruit and vegetables in achieving the observed health benefits. There are thousands of phytochemicals present in whole foods. These compounds differ in molecular size, polarity, and solubility, which may affect the bioavailability and distribution of each phytochemical in different macromolecules, subcellular organelles, cells, organs, and tissues. This balanced natural combination of phytochemicals present in fruit and vegetables cannot simply be mimicked by pills or tablets.

Research progress in antioxidant and bioactive compounds has boosted the dietary supplement and nutraceutical industries. The use of dietary supplements is growing, especially among baby-boomer consumers. However, many of these dietary supplements have been developed based on the research results derived from biochemical/chemical analyses and studies, in vitro cell culture studies, and in vivo animal experiments, but without human intervention studies. The health benefits of natural phytochemicals at the low levels present in fruit and vegetables does not mean that these compounds are more effective or safe when they are consumed at a higher dose, even in a pure dietary supplement form. Generally speaking, higher doses increase the risk of toxicity. The basic principle of toxicology is that any compound can be toxic if the dose is high enough, and dietary supplements are no exception. Therefore, a thorough understanding of the efficacy and long-term safety of many dietary supplements needs further investigation.

It is also important to differentiate a pharmacological dose from a physiological (or nutritional) dose. Pharmacological doses are used clinically to treat specific diseases in certain situations, and need a doctor's prescription; physiological (or nutritional) doses are used to improve or maintain optimal health, such as in dietary supplements. In the case of antioxidant nutrients, the proper physiological (or nutritional) dose should follow the recommended dietary allowances. The pharmacological dose is not equal to the physiological (or nutritional) dose, and, in some cases, can be toxic for long-term use. We do not have recommended daily allowances for phytochemicals. Therefore, it is not wise to take mega-doses of purified phytochemicals as supplements before the appearance of strong supporting scientific evidence.

5. SUMMARY

Dietary modification by increasing the consumption of a wide variety of fruit, vegetables, and whole grains daily is a practical strategy for consumers to optimize their health and reduce the risk of chronic diseases. Use of dietary supplements, functional foods, and nutraceuticals is increasing as industry is responding to consumers' demands. However, there is a need for more information about the health benefits and possible risks of dietary supplements so as to ensure their efficacy and safety. Phytochemical extracts from fruit and vegetables have strong antioxidant and antiproliferative activities, and the major part of total antioxidant activity is from the combination of phytochemicals. The additive and synergistic effects of phytochemicals in fruit and vegetables are responsible for their potent antioxidant and anticancer activities. The benefit of a diet rich in fruit, vegetables, and whole grains is attributed to the complex mixture of phytochemicals present in these and other whole foods. This explains why no single antioxidant can replace the combination of natural phytochemicals in fruit and vegetables and achieve their health benefits. Therefore, the evidence suggests that antioxidants are best acquired through whole food consumption, not from expensive dietary supplements. Further research on the health benefits of phytochemicals in whole foods is warranted.

REFERENCES

1. Temple NJ. Antioxidants and disease: More questions than answers. Nutr Res 2000; 20:449–459.
2. Willett WC. Diet and health: what should we eat. Science 1994; 254:532–537.
3. Willett WC. Balancing life-style and genomics research for disease prevention. Science 2002; 296:695–698.
4. Doll R, Peto R. Avoidable risks of cancer in the United States. J Natl Cancer Inst 1981; 66:1197–1265.
5. Willett WC. Diet, nutrition, and avoidable cancer. Environ Health Perspect 1995; 103:165–170.
6. National Academy of Sciences. Committee on Diet, Nutrition, and Cancer, Assembly of Life Sciences, National Research Council. Diet, nutrition, and cancer. National Academy Press, Washington, DC, 1982.
7. National Academy of Sciences. Committee on Diet and Health, National Research Council. 1989. Diet and health: implications for reducing chronic disease risk. National Academy Press, Washington, DC, 1989.
8. Liu RH. Health benefits of fruits and vegetables are from additive and synergistic combination of phytochemicals. Am J Clin Nutr 2003; 78:517S–520S.
9. Ames BN, Gold LS. Endogenous mutagens and the causes of aging and cancer. Mutat Res 1991; 250:3–16.
10. Sun J, Chu Y-F, Wu X, Liu RH. Antioxidant and antiproliferative activities of fruits. J Agric Food Chem 2002; 50:7449–7454.
11. Chu Y-F, Sun J, Wu X, Liu RH. Antioxidant and antiproliferative activities of vegetables. J Agric Food Chem 2002; 50:6910–6916.
12. Hollman PCH, Arts ICW. Flavonols, flavones and flavanols - nature, occurrence and dietary burden. J Sci Fd Agric 2000; 80:1081–1093.
13. Hollman PCH, Katan MB. Dietary flavonoids: intake, health effects and bioavailability. Food Chem Toxicol 1999; 37:937–942.
14. Kuhnau J. The flavonoids. A class of semi-essential food components: their role in human nutrition. World Rev Nutr Diet 1976; 24:117–191.
15. Hertog MGL, Hollman PCH, Katan MB, Kromhout D. Intake of potentially anticarcinogenic flavonoids and their determinants in adults in The Netherlands. Nutr Cancer 1993a; 20:21–29.
16. Adom KK, Liu RH. Antioxidant activity of grains. J Agric Food Chem 2002; 50:6182–6187.
17. Dewanto V, Wu X, Liu RH. Processed sweet corn has higher antioxidant activity. J Agric Food Chem 2002; 50:4959–4964.
18. Britton G. Structure and properties of carotenoids in relation to function. FASEB J 1995; 9:1551–1558.
19. Liu RH, Hotchkiss JH. Potential genotoxicity of chronically elevated nitric oxide: A review. Mutat Res 1995; 339:73–89.
20. Ames BN, Shigenaga MK, Gold LS. DNA lesions, inducible DNA repair, and cell division: the three key factors in mutagenesis and carcinogenesis. Environ Health Perspect 1993; 101(Suppl 5):35–44.
21. Wang H, Cao GH, Prior RL. Total antioxidant capacity of fruits. J Agric Food Chem 1996; 44:701–705.
22. Vinson JA, Hao Y, Su X, Zubik L, Bose P. Phenol antioxidant quantity and quality in foods: fruits. J Agric Food Chem 2001; 49:5315–5321.
23. Adom KK, Sorrells ME, Liu RH. Phytochemicals and antioxidant activity of wheat varieties. J Agric Food Chem 2003; 51:7825–7834.
24. Block G, Patterson B, Subar A. Fruit, vegetables, and cancer prevention: a review of the epidemiological evidence. Nutr Cancer 1992; 18:1–29.
25. Knekt P, Jarvinen R, Seppanen R, et al. Dietary flavonoids and the risk of lung cancer and other malignant neoplasms. Am J Epidemiol 1997; 146:223–230.
26. Le Marchand L, Murphy SP, Hankin JH, Wilkens LR, Kolonel LN. Intake of flavonoids and lung cancer. J Natl Cancer Inst 2000; 92:154–160.
27. Boyle SP, Dobson VL, Duthie SJ, Kyle JAM, Collins AR. Absorption and DNA protective effects of flavonoid glycosides from an onion meal. Eur J Nutr 2000; 39:213–223.

28. Dragsted LO, Strube M, Larsen JC. Cancer-protective factors in fruits and vegetables: biochemical and biological background. Pharmacol Toxicol 1993; 72:116–135.
29. Waladkhani AR, Clemens MR. Effect of dietary phytochemicals on cancer development. Int J Mol Med 1998; 1:747–753.
30. Hertog MGL, Feskens EJM, Hollman PCH, Katan MB, Kromhout D. Dietary antioxidant flavonoids and risk of coronary heart disease: The Zutphen Elderly Study. Lancet 1993b; 342:1007–1011.
31. Hertog MGL, Kromhout D, Aravanis C, et al. Flavonoid intake and long-term risk of coronary heart disease and cancer in the Seven Countries Study. Arch Intern Med 1995; 155:381–386.
32. Knekt P, Jarvinen R, Reunanen A, Maatela J. Flavonoid intake and coronary mortality in Finland: a cohort study. Br Med J 1996; 312:478–481.
33. Arai Y, Watanabe S, Kimira M, Shimoi K, Mochizuki R, Kinae N. Dietary intakes of flavonols, flavones and isoflavones by Japanese women and the inverse correlation between quercetin intake and plasma LDL cholesterol concentration. J Nutr 2000; 131:2243–2250.
34. Joshipura KJ, Hu FB, Manson JE, et al. The effect of fruit and vegetable intake on risk for coronary heart disease. Ann Intern Med 2001; 134:1106–1114.
35. Liu S, Manson JE, Lee I-M, et al. Fruit and vegetable intake and risk of cardiovascular disease: the Women's Health Study. Am J Clin Nutr 2000; 72:922–928.
36. Bazzano LA, He J, Ogden LG, et al. Fruit and vegetable intake and risk of cardiovascular disease in US adults: the first National Health and Nutrition Examination Survey. Epidemiologic Follow-up Study. Am J Clin Nutr 2002; 76:93–99.
37. Berliner J, Leitinger N, Watson A, Huber J, Fogelman A, Navab M. Oxidized lipids in atherogenesis: formation, destruction and action. Thromb Haemost 1997; 78:195–199.
38. Witztum JL, Berliner JA. Oxidized phospholipids and isoprostanes in atherosclerosis. Curr Opin Lipidol 1998; 9:441–448.
39. Sanchez-Moreno C, Jimenez-Escrig A, Saura-Calixto F. Study of low-density lipoprotein oxidizability indexes to measure the antioxidant activity of dietary polyphenols. Nutr Res 2000; 20:941–953.
40. Ridker PM, Rifai N, Rose L, Buring JE, Cook NR. Comparison of C-reactive protein and low-density lipoprotein cholesterol levels in the prediction of first cardiovascular events. N Engl J Med 2002; 347:1557–1565.
41. Libby P, Ridker PM, Maseri A. Inflammation and atherosclerosis. Circulation 2002; 105:1135–1143.
42. Ommen GS, Goodman GE, Thomquist MD, Barnes J, Cullen MR. Effects of a combination of Œ≤-carotene and vitamin A on lung cancer and cardiovascular disease. N Engl J Med 1996; 334:1150–1155.
43. Stephens NG, Parsons A, Schofield PM, Kelly F, Cheeseman K, Mitchinson MJ. Randomized controlled trial of vitamin E in patients with coronary disease: Cambridge Heart Antioxidant Study (CHAOS). Lancet 1996; 347:154–160.
44. Yusuf S, Dagenais G, Pogue J, Bosch J, Sleight P. Vitamin E supplementation and cardiovascular events in high-risk patients. The Heart Outcomes Prevention Evaluation Study Investigators. N Engl J Med 2000; 342:154–160.
45. Hennekens CH, Buring JE, Manson JE, Stampfer M, Rosner B. Lack of effect of long-term supplementation with Œ≤-carotene on the incidence of malignant neoplasms and cardiovascular disease. N Engl J Med 1996; 334:1145–1149.
46. Greenberg ER, Baron JA, Stuckel TA, Stevens MM, Mandel JS. A clinical trial of β-carotene to prevent basal cell and squamous cell cancers of the skin. N Engl J Med 1990; 323:789–795.
47. The Alpha-Tocopherol, Beta Carotene Cancer Prevention Study Group. The effect of vitamin E and β-carotene on the incidence of lung cancer and other cancers in male smokers. N Engl J Med 1994; 330:1029–1035.
48. The HOPE Investigators. Vitamin E supplementation and cardiovascular events in high-risk patients. N Engl J Med 2000; 342:154–160.
49. GISSI-Prevenzione Investigators. Dietary supplementation with n-3 polyunsaturated fatty acids and vitamin E after myocardial infarction: results of the GISSI-Prevenzione trial. Lancet 1999; 354:447–455.
50. Miller ER, Pastor-Barriuso R, Dalal D, Riemersma RA, Appel LJ, Guallar E. Meta-analysis: high-dosage vitamin E supplementation may increase all-cause mortality. Ann Intern Med 2005; 142:37–46.
51. Blot WJ, Li JY, Taylor PR, et al. Nutrition intervention trials in Linxian, China: supplementation with specific vitamin/mineral combinations, cancer incidence, and disease-specific mortality in the general population. J Natl Cancer Inst 1993; 85:1483–1492.

52. Salonen JT, Nyyssonen K, Salonen R, et al. Antioxidant supplementation in artherosclerosis prevention (ASAP) study: a randomized trial of the effect of vitamins E and C on 3-year progression of carotid atherosclerosis. J Intern Med 2000; 248:377–386.

53. Eberhardt MV, Lee CY, Liu RH. Antioxidant activity of fresh apples. Nature 2000; 405:903, 904.

54. Temple NJ, Gladwin KK. Fruits, vegetables, and the prevention of cancer: research challenges. Nutrition 2003; 19:467–470.

11 Herbs as Useful Adjuncts to Manage Chronic Diseases

Winston J. Craig

KEY POINTS

- Ethnic dishes that have become popular in recent years use a variety of interesting herbs and spices that provide healthful substances in addition to their unique flavors.
- A variety of common herbal products are available for the treatment of cardiovascular problems, for improving glycemic control, enhancing immune function, and providing cancer chemopreventive activity.
- More clinical trials are needed to validate the activity of those herbs that show promise for the prevention or treatment of chronic diseases. Some herbal products are not standardized and provide highly variable amounts of active components.
- Most of the herbs that are promoted to promote weight loss are ineffective, unreliable, or unsafe.
- Because there are a number of herb–drug interactions, it is imperative that primary health care providers be aware of these interactions, and that they know what herbal products their clients are taking, how much, and how often.

1. INTRODUCTION

Plants have played a significant role in maintaining the health and improving the quality of human life for thousands of years. The majority of the earth's inhabitants rely on traditional medicine for their primary health care needs, and a major part of this therapy involves the use of plants, plant extracts, or their active principles. For centuries American Indians have used a number of native herbs for medicinal purposes. During the past decade, many more Americans have turned to herbal remedies for the treatment of a variety of medical conditions including coughs and colds, insomnia, digestive problems, headache, premenstrual syndrome, prostate problems, anxiety, and depression. The increasing use of herbs in the United States has been fueled by the high cost of drugs, the fear of side effects experienced with conventional drugs, and the desire to take more personal responsibility for one's health in a way that is perceived as more natural. The use of herbal preparations for health promotion and disease treatment has remained

From: *Nutritional Health: Strategies for Disease Prevention, Second Edition*
Edited by: N. J. Temple, T. Wilson, and D. R. Jacobs © Humana Press Inc., Totowa, NJ

popular in the Third World because of their low price and local accessibility in contrast to the high cost of Western pharmaceutical derivatives.

Some of the more popular herbs in use today include echinacea, ginkgo, garlic, ginseng, goldenseal, saw palmetto, St. John's wort, chamomile, cranberry, aloe vera, kava, valerian, milk thistle, and feverfew. Recently, research has validated the usefulness of Echinacea for stimulating the immune function; saw palmetto berries and stinging nettle for the treatment of benign prostatic hypertrophy; hops, passionflower, and valerian for the treatment of insomnia; St. John's wort for anxiety and depression; chamomile for its anti-inflammatory effects; cranberry for urinary tract infections; aloe vera for healing burns and wounds; kava for anxiety disorders; milk thistle to protect and restore liver function; and feverfew for the relief of migraine headaches (1).

2. UNIQUE HERBAL FLAVORS AND USES

Herbs and spices can be defined as fragrant, aromatic, or pungent edible plant substances (bark, buds, bulbs, flowers, leaves, fruit, seeds, rhizomes, and roots) that contribute flavor to food (including beverages). Herbal teas have become very popular as an alternative to caffeinated beverages. Dried herbs usually smell and taste somewhat differently from their fresh counterparts. The drying process usually causes a loss or change in the volatile oil of the plant material. Hence, the nonvolatile components become concentrated, resulting in the domination of bitter elements. Furthermore, the flavor of most dried herbs diminishes with time.

Culinary herbs and spices have been used since antiquity to flavor and preserve food. The ability of herbs and spices to delay food spoilage is owing in large part to their rich content of antioxidants. The aromatic ingredients of their essential oils and oleoresins (mixtures of terpenes, such as thymol, menthol, carvone, cineole, etc.) provide the unique flavors associated with different herbs, whereas their pungency is caused by their alkaloids (such as piperine in black pepper and capsaicin in red pepper). In addition, some herbs, such as saffron, paprika, and turmeric, are used to add color to food.

With the current emphasis on eating more healthful diets that are low in fat and salt, people are turning to various herbs and spices to flavor their food. This trend is in line with the recommendations of various government health agencies and professional health organizations. The culinary herbal seasonings that can be safely used to enhance the flavor of vegetables, soups, stews, and pasta dishes include basil, caraway, cilantro, coriander, cumin, dill, fennel, ginger, marjoram, oregano, parsley, pepper, rosemary, sage, and thyme. Sometimes these herbs are blended together, as in Italian seasoning, to give a richer, more pleasing aroma and flavor to the food.

During the past two centuries immigrants to the United States brought with them their own culture and ethnic dishes resulting in the highlighting of new flavors. The present popularity of Italian, Mexican, Indian, and other ethnic dishes has resulted in an increased use of herbal seasonings. For example, oregano is essential in the preparation of Italian and Spanish food and is commonly used to flavor pizza. Chili pepper is commonly used in many Italian, Mexican, and Indian dishes. Italians use sweet basil for flavoring beans and many of their tomato dishes. Thyme has a prominent place in French cuisine, whereas rosemary is a common ingredient in Italian and French dishes. For centuries, garlic has been used in Mediterranean, Indian, and Oriental dishes. Many

Americans are now using garlic in a variety of dips, vegetable dishes, soups, and some baked goods. Similarly, onions or dehydrated onion can be used to enhance the flavor of most vegetables, salads, soups, gravies, and many entrees.

A number of the culinary herbs contain physiologically active compounds that make them useful in treating certain disorders, or generally to promote health. In this fashion, the herb can provide a typical drug-like action. For example, fennel and various mints have been successfully used to treat coughs and colds; ginger is effective as an antiemetic for preventing nausea and vomiting associated with motion sickness, as well as for morning sickness; licorice root can help heal stomach and duodenal ulcers; and peppermint has found use in the treatment of irritable bowel syndrome (1,2). These physiological effects of herbs are parallel to those observed with some conventional medicines, but without the undesirable side effects.

Many commonly consumed plant foods, such as broccoli, carrots, citrus, grapes, soy, and tomatoes, contain physiologically active phytochemicals or phytonutrients that promote health and protect against chronic diseases (3,4). This has given rise to the term "functional foods" to designate those foods that provide health benefits beyond basic nutrition (5). However, the distinction between a basic nutrient and a phytochemical is increasingly blurred. This situation is highlighted when substances, such as soluble fiber and linolenic acid, provide a variety of health-promoting properties (see Table 1) in addition to their traditional roles in normal digestion and metabolism. This has led some people to look on food not only as a source of nutrients but also as medicine.

3. HERBS FOR IMPROVED CARDIOVASCULAR FUNCTION

Atherosclerosis is a complex series of events that involves intracellular accumulation of oxidized cholesterol and a cascade of inflammatory processes. Various botanical products can interfere with the development of cardiovascular disease (CVD) at different stages in the process. Some herbal substances can inhibit cholesterol absorption; have antioxidant activity and thereby reduce the oxidation of low-density lipoprotein (LDL) cholesterol; inhibit the activity of 3-hydroxy-3-methylglutaryl coenzyme A (HMG-CoA) reductase and thereby limit cholesterol synthesis in the cell; contain anti-inflammatory substances; inhibit platelet aggregation and thereby decrease the risk of blood clots; and improve endothelial function (6).

A plant-based diet, rich in whole grains, fruits, vegetables, and legumes, modest in nuts and low in saturated fat along with a regular aerobic exercise program, is recommended for anyone with an elevated risk of CVD. In addition, there are herbs that appear to provide help for persons with hyperlipidemia, an abnormal tendency to form blood clots, impaired blood flow, or other cardiovascular problems (7).

Policosanols appear to be a promising resource for preventing CVD. Policosanols are a mixture of high-molecular-weight aliphatic alcohols derived from sugar cane (*Saccharum officinarum* L.) wax. The mixture of aliphatic alcohols contains 24–34 carbons and is mostly octacosanol. Policosanols exhibit hypocholesterolemic effects comparable to that of the statins, except that the effects are achievable with much smaller doses of policosanols. The maximum effect of policosanols on lipid profiles appears to be reached with the use of only 10 mg/d. When administered to animals, policosanols reduce platelet aggregation, endothelial damage, and foam cell formation (8). Furthermore, policosanols effectively

Table 1
Commonly Used Health-Promoting Herbs, Their Functions, and Active Components

Physiological function	Herb or herbal extract	Active components
Lowers total and low-density lipoprotein (LDL) cholesterol	Policosanols	Octacosanol, other long-chain alcohols
	Phytosterols	β-Sitosterol, other sterols/stanols
	Garlic	Disulphides
	Psyllium	soluble fiber
	Flaxseed	Soluble fiber, phytosterols
	Fenugreek	Soluble fiber, saponins
	Red yeast rice	Monacolins
	Guggulipid	Guggulsterones
	Lemon grass oil	Terpenoids
Inhibits LDL oxidation	Green tea	Catechins
	Black tea	Theaflavins
	Licorice root	Glabridin
	Grape seed	Proanthocyanidins
	Pine bark	Pycnogenols
Inhibits blood clots	Garlic	Ajoenes, vinyldithiins, diallyl trisulfide
	Onions	Alpha-sulfinyl disulfides
	Flaxseed	Linolenic acid
	Ginger	Diterpene dialdehydes
	Asian ginseng	
	Hawthorn	Proanthocyanidins
	Evening primrose oil	Linolenic acid
Improves circulation or vascular function/arterial compliance	Green tea	Epicatechins
	Ginkgo biloba	Flavonoids, terpenoids
	Hawthorn	Flavonoids
	Horse chestnut	Escin
	Red clover	Isoflavones
Improves glycemic control or insulin utilization	Bitter melon	Steroids, polypeptide
	Fenugreek	Soluble fiber, saponins
	Gurmar	
	Flaxseed	Soluble fiber
	Psyllium	Soluble fiber
	American ginseng	Polysaccharides
	Cinnamon	Chalcone polymers
	Ivy gourd	
Enhances immune function	Echinacea	Isobutylamides, flavonoids
	Garlic	
	Cat's claw	Flavonoids, terpenoids
	Licorice root	Glycyrrhizin, chalcones
	Astragalus	Saponins
	Blackcurrant seed	
Cancer chemopreventive activity	Garlic	Sulfides, disulfides, and trisulfides
	Onions, chives, leeks	Disulfides and trisulfides
	Lamiaceae herbs (mint family)	Terpenoids, flavonoids, ursolic acid
	Apiaceae herbs (carrot family)	Coumarins, phthalides, terpenoids, polyacetylenes
	Licorice root	Glycyrrhizin, chalcones
	Green tea	Catechins
	Flaxseed	Lignans
	Ginger	Curcuminoids, gingerols, diarylheptanoids
	Turmeric	Curcuminoids
	Asian ginseng	Ginsenosides

lower the total cholesterol and LDL cholesterol levels by 13–23% and 19–31%, respectively, in human studies, and raise the high-density lipoprotein (HDL) cholesterol levels by 8–25%, without changing the triglyceride levels *(8)*. Policosanols appear to be well tolerated. They are believed to improve lipid profiles by decreasing hepatic cholesterol synthesis and enhancing LDL clearance *(8)*.

Plant sterol or stanol esters have become popular additives to margarines and other foodstuffs to help cardiovascular patients control their blood lipids. Plant sterols (phytosterols) and their Δ-5 hydrogenated derivatives (plant stanols) are derived from either wood pulp or vegetable oils. The esterification of phytosterol long-chain fatty acids increases their fat solubility about 10-fold. The phytosterol mixture is mostly β-sitosterol with lesser amounts of stigmasterol and campesterol. Recent data suggest that approx 1.6 g/d of plant sterol esters provides an LDL cholesterol reduction of about 10% *(9)*, whereas triglyceride and HDL cholesterol levels remain unchanged. There is little difference between the hypolipidemic effect of the plant sterol esters and stanol esters. These compounds inhibit the absorption of intestinal cholesterol, including the recirculating endogenous biliary cholesterol, a key step in the elimination of cholesterol *(10)*. Ingesting phytosterols in a single daily dose or between meals are equally effective methods *(11)*. The cholesterol-lowering effect of phytosterols esters is influenced by the food matrix. Serum LDL cholesterol levels decreased less when the phytosterols were given with bread or cereals than with milk *(12)*. Phytosterol-fortified orange juice was also shown to be an effective system for reducing LDL cholesterol levels *(13)*. Plant sterol and stanols are both safe and effective hypolipidemic agents. They do not affect plasma levels of vitamins A, D, and E, lycopene, and α-carotene, but do cause a reduction in β-carotene levels *(14)*.

Garlic (*Allium sativum* L.) has been used therapeutically for many centuries. The compound producing much of the activity of garlic is allicin, which is released when intact cells of a clove are cut or crushed. Allicin inhibits the growth of a wide variety of bacteria, molds, yeasts (including *Candida*), and viruses. The regular use of garlic can also be useful in lowering the risk of heart attacks and strokes because it lowers both total and LDL cholesterol levels and triglyceride levels, without affecting HDL cholesterol levels *(15,16)*. On average, consuming one-half to one clove of garlic per day for 3–6 mo reduces hypercholesterolemia by about 10% of its initial value *(16)*. Garlic also increases fibrinolytic activity and inhibits platelet aggregation caused by a variety of sulfur compounds *(15,17)*. Different forms of garlic exhibit various levels of activity. Dehydrated garlic powder, steam-distilled garlic oil, and garlic oil macerate, do not possess the bioactivity displayed by aged garlic extract, which is rich in water-soluble compounds. It appears to be the water-soluble compounds, such as *S*-allylcysteine, *S*-ethylcysteine, and saponins, rather than the lipid-soluble compounds, such as diallyl sulfide and diallyl disulfide, that are responsible for the cholesterol-lowering activity of garlic *(18,19)*. The odor-modified aged garlic extract (Kyolic) has been found to be just as effective as fresh garlic for lowering blood cholesterol levels *(20)*. The results of a meta-analysis suggest that garlic may also be useful for patients with mild hypertension *(21)*.

Onions (*Allium cepa* L.) contain many compounds that are identical or similar to those found in garlic. However, garlic is considered a more potent herb because it contains about three times the level of sulfur compounds found in onions. Onions are considered anticlotting agents because they possess substances with fibrinolytic activity and can suppress platelet aggregation *(15,17,22)*. A whole family of α-sulfinyl disulfides isolated from onions have been shown to strongly inhibit platelet aggregation *(22)*. However, onion consumption has not been linked to modifications of the plasma lipid profile.

Diets rich in soluble fiber are also known to influence the lipid profile. Psyllium (*Plantago psyllium*), the major component of Metamucil, is a rich source of soluble fiber in the diet and hypercholesterolemic patients have experienced decreases in total and LDL cholesterol levels of about 10–15 mg/dL (0.26–0.4 mmol/L) and 11–13 mg/dL (0.28-0.34 mmol/L), respectively *(23)*. In a meta-analysis of 12 studies, hypercholesterolemic adults experienced decreases in total cholesterol and LDL cholesterol levels of 0.31 and 0.35 mmol/L (5 and 9%), respectively, without changes in HDL cholesterol levels, after consumption of a psyllium-enriched cereal for an average of 42 d *(24)*. The regular use of ground flaxseed (*Linum usitatissimum*) can also lower both total cholesterol and LDL cholesterol levels about 10%, as well as producing a substantial decrease in platelet aggregation, without altering HDL cholesterol and triglyceride levels *(25,26)*. Flax has a very low saturated fat content, and a high content of polyunsaturated fat and phytosterols, in addition to its soluble fiber content.

Other herbal products have also been shown to exert various effects on cardiovascular risk factors. In clinical trials, subjects who were fed fenugreek (*Trigonella foenum-graecum*) seeds for up to 3 mo experienced a reduction in total serum cholesterol levels between 15 and 33% *(27–30)*. Fenugreek is a legume cultivated in India and the Mediterranean region. Mild gastrointestinal symptoms are commonly associated with its use. Clinical trials with guggul (*Commiphora mukul*) involving more than 200 patients with hyperlipidemia revealed significant reductions in total cholesterol levels of about 20–25% and significant drops in LDL cholesterol, but no changes in HDL levels *(31,32)*. The bioactive compounds in guggul were recently identified as the guggulsterones, potent antagonists of nuclear hormone receptors involved in cholesterol metabolism. A recent study conducted in Philadelphia was unable to verify the hypolipidemic action of guggulipid after 8 wk of therapy *(33)*. Mild adverse symptoms, including rash, nausea, and loose stools, often accompany the use of guggul. Two randomized trials, involving over 150 hypercholesterolemic subjects, revealed cholesterol-reducing effects (both total and LDL cholesterol levels) of using artichoke (*Cynara scolymus*) leaf extract for 6–12 wk *(34)*. Tolerance for the artichoke product was good, but more rigorous clinical trials are needed to assess the long-term effectiveness of artichoke.

Red yeast rice is another product that has become popular for lowering blood lipids. It is the product of fermentation of rice using the yeast *Monascus purpureus*. Red yeast rice has been used in foods and medicines for 12 centuries in China. It is also used as a coloring and flavoring agent in food. Four randomized, clinical trials involving nearly 700 subjects with hyperlipidemia, found that the use of red yeast rice was associated with a 16–31% reduction in total cholesterol and a 22–32% reduction in LDL cholesterol levels, after 8–12 wk *(31)*. In addition to natural pigments, red yeast rice also contains a family of monacolins, with the principal one being lovastatin. These metabolites possess HMG-CoA reductase-inhibitory activity *(35)*. Other changes resulting from the use of a red yeast extract (Xuezhikang), which would be associated with a lower risk of coronary heart disease, are the significant reductions in Lp(a), postprandial triglyceride levels, and high-sensitivity C-reactive protein levels observed in heart patients taking the extract for 6 wk *(36)*. Adverse reactions to the rice are well-known and include heartburn, dizziness, and flatulence. Standardized manufacturing practices need to be established for Chinese red yeast rice supplements to ensure all of the active monacolins are present and to ensure the absence of unwanted toxic byproducts, such as citrinin *(37)*.

Blood cholesterol levels may also be reduced by the oils of lemon grass (*Cymbopogon citratus*) *(38)* and evening primrose (*Oenothera biennis*) *(39)*, and by the terpenoids found in *Lamiaceae* (mint family) and *Apiaceae* (parsley family) herbs *(40)*. Although preliminary trials suggest that cholesterol levels may be decreased by yarrow (*Achillea wilhelmsii*), holy basil (*Ocimum sanctum*), and arjun (*Terminalia arjuna*) *(31)*, additional clinical trials are needed to establish the efficacy of these herbs. Asian ginseng (*Panax ginseng*) is reported to inhibit platelet aggregation and increase blood clotting times *(41)*. Many herbs also contain a variety of antioxidant phenolic compounds such as caffeic acid, ferulic acid, and ellagic acid, which can inhibit atherosclerosis *(42)*.

Flavonoids are plant pigments responsible for the colors of flowers, fruits, and some leaves *(43)*. Flavonoids have extensive biological properties that promote human health and help reduce the risk of disease. Suggested activities include the extension of the activity of vitamin C, acting as antioxidants, protection of LDL cholesterol from oxidation, inhibition of platelet aggregation, as well as anti-inflammatory and antitumor activity *(44,45)*. In the Zutphen study it was shown that flavonoid intake from fruit, vegetables, and herbs was inversely associated with heart disease mortality, and incidence of heart attack and stroke for a 5- and 15-yr period, respectively. Those in the highest tertile of flavonoid intake had a 68% lower risk of mortality from heart disease (after adjustment for potential confounders) compared with those in the lowest tertile of flavonoid intake *(46)*. Those in the highest quartile of flavonoid intake had a 73% lower risk of stroke compared with those in the lowest quartile *(47)*. In a prospective study of postmenopausal women in Iowa, total flavonoid intake was associated with a 38% decreased risk of coronary heart disease mortality (for the highest pentile of flavonoid intake vs the lowest) but no association was observed between flavonoid intake and stroke mortality *(48)*. Among the commonly consumed herbs, there are a number that contain substantial levels of flavonoids. These include chamomile, dandelion, ginkgo, green and black tea, hawthorn, licorice, passionflower, milk thistle, onions, rosemary, sage, and thyme *(43)*.

Anthocyanins are the water-soluble pigments responsible for the red, pink, mauve, purple, blue, and violet color of most flowers and fruits. They are useful for the treatment of vascular disorders and symptoms associated with capillary and venous fragility *(43)*. Grape seeds (*Vitis vinifera* L.) are a good source of proanthocyanidins—polyphenolics that provide protection against LDL oxidation and show good promise for the treatment of vascular disorders, such as inadequate circulation *(43,49)*. Similar compounds are found in the bark of the French maritime pine, *Pinus maritima*, and are marketed as pycnogenol. An extract of horse chestnut seeds contains escin, a triterpene glycoside that is also useful for chronic venous insufficiency *(50)*.

Ginkgo biloba and hawthorn appear to exert their cardiovascular effects by acting as vasodilators. *G. biloba* leaf extract appears to be somewhat effective, especially in geriatric patients, against conditions, such as memory loss, dizziness, depression, confusion, and other ailments. These conditions often respond to the vasodilation and improved cerebral blood flow induced by the *Ginkgo* extract that contains flavone glycosides and diterpenoids (gingkolides) *(1,51,52)*. The leaves, fruits, and flowers of hawthorn (*Crataegus* spp.) can improve coronary blood flow and have been suggested to improve the pumping capacity of the heart, increase the integrity of the blood vessel wall, improve oxygen use, and reduce the tendency for angina *(53)*. Proanthocyanidins, the active principles in the flower heads of hawthorn (*Crataegus oxyacantha*), are known to inhibit platelet aggregation *(54)*. Clinical studies show promise that various *Crataegus* species are useful adjuncts for the treatment of left ventricular dysfunction *(55)* and congestive heart failure *(56,57)*. Recently, a 22–23% reduction occurred in the total cholesterol and triglyceride levels of rabbits fed hawthorn fruit for 12 wk *(58)*. In addition to hawthorn, coenzyme Q_{10} (CoQ_{10}) has promise as a safe and effective approach to treating chronic heart failure *(59)*. Clinical trials have shown that CoQ_{10} supplements improve clinical parameters including reduced frequency of hospitalization, improved exercise tolerance, and improved hemodynamic parameters.

LDL oxidation is believed to play a key role in atherosclerosis. Plants contain a variety of antioxidants that can offer defense against LDL oxidation. LDL cholesterol isolated from 10 normolipidemic subjects, who consumed licorice root extract for 2 wk, was more resistant to oxidation than LDL isolated before the licorice was consumed. When a licorice extract (free of glycyrrhizinic acid) or glabridin, a flavonoid found in licorice, was fed to apo-E deficient mice, they also experienced a reduced susceptibility of their LDL cholesterol to oxidation and a reduction in the extent of atherosclerotic lesions compared with the control mice *(60)*. The use of licorice had no effect on either the total or LDL cholesterol levels, and blood coagulation was unaffected. Because glabridin was found to be less active than the whole licorice extract, it is thought that licorice contains a number of other antioxidants, including licochalcones and other polyphenols.

LDL oxidation is also inhibited by tea flavonoids—the catechins from green tea or the theaflavins (catechin dimers) from black tea *(61)*. Of the catechins, epigallocatechin gallate appears to provide the most protection, although the theaflavins exert stronger inhibitory effects than the catechins. Regular use of tea has been associated with lower heart disease rates. In one prospective study in Japan, the relative risk of death from CVD was 0.58 for men, and 0.82 for women consuming over 10 cups per day of green tea compared with those consuming less than 3 cups per day *(62)*. The protective effect of tea may result from the ability of the catechins and similar compounds to reduce intestinal cholesterol absorption, as well as lower blood coagulability and inhibit proliferation of human aortic smooth muscle cells *(63)*. Animal experiments have revealed that epigallo-catechin-3-gallate, the major constituent of green tea, induces endothelial-dependent vasodilation caused primarily by the synthesis of nitric oxide *(64)*. Several epidemiological studies have suggested that drinking either green or black tea may lower blood cholesterol and provide a measure of protection against CVD. In a randomized, clinical trial in China, 240 adults with mild-to-moderate hypercholesterolemia were given 375 mg/d of a theaflavin-enriched green tea extract or a placebo. Those receiving the tea extract experienced an 11.3 and 16.4% drop in total and LDL cholesterol levels, respectively, for 12 wk, whereas HDL and triglyceride levels were unchanged *(65)*.

4. BLOOD SUGAR MODIFICATION

Diabetes mellitus is a disease characterized by elevated blood sugar levels. A more general discussion is provided in Chapters 4 and 5. The unregulated blood sugar may result from either a lack of insulin or a reduction in its effectiveness. Careful dietary habits and regular exercise are essential components in the management of type 2 diabetes (noninsulin-dependent diabetes). In addition, there are some herbs that may be useful therapeutically. These herbs may lower blood glucose levels or improve the body's ability to release and use insulin.

A variety of botanical products with purported hypoglycemic activity have been used in Chinese traditional medicine *(66,67)*, the Ayurveda traditional health care system of India *(68,69)*, Native American Indian traditional medicine, and other traditional healing systems throughout the world *(70–72)*. These traditional medicines are not readily available in the West and few of them have been clinically tested in randomized human trials. Nevertheless, herbal products are commonly used in America for a variety of disorders. A national survey found that one-third of respondents with diabetes use complementary and alternative medicine, including herbal treatments, to treat the condition *(73)*. Recently, Yeh et al. *(74)* provided a comprehensive review of clinical trials that involve the use of herbal supplements commonly promoted for glycemic control in diabetes.

Ivy gourd (*Coccinia indica*) is a creeping plant that grows wild on the Indian subcontinent. A double-blind, 6-wk study, involving 32 persons with untreated type 2 diabetes, demonstrated significantly improved glycemic control with the use of powdered dried ivy gourd leaves, without any adverse effects *(75)*. In a 12-wk trial, blood glucose reductions were observed in patients with type 2 diabetes who consumed the dried leaves of ivy gourd *(76)*. Further research needs to be done to identify the hypoglycemic agent in this plant.

Bitter melon, balsam pear, or karela (*Momordica charantia*) is a green, cucumber-shaped tropical fruit with a bitter taste and gourd-like bumps that is eaten unripe like a vegetable. It is used traditionally throughout India, Sri Lanka, Africa, South America, and the West Indies as a diabetic remedy and is available in the United States in Asian food stores. Clinical trials have revealed that the use of the bitter melon extract can effectively lower blood sugar levels and improve glucose tolerance in persons with type 2 diabetes *(77)*. Bitter melon contains a mixture of steroidal glycosides, which have a potent hypoglycemic effect, and a polypeptide that mimics insulin activity *(78)*.

The consumption of fenugreek seeds (*T. foenum-graecum*) can also lower blood sugar levels in diabetics. Research in India found that glucose tolerance improved, urinary glucose excretion decreased 70%, and insulin responses were reduced in diabetics after defatted fenugreek was used for 10 d *(27)*. As mentioned earlier, fenugreek induces a reduction in total serum cholesterol and this is important for a diabetic who has hyperlipidemia. Fenugreek contains a high level of soluble fiber, and hence it will delay gastric emptying and slow glucose absorption. A daily use of 25–100 g of fenugreek seeds could serve as an effective supportive therapy in the management of diabetes.

Although there are different varieties of ginseng (Korean, Japanese, American, and Siberian), it is mostly American ginseng (*Panax quiquefolius*) that has been used in clinical trials. For centuries, ginseng has been used to treat diabetes by practitioners of traditional Chinese medicine. In a double-blind, placebo-controlled study, patients with type 2 diabetes who took 200 mg of American ginseng daily for 8 wk experienced improved fasting blood glucose levels and improved glycated hemoglobin levels *(79)*. A more recent study using a combination of American ginseng and Konjac-mannan produced similar results *(80)*. Other short-term metabolic trials using *P. quiquefolius* lowered postprandial glucose levels in support of its hypoglycemic activity *(74)*. Antihyperglycemic activity is not limited to the root of American ginseng, because there is substantial activity in the leaves and berries *(81,82)*. A polysaccharide fraction of the berries provides antihyperglycemic activity in *P. quiquefolius (83)*. The high variability in the quality of ginseng products casts some doubt regarding their reliability for treating type 2 diabetes *(84)*.

Prickly pear cactus, *Opuntia streptacantha* and other *Opuntia* ssp. originally native to Mexico and now grown in Mediterranean regions, the arid regions of Western United States, and throughout Latin America. In Mexican traditional medicine, prickly pear cactus (or "nopal" as it was known to the Aztecs) was used for treatment of diabetes and high cholesterol. Today, nopal is commonly used by Mexican Americans, as well as Pima Indians, for the treatment of type 2 diabetes. The hypoglycemic action of nopal, a good source of soluble fiber, has been well documented for patients with type 2 diabetes *(85)*. Extracts of *O. streptacantha* decreased postprandial glucose and hemoglobin A_{1C} levels when orally administered to animals with experimentally induced diabetes, as well as to healthy animals with physiological hyperglycemia *(86)*. In patients with type 2 diabetes, the ingestion of broiled nopal stems produced a significant 18% reduction of blood glucose and a 50% reduction in serum insulin levels *(87)*. The use of prickly pear cactus can also improve platelet function and lower blood cholesterol levels *(88–90)*. No side effects have been reported. Long-term trials are needed to establish its use as a hypoglycemic agent.

Gurmar (*Gymnema sylvestre*), a native plant of the forests of India, has been effectively used in the management of diabetes (types 1 and 2). The leaves of this climbing vine contain certain components that block the sensation of sweetness when applied to the tongue. An extract of the leaves of *Gymnema* reduces insulin requirements (or oral hypoglycemic drug dosage), improves fasting blood glucose levels, and improves blood glucose control by enhancing the action of insulin and possibly by rejuvenating the dysfunctional β-cells of the pancreas *(91,92)*. It may also produce lower levels of blood cholesterol and triglycerides. These effects are seen in diabetics only, and not in healthy volunteers.

Aloe vera, a native of North Africa, is a cactus-like plant belonging to the Lily family. The dried sap of *A. vera* is a traditional remedy for diabetes in the Arabian peninsula *(74)*. Animal feeding experiments have given somewhat inconsistent results, possibly owing to the fact that different parts of the plant were used. *A. vera* leaf pulp, rich in the water soluble fiber glucomannan, had hypoglycemic activity in both type 1 and 2 diabetic rats, whereas a leaf gel extract was found to be hyperglycemic *(93)*. Human clinical trials report improved fasting blood glucose and HbA_{1c} levels from use of *Aloe* products by persons with type 2 diabetes *(74,94)*. No adverse effects are seen with the use of *A. vera*.

Animal experiments suggest that holy basil (*O. sanctum*) has hypoglycemic properties *(74)*. A clinical trial using holy basil showed a significant 17.6 and 7.3% drop in fasting blood glucose and postprandial blood glucose levels, respectively, compared with placebo *(95)*. Flaxseed and psyllium may also provide benefits to diabetics. Because flaxseed (*L. usitatissimum*) is very rich in soluble fiber, it is also a candidate for the management of abnormal glucose levels. Subjects consuming bread containing 25% flaxseed meal showed an almost 30% improvement in a glucose tolerance test compared with those who ate plain bread *(26)*. Men with type 2 diabetes who took 5 g of psyllium

(*P. psyllium*) twice a day for 8 wk experienced an 11% drop in daily blood glucose levels in addition to a 13% drop in LDL cholesterol levels *(96)*.

Cinnamon (*Cinnamomum cassia*) consists of the dried bark of an evergreen tree that grows in Asia (Sri Lanka, Indonesia, the Seychelles, and India), the West Indies, and South America. The bark has a characteristic pleasant aromatic odor and a pungent, spicy taste. Cinnamon activates insulin receptor kinase and inhibits insulin receptor phosphatase, thereby improving insulin receptor function and thence increasing insulin sensitivity *(97)*. The biologically active compounds in cinnamon were recently shown to be chalcone polymers *(98)*. In a recent study in Pakistan involving 60 subjects with type 2 diabetes, the consumption of 1, 3, or 6 g/d of cinnamon produced an 18–29% reduction in mean fasting serum glucose levels after 40 d *(99)*. In addition, total cholesterol and LDL cholesterol levels dropped 12–26% and 7–27%, respectively. Cinnamon appears to be a safe and effective product for persons with type 2 diabetes.

Preliminary studies have reported antihyperglycemic activity or improved glucose tolerance from a number of other herbs including garlic (*A. sativum*), onions (*A. cepa*), bay leaf (*Laurus nobilis*), fig leaf (*Ficus carica*), and cloves (*Syzigium aromaticum*) *(74,98,100)*. Further research is needed to validate these findings and discover if there is any clinical significance to the hypoglycemic effects of these herbs.

5. HELP FOR THE IMMUNE SYSTEM

Echinacea, licorice, cat's claw, and garlic are some of the herbal products that may help enhance the immune system *(1,43)*. In the early 1900s, echinacea (purple coneflower) was the major plant-based antimicrobial medicine in use, but with the development of sulfa drugs its use rapidly declined. Echinacea is known to promote the activity of lymphocytes, increase phagocytosis, and induce interferon production *(1)*. It appears to be useful in moderating the symptoms of the common cold, flu, and sore throat. However, not all studies have shown that echinacea extracts significantly decrease the incidence, duration, or severity of colds and respiratory infections *(101)*. The immuno-enhancing activity of echinacea is believed to come from certain polysaccharides and isobutylamides *(43)*.

Glycyrrhizin, a sweet tasting triterpenoid saponin in licorice root (*Glycyrrhiza glabra* L.), and its aglycone (glycyrrhetinic acid) have been reported to augment interferon activity and natural-killer cell activity *(102)*. The chalcones in licorice also possess antiviral activity against the HIV, whereas glycyrrhizin possesses noticeable anti-inflammatory and antiallergic properties *(103)*.

For more than 2000 yr the Peruvian Indians have used two species of cat's claw, *Uncaria guianesis* and *Uncaria tomentosa* for medicinal purposes. Today, preparations of the bark from the root and stalk of these plants are attracting much attention in the West because of their immunostimulant properties and their potential to help fight AIDS and leukemia *(104,105)*. Extracts of cat's claw are reported to stimulate T-cells, macrophages, and other components of the immune system. Extracts are also reported to have antimutagenic and anti-inflammatory properties *(104,105)*. Recently, blackcurrant seed oil, an oil rich in linolenic acids, has been shown to have a moderate immune-enhancing effect because of its effect on prostaglandin metabolism *(106)*.

Garlic preparations have also been reported to stimulate the immune system of patients with AIDS *(107)*. Garlic can increase the number of helper cells and killer cell activity, as well as improve AIDS-related conditions such as diarrhea and fungal and viral infections *(108)*. Validation of the immunostimulant activities of garlic may be of particular importance for the treatment of AIDS in developing countries, where a lack of hard currency may limit access to Western drugs and medicine.

6. HERBS WITH CANCER CHEMOPREVENTIVE ACTIVITY

A number of commonly used herbs have been identified as possessing cancer-protective properties. These include members of the *Allium* sp. (garlic, onions, chives, and leeks), members of the mint family (basil, mints, oregano, rosemary, sage, sweet savory, and thyme), turmeric, ginger, licorice root, green tea, flax, and members of the *Apiaceae* (carrot) family, such as anise, caraway, celery, chervil, cilantro, coriander, cumin, dill, fennel, and parsley *(109)*.

Unique cancer chemoprotective phytochemicals have been identified in all of these herbs. In addition, many herbs contain a variety of phytosterols, terpenoids, flavonoids, saponins, and carotenoids, which also have cancer chemoprotective activity *(110)*. These beneficial substances act as antioxidants, immune system stimulants, inhibit the formation of DNA adducts from carcinogens, inhibit hormonal actions and metabolic pathways associated with the development of cancer, or induce protective phase I or II detoxification enzymes such as glutathione-*S*-transferase *(110–115)*.

Examples of phytochemicals that stimulate glutathione-*S*-transferase activity include the phthalides in the *Apiaceae* herbs, the sulfides in garlic and onions, curcumin in turmeric and ginger, and terpenoids, such as limonene, geraniol, cineole, α-pinene, and carvone found in commonly used culinary herbs *(110,111,114)*. Rosemary and sage contain the antioxidant diterpenoids (rosmanol, carnosol, rosmarinic acid, carnosic acid, epirosmanol, and isorosmanol) and ursolic acid, a triterpenoid with antitumor activity *(112)*.

Garlic (*A. sativum*) has been shown to reduce the development of bladder, skin, stomach, and colon cancer *(20,116)*. In a review of case–control and cohort studies of all types of cancer, 27 out of 34 studies revealed an inverse association between cancer and the consumption of allium vegetables *(117)*. A prospective study in Iowa revealed that risk of colon cancer was 32% less in those in the highest quartile of garlic consumption compared with those in the lowest quartile *(118)*. Garlic can inhibit the formation of nitrosamines, which are potent carcinogens, and also inhibit the formation of DNA adducts *(119)*. The rich content of sulfides, disulfides, and trisulfides in garlic also helps to explain its cancer chemopreventive properties. In China, those in the highest quartile of intake of garlic, onions, and other allium herbs have a risk of stomach cancer that is 40% less than those in the lowest quartile *(120)*. Case–control studies in Greece have also shown a high consumption of garlic, onion, and other allium herbs to be protective against stomach cancer *(110)*. Finally, a Dutch study revealed that cancer in the noncardia section of the stomach for those consuming the highest level of onions (at least half an onion a day) was about 50% lower than that in persons consuming no onions *(121)*.

Flaxseed, turmeric, and ginger have all been suggested to prevent cancer proliferation. Flaxseed (*L. usitatissimum*) contains a rich supply of lignans. Metabolites of these lignans act as phytoestrogens by binding to estrogen receptors and inhibiting the growth of estrogen-stimulated breast cancer *(122)*. Turmeric (*Curcuma longa*) contains phenolic compounds that inhibit cancer development, as well as having antimutagenic activity. Turmeric has been shown to suppress the development of stomach, breast, lung, and skin tumors *(123)*. Its activity is largely caused by its content of the antioxidant curcumin. Ginger also contains curcumin in addition to a dozen powerful antioxidant phenolic compounds, known as gingerols and diarylheptanoids *(113)*.

Carotenoid pigments are also effective antioxidants that quench free radicals, provide protection against oxidative damage to cells, and stimulate immune function. Persons with high levels of serum carotenoids typically have a reduced risk of cancer *(124)*. Carotenoids are the pigments found in rose hips, paprika, and the green, leafy herbs. However, studies using β-carotene supplements have not provided the expected health benefits, and in some cases have produced adverse effects such as an increased risk of lung cancer and overall mortality in smokers *(125,126)*. These findings suggest that although the consumption of carotenoid-rich fruits and vegetables promotes health, caution should be exercised in the use of β-carotene supplements.

Polyphenolics in green tea (*Camellia sinensis*) are known to possess antimutagenic and anticancer activity. Some evidence suggests a protective effect of tea against cancer of the stomach and colon *(61)*. Tumor incidence and average tumor yield in rats with chemically induced colon carcinogenesis was significantly reduced when the rats received (–)-epigallocatechin gallate, a major polyphenolic constituent of green tea *(127)*. Extracts of both black and green tea have significantly inhibited leukemia and liver tumor cells *(128)*. Extracts of gotu kolu (*Centella asiatica*) were recently shown to be very effective in killing cultured tumor cells. *Centella* appears to have selective toxicity against tumor cells as it lacked toxicity towards human lymphocytes. In follow-up studies, *Centella* extract more than doubled the life-span of mice with tumors, and showed a remarkable lack of toxicity even at high doses *(129)*. *Centella* is also therapeutic for the treatment of ulcers, wounds, and eczema.

Recent Korean studies suggest that ginseng (*P. ginseng*) may also lower the risk of cancer in humans *(130)*. Ginseng extract and powder has been found to be more effective than fresh sliced ginseng, the juice, or a ginseng tea, in reducing the risk of cancer *(131)*. In a case–control study, the incidence of human cancer was seen to steadily decrease with duration of ginseng use and total lifetime use of ginseng. Those who had taken ginseng for 1 yr had 36% less risk of cancer than nonusers, whereas those who used ginseng for 5 yr or more had 69% less risk *(132)*. Ginseng seems to be most protective against cancer of the ovaries, larynx, pancreas, esophagus, and stomach but less effective against breast, cervical, bladder, and thyroid cancer. The protective properties of ginseng root are believed to be partly caused by its content of ginsenosides, a family of triterpene saponins *(43)*.

7. HERBAL SUPPLEMENTS FOR WEIGHT REDUCTION

There is a plethora of over-the-counter weight-loss aids available today. Most of the herbal and nutritional supplements recommended for weight loss or to increase the proportion of lean body mass of a person are sold with claims of effectiveness. However, the amount of evidence supporting these claims varies substantially, and for many supplements the evidence is rather weak *(133)*. For some of the products there are additional safety concerns.

The plant *Ephedra sinica* is commonly known as "ma huang." In clinical trials this plant, and its active component ephedrine, have been shown (especially when combined with caffeine) to provide a modest weight loss of about 1 kg/mo *(133)*. However, these supplements are associated with a threefold increase in the risk of high blood pressure, stroke, heart palpitations, and psychiatric and gastrointestinal problems. Owing to these safety issues, the FDA has taken regulatory actions to restrict the use of these supplements. Many companies are now substituting an extract of bitter orange (*Citrus aurantium*) peel in place of ephedra in their "ephedra-free" formulations. Some studies suggest bitter orange helps in weight loss and increases thermogenesis to some extent *(134)*. However, bitter orange contains *m*-synephrine (phenylephrine), a stimulant that can cause adverse cardiovascular reactions *(135)*. Glucomannan, is another effective weight-loss herbal supplement, but in this case it comes without any adverse effects. Glucomannan is a soluble fiber isolated from Konjac root, derived from the plant *Amorphophallus Konjac* C. Koch. In a randomized clinical trial, obese subjects given 3 g/d of glucomannan experienced significantly greater weight loss than those in the placebo group *(136)*.

Other herbal products that have shown conflicting results in weight loss clinical trials include extracts of *Garcinia cambogia* (containing hydroxycitric acid, a suppressant of fatty acid synthesis), chitosan (derived from the exoskeleton of crustaceans), and yohimbe, the ground bark of the African evergreen *Pausinystalia yohimbe (133)*. Adverse reactions to these herbal products are usually only minor in nature, but the evidence for their effectiveness is not compelling. When Yerba mate (*Ilex paraguariensis*) is combined with another caffeine-rich South American herb, guarana (*Paullinia cupana*), the resulting mixture was found to be effective in reducing the body weight of overweight patients *(137)*. Despite their popularity, neither guar gum, a soluble fiber from the Indian cluster bean (*Cyamopsis tetragonolbus*), nor psyllium, a water-soluble fiber from the seeds of *Plantago ovata*, were found to be effective weight-loss agents *(133)*.

8. CONCERNS WITH HERBAL USAGE

When taking clinical histories health practitioners often fail to ask patients about their use of herbal products. In addition, patients may not volunteer this information because they do not realize its importance. Furthermore, patients may not wish to frustrate the health practitioner by telling them they are self-medicating with botanical materials or herbal supplements. Because herbs can often enhance or negate the effect of a conventional drug, it is important for physicians to know which herbs their patients take, how much, and how often. There are a number of possible drug–herb interactions to be considered *(138)*. For example, nonsteroidal anti-inflammatory drugs may negate the usefulness of feverfew in the treatment of migraine headaches; ginkgo, garlic, ginger, and ginseng should not be used concomitantly with warfarin because they may alter bleeding time; immunostimulants, such as echinacea, should not be given with immunosuppressants, such as corticosteroids; evening primrose oil should not be used with an anticonvulsant because it may lower the seizure threshold; excessive sedation may result when kava and barbiturates are used together; and licorice may offset the effect of spironolactone.

Another problem with the use of herbs or herbal extracts is the fact that the contents of many are not standardized so that the dose of a particular active ingredient is unknown

(1). The phytochemical content of an herb can vary from plant to plant based on where the herb was grown, the light conditions, and the maturity of the plant when harvested. The level of phytochemicals can vary greatly even between cultivars of the same species. Furthermore, different parts of an herb usually contain different amounts of the active ingredient *(44,139)*. Methods of preparation of the herbal extract also influence the activity of the final product for the consumer. The level of ginsenosides has been found to vary as much as 60-fold among 10 common brands of ginseng on the market *(140)*. Occasionally, there are also some reports of adulteration of herbal products. For example, echinacea is sometimes adulterated with the inactive root of wild quinine, *Parthenium integrifolium*, for reasons of cost.

9. CONCLUSIONS

A variety of commonly used herbs containing different phytochemicals have the potential for use in the treatment of chronic diseases. Some of these herbs provide assistance in the treatment of hypercholesterolemia; some provide protection against cancer; some help with blood sugar control, whereas others are known to stimulate the immune system. Furthermore, a diet in which culinary herbs are generously used to flavor the food will provide a variety of active phytochemicals that promote health and protect against chronic diseases. Herbs have been described as both a friend of physicians and the praise of cooks *(141)*. Although the discriminate use of some herbal products is safe and some therapeutic benefits may be derived from their proper usage, the indiscriminate or excessive use of herbs can be unsafe *(1)*.

REFERENCES

1. Tyler V. Herbs of Choice. The Therapeutic Use of Phytomedicinals. Haworth Press, New York, 1994.
2. Dew MJ, Evans BK, Rhodes J. Peppermint oil for the irritable bowel syndrome: a multicentre trial. Br J Clin Pract 1984; 38:394–398.
3. Beecher GR. Phytonutrients' role in metabolism: effects of resistance to degenerative processes. Nutr Rev 1999; 57:S3–S6.
4. Craig WJ. Phytochemicals: guardians of our health. J Am Diet Assoc 1997; 97:S199–S204.
5. Thomson C, Bloch AS, Hasler CM. Position of the American Dietetic Association: functional foods. J Am Diet Assoc 1999; 99:1278–1285.
6. Heber D. Herbs and atherosclerosis. Curr Atheroscler Rep 2001; 3:93–96.
7. Fugh-Berman A. Herbs and dietary supplements in the prevention and treatment of cardiovascular disease. Prev Cardiol 2000; 3:24–32
8. Varady KA, Wang Y, Jones PJH. Role of policosanols in the prevention and treatment of cardiovascular disease. Nutr Rev 2003; 61:376–383.
9. Lichtenstein AH. Plant sterols and blood lipid levels. Curr Opin Clin Nutr Metab Care 2002; 5:147–152.
10. Ostlund RE Jr. Phytosterols in human nutrition. Annu Rev Nutr 2002; 22:533–549.
11. Quilez J, Garcia-Lorda P, Salas-Salvado J. Potential uses and benefits of phytosterols in diet: present situation and future directions. Clin Nutr 2003; 22:343–351.
12. Clifton PM, Noakes M, Sullivan D, et al. Cholesterol-lowering effects of plant sterol esters differ in milk, yoghurt, bread and cereal. Eur J Clin Nutr 2004; 58:503–509.
13. Devaraj S, Jialal I, Vega-Lopez S. Plant sterol-fortified orange juice effectively lowers cholesterol levels in mildly hypercholesterolemic healthy individuals. Arterioscler Thromb Vasc Biol 2004; 24: e25–e28.
14. Katan MB, Grundy SM, Jones P, Law M, Miettinen T, Paoletti R, Stress Workshop Participants. Efficacy and safety of plant stanols and sterols in the management of blood cholesterol levels. Mayo Clin Proc 2003; 78:965–978.

15. Kleijnen J, Knipschild P, ter Riet GT. Garlic, onions and cardiovascular risk factors. A review of the evidence from human experiments with emphasis on commercially available preparations. Br J Clin Pharmacol 1989; 28:535–544.

16. Warshafsky S, Kramer RS, Sivak SL. Effect of garlic on total serum cholesterol: a meta-analysis. Ann Intern Med 1993; 119:599–605.

17. Kendler BS. Garlic (Allium sativum) and onion (Allium cepa): A review of their relationship to cardiovascular disease. Prev Med 1987; 16:670–685.

18. Yeh YY, Liu L. Cholesterol-lowering effect of garlic extracts and organosulfur compounds: human and animal studies. J Nutr 2001; 131:989S–993S.

19. Matsuura H. Saponins in garlic as modifiers of the risk of cardiovascular disease. J Nutr 2001; 131: 1000S–1005S.

20. Dauusch JG, Nixon DW. Garlic: A review of its relationship to malignant disease. Prev Med 1990; 19:346–361.

21. Silagy CA, Neil HA. A meta-analysis of the effect of garlic on blood pressure. J Hypertens 1994; 12:463–468.

22. Kawakishi S, Morimitsu Y. Sulfur chemistry of onions and inhibitory factors of the arachidonic acid cascade. In: Huang MT, Osawa T, Ho CT, Rosen RT, eds. Food Phytochemicals for Cancer Prevention. I. Fruits and Vegetables. American Chemical Society, Washington DC, 1994, pp. 120–127.

23. Sprecher DL, Harris BV, Goldberg AC, et al. Efficacy of psyllium in reducing serum cholesterol levels in hypercholesterolemic patients on high- or low-fat diets. Ann Intern Med 1993; 119:545–554.

24. Olson BH, Anderson SM, Becker MP, et al. Psyllium-enriched cereals lower blood total cholesterol and LDL cholesterol, but not HDL cholesterol, in hypercholesterolemic adults: results of a meta-analysis. J Nutr 1997; 127:1973–1980.

25. Bierenbaum ML, Reichstein R, Walkins T. Reducing atherogenic risk in hyperlipemic humans with flax seed supplementation: a preliminary report. J Am Coll Nutr 1993; 12:501–504.

26. Cunnane SC, Ganguli S, Menard C, et al. High alpha-linolenic acid flaxseed (Linum usitatissimum): some nutritional properties in humans. Br J Nutr 1993; 69:443–453.

27. Sharma RD, Raghuram TC. Hypoglycaemic effect of fenugreek seeds in non-insulin dependent diabetic subjects. Nutr Res 1990; 10:731–739.

28. Singh RB, Niaz MA, Rastogi V, Postiglione A, Rastogi SS. Hypolipidemic and antioxidant effects of fenugreek seeds and triphala as adjuncts to dietary therapy in patients with mild to moderate hypercholesterolemia. Perfusion 1998; 11:124–130.

29. Prasanna M. Hypolipidemic effect of fenugreek: a clinical study. Indian J Pharmacol 2000; 32:34–36.

30. Sharma RD, Raghuram TC, Rao NS. Effect of fenugreek seeds on blood glucose and serum lipids in type I diabetes. Eur J Clin Nutr 1990; 44:301–306.

31. Thompson Coon JS, Ernst E. Herbs for serum cholesterol reduction: a systematic view. J Fam Pract 2003; 52:468–478.

32. Nityanand S, Srivastava JS, Asthana OP. Clinical trials with gugulipid, a new hypocholesterolemic agent. J Assoc Physicians India 1989; 37:323–328.

33. Szapary PO, Wolfe ML, Bloedon LT. Guggulipid for the treatment of hypercholesterolemia: a randomized controlled trial. JAMA 2003; 290:765–772.

34. Pittler MH, Thompson CO, Ernst E. Artichoke leaf extract for treating hypercholesterolaemia. Cochrane Database Syst Rev 2002; (3):CD003335.

35. Hendler SS, Rorvik D, eds. PDR for Nutritional Supplements. Medical Economics Company, Montvale, NJ, 2001.

36. Liu L, Zhao SP, Cheng YC, Li YL. Xuezhikang decreases serum lipoprotein (a) and C-reactive protein concentrations in patients with coronary heart disease. Clin Chem 2003; 49:1347–1352.

37. Herber D, Lembertas A, Lu QY, Bowerman S, Go VL. An analysis of nine proprietary Chinese red yeast rice dietary supplements: implications of variability in chemical profile and contents. J Altern Complement Med 2001; 7:133–139.

38. Elson CE, Underbakke GL, Hanson P, Shrago E, Wainberg RH, Qureshi AA. Impact of lemongrass oil, an essential oil, on serum cholesterol. Lipids 1989; 24:677–679.

39. Sugano M, Ide T, Ishada T, Yoshida K. Hypocholesterolemic effect of gamma-linolenic acid as evening primrose oil in rats. Ann Nutr Metab 1986; 30:289–299.

40. Case GL, He L, Mo H, Elson CE. Induction of geranyl pyrophosphate pyrophosphatase activity by cholesterol-suppressive isoprenoids. Lipids 1995; 30:357–359.

41. Park HJ, Rhee MH, Park KM, Nam KY, Park KH. Effect of non-saponin fraction from Panax ginseng on cGMP and thromboxane A2 in human platelet aggregation. J Ethnopharmacol 1995; 49:157–162.

42. Decker EA. The role of phenolics, conjugated linoleic acid, carnosine, and pyrroloquinoline quinone as nonessential dietary antioxidants. Nutr Rev 1995; 53:49–58.

43. Bruneton J. Pharmacognosy, Phytochemistry, Medicinal Plants. C.K. Lavoisier Publishers, Paris, 1995.

44. Manach C, Regerat F, Texier O, Agullo G, Demigne C, Remesy C. Bioavailability, metabolism and physiological impact of 4-oxo-flavonoids. Nutr Res 1996; 16:517–544.

45. Cook NC, Samman S. Flavonoids - chemistry, metabolism, cardioprotective effects, and dietary sources. J Nutr Biochem 1996; 7:66–76.

46. Hertog MGL, Feskens EJM, Hollman PC, Katan MB, Kromhout D. Dietary antioxidant flavonoids and risk of coronary heart disease. Lancet 1993; 342:1007–1011.

47. Keli SO, Hertog MG, Feskins EJ, Kromhout D. Dietary flavonoids, antioxidant vitamins, and incidence of stroke: the Zutphen study. Arch Intern Med 1996; 156:637–642.

48. Yochum L, Kushi LH, Meyer K, Folsom AR. Dietary flavonoid intake and risk of cardiovascular disease in postmenopausal women. Am J Epidemiol 1999; 149:943–949.

49. Nuttall SL, Kendall MJ, Bombardelli E, Morazzoni P. An evaluation of the antioxidant activity of a standardized grape seed extract, Leucoselect. J Clin Pharm Ther 1998; 23:385–389.

50. Pittler MH, Ernst E. Horse-chestnut seed extract for chronic venous insufficiency. A criteria-based systematic review. Arch Dermatol 1998; 134:1356–1360.

51. Kleijnen J, Knipschild P. Gingko biloba for cerebral insufficiency. Br J Clin Pharmacol 1992; 34:352–358.

52. Curtis-Prior P, Vere D, Fray P. Therapeutic value of Ginkgo biloba in reducing symptoms of decline in mental function. J Pharm Pharmacol 1999; 51:535–541.

53. Rigelsky JM, Sweet BV. Hawthorn: pharmacology and therapeutic uses. Am J Health Syst Pharm 2002; 59:417–422.

54. Vibes J, Lasserre B, Gleye J, Declume C. Inhibition of thromboxane A2 biosynthesis in vitro by the main components of Crataegus oxyacantha (Hawthorn) flower heads. Prostaglandins Leukot Essent Fatty Acids 1994; 50:173–175.

55. Fong HH, Bauman JL. Hawthorn. J Cardiovasc Nurs 2002; 16(4):1–8.

56. Pittler MH, Schmidt K, Ernst E. Hawthorn extract for treating chronic heart failure: meta-analysis of randomized trials. Am J Med 2003; 114:665–674.

57. Eaton LJ, Kinkade S. Hawthorn extract improves chronic heart failure. J Fam Pract 2003; 52:753, 754.

58. Zhang Z, Ho WK, Huang Y, James AE, Lam LW, Chen ZY. Hawthorn fruit is hypolipidemic in rabbits fed a high cholesterol diet. J Nutr 2002; 132:5–10.

59. Motensen SA. Overview on coenzyme Q10 as adjunctive therapy in chronic heart failure. Rationale, design and end-points of "Q-symbio"—a multinational trial. Biofactors 2003; 18:79–89.

60. Fuhrman B, Buch S, Vaya J, et al. Licorice extract and its major polyphenol glabridin protect low-density lipoprotein against lipid peroxidation: in vitro and ex vivo studies in humans and in atherosclerotic aoplipoprotein E-deficient mice. Am J Clin Nutr 1997; 66:267–275.

61. Ishikawa T, Suzukawa M, Ito T, et al. Effect of tea flavonoid supplementation on the susceptibility of low-density lipoprotein to oxidative modification. Am J Clin Nutr 1997; 66:261–266.

62. Nakachi K, Matsuyama S, Miyake S, Suganuma M, Imai K. Preventive effects of drinking green tea on cancer and cardiovascular disease: epidemiological evidence for multiple targeting prevention. Biofactors 2000; 13:49–54.

63. Dreosti IE. Bioactive ingredients: antioxidants and polyphenols in tea. Nutr Rev 1996; 54:S51–S58.

64. Lorenz M, Wessler S, Follmann E, et al. A constituent of green tea, epigallocatechin -3-gallate, activates endothelial nitric oxide synthase by a phosphatidylinositol-3-OH-kinase-, cAMP-dependent

protein kinase-, and Akt-dependent pathway and leads to endothelial-dependent vasorelaxation. J Biol Chem 2004; 279:6190–6195.

65. Maron DJ, Lu GP, Cai NS, et al. Cholesterol-lowering effect of a theaflavin-enriched green tea extract: a randomized controlled trial. Arch Intern Med 2003; 163:1448–1453.

66. Jia W, Gao W, Tang L. Antidiabetic herbal drugs officially approved in China. Phytother Res 2003; 17:1127–1134.

67. Li WL, Zheng HC, Bukuru J, De Kimpe N. Natural medicines used in the traditional Chinese medical system for therapy of diabetes mellitus. J Ethnopharmacol 2004; 92:1–21.

68. Elder C. Ayurveda for diabetes mellitus: a review of biomedical literature. Altern Ther Health Med 2004; 10:44–50.

69. Grover JK, Yadav S, Vats V. Medicinal plants of India with anti-diabetic potential. J Ethnopharmacol 2002; 81:81–100.

70. Al-Rowais NA. Herbal medicine in the treatment of diabetes mellitus. Saudi Med J 2002; 23:1327–1331.

71. Newairy AS, Mansor HA, Yousef MI, Sheweita SA. Alterations of lipid profile in plasma and liver of diabetic rats: effect of hypoglycemic herbs. J Environ Sci Health B 2002; 37:475–484.

72. Yaniv Z, Dafni A, Friendman J, Palevitch D. Plants used for the treatment of diabetes in Israel. J Ethnopharmacol 1987; 19:145–151.

73. Yeh GY, Eisenberg DM, Davis RB, Philips RS. Complementary and alternative medicine use among patients with diabetes mellitus: results of a national survey. Am J Public Health 2002; 92:1648–1652.

74. Yeh GY, Eisenberg DM, Kaptchuk TJ, Philips RS. Systematic review of herbs and dietary supplements for glycemic control in Diabetes. Diabetes Care 2003; 26:1277–1298.

75. Azad Khan AK, Akhatar S, Mahtab H. Coccinia indica in the treatment of patients with diabetes mellitus. Bangladesh Med Res Counc Bull 1979; 5:60–66.

76. Kamble SM, Jyotishi GS, Kamlakar PL, Vaidya SM. Efficacy of Coccinia indica W. & A in diabetes mellitus. J Res Ayurveda Siddha 1996; XVII:77–84.

77. Srivastava Y, Venkatakrishna-Bhatt H, Verma Y, Venkaiah, K, Raval BH. Antidiabetic and adaptogenic properties of Momardica charantia extract: an experimental and clinical evaluation. Phytother Res 1993; 7:285–289.

78. Marles RJ, Farnsworth NR. Antidiabetic drugs and their active constituents. Phytomedicine 1995; 2:137–189.

79. Sotaniemi EA, Haapakoski E, Rautio A. Ginseng therapy in non-insulin-dependent diabetic patients. Diabetes Care 1995; 118:1373–1375.

80. Vuksan V, Sievenpiper JL, Xu Z, et al. Konjac-Mannan and American ginseng: emerging alternative therapies for type 2 diabetes mellitus. J Am Coll Nutr 2001; 20(5 Suppl):370S–380S.

81. Xie JT, Mehendale SR, Wang A, et al. American ginseng leaf: ginsenoside analysis and hypoglycemic activity. Pharmacol Res 2004; 49:113–117.

82. Xie JT, Aung HH, Wu JA, Attel AS, Yuan CS. Effects of American ginseng berry extract on blood glucose levels in ob/ob mice. Am J Chin Med 2002; 30:187–194.

83. Xie JT, Wu JA, Mehendale S, Aung HH, Yuan CS. Anti-hyperglycemic effect of the polysaccharides fraction from American ginseng berry extract in ob/ob mice. Phytomedicine 2004; 11:182–187.

84. Sievenpiper JL, Arnason JT, Vidgen E, Leiter LA, Vuksan V. A systematic quantitative analysis of the literature of the high variability in ginseng (Panax spp.): should ginseng be trusted in diabetes? Diabetes Care 2004; 27:839, 840.

85. Frati AC, Gordillo BE, Altamirano P, et al. Influence of nopal intake upon fasting glycemia in type II diabetes and healthy subjects. Arch Invest Med (Mex) 1991; 22:51–56.

86. Ibanez-Camacho R, Roman-Ramos R. Hypoglycemic effect of Opuntia cactus. Arch Invest Med (Mex) 1979; 10:223–230.

87. Frati-Munari AC, Gordillo BE, Altamirano P, Ariza CR. Hypoglycemic effect of Opuntia streptacantha Lemaire in NIDDM. Diabetes Care 1988; 11:63–66.

88. Wolfram R, Budinsky A, Efthimiou Y, Stomatopoulos J, Oguogho A, Sinzinger H. Daily prickly pear consumption improves platelet function. Prostaglandins Leukot Essent Fatty Acids 2003; 69:61–66.

89. Wolfram RM, Kritz H, Efthimiou Y, Stomatopoulos J, Sinzinger H. Effect of prickly pear (Opuntia robusta) on glucose- and lipid-metabolism in non-diabetics with hyperlipidemia—a pilot study. Wien Klin Wochenschr 2002; 114:840–846.

90. Budinsky A, Wolfram R, Oguogho A, Efthimiou Y, Stamatopoulos Y, Sinzinger H. Regular ingestion of Opuntia robusta lowers oxidation injury. Prostaglandins Leukot Essent Fatty Acids 2001; 65:45–50.

91. Shanmugasundaram ERB, Rajeswari G, Baskaran K, Rajesh Kumar BR, Shanmugasundaram KR, Arhmath BK. Use of Gymnema sylvestre leaf extract in the control of blood glucose in insulin-dependant diabetes mellitus. J Ethnopharmacol 1990; 30:281–294.

92. Baskaran K, Kizar Ahamath B, Shanmugasundaram KR, Shanmugasundaram ER. Antidiabetic effect of a leaf extract from Gymnema sylvestre in non-insulin dependent diabetes mellitus patients. J Ethnopharmacol 1990; 30:295–305.

93. Okyar A, Can A, Akev N, Baktir G, Sutlupinar N. Effect of Aloe vera leaves on blood glucose level in type I and type II diabetic rat models. Phytother Res 2001; 15:157–161.

94. Ghannam N, Kingston M, Al-Meshaal IA, Tariq M, Parman NS, Woodhouse N. The antidiabetic activity of aloes: preliminary clinical and experimental observations. Horm Res 1986; 24:288–294.

95. Agrawal P, Rai V, Singh RB. Randomized placebo-controlled, single blind trial of holy basil leaves in patients with noninsulin-dependent diabetes mellitus. Int J Clin Pharmacol Ther 1996; 34:406–409.

96. Anderson JW, Allgood LD, Turner J, Oeltgen PR, Daggy, BP. Effects of psyllium on glucose and serum lipid responses in men with type 2 diabetes and hypercholesterolemia. Am J Clin Nutr 1999; 70:466–473.

97. Imparl-Radosevich J, Deas S, Polansky MM, et al. Regulation of PTP-1 and insulin receptor kinase by fractions from cinnamon: implications for cinnamon regulation of insulin signalling. Horm Res 1998; 50:177–182.

98. Broadhurst CL, Polansky MM, Anderson RA. Insulin-like biological activity of culinary and medicinal plant aqueous extracts in vitro. J Agric Food Chem 2000; 48:849–852.

99. Khan A, Safdar M, Ali Khan MM, Khattak KN, Anderson RA. Cinnamon improves glucose and lipids of people with type 2 diabetes. Diabetes Care 2003; 26:3215–3218.

100. Khan A, Bryden NA, Polansky MM, Anderson RA. Insulin potentiating factor and chromium content of selected foods and spices. Biol Trace Elem Res 1990; 24:183–188.

101. Grimm W, Muller HH. A randomized controlled trial of the effect of fluid extract of Echinacea purpurea on the incidence and severity of colds and respiratory infections. Am J Med 1999; 106:138–143.

102. Abe N, Ebina T, Ishida N. Interferon induction by glycyrrhizin and glycyrrhetinic acid in mice. Microbiol Immunol 1982; 26:535–539.

103. Shibata S. Antitumor-promoting and anti-inflammatory activities of licorice principles and their modified compounds. In: Huang MT, Osawa T, Ho CT, Rosen RT, eds. Food Phytochemicals for Cancer Prevention II. Teas, Spices and Herbs. American Chemical Society, Washington DC, 1994, pp. 308–321.

104. Rizzi R, Re F, Bianchi A, De Feo V, de Simone F, Bianchi L, Stivala LA. Mutagenic and antimutagenic activities of Uncaria tomentosa and its extracts. J Ethnopharmacol 1993; 38:63–77.

105. Aquino R, De Feo V, De Simone F, Pizza C, Cirino G. Plant metabolites. New compounds and anti-inflammatory activity of Uncaria tomentosa. J Nat Prod 1991; 54:453–459.

106. Wu D, Meydani M, Leka LS, et al. Effect of dietary supplementation with black currant seed oil on the immune response of healthy elderly subjects. Am J Clin Nutr 1999; 70:536–543.

107. Burger RA, Warren RP, Lawson LD, Hughes BG. Enhancement of in vitro human immune function by Allium sativum L (garlic) fractions. Int J Pharmacogn 1993; 31:169–174.

108. Abdullah TH, Kirkpatrick DV, Carter J. Enhancement of natural killer cell activity in AIDS with garlic. Deutsch Zeishrift fur Oncology 1989; 21:52, 53.

109. Caragay AB. Cancer-preventative foods and ingredients. Food Tech 1992; 46(4):65–68.

110. Huang MT, Ferraro T, Ho CT. Cancer chemoprevention by phytochemicals in fruits and vegetables. An overview. In: Huang MT, Osawa T, Ho CT, Rosen RT, eds. Food Phytochemicals for Cancer Prevention I. Fruits and Vegetables. American Chemical Society, Washington DC, 1994, pp. 2–16.

111. Bisset NG, ed. Herbal Drugs and Phytopharmaceuticals. A Handbook for Practice on a Scientific Basis. Medpharm Scientific Publishers, Stuttgart, 1994.

112. Ho CT, Ferraro T, Chen Q, Rosen RT, Huang MT. Phytochemicals in teas and rosemary and their cancer-preventive properties. In: Huang MT, Osawa T, Ho CT, Rosen RT, eds. Food Phytochemicals for Cancer Prevention II. Teas, Spices and Herbs. American Chemical Society, Washington DC, 1994, pp. 2–19.

113. Kikuzaki H, Nakatani N. Antioxidant effects of some ginger constituents. J Food Sci 1993; 58:1407–1410.

114. Nakatani N. Chemistry of antioxidants from Labiatae herbs. In: Huang MT, Osawa T, Ho CT, Rosen RT, eds. Food Phytochemicals for Cancer Prevention II. Teas, Spices and Herbs. American Chemical Society, Washington DC, 1994, pp. 144–153.

115. Steinmetz KA, Potter JD. Vegetables, fruit, and cancer, II. Mechanisms. Cancer Causes Control 1991; 2:427–442.

116. Lau BHS, Tadi PP, Tosk JM. Allium sativum (garlic) and cancer prevention. Nutr Res 1990; 10:937–948.

117. Steinmetz KA, Potter JD. Vegetables, fruit, and cancer prevention: a review. J Am Diet Assoc 1996; 96:1027–1039.

118. Steinmetz KA, Kushi LH, Bostick RM, Folsom AR, Potter JD. Vegetable, fruit, and colon cancer in the Iowa women's health study. Am J Epidemiol 1994; 139:1–15.

119. Milner JA. Garlic: its anticarcinogenic and antitumorigenic properties. Nutr Rev 1996; 54(11):S82–S86.

120. You WC, Blot WJ, Chang YS, et al. Allium vegetables and reduced risk of stomach cancer J Natl Cancer Inst 1989; 81:162–164.

121. Dorant E, van den Brandt PA, Goldbohm RA, Sturmans F. Consumption of onions and a reduced risk of stomach carcinoma. Gastroenterology 1996; 110:12–20.

122. Serraino M, Thompson LU. The effect of flaxseed supplementation on the initiation and promotional stages of mammary tumorigenesis. Nutr Cancer 1992; 17:153–159.

123. Nagabhushan M, Bhide SV. Curcumin as an inhibitor of cancer. J Am Coll Nutr 1992; 11:192–198.

124. Van Poppel G, Goldbohm RA. Epidemiologic evidence for beta-carotene and cancer prevention. Am J Clin Nutr 1995; 62:1393S–1402S.

125. Lee I, Cook NR, Manson JE, Buring JE, Hennekens CH. Beta-carotene supplementation and incidence of cancer and cardiovascular disease: the Women's health study. J Natl Cancer Inst 1999; 91:2102–2106.

126. Albanes D. Beta-carotene and lung cancer: a case study. Am J Clin Nutr 1999; 91:2102–2106.

127. Anon. D-Limonene, an anticarcinogenic terpene. Nutr Rev 1988; 46:363–365.

128. Lea MA, Xiao Q, Sadhukhan AK, Cottle S, Wang ZY, Yang CS. Inhibitory effects of tea extracts and (-)-epigallocatechin gallate on DNA synthesis and proliferation of hepatoma and erythroleukemia cells. Cancer Lett 1993; 68:231–236.

129. Babu TD, Kuttan G, Padikkala J. Cytotoxic and anti-tumor properties of certain taxa of Umbelliferae with special reference to Centella asiatica urban. J Ethnopharmacol 1995; 48:53–57.

130. Yun TK. Experimental and epidemiological evidence of the cancer-preventive effects of Panax ginseng CA Meyer. Nutr Rev 1996; 54(11):S71–S81.

131. Yun TK, Choi SY. A case-control study of ginseng intake and cancer. Int J Epidemiol 1990; 19:871–876.

132. Yun TK, Choi SY. Preventive effect of ginseng intake against various human cancers: a case-control study on 1987 pairs. Cancer Epidemiol Biomarkers Prev 1995; 4:401–408.

133. Pittler MH, Ernst E. Dietary supplements for body-weight reduction: a systematic review. Am J Clin Nutr 2004; 79:529–536.

134. Preuss HG, DiFerdinando D, Bagchi M, Bagchi D. Citrus aurantium as a thermogenic, weight-reduction replacement for ephedra: an overview. J Med 2002; 33:247–264.

135. Nykamp DL, Fackih MN, Compton AL. Possible association of acute lateral-wall myocardial infarction and bitter orange supplement. Ann Pharmacother 2004; 38:812–816.

136. Walsh DE, Yaghoubian V, Behforooz A. Effect of glucomannan on obese patients: a clinical study. Int J Obes 1983; 8:289–293.

137. Anderson T, Fogh J. Weight loss and delayed gastric emptying following a South American herbal preparation in overweight patients. J Hum Nutr Dietet 2001; 14:243–250.

138. Miller LG. Herbal medicinals. Selected clinical considerations focusing on known or potential drug-herb interactions. Arch Intern Med 1998; 158:2200–2211.

139. Bravo L. Polyphenols: chemistry, dietary sources, metabolism, and nutritional significance. Nutr Rev 1998; 56:317–333.

140. Ansley D, ed. Ginseng. Much ado about nothing? Consumer Reports 1995; 60:699.

141. Farrell KT. Spices, Condiments and Seasonings. AVI Publishing Company, Westport, CT, 1985, pp. 17.

12

What Are the Health Implications of Alcohol Consumption?

Eric Rimm and Norman J. Temple

KEY POINTS

- An alcoholic drink is generally considered to contain 12.5–13 g of alcohol (ethanol); this amount is found in 12-oz (356 g) beer, 4–5-oz (118–148 g) wine, or 1.5 oz (42 g) of distilled spirits. The US Department of Agriculture defines moderate alcohol consumption as two drinks per day for men or one drink per day for women.
- Alcohol creates many social problems, such as violence and accidents, as well as negative health effects, most notably those related to cancer and fetal alcohol syndrome.
- Although persons with alcoholism should perhaps never drink, moderate alcohol consumption is associated with significant protective effects with respect to cardiovascular disease (especially coronary heart disease), several other diseases, and overall mortality.
- The alcohol intake associated with the lowest overall mortality is 0.7–1.3 drinks per day in men and approx 0.3 drinks per day in women, but this is probably an underestimate.

1. INTRODUCTION

The harmful effects of alcohol are far better known that the beneficial effects. This is scarcely surprising: it requires no training in epidemiology to recognize the devastating harm that often comes with both drunkenness and chronic alcohol abuse. However, findings that have emerged in recent years have uncovered several surprising associations between moderate intake of alcohol and enhanced health and well-being.

In this chapter we use the American definition of a drink, namely 12.5–13.0 g of alcohol. This quantity of alcohol is approximately the amount contained in 12 oz (356 g) of regular beer, 4–5 oz (118–148 g) of wine, or 1.5 oz (42 g) of spirits. We also use the US Department of Agriculture dietary guidelines' definition of moderate alcohol consumption as up to two drinks a day for men and one drink a day for women.

2. HARMFUL EFFECTS OF ALCOHOL

2.1. Accidents, Violence, and Suicide

It is well established that abuse of alcohol is associated with accidents, violence, and suicide. The most dramatic evidence of this has come from Russia. Between 1984 and

From: *Nutritional Health: Strategies for Disease Prevention, Second Edition*
Edited by: N. J. Temple, T. Wilson, and D. R. Jacobs © Humana Press Inc., Totowa, NJ

1994 there was both serious economic decline and great political turmoil. During this period, life expectancy fell by 4 yr in men and by 2 yr in women. A major factor in this was apparently widespread alcohol abuse, particularly binge drinking, which led to large increases in deaths from accidents, homicide, and suicide, as well as cardiovascular disease *(1,2)*. Alcohol may also be an important factor in the substantial increase in mortality during the period from 1992 to 2001 *(3)*. Other investigators, however, postulate that the importance of alcohol as a cause of the rise in mortality rates in Russia has been exaggerated, especially in women *(4)*.

In the United States in 2003 the driver's blood alcohol level was a factor in about 14,260 of fatal crashes, or about 25% of all fatal crashes. This is a decrease of 38% compared with 1982 when the driver's blood alcohol level was a factor in about 41% of fatal crashes *(5)*. Stricter enforcement of existing legal codes and the passage of new laws have been suggested as promoting these beneficial changes.

2.2. Chronic Alcohol Abuse

For many persons, years of alcohol abuse eventually leads to chronic health and nutritional problems. Alcohol is rich in calories and typically devoid in nutrients, especially alcohol- and sugar-rich hard liquors. The body often compensates for the high caloric intake by decreasing the stimulus to eat regular nutrient-rich foods. As a result, there is a high probability of malnutrition, especially of folate and thiamin. The thiamin deficiency associated with alcohol abuse is known as Wernicke-Korsakoff syndrome. Liver disease is also a likely result with a downward spiral from fatty liver, to alcoholic hepatitis, and, eventually, to cirrhosis.

2.3. Fetal Alcohol Syndrome

Pregnancy is another situation where alcohol misuse can have tragic consequences. This alcohol misuse induces fetal alcohol syndrome (FAS). FAS encompasses a variety of symptoms including prenatal and postnatal growth retardation, abnormal facial features, and an increased frequency of major birth defects. Children born with FAS never recover.

A subclinical form of FAS is known as fetal alcohol effects (FAE). Children with FAE may be short or have only minor facial abnormalities, or develop learning disabilities, behavioral problems, or motor impairments.

FAS occurs at a level of alcohol intake that in a nonpregnant woman would not be considered alcohol abuse. Four drinks per day pose a real threat of FAS, although one or two drinks per day may still retard growth; the epidemiological data are weaker and somewhat inconsistent at these lower levels of consumption. Although women who have an occasional drink during pregnancy should not fear they are doing irreparable harm to their fetus, it is now generally accepted that any woman who is or may become pregnant should abstain from alcohol.

2.4. Cancer

Alcohol much increases the risk of cancer of the mouth, throat, and esophagus *(6,7)*. It also acts as a cocarcinogen with cigarette smoke *(8)*. It is likely that among heavy consumers the alcohol or one of its metabolites, acetaldehyde, is directly toxic to mucosal epithelial cells. Alcohol also increases the risk of cancer of the liver, ovary, and breast *(6,7,9)*.

The risk ratio (RR) with an alcohol intake of four drinks per day is estimated to be 1.9–3.1 for cancer of the mouth, throat, and esophagus, 1.6 for breast cancer, and 1.1–1.4 for cancer of the stomach, colon-rectum, liver, and ovary *(7,9)*. For all cancer combined a significant risk is seen starting at an alcohol intake of two drinks per day, with a RR of 1.22 at four drinks per day *(7)*. For breast cancer, it is less likely that ethanol is directly toxic because the increase has been seen at relatively low levels. It is more likely that alcohol influences circulating estrogen levels, which may impact on disease occurrence *(10,11)*.

Emerging evidence also indicates that alcohol, even in moderation, may suppress circulating folate levels, which could impact on DNA synthesis and gene expression. Several recent large prospective studies of breast cancer show that an adequate intake of folate ameliorated the carcinogenic action of alcohol *(12–14*; *see* Fig. 1). As with breast cancer, the effect of alcohol on colon cancer *(15)* and on total risk of cancer *(16)* may be muted or eliminated completely if the diet has sufficient folate or methionine (both methyl donors). The relationship between alcohol and cancer is further discussed in Chapter 9.

2.5. Obesity

Alcohol, of course, is a source of calories (7 kcal/g). It is important to remember that alcoholic beverages also contain carbohydrates that add additional calories. A half liter of wine contains about 350 kcal whereas three cans of beer supply about 250–450 kcal, clearly enough to tip the energy balance well into positive territory. These numbers explain the popularity of low-calorie "light beers." It is predictable, therefore, that alcohol consumption should be associated with excess weight gain. However, as so often happens in nutrition, predictions collapse in the face of reality. A solid body of evidence, mostly from cross-sectional studies, has demonstrated that alcohol intake actually has an inverse association with body mass index (an index of weight relative to height) *(17–19)*. However, when diet, physical activity, and other lifestyle factors are not examined prospectively, it can be difficult to interpret whether the association is causal. In a cohort study of 16,600 men aged 40–75 yr, change in alcohol intake was not associated with change in waist circumference over 9 yr of follow-up *(20)*. Intervention studies are inconclusive although Cordain et al. *(21)* reported that when men consumed 35 g of alcohol per day (a little less than three glasses of wine) for a period of 6 wk, this did not affect body weight. A follow-up study confirmed this when overweight women consumed 25 g of alcohol per day, 5 d/wk, for 10 wk *(22)*. It is feasible that an increase in basal metabolic rate caused by moderate alcohol consumption may offset the additional calories from consuming alcohol-containing beverages *(23)*. At present, therefore, there is sparse evidence to establish alcohol as a risk factor for weight gain. However, more longitudinal studies of alcohol and weight gain are needed.

3. PROTECTIVE EFFECTS OF ALCOHOL

3.1. Coronary Heart Disease

A convincing body of evidence suggests that the risk of coronary heart disease (CHD) is reduced by 10–40% in persons who consume alcohol in moderation *(23,24)*. In some populations this association can be skewed if individuals at higher risk for CHD reduce or eliminate alcohol consumption because of a diagnosis of a related chronic disease (e.g.,

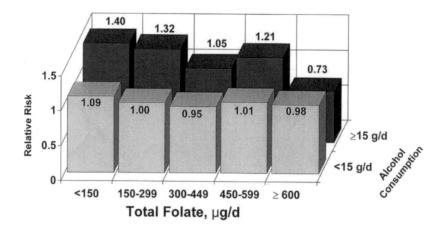

Fig. 1. Multivariate relative risk of breast cancer by total folate intake and alcohol consumption. The reference group for all comparisons was women who consumed 150 g/d of total folate and fewer than 15 g/d of alcohol.

hypertension or diabetes). This is frequently described as the "sick quitter" syndrome and can create a spurious artificial inverse association between alcohol and CHD *(26)*. Because conditions such as hypertension and diabetes increase the risk of CHD by two- to three-fold, a study that does not take these conditions into account may find that moderate drinkers have as much as 50–70% less heart disease. However, even in large cohort studies where "sick quitters" are removed or moderate drinkers are compared to lifelong abstainers, alcohol has been found to have strong cardiovascular benefit *(25,27)*.

There has been much speculation that wine may be more potent than beer or spirits in preventing CHD. This is largely based on findings from ecological studies (i.e., countries, such as France with a high intake of wine tend to have relatively low rates of CHD) *(24)*. It has been repeatedly shown that such associations can easily be spurious. This is indicated by the findings from case–control and cohort studies: these show no clear trend for one type of alcohol to be more consistently associated with protection from CHD *(24, 25)*. Where one type of alcohol does manifest a stronger association than other types, this is likely owing to confounding by such factors as smoking and drinking pattern or to differences in other lifestyle factors, such as eating patterns or physical activity.

Short-term experimental studies have helped to explain the mechanisms by which alcohol prevents CHD *(28)*. First and foremost, it causes an increased level of high-density lipoprotein (HDL)-cholesterol. This explains about half of the association between alcohol and CHD. Another protective mechanism is that alcohol exerts an antithrombotic action by reducing hepatic production of fibrinogen and other clotting proteins. There is also some evidence indicating that alcohol may lower low-density lipoprotein (LDL)-cholesterol levels *(29)*, but findings have not been consistent.

Alcohol has been reported to elevate the blood homocysteine level, a relatively new predictor of CHD. This was seen with 6 wk of consumption of a moderate level of alcohol (30 g/d) *(30)*. Red wine and beer had a greater effect than spirits in this regard. This action of alcohol would be predicted to partly counter its protective benefit on CHD.

As with cancer there is a suggestion of an alcohol–folate interaction: the beneficial effects of alcohol on CHD may be strongest among those with folate-sufficient diets *(31,32)*. Because alcohol may suppress folate levels leading to a subsequent increase in homocysteine, individuals with high intakes of folate may benefit the most from a moderate intake of alcohol because they will have low levels of homocysteine from the extra folate yet still reap the beneficial effects of alcohol on lipids, coagulation factors, and insulin sensitivity.

Recent findings from the Physicians' Health Study reveal a genetic component to the relationship between alcohol intake and risk of CHD (33). The enzyme alcohol dehydrogenase is crucial to the metabolism of alcohol. Approximately 15% of the population is homozygous (or has two copies of the gene) for the form of the gene that induces a slow rate of metabolism of alcohol. Slow metabolizers have higher plasma HDL-cholesterol levels than fast metabolizers and also, among those who drink moderately in the Physicians' Health Study, have a dramatically lower risk of CHD. This is one of the first diet–gene interactions to be reported in the literature and provides strong evidence that the ethanol component of alcohol-containing beverages is responsible for the benefit rather than other components in wine, beer, or spirits.

3.2. Blood Pressure and Stroke

A relatively high alcohol intake (more than four drinks per day) has been shown to be associated with elevated blood pressure *(9,34,35)* and an increased risk of stroke *(9,36)*. However, recent evidence from cohort studies suggest that the association between alcohol and hypertension may be J-shaped such that light and moderate drinkers have a modestly reduced risk of developing the condition; however, the exact mechanism for this effect is unknown *(37)*. Although the results of large epidemiological studies have not been consistent, the data as a whole indicate that there is also a J-shaped relationship between alcohol intake and risk of stroke *(36)*. This relationship is considerably more pronounced in women. The protective effect of moderate consumption of alcohol is stronger for ischemic rather than hemorrhagic stroke. More work is needed to determine if drinking patterns influence risk of stroke (i.e., frequent consumption of small amounts of alcohol vs binge drinking).

3.3. Impotence

The relationship between excessive alcohol intake and poor erectile function is well known. As Shakespeare put it: "It provokes the desire, but takes away from the performance" (Macbeth). But, as in the case of alcohol and blood pressure, recent findings have revealed an apparently beneficial effect, or at least no ill effects, of moderate alcohol consumption. Preliminary data from the Health Professionals' Follow-up Study, a prospective cohort study of more than 50,000 US male health professionals, show a modest U-shaped relationship between alcohol intake and erectile dysfunction. Like CHD, the strongest risk reduction was among those who consumed one to two drinks per day *(38)*. Although erectile dysfunction was originally thought to be purely pyschogenic in nature, 80–90% is likely caused by biological factors that may share a similar profile to atherosclerosis.

3.4. Gallstones

Most studies that have examined this question have reported a protective association between alcohol and risk of gallstones. For instance, Leitzmann et al. *(39)* observed that men who consume alcohol frequently (5–7 d/wk) have a reduced risk of gallstones but not those who consume alcohol less frequently (1–2 d/wk). These findings indicate that frequency of alcohol consumption rather than quantity is the critical factor.

3.5. Bone Health

Although findings are not consistent, several studies have reported that compared with nondrinking, moderate alcohol intake is associated with higher bone mineral density, especially in postmenopausal women *(40–42)*. This suggests that alcohol may help prevent osteoporosis. However, as osteoporosis is so dependent on lifetime diet, physical activity, obesity, and other factors, it is probable that alcohol does not play an important role. In contrast to the situation with osteoporosis, high levels of drinking cause loss of balance and falls leading to an increased risk of hip or wrist fracture.

3.6. Hearing Loss

A cross-sectional study of subjects aged 50–91 yr reported that moderate alcohol intake was associated with better hearing *(43)*. Again, like bone health, many other environmental and genetic effects play a more important role in the etiology of hearing loss.

3.7. Cognitive Function and Dementia

It is well-known that heavy drinking has a damaging effect on brain function. Nevertheless, alcohol manifests a J-shaped relationship with the decline in brain function with aging. In several studies, mostly carried out on older adults, moderate consumption of alcohol was associated with enhanced cognitive ability or a slower rate of decline with aging. This effect is generally more pronounced in women *(44–46)*. Although results have not been entirely consistent, several cohort studies have reported a protective association between moderate alcohol consumption and the development of dementia (mainly Alzheimer's disease) *(47–49)*.

3.8. Benign Prostatic Hyperplasia

A cohort study reported that moderate alcohol intake (2.5–4 drinks per day) was associated with a reduced risk of benign prostatic hyperplasia (RR of 0.59) *(50)*. The mechanisms for this action are more speculative, but may include the effects of alcohol on steroid hormone levels.

3.9. Diabetes

Cohort studies have suggested that alcohol may be protective against type 2 diabetes. Moderate consumers have a 33–56% reduced risk of developing the condition *(51)*. Interestingly, several studies have suggested that moderate consumption of alcohol among men and women with type 2 diabetes is also associated with a much-reduced risk of subsequent CHD *(52–55)*, the number one killer of diabetics.

3.10. Lung Disease

Alcohol may also be protective against chronic obstructive pulmonary disease. A cohort study of middle-aged men in Finland, Netherlands, and Italy revealed a protective association between alcohol intake and risk of death from chronic obstructive pulmonary disease *(56)*. The lowest risk was seen at an intake of up to about three drinks per day. Alcohol intake has also been observed to manifest a protective association with emphysema in smokers *(57)*.

4. EFFECT OF ALCOHOL ON TOTAL MORTALITY

When intake is moderate, the beneficial health effects of alcohol on the cardiovascular system outweigh most detrimental effects. As a result, the net effect of alcohol on total mortality is a J-shaped curve with minimum mortality associated with a moderate intake of alcohol but with a rising curve as consumption increases. A major study by the American Cancer Society reported that in each sex, persons consuming one drink daily had a risk of death from all causes about 20% lower than those of nondrinkers *(6)*. To put this in perspective, among American men and women aged 35–69 yr, a moderate consumption of alcohol prevents approximately one death for every six deaths caused by smoking *(6)*.

The alcohol intake corresponding to the nadir for mortality is still unclear but in people aged 50–80 yr is around 0.7–1.2 drinks per day in men and 0.3 drinks per day in women *(58)*. However, as this is based on self-reported intake, which represents a substantial underestimation, the true nadir is almost certainly higher *(58)*.

The benefits of alcohol are most apparent in the middle-aged and elderly. This is because alcohol reduces risk of CHD and stroke, the first and third leading cause of death, respectively, in that age group. By contrast the leading cause of death in Americans under age 40 yr is accidents, with homicide and suicide also being major causes, especially in males. These are all associated with alcohol. This age effect is illustrated by a report from the Nurses' Health Study. A moderate intake of alcohol has a protective relationship with total mortality in women aged over 50 yr (RR is 0.80–0.88) but is associated with a doubling of the risk of death in those aged 34–39 yr *(59)*. Similar findings were reported from England and Wales. A net favorable mortality outcome was seen only in men over age 55 yr and women over 65 yr *(60)*.

5. DRINKING PATTERNS

More recently, research has focused on the importance of the pattern of drinking on the risk of health outcomes. Not surprisingly, alcohol is most protective when consumed in small regular amounts rather than binge or episodic drinking. This was demonstrated in cohort studies in the United States *(61)* and Finland *(62)*. People who engaged in occasional heavy drinking had a higher risk of death than persons with the same alcohol intake but who did not engage in binge drinking. Similar observations were made on cardiovascular disease in Canada. The data from that study revealed that although alcohol consumption has a protective association with both CHD and hypertension, binge drinking increases the risk of both, especially in men *(63)*. In a recent study of US male health professionals, frequency of consumption (days per week) was more important than quantity consumed. Men who consumed alcohol at least 5 d/wk had the lowest risk of both type 2 diabetes *(64)* and myocardial infarction *(25)*, regardless of the total amount consumed. These findings are hardly surprising: many dietary components cause no harm in small, frequent doses but are toxic when a large dose is taken.

6. CONCLUSION

Clearly, alcohol can do much good but also much harm. It is important to bear in mind that the harmful effects of alcohol frequently occur at a much younger age than the benefits. Consequently, if the effects of alcohol are measured in terms of quality years of life (lost or gained), then the harm done to one (usually younger) person by alcohol may be far greater than the benefit gained by another (usually older) person.

The large majority of the harmful effects of alcohol can be avoided by sensible drinking, by drinking in moderation, and by the avoidance of alcohol when driving. For the person who can drink sensibly and can avoid alcohol's negative side, alcohol can be of considerable benefit. Like so much else in life, it's a matter of balance. Although alcohol should perhaps not be prescribed *(65)*, neither should it be proscribed.

Researchers in Australia estimated that for people aged over 60 yr, the cost per life year gained by moderate consumption of alcohol was A $5700 in men and A $19,000 in women *(66)*. This translates to about US $4900 in men and US $16,300 in women in 2005 dollars. On this basis alcohol can be considered a cost-effective medication. For instance, it is many times more cost-effective than is medication with statins for treatment of hypercholesterolemia *(67)*.

The findings discussed in this chapter have implications for public health policy. But what are these implications? One possible policy is the following: all adults aged over 40 yr should be encouraged to consume moderate amounts of alcohol daily, unless there is a specific reason to the contrary, such as religion, medication use, or a history of alcohol abuse. The problem with such a policy is the risk of causing a rise in the prevalence of alcohol abuse. Typically, about 5–10% of people in any society where alcohol is available become abusers of the beverage. The actual proportion is related to the mean alcohol intake: the higher the mean alcohol intake, the higher is the proportion of alcohol abusers *(68)*. Thus, a policy that encourages greater use of alcohol will likely also lead to more problems associated with abuse.

Arguably, the most prudent policy is one that explains that alcohol in moderation will likely have several health benefits for people in middle age and older, while also stressing the hazards of abuse.

REFERENCES

1. Leon DA, Chenet L, Shkolnikov VM, et al. Huge variation in Russian mortality rates 1984–94: artefact, alcohol, or what? Lancet 1997; 350:383–388.
2. Walberg P, McKee M, Shkolnikov V, Chenet L, Leon DA. Economic change, crime, and mortality crisis in Russia: regional analysis BMJ 1998; 317:312–318.
3. Men T, Brennan P, Boffetta P, Zaridze D. Russian mortality trends for 1991–2001: analysis by cause and region. BMJ 2003; 327:964.

4. Malyutina S, Bobak M, Kurilovitch S, et al. Relation between heavy and binge drinking and all-cause and cardiovascular mortality in Novosibirsk, Russia: a prospective cohort study. Lancet 2002; 360: 1448–1454.

5. Report HS 809 772 from Department of Transportation. Available at website: www-nrd.nhtsa.dot.gov/departments/nrd-30/ncsa/. Last accessed December 28, 2004.

6. Thun MJ, Peto R, Lopez AD, et al. Alcohol consumption and mortality among middle-aged and elderly U.S. adults. N Engl J Med 1997; 337:1705–1714.

7. Bagnardi V, Blangiardo M, Vecchia CL, Corrao G. A meta-analysis of alcohol drinking and cancer risk. Br J Cancer 2001; 85:1700–1705.

8. World Cancer Research Fund/American Institute for Cancer Research. Food, Nutrition and the Prevention of Cancer: A Global Perspective. American Institute for Cancer Research, Washington, DC, 1997.

9. Corrao G, Bagnardi V, Zambon A, La Vecchia C. A meta-analysis of alcohol consumption and the risk of 15 diseases. Prev Med 2004; 38:613–619.

10. Hankinson SE, Willett WC, Manson JE, et al. Alcohol, height, and adiposity in relation to estrogen and prolactin levels in postmenopausal women. J Natl Cancer Inst 1995; 87:1297–1302.

11. Dorgan JF, Baer DJ, Albert PS, et al. Serum hormones and the alcohol-breast cancer association in postmenopausal women. J Natl Cancer Inst 2001; 93:710–715.

12. Zhang S, Hunter DJ, Hankinson SE, et al. A prospective study of folate intake and the risk of breast cancer. JAMA 1999; 281:1632–1637.

13. Sellers TA, Kushi LH, Cerhan JR, et al. Dietary folate intake, alcohol, and risk of breast cancer in a prospective study of postmenopausal women. Epidemiology 2001; 12:420–428.

14. Rohan TE, Jain MG, Howe GR, Miller AB. Dietary folate consumption and breast cancer risk. J Natl Cancer Inst 2000; 92:266–269.

15. Giovannucci E, Rimm EB, Ascherio A, Stampfer MJ, Colditz GA, Willett WC. Alcohol, low-methionine–low-folate diets, and risk of colon cancer in men. J Natl Cancer Inst 1995; 87:265–273.

16. Jiang R, Hu FB, Giovannucci EL, et al. Joint association of alcohol and folate intake with risk of major chronic disease in women. Am J Epidemiol 2003; 158:760–771.

17. Colditz GA, Giovannucci E, Rimm EB, et al. Alcohol intake in relation to diet and obesity in women and men. Am J Clin Nutr 1991; 54:49–55.

18. Williamson DF, Forman MR, Binkin NJ, Gentry EM, Remington PL, Trowbridge FL. Alcohol and body weight in United States adults. Am J Public Health 1987; 7:1324–1330.

19. Hellerstedt WL, Jeffery RW, Murray DM. The association between alcohol intake and adiposity in the general population. Am J Epidemiol 1990; 132:594–611.

20. Koh-Banerjee P, Chu NF, Spiegelman D, et al. Prospective study of the association of changes in dietary intake, physical activity, alcohol consumption, and smoking with 9-y gain in waist circumference among 16,587 US men. Am J Clin Nutr 2003; 78:719–727.

21. Cordain L, Bryan ED, Melby CL, Smith MJ. Influence of moderate daily wine consumption on body weight regulation and metabolism in healthy free-living males. J Am Coll Nutr 1997; 16:134–139.

22. Cordain L, Melby CL, Hamamoto AE, et al. Influence of moderate chronic wine consumption on insulin sensitivity and other correlates of syndrome X in moderately obese women. Metabolism 2000; 49:1473–1478.

23. Klesges R, Maaler CZ, Klesges LM. Effect of alcohol intake on resting energy expenditure in young women social drinkers. Am J Clin Nutr 1994; 59:805–809.

24. Rimm EB, Klatsky A, Grobbee D, Stampfer MJ. Review of moderate alcohol consumption and reduced risk of coronary heart disease: is the effect due to beer, wine, or spirits? BMJ 1996; 312:731–736.

25. Mukamal KJ, Conigrave KM, Mittleman MA, et al. Roles of drinking pattern and type of alcohol consumed in coronary heart disease in men. N Engl J Med 2003; 348:109–118.

26. Shaper AG, Wannamethee G, Walker M. Alcohol and mortality in British men: explaining the U-shaped curve. Lancet 1988; 2:1267–1273.

27. Rimm E. Alcohol and cardiovascular disease. Curr Atheroscler Rep 2000; 2:529–535.

28. Rimm EB, Williams P, Fosher K, Criqui M, Stampfer MJ. Moderate alcohol intake and lower risk of coronary heart disease: meta-analysis of effects on lipids and haemostatic factors. BMJ 1999; 319:1523–1528.

29. Castelli, WP, Doyle, JT, Gordon, T, et al. Alcohol and blood lipids: the cooperative lipoprotein phenotyping study. Lancet 1977; 2:153–157.

30. Bleich S, Bleich K, Kropp S, et al. Moderate alcohol consumption in social drinkers raises plasma homocysteine levels: a contradiction to the "French Paradox"? Alcohol 2001; 36:189–192.

31. Rimm EB, Willett WC, Hu FB, et al. Folate and vitamin B6 from diet and supplements in relation to risk of coronary heart disease among women. JAMA 1998; 279:359–364.

32. Koehler KM, Baumgartner RN, Garry PJ, Allen RH, Stabler SP, Rimm EB. Association of folate intake and serum homocysteine in elderly persons according to vitamin supplementation and alcohol use. Am J Clin Nutr 2001; 73:628–637.

33. Hines LM, Stampfer MJ, Ma J, et al. Genetic variation in alcohol dehydrogenase and the beneficial effect of moderate alcohol consumption on myocardial infarction. N Engl J Med 2001; 344:549–555.

34. Ascherio A, Rimm EB, Giovannucci EL, et al. A prospective study of nutritional factors and hypertension among US men. Circulation 1992; 86:1475–1484.

35. Puddey IB, Beilin LJ, Vandongen R, Rouse IL, Rogers P. Evidence for a direct effect of alcohol consumption on blood pressure in normotensive men. A randomized controlled trial. Hypertension 1985; 7:707–713.

36. Reynolds K, Lewis B, Nolen JD, Kinney GL, Sathya B, He J. Alcohol consumption and risk of stroke: a meta-analysis. JAMA 2003; 289:579–588.

37. Thadhani R, Camargo CA Jr, Stampfer MJ, Curhan GC, Willett WC, Rimm EB. Prospective study of moderate alcohol consumption and risk of hypertension in young women. Arch Intern Med 2002; 162:569–574.

38. Rimm EB, Bacon C, Giovannucci E, Kawachi I. Waist circumference, physical activity, and alcohol consumption in relation to erectile dysfunction among US male health professionals. Annual Meeting of the American Urological Association, May 2, 2000, Atlanta, GA.

39. Leitzmann MF, Giovannucci EL, Stampfer MJ, et al. Prospective study of alcohol consumption patterns in relation to symptomatic gallstone disease in men. Alcohol Clin Exp Res 1999; 23:835–841.

40. Rapuri PB, Gallagher JC, Balhorn KE, Ryschon KL. Alcohol intake and bone metabolism in elderly women. Am J Clin Nutr 2000; 72:1206–1213.

41. Feskanich D, Korrick SA, Greenspan SL, Rosen HN, Colditz GA. Moderate alcohol consumption and bone density among postmenopausal women. J Women's Health 1999; 8:65–73.

42. Macdonald HM, New SA, Golden MH, Campbell MK, Reid DM. Nutritional associations with bone loss during the menopausal transition: evidence of a beneficial effect of calcium, alcohol, and fruit and vegetable nutrients and of a detrimental effect of fatty acids. Am J Clin Nutr 2004; 79:155–165.

43. Popelka MM, Cruikshanks KJ, Wiley TL, et al. Moderate alcohol consumption and hearing loss: a protective effect. J Am Geriatr Soc 2000; 48:1273–1278.

44. Britton A, Singh-Manoux A, Marmot M. Alcohol consumption and cognitive function in the Whitehall II Study. Am J Epidemiol 2004; 160:240–247.

45. Leroi I, Sheppard JM, Lyketsos CG. Cognitive function after 11.5 years of alcohol use: relation to alcohol use. Am J Epidemiol 2002; 156:747–752.

46. Kalmijn S, van Boxtel MP, Verschuren MW, Jolles J, Launer LJ. Cigarette smoking and alcohol consumption in relation to cognitive performance in middle age. Am J Epidemiol 2002; 156:936–944.

47. Ruitenberg A, van Swieten JC, Witteman JC, et al. Alcohol consumption and risk of dementia: the Rotterdam Study. Lancet 2002; 359:281–286.

48. Huang W, Qiu C, Winblad B, Fratiglioni L. Alcohol consumption and incidence of dementia in a community sample aged 75 years and older. J Clin Epidemiol 2002; 55:959–964.

49. Mukamal KJ, Kuller LH, Fitzpatrick AL, Longstreth WT Jr, Mittleman MA, Siscovick DS. Prospective study of alcohol consumption and risk of dementia in older adults. JAMA 2003; 289:1405–1413.

50. Platz EA, Rimm EB, Kawachi I, et al. E. Alcohol consumption, cigarette smoking, and risk of benign prostatic hyperplasia. Am J Epidemiol 1999; 149:106–115.

51. Howard AA, Arnsten JH, Gourevitch MN. Effect of alcohol consumption on diabetes mellitus: a systematic review. Ann Intern Med 2004; 140:211–219.

52. Tanasescu M, Hu FB, Willett WC, Stampfer MJ, Rimm EB. Alcohol consumption and risk of coronary heart disease among men with type 2 diabetes mellitus. J Am Coll Cardiol 2001; 38:1836–1842.

53. Ajani UA, Gaziano JM, Lotufo PA, et al. Alcohol consumption and risk of coronary heart disease by diabetes status. Circulation 2000; 102:500–505.

54. Solomon CG, Hu FB, Stampfer MJ, et al. Moderate alcohol consumption and risk of coronary heart disease among women with type 2 diabetes mellitus. Circulation 2000; 102:494–499.

55. Valmadrid CT, Klein R, Moss SE, Klein BE, Cruickshanks KJ. Alcohol intake and the risk of coronary heart disease mortality in persons with older-onset diabetes mellitus. JAMA 1999; 282:239–246.

56. Tabak C, Smit HA, Rasanen L, et al. Alcohol consumption in relation to 20-year COPD mortality and pulmonary function in middle-aged men from three European countries. Epidemiology 2001; 12:239–245.

57. Pratt PC, Vollmer RT. The beneficial effect of alcohol consumption on the prevalence and extent of centrilobular emphysema. Chest 1984; 85:372–377.

58. White IR. The level of alcohol consumption at which all-cause mortality is least. J Clin Epidemiol 1999; 52:967–975.

59. Fuchs CS, Stampfer MJ, Colditz GA, et al. Alcohol consumption and mortality among women. N Engl J Med 1995; 332:1245–1250.

60. Britton A, McPherson K. Mortality in England and Wales attributable to current alcohol consumption. J Epidemiol Community Health 2001; 55:383–388.

61. Rehm J, Greenfield TK, Rogers JD. Average volume of alcohol consumption, patterns of drinking, and all-cause mortality: results from the US National Alcohol Survey. Am J Epidemiol 2001; 153:64–71.

62. Laatikainen T, Manninen L, Poikolainen K, Vartiainen E. Increased mortality related to heavy alcohol intake pattern. J Epidemiol Community Health 2003; 57:379–384.

63. Murray RP, Connett JE, Tyas SL, Bond R, Ekuma O, Silversides CK, Barnes GE. Alcohol volume, drinking pattern, and cardiovascular disease morbidity and mortality: is there a U-shaped function? Am J Epidemiol 2002; 155:242–248.

64. Conigrave KM, Hu BF, Camargo CA Jr, Stampfer MJ, Willett WC, Rimm EB. A prospective study of drinking patterns in relation to risk of type 2 diabetes among men. Diabetes 2001; 50:2390–2395.

65. Wannamethee SG, Shaper AG. Taking up regular drinking in middle age: effect on major coronary heart disease events and mortality. Heart 2002; 87:32–36.

66. Simons LA, McCallum J, Friedlander Y, Ortiz M, Simons J. Moderate alcohol intake is associated with survival in the elderly: the Dubbo Study. Med J Australia 2000; 173:121–124.

67. Thompson A, Temple NJ. The case for statins: has it really been made? J R Soc Med 2004; 97:461–464 .

68. Colhoun H, Ben-Shlomo Y, Dong W, Bost L, Marmot M. Ecological analysis of collectivity of alcohol consumption in England: importance of average drinker. BMJ 1997; 314:1164–1168.

13 Diet in the Prevention and Treatment of Obesity

Sahaspahorn Paeratakul*, George A. Bray, and Barry M. Popkin

KEY POINTS

- Diet composition plays a critical role in total energy management; current thinking is that different diets might work better for some individuals than others.
- Fat is the most energy dense macronutrient. One gram of fat provides 9 kcal of energy compared with 4 kcal/g for carbohydrate and protein.
- Fat intake is poorly regulated whereas food volume appears to be better regulated. Extensive studies show it is difficult to gain weight if a low-fat diet is consumed combined with a higher complex carbohydrate (high fiber) intake.
- A large body of animal, clinical, and epidemiological data shows that higher fat foods are less expensive, palatable, and easily consumed in excess of needs.
- Recent clinical trials show that a low-carbohydrate, high-protein diet can reduce body weight in the short term, but longer-term results are equivocal.

1. INTRODUCTION

Current theories regarding the role of diet in human obesity have evolved around the role of portion size and macronutrient composition of diet and their effect on weight gain, weight loss, and weight maintenance. Portion sizes containing various amounts of fat, protein, and carbohydrate contribute to the total energy intake. Of these macronutrients, dietary fat has been most strongly implicated in the development of obesity. In this chapter, we review the role of portion size and diet composition, particularly dietary fat, in the regulation of food intake and body weight. Understanding this role is necessary for answering two important questions: could the reduction of fat intake, independent of portion control, be effective in slowing the rate at which obesity develops or in reducing obesity in the industrialized countries where the diet is usually high in fat?, and conversely, can obesity be prevented in a population where diet is traditionally low in fat by stopping the progression toward a high-fat, Western-style diet that has been observed in many developing countries?

---

*Deceased.

From: *Nutritional Health: Strategies for Disease Prevention, Second Edition*
Edited by: N. J. Temple, T. Wilson, and D. R. Jacobs © Humana Press Inc., Totowa, NJ

2. DIET AND THE PREVENTION OF OBESITY

2.1. Portion Size

Portion sizes have been increasing steadily for the past 50 yr *(1)*. For example, the hamburger at Burger King went from 2.8 oz and 202 kcal in 1954 to 4.3 oz and 310 kcal in 2004, an increase of more than 50%. A serving of McDonald's fries increased even more going from 2.4 oz and 210 kcal in 1955 to 7 oz and 610 kcal in 2004. A Hershey's chocolate bar in 1900 had 297 kcal compared with 1000 kcal in a 7-oz bar in 2004. Coca-Cola in 1916 had a 6.5-oz bottle with 79 calories compared with the widely sold 16-oz bottle containing 194 kcal in 2004. Many other examples demonstrate clearly that the portion sizes available in grocery stores and the sizes served in restaurants have increased *(1)*. When we are offered larger portion sizes, either in a laboratory *(2)* or in a restaurant setting *(3)*, we tend to eat more. These interacting effects of tending to eat more when larger portions are offered and the larger portion sizes that are widely available have played a key role in the rising energy intake reported by the Economic Research Service of the US Department of Agriculture *(4)*.

2.2. Dietary Fat Intake and the Development of Obesity

Some researchers argue that fat intake is not associated with body weight independently of total energy intake, and that simply reducing fat intake is not the best solution to prevent or reverse obesity *(5,6)*. However, it is important to place the role of dietary fat in its proper context and fat intake must be seen through its effects on total energy intake. For example, it is well-known that a high-fat diet is highly palatable, and this often leads to passive overconsumption: the unintentionally higher intake of high-fat foods compared to low-fat foods. Moreover, high-fat diets are less satiating and the thermic effect of dietary fat is low. In contrast, a diet rich in complex carbohydrate or protein induces greater satiety and tends to be associated with lower total energy intake. Because the amount, as well as composition, of food consumed may influence energy intake and hence body weight, the control of energy intake through manipulation of diet composition may be an approach to prevent obesity. In this chapter, we first discuss the role of dietary fat in obesity. Evidence from experimental, clinical, and epidemiological studies is presented. We then discuss the role of low-fat diets in preventing obesity, and the potential of dietary manipulation as a strategy for obesity control. Although the focus is on dietary fat, the role of carbohydrate and protein in obesity is also examined. Finally, we summarize the more recent issues related to obesity such as the role of different types of fat and fatty acids, fat substitutes, energy density, diet quality and dietary patterns, and popular diets, such as the low-carbohydrate diet, which many believe to be an effective weight-control strategy.

The human body has the ability to adjust the metabolic fuel mix it oxidizes so that carbohydrate and protein metabolism is tightly regulated and the body can achieve carbohydrate and protein balance quickly. However, the body has a poor regulatory mechanism for fat use and has an almost unlimited ability to store fat. There are several ways in which a high-fat diet may contribute to the development of obesity. We begin with evidence from animal experiments, clinical studies, and controlled trials and then we discuss results from population studies.

2.2.1. ANIMAL EXPERIMENTS

As a rule, experimental animals eating low-fat diets do not become obese. The major exceptions are animals with genetic forms of obesity or neuroendocrine disorders, and animals treated with drugs or certain peptides. Although experimental obesity induced by a low-fat diet is the exception, development of obesity in animals eating high-fat diets is the expected outcome *(7,8)*. The susceptibility or resistance of animals to obesity when eating high-fat diets has a strong genetic component. Some strains of mice and rats are exquisitely susceptible to developing obesity when eating high-fat or high-fat, high-carbohydrate diets, whereas other strains of mice (SWR) and rats (S5B/Pl) are resistant to developing obesity when fed similar diets. The finding that genetic susceptibility may predispose the development of obesity when exposed to a high-fat diet is also seen in humans and has important implications.

2.2.2. CLINICAL STUDIES

It is the slow but continual overconsumption of energy relative to needs that leads to obesity. As noted in the following sections, an increase in dietary fat content increases the tendency to overconsume. When fat intake increases, the body reacts in one of two ways to maintain energy balance. On one hand, the extra fat in the diet can be oxidized by the body. Alternatively, the increased dietary fat can be sensed by the body in such a way that the subsequent intake of foods is reduced and the energy balance is maintained. Over the past few decades in the United States, there has been a reduction in the proportion of energy from fat but not in total fat, and moreover, this reduction has been offset by increased intake of carbohydrates *(9)*. A number of factors are responsible for these changes, including increased portion sizes, increased intake of alcohol and fatty foods on weekends, increased snacking, and increased consumption of away-from-home, higher energy density foods *(10–13)*.

2.2.2.1. Fat Oxidation on a High-Fat Diet

The possibility that a high-fat diet may stimulate fat oxidation and increase metabolism of excess dietary fat has been tested in several studies. However, results show that when fat is added to a meal, there is no corresponding increase in fat oxidation *(14,15)*. This is in contrast with studies that show that adding carbohydrate to the diet is paralleled by an increase in carbohydrate oxidation. Because fat intake does not stimulate fat oxidation, the maintenance of energy balance when consuming a high-fat diet can be achieved only by a reduction in fat intake.

2.2.2.2. Overfeeding Study

The metabolic effect of the transition from a low-fat to a high-fat diet or *vice versa* in individuals housed in a respiratory chamber has been studied by several investigators *(16,17)*. Overfeeding results in glycogen stores being rapidly filled and, next, to the extent that there is excess dietary protein, the protein stores are also filled. Beyond this point, overfeeding results in metabolism of the available carbohydrate with any excess being converted to body fat. Careful overfeeding and underfeeding can also shift the energy expenditure: when the body weight of obese volunteers increases after overeating, the energy expenditure increases; when the body weight decreases below baseline weight, energy expenditure decreases *(18)*. In most studies, however, the subjects were in positive energy balance because respiratory chambers restricted their energy expenditure, and thus it was difficult to match energy intake and energy expenditure.

Because obesity may modify the metabolic response to a diet, postobese individuals usually regain weight and are therefore good candidates for studying what forces drive body weight upward. Specifically, it appears that postobese subjects are unable to metabolize excess dietary fat and have a smaller rise in energy expenditure when fed a high-fat meal than never-obese control subjects *(19)*. A defect in the ability to oxidize fat by formerly obese individuals and by obese individuals overfed fat while in a respiratory chamber suggests that consistent consumption of a diet high in fat, rather than in carbohydrate, results in the gradual accumulation of fat until the body has reached a new plateau of weight maintenance *(20)*.

2.2.2.3. Passive Overconsumption of Fat

Unlike protein and carbohydrate, fat stimulates excess energy intake through its high palatability and lack of satiating power *(21)*. Periodic exposure to a high-fat meal, particularly when hungry, may be sufficient to lead to overconsumption of energy that is not compensated by the body (i.e., by eating less at subsequent meals) *(22)*. Several approaches have been used to examine the effect of macronutrients on satiety and on subsequent food intake. One question that remains unclear is whether the degree of reduction in subsequent food intake after ingestion of a high-fat meal is similar to that after ingestion of high-carbohydrate or high-protein meals. There is limited understanding of the compensatory mechanisms that link diet composition to energy balance. Overfeeding studies that compare high-fat with high-carbohydrate diets indicate that metabolic adaptations to changes in fat in the diet are slow whereas adjustment to carbohydrate is almost immediate *(14,17,19,23,24)*. However, it appears that the ability to reduce food intake to compensate for the food eaten earlier is impaired when the subsequent foods are high in fat *(25,26)* and especially when they are high in both fat and sugar *(27,28)*. These findings point to one reason why sweet, high-fat foods are problematic for obesity: people tend to overconsume them rather than compensate for them.

2.2.3. Epidemiological Studies

Ecological studies are the most basic type of epidemiological investigation. They do not indicate causal relationships but they provide an insight to the diet–disease relationship in different populations. Figure 1 shows the association of the proportion of energy from fat (obtained from national food balance data) with the prevalence of overweight (body mass index [BMI] of 25 kg/m^2 or greater) among the adult participants of nationally representative surveys from 20 countries. A weighted regression analysis shows a significant positive association between fat consumption and the proportion of the population who are overweight. This suggests that a public health strategy to halt the tendency toward a high-fat diet in many countries where the diet is traditionally low in fat may be an effective way to prevent the increase in obesity already observed in these countries. Migration studies provide additional evidence. Reanalysis of the Ni-Hon-San migration study, where 8006 Japanese men living in Honolulu were compared with 2183 men living in Hiroshima and Nagasaki, shows that although the total energy intake was only slightly higher in Honolulu than Hiroshima and Nagasaki, the percentage of energy from fat was two times greater in Honolulu *(30)*. The mean BMI and subscapular skinfold thickness were both greater in men living in Honolulu and more of these men were obese.

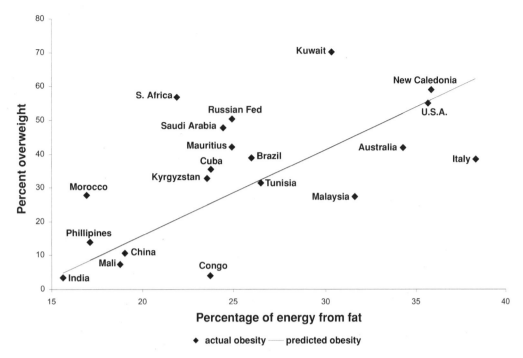

Fig. 1. The relationship between the percentage of the population that is overweight and the percentage of energy intake from fat. (Reproduced with permission from ref. *29*. © The American Journal of Clinical Nutrition and the American Society for Clinical Nutrition.)

The Leeds Fat Study shows that when the frequency distribution of BMI among individuals who consumed a higher-fat diet (>45% of energy) was plotted, the tail was skewed to the right and the proportion of obese individuals was about 19 times higher as compared with those who consumed a lower-fat diet (<35% of energy) *(28)*. However, there were also a number of individuals who consumed a higher-fat diet but had a normal BMI, suggesting that other factors, including the genetic susceptibility, may play a role. Another study used time-trend analysis to examine obese individuals and their past diet. Among 377,200 Danish military recruits from the years 1943 to 1974, there was a marked parallel between the percentage of energy from fat and the subsequent development of obesity *(31)*. Studies conducted among the Pima Indians in the United States produced similar results *(32)*.

Our longitudinal survey in China also suggests that an increase in fat intake led to an increase in body weight *(33,34)*. The results are presented in Table 1. Note that the potential confounders of the diet–BMI relationship (e.g., age, sex, physical activity, and smoking) were taken into account. To test the hypothesis that fat has an independent effect on body weight, the effect of change in absolute amount of energy from fat was examined while controlling for the effect of change in energy from the nonfat sources (i.e., protein and carbohydrate). A significant effect of fat intake on BMI was found: a 100-kcal increase in fat intake was associated with about a 0.05- and 0.01-BMI units increase in BMI in adolescents and adults, respectively. In contrast, a 100-kcal increase in protein and carbohydrate intake combined was associated with an increase of only 0.01 and 0.0007 BMI units in adolescents and adults, respectively. Similar results were seen

Table 1
Analysis of Dietary Modification as a Predictor of Change
in Body Mass Index Using the China Health and Nutrition Survey[a]

	Adolescents[b] 10–18 yr old (n = 742)	Adults[c] 20–45 yr old (n = 6667)
Predictors	Coefficient ± SE	Coefficient ± SE
(a) Change in energy from fat	0.0005 ± 0.0003^d	0.0001 ± 0.00005^d
Change in energy from nonfat	0.0001 ± 0.0001	0.000007 ± 0.00003
(b) Change in percent energy from fat	0.01 ± 0.008^e	0.003 ± 0.002^e
Change in total energy	0.0002 ± 0.0001^e	0.00002 ± 0.00002

[a]1991 and 1993 survey used for adolescents and 1991, 1992, and 1993 used for adults.
[b]Adjusted for age in years, gender, and residence.
[c]Adjusted for age in years, gender, residence, smoking, and physical activity.
[d]$p < 0.05$.
[e]$p < 0.10$.
SE, standard error.

when fat intake was expressed as a *percentage* of total energy intake while controlling for total energy intake. These findings suggest that energy from fat may have a greater effect on body weight than energy from nonfat sources. They are consistent with the view that the increase in fat intake may put a significant fraction of the population at risk of obesity, especially those who are genetically predisposed to the condition *(7,8,35,36)*. Obviously, the association between a high intake of fat and subsequent obesity is compounded by other factors, most notably the declining trend in physical activity.

2.3. Carbohydrate Intake and Obesity

2.3.1. ANIMAL STUDIES

Some older literature shows clearly that giving animals solutions of sucrose to drink increases their intake of carbohydrate. Failure to adequately suppress intake of other nutrients increases body fat *(37)*.

2.3.2. CLINICAL STUDIES

Several clinical studies show that the compensation for consumption of calorically sweetened beverages is inadequate. In single meal tests, providing a calorically sweetened beverage does not reduce the intake of nonbeverage foods, and total intake is slightly increased *(38)*. In a 3-wk crossover study, the intake of beverages sweetened with high-fructose corn syrup increased body weight compared to beverages sweetened with aspartame *(39)*. A slightly longer study showed that for more than 10 wk subjects drinking a defined amount of sucrose-sweetened soft drinks gained about 1.5 kg compared with a loss of 1.5 kg when the beverages were sweetened with aspartame *(40)*. In a third observational study, Schulze et al. *(41)* noted that for 5 yr individuals who drank more calorie-sweetened soft drinks did not reduce their intake of other foods and experienced a significant weight gain. The intake of sweetened beverages in children is a predictor of future weight gain *(42)*, as it is in adults *(41)*.

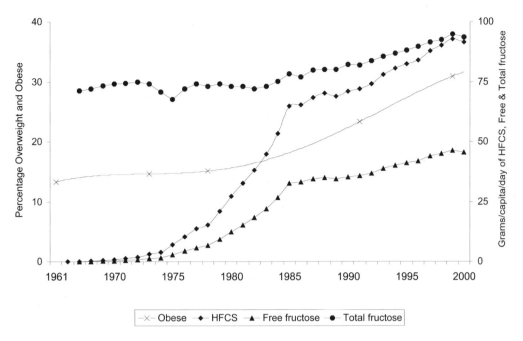

Fig. 2. Relationship of changing intake of total fructose, free fructose, high-fructose corn syrup and body mass index in the United States between 1960 and 2000. (Reproduced with permission from ref. *43.* © The American Journal of Clinical Nutrition and the American Society for Clinical Nutrition.)

The changing pattern of sweeteners used to sweeten soft drinks in the United States and several parts of the world is shown in Fig. 2 *(43).* From its introduction in 1970, high-fructose corn syrup has now replaced more than half of the sugar intake. Separating the fructose from the glucose changes the sweetness characteristics of these beverages, and we believe this may play a role in the increased preference for larger portion sizes of sweetened beverages *(43).*

3. DIETARY TREATMENT OF OBESITY

There is an important difference between preventing weight gain and producing weight loss. The slow increases in body weight that result in obesity in some people can be modified by environmental factors including portion control and dietary macronutrients. For weight loss, on the other hand, restriction of caloric intake is the most effective treatment. Numerous diets manipulating various macronutrients, as well as controlling portion size, have been proposed. In the next few paragraphs we will review some of the data on portion control and macronutrient manipulation. However, it should be pointed that when calorie intake is held constant, the rate of weight loss is uninfluenced by the composition of the diet that is fed in a metabolic ward *(44).* Rather, it is the "adherence" to the diet that makes the difference, and if any effects result from macronutrient manipulation, it is in the ease with people can "adhere" to a diet over an extended period of time *(45).*

3.1. Portion Size and Energy Density

Reducing the energy density of foods by increasing the water content or reducing the fat content are two strategies that can be used so as to reduce energy intake. This approach has been applied in a book called *Volumetrics* written for the public by Dr. Barbara Rolls *(46)*. The other strategy has been to use "portion-controlled" foods, such as beverages, bars, or frozen foods. There are published data showing that the use of these strategies can have a long-term effect of modest proportions on the control of body weight *(47)*.

3.2. Can a Reduction in Dietary Fat Prevent or Reverse Obesity?

3.2.1. ANIMAL EXPERIMENTS

Two major findings from animal experiments are noteworthy: first, a high-fat diet induces an increase in the number of fat cells or adipocytes, and second, replacing a high-fat with a low-fat diet may, but not always, reverse obesity. Lemonnier *(48)* was the first to show that feeding mice a high-fat diet increases the number of adipocytes, with the intra-abdominal depot showing the greatest response. Subsequently, this has been shown in both mice and rats by others *(49,50)*. Switching from a high-fat to a low-fat diet might be expected to reverse fat-induced obesity, unless the number of adipocytes increases in which case weight reduction may be incomplete. For example, when mice were switched from a high-fat to a low-fat diet, the number of adipocytes did not decrease and even when the fat cells returned to their normal size, the animals were still obese *(51)*. Rolls and associates *(52)* showed that rats fed a high-fat diet did not return to their baseline weight when switched to a lower-fat diet. In addition, the animals switched to a low-fat diet after having been fed a high-fat diet for a relatively short period (4 mo) reduced their weight to levels similar to that of the control animals not fed the high-fat diet *(51)*. However, when fed with a high-fat diet for a longer period (7 mo), the animals did not reduce their weight to the control levels. Others also reported that body weight did not return to the level of control animals maintained on a low-fat diet throughout the study *(53,54)*. The extent to which genetic factors are involved in the size or number of fat cells and in this reversal process has not yet been determined, but they are likely to play an important role. These data suggest that the increase in fat intake may be particularly important in inducing obesity, whereas a reduction in dietary fat has less of an effect on weight loss.

3.2.2. EFFECT OF FAT REDUCTION ON WEIGHT LOSS IN NONOBESE SUBJECTS

We have reviewed several clinical trials that involved manipulation of diet composition, mostly through the reduction of fat *(29)*. Although weight reduction was not the primary objective of these studies, the subjects that were placed on a low-fat diet nonetheless lost weight *(55–74)*. Typically, greater weight loss was seen in short-term studies (<6 mo) compared with longer studies. The magnitude of weight loss depends on the initial body weight, and patient compliance is the crucial factor *(75)*. Weight-loss maintenance generally declines with long-term interventions *(60,61)*. However, this may be partially attributed to the fact that weight reduction or weight maintenance was not specifically emphasized in these studies. In any case, decreasing total fat in the diet without intentionally restricting food intake resulted in lower total energy intake in nonobese individuals, and approx 12% of the initial reduction in energy intake was not compensated for by those on low-fat, *ad libitum* regimens.

3.2.3. Effect of Fat Reduction on Weight Loss in Overweight Subjects

Several intervention trials have examined the effect of a low-fat diet with or without energy restriction in overweight subjects (68,71,73,76–89). The rate of weight loss was generally greater when the low-fat diet was combined with reduction in total energy intake. These studies show that apart from energy restriction, a low-fat diet alone is effective in inducing weight loss in overweight subjects, with an observed mean weight loss of about 1.8 kg/mo. Although the rate of weight loss on an *ad libitum*, low-fat, high-carbohydrate diet may not be as rapid as that induced by energy restriction (calorie counting), the diet has been found to provide greater satiety and subsequently the compensation for the decrease in energy intake is not complete (i.e., energy intake remains decreased) (52,74,84,85). When a low-fat diet is consumed, total energy intake is often unintentionally reduced, even in studies where the goal is to keep it constant (77). Among obese subjects, about 23% of the initial reduction in total energy intake is not compensated for. Despite the fact that compliance tends to decrease over time, a low-fat, high-carbohydrate diet is still one of the most effective tools in weight maintenance (66,75). Consumption of reduced-fat products leads to lower energy consumption, suggesting that this may make it easier to maintain a long-term energy deficit and hence slow down the rate of weight gain or regain (90). In at least one study, an *ad libitum*, low-fat, high-carbohydrate diet was shown to be more effective than energy restriction alone in maintaining weight loss during 1 yr (75). This may be owing to the fact that simple energy restriction is often associated with extremely poor compliance (85).

3.3. Low-Carbohydrate Diets

The initial popular low-carbohydrate diet was written in 1863 by William Banting, an undertaker who lost 50 lb using this type of diet (91). Before beginning his diet he had become so fat that he had to walk down stairs backward for fear of falling. He was so proud of his success using a diet given to him by a Dr. Harvey that he published a small pamphlet that became the first best-selling diet book. There have been many reincarnations of the low-carbohydrate diet, but the one currently sweeping the market is the Atkins Diet. This diet strategy has been studied in several clinical trials (92–95). In these studies the low-carbohydrate diets produced more weight loss for the first 6 mo but not thereafter. This is discussed in more detail in Chapter 14.

3.4. Low-Fat Diets

A number of studies have also been done comparing low-fat diets. In Fig. 3 we summarize the studies of the effect of fat reduction on body weight. The data depict the relation between the percent reduction in fat energy and the resultant weight change (isoenergetic studies were not included). The main explanatory variable is the change in percentage of energy from fat. The covariates analysis included gender, mean initial body weight, and age of the subjects; the difference in size of the studies was allowed for. As expected the regression model reveals that more weight was lost by those with a higher initial weight. The slope of the regression line suggests that a 10% decrease in fat (e.g., from 36 to 26% of total energy) is associated with weight loss of 32 g/d among obese subjects and 9.9 g/d for all studies combined. Although the results are not statistically significant, they reiterate the importance of dietary fat reduction in obesity. A subsequent

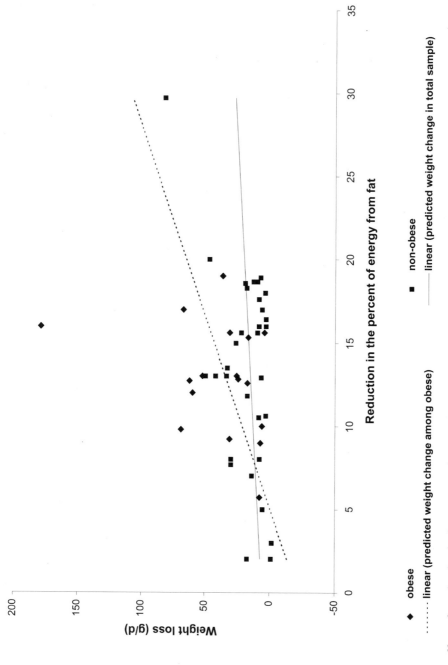

Fig. 3. The effect of a reduction in the percent of energy from fat on grams of weight loss per day. (Reproduced with permission from ref. 29. © The American Journal of Clinical Nutrition and the American Society for Clinical Nutrition.)

meta-analysis of the effect of changes in fat intake on weight loss showed comparable results (Astrup A, correspondence with author)).

A meta-analysis of randomized placebo-controlled trials concluded that low-fat diets produce weight loss, but not more so than control diets *(96)*. When low-fat diets were prepared using complex carbohydrates, the weight loss was not different than when simple carbohydrates predominated *(97)*. However, using a higher protein level combined with a low-fat diet increased the weight loss compared to a low-protein diet at the same fat intake. Thus the macronutrient composition may play a role in the adherence to diets and in the ease with which overweight individuals can follow them.

3.5. Low-Fat Substitutes

There is a growing interest in the role of fat substitutes and energy density of the diet as strategies for enhancing weight loss.

3.5.1. FAT SUBSTITUTES

Fat substitutes, such as sucrose polyester (e.g., Olestra®), have been used to facilitate research on the degree to which covert changes in the diet alter total energy intake and macronutrient selection. Short-term studies of the substitution of indigestible fat substitutes for dietary fat show two patterns of adaptation. When 20 or 30 g of Olestra was substituted for fat in a single breakfast meal, there was energy compensation over the next 24–36 h in healthy young men *(98,99)*. When fat intake was lowered from 40 to 30% of energy by substituting Olestra for fat at the noon or evening meals, there was no energy compensation during the next 24 h *(100)*. However, when Olestra substitution lowered the fat intake from 30 to nearly 20% of energy over three meals, healthy subjects felt less satisfied and compensated for nearly 75% of the energy deficit over the next day *(101)*. In longer-term experiments lasting 2 wk or 3 mo, the substitution of Olestra for about one-third of the fat in all meals containing 40% of energy from fat reduced energy intake by about 15% for the same weight of food. In each experiment, there was only partial compensation for energy, suggesting that when the energy density of the diet was altered, the subjects continued to eat the same amount of food even though it provided less metabolizable energy. Mean weight loss in the 2-wk experiment was 1.5 kg and in the 3-mo experiment was nearly 5 kg, which was significantly greater than the weight loss in the control group *(101,102)*.

3.5.2. ENERGY DENSITY

Energy density is also determined by the water content of foods, which account for much of the total food amount *(103)*. Free-living individuals tend to consume a fairly constant weight or volume of food notwithstanding its energy content, although this may be compensated for at later meals. Apart from complex carbohydrate, an increase in the water or dietary fiber content of food may lead to satiety and lower energy intake *(103)*. It has been shown that a sizeable amount of energy-diluted food may lead to short-term satiety and the incomplete compensation for lost calories *(104)*. When healthy, normal weight women were fed with test meals that provided a similar macronutrient content and composition but had a different water content, the amount of the food eaten was unaffected by the energy density of the meals. Accordingly, significantly less energy was consumed from meals having a higher water content *(105)*.

A practical role for the effect of energy density may be seen in comparing the types of foods eaten on days when a fast food meal is eaten as compared to days when no fast food meals are eaten *(106)*. During the day when a fast-food meal is eaten, there is a smaller intake of cereals, green vegetables, and milk, and an increased intake of fried potatoes and soft drinks. These observations support the difficulty that the body has in adapting to the high fat and high energy density of many components of the current Western diet.

4. CONCLUSIONS

The role of portion size and diet composition, particularly dietary fat intake, in the development and control of obesity is complex. Portion sizes have been increasing steadily over the past 50 yr, thereby providing easy access to excessive energy intake. In addition, there is evidence that an increase in fat intake in developing countries is associated with an increase in body weight, and may play a role in maintaining or augmenting obesity in genetically susceptible people in countries with a higher fat intake. Reduction in portion size through using portion-controlled meals or foods with lower energy density is one strategy for losing weight. Reduction of fat intake is also a practical way to prevent weight gain, and when coupled with regular exercise, induces a sustainable weight loss. Reduction of fat intake may be accomplished by replacing dietary fat with complex carbohydrate, fruits, and vegetables. Reduction in fat intake alone should not be expected to entirely reverse the development of obesity. Instead, this should be seen as a means to reduce the energy density of the diet and hence the total energy intake.

The increasing prevalence of obesity in many developing countries can be explained in part by the increase in availability of high-fat foods and the adoption of the so-called affluent or Western-style diet. In these countries, limiting further increases in fat intake may be an effective strategy to prevent obesity. In the industrialized countries where fat intake is relatively high, reductions in both fat intake, as well as total energy intake, may be warranted.

Reduction in carbohydrate intake produces weight loss for more than 6 mo that in some trials is greater than the control diet, but this difference is usually not maintained. Low-fat diets also produce weight loss, but not more than the control diets. Thus, treatment of obesity using portion control and lowered energy density appears to be as effective as manipulation of macronutrient intake.

REFERENCES

1. Nielsen SJ, Popkin BM. Patterns and trends in portion sizes, 1977–1998. JAMA 2003; 289:450–453.
2. Rolls BJ, Morris EL, Roe LS. Portion size of food affects energy intake in normal-weight and overweight men and women. Am J Clin Nutr 2002; 76:1207–1213.
3. Diliberti N, Bordi PL, Conklin MT, Roe LS, Rolls BJ. Increased portion size leads to increased energy intake in a restaurant meal. Obes Res 2004; 12:562–568.
4. Putnam J, Allshouse JE. Food consumption, prices and expenditures, 1970–97. U.S. Department of Agriculture Economic Research Service, April 1999, p. 965.
5. Willett WC. Is dietary fat a major determinant of body fat? Am J Clin Nutr 1998; 67(3 Suppl): 556S–562S.
6. Katan MB, Grundy SM, Willett WC. Should a low-fat, high-carbohydrate diet be recommended for everyone? Beyond low-fat diets. N Engl J Med 1997; 337:563–566; discussion 566, 567.
7. Bray GA, Fisler J, York DA. Neuroendocrine control of the development of obesity: understanding gained from studies of experimental animal models. Front Neuroendocrinol 1990; 11:128–181.

8. West DB, York B. Dietary fat, genetic predisposition, and obesity: lessons from animal models. Am J Clin Nutr 1998; 67(3 Suppl):505S–512S.

9. Chanmugam P, Guthrie JF, Cecilio S, Morton JF, Basiotis PP, Anand R. Did fat intake in the United States really decline between 1989–1991 and 1994–1996? J Am Diet Assoc 2003; 103:867–872.

10. Haines PS, Hama MY, Guilkey DK, Popkin BM. Weekend eating in the United States is linked with greater energy, fat, and alcohol intake. Obes Res 2003; 11:945–949.

11. Nielsen SJ, Popkin BM. Patterns and trends in food portion sizes, 1977-1998. JAMA 2003; 289:450–453.

12. Nielsen SJ, Popkin BM. Changes in beverage intake between 1977 and 2001. Am J Prev Med 2004; 27:205–210.

13. Nielsen SJ, Siega-Riz AM, Popkin BM. Trends in energy intake in U.S. between 1977 and 1996: similar shifts seen across age groups. Obes Res 2002; 10:370–378.

14. Flatt JP, Ravussin E, Acheson KJ, Jequier E. Effects of dietary fat on postprandial substrate oxidation and on carbohydrate and fat balances. J Clin Invest 1985; 76:1019–1024.

15. Bennett C, Reed GW, Peters JC, Abumrad NN, Sun M, Hill JO. Short-term effects of dietary-fat ingestion on energy expenditure and nutrient balance. Am J Clin Nutr 1992; 55:1071–1077.

16. Schrauwen P, van Marken Lichtenbelt WD, Saris WH, Westerterp KR. Changes in fat oxidation in response to a high-fat diet. Am J Clin Nutr 1997; 66:276–282.

17. Hill JO, Peters JC, Reed GW, Schlundt DG, Sharp T, Greene HL. Nutrient balance in humans: effects of diet composition. Am J Clin Nutr 1991; 54:10–17.

18. Leibel RL, Rosenbaum M, Hirsch J. Changes in energy expenditure resulting from altered body weight. N Engl J Med 1995; 332:621–628.

19. Astrup A, Buemann B, Christensen NJ, Toubro S. Failure to increase lipid oxidation in response to increasing dietary fat content in formerly obese women. Am J Physiol Apr 1994; 266(4 Pt 1): E592–599.

20. Horton TJ, Drougas H, Brachey A, Reed GW, Peters JC, Hill JO. Fat and carbohydrate overfeeding in humans: different effects on energy storage. Am J Clin Nutr 1995; 62:19–29.

21. Astrup A, Toubro S, Raben A, Skov AR. The role of low-fat diets and fat substitutes in body weight management: what have we learned from clinical studies? J Am Diet Assoc 1997; 97 (7 Suppl):S82–S87.

22. Lawton CL, Burley VJ, Wales JK, Blundell JE. Dietary fat and appetite control in obese subjects: weak effects on satiation and satiety. Int J Obes Relat Metab Disord 1993; 17:409–416.

23. Abbott WG, Howard BV, Christin L, et al. Short-term energy balance: relationship with protein, carbohydrate, and fat balances. Am J Physiol 1988; 255(3 Pt 1):E332–E337.

24. Thomas CD, Peters JC, Reed GW, Abumrad NN, Sun M, Hill JO. Nutrient balance and energy expenditure during ad libitum feeding of high-fat and high-carbohydrate diets in humans. Am J Clin Nutr 1992; 55:934–942.

25. Sparti A, Windhauser MM, Champagne CM, Bray GA. Effect of an acute reduction in carbohydrate intake on subsequent food intake in healthy men. Am J Clin Nutr 1997; 66:1144–1150.

26. Tremblay A, Lavallee N, Almeras N, Allard L, Despres JP, Bouchard C. Nutritional determinants of the increase in energy intake associated with a high-fat diet. Am J Clin Nutr 1991; 53:1134–1137.

27. Green SM, Blundell JE. Effect of fat- and sucrose-containing foods on the size of eating episodes and energy intake in lean dietary restrained and unrestrained females: potential for causing overconsumption. Eur J Clin Nutr 1996; 50:625–635.

28. Blundell JE, Macdiarmid JI. Passive overconsumption. Fat intake and short-term energy balance. Ann NY Acad Sci 1997; 827:392–407.

29. Bray GA, Popkin BM. Dietary fat intake does affect obesity! Am J Clin Nutr 1998; 68:1157–1173.

30. Curb JD, Marcus EB. Body fat and obesity in Japanese Americans. Am J Clin Nutr 1991; 53(6 Suppl): 1552S–1555S.

31. Sonne-Holm S, Sorensen TI. Post-war course of the prevalence of extreme overweight among Danish young men. J Chronic Dis 1977; 30:351–358.

32. Price RA, Charles MA, Pettitt DJ, Knowler WC. Obesity in Pima Indians: large increases among post-World War II birth cohorts. Am J Phys Anthropol 1993; 92:473–479.

33. Popkin BM, Paeratakul S, Zhai F, Ge K. Dietary and environmental correlates of obesity in a population study in China. Obes Res 1995; 3 Suppl 2:135s–143s.

34. Paeratakul S, Popkin BM, Keyou G, Adair LS, Stevens J. Changes in diet and physical activity affect the body mass index of Chinese adults. Int J Obes Relat Metab Disord 1998; 22:424–431.

35. Lissner L, Heitmann BL. Dietary fat and obesity: evidence from epidemiology. Eur J Clin Nutr 1995; 49:79–90.

36. Heitmann BL, Lissner L, Sorensen TI, Bengtsson C. Dietary fat intake and weight gain in women genetically predisposed for obesity. Am J Clin Nutr 1995; 61:1213–1217.

37. Teague RJ, Kanarek R, Bray GA, Glick Z, Orthen-Gambill N. Effect of diet on the weight of brown adipose tissue in rodents. Life Sci 1981; 29:1531–1536.

38. Rolls BJ, Kim S, Fedoroff IC. Effects of drinks sweetened with sucrose or aspartame on hunger, thirst and food intake in men. Physiol Behav 1990; 48:19–26.

39. Tordoff MG, Alleva AM. Effect of drinking soda sweetened with aspartame or high-fructose corn syrup on food intake and body weight. Am J Clin Nutr 1990; 51:963–969.

40. Raben A, Vasilaras TH, Moller AC, Astrup A. Sucrose compared with artificial sweeteners: different effects on ad libitum food intake and body weight after 10 wk of supplementation in overweight subjects. Am J Clin Nutr 2002; 76:721–729.

41. Schulze MB, Manson JE, Ludwig DS, et al. Sugar-sweetened beverages, weight gain, and incidence of type 2 diabetes in young and middle-aged women. JAMA 2004; 292:927–934.

42. Ludwig DS, Peterson KE, Gortmaker SL. Relation between consumption of sugar-sweetened drinks and childhood obesity: a prospective, observational analysis. Lancet 2001; 357:505–508.

43. Bray GA, Nielsen SJ, Popkin BM. Consumption of high-fructose corn syrup in beverages may play a role in the epidemic of obesity. Am J Clin Nutr 2004; 79:537–543.

44. Kinsell LW, Gunning B, Michaels GD, Richardson J, Cox SE, Lemon C. Calories Do Count. Metabolism 1964; 13:195–204.

45. Lyon XH, Di Vetta V, Milon H, Jequier E, Schutz Y. Compliance to dietary advice directed towards increasing the carbohydrate to fat ratio of the everyday diet. Int J Obes Relat Metab Disord 1995; 19:260–269.

46. Rolls BJ, Barnett RA. Volumetrics: Feel Full on Fewer Calories. 1st ed. Harper Collins, New York, 2000.

47. Flechtner-Mors M, Ditschuneit HH, Johnson TD, Suchard MA, Adler G. Metabolic and weight loss effects of long-term dietary intervention in obese patients: four-year results. Obes Res 2000; 8:399–402.

48. Lemonnier D. Effect of age, sex, and site on the cellularity of adipose tissue in mice and rats rendered obese by a high-fat diet. J Clin Invest 1972; 51:2907–2915.

49. Faust IM, Johnson PR, Stem JS, Hirsch J. Diet-induced adipocyte number increase in adult rats: a new model of obesity. Am J Physiol 1978; 235:E279–E286.

50. Hill JO. Body weight regulation in obese and obese-reduced rats. Int J Obes 1990; 14 Suppl 1:31–45; discussion 45–37.

51. Hill JO, Lin D, Yakubu F, Peters JC. Development of dietary obesity in rats: influence of amount and composition of dietary fat. Int J Obes Relat Metab Disord 1992; 16:321–333.

52. Rolls DJ, Rowe E, Turner RC. Persistent obesity in rats following a period of consumption of a mixed, high energy diet. J Physiol (Lond) 1980; 298:415–427.

53. Harris RB, Kasser TR, Martin RJ. Dynamics of recovery of body composition after overfeeding, food restriction or starvation of mature female rats. J Nutr 1986; 116:2536–2546.

54. Uhley VE, Jen KL. Changes in feeding efficiency and carcass composition in rats on repeated high-fat feedings. Int J Obes 1989; 13:849–856.

55. Lissner L, Levitsky DA, Strupp BJ, Kalkwarf HJ, Roe DA. Dietary fat and the regulation of energy intake in human subjects. Am J Clin Nutr 1987; 46:886–892.

56. Kendall A, Levitsky DA, Strupp BJ, Lissner L. Weight loss on a low-fat diet: consequence of the imprecision of the control of food intake in humans. Am J Clin Nutr 1991; 53:1124–1129.

57. Boyar AP, Rose DP, Loughridge JR, et al. Response to a diet low in total fat in women with postmenopausal breast cancer: a pilot study. Nutr Cancer 1988; 11:93–99.

58. Lee-Han H, Cousins M, Beaton M, et al. Compliance in a randomized clinical trial of dietary fat reduction in patients with breast dysplasia. Am J Clin Nutr 1988; 48:575–586.

59. Boyd NF, Cousins M, Beaton M, Kriukov V, Lockwood G, Tritchler D. Quantitative changes in dietary fat intake and serum cholesterol in women: results from a randomized, controlled trial. Am J Clin Nutr 1990; 52:470–476.

60. Bloemberg BP, Kromhout D, Goddijn HE, Jansen A, Obermann-de Boer GL. The impact of the Guidelines for a Healthy Diet of The Netherlands Nutrition Council on total and high density lipoprotein cholesterol in hypercholesterolemic free-living men. Am J Epidemiol 1991; 134:39–48.

61. Sheppard L, Kristal AR, Kushi LH. Weight loss in women participating in a randomized trial of low-fat diets. Am J Clin Nutr 1991; 54:821–828.

62. Singh RB, Rastogi SS, Verma R, et al. Randomised controlled trial of cardioprotective diet in patients with recent acute myocardial infarction: results of one year follow up. BMJ 1992; 304:1015–1019.

63. Hunninghake DB, Stein EA, Dujovne CA, et al. The efficacy of intensive dietary therapy alone or combined with lovastatin in outpatients with hypercholesterolemia. N Engl J Med 1993; 328:1213–1219.

64. Kasim SE, Martino S, Kim PN, et al. Dietary and anthropometric determinants of plasma lipoproteins during a long-term low-fat diet in healthy women. Am J Clin Nutr 1993; 57:146–153.

65. Schaefer EJ, Lichtenstein AH, Lamon-Fava S, et al. Body weight and low-density lipoprotein cholesterol changes after consumption of a low-fat ad libitum diet. JAMA 1995; 274:1450–1455.

66. Westerterp KR, Verboeket-van de Venne WP, Westerterp-Plantenga MS, Velthuis-te Wierik EJ, de Graaf C, Weststrate JA. Dietary fat and body fat: an intervention study. Int J Obes Relat Metab Disord 1996; 20:1022–1026.

67. Raben A, Jensen ND, Marckmann P, Sandstrom B, Astrup A. Spontaneous weight loss during 11 weeks' ad libitum intake of a low fat/high fiber diet in young, normal weight subjects. Int J Obes Relat Metab Disord 1995; 19:916–923.

68. Prewitt TE, Schmeisser D, Bowen PE, et al. Changes in body weight, body composition, and energy intake in women fed high- and low-fat diets. Am J Clin Nutr 1991; 54:304–310.

69. Baer JT. Improved plasma cholesterol levels in men after a nutrition education program at the worksite. J Am Diet Assoc 1993; 93:658–663.

70. Weststrate JA, van het Hof KH, van den Berg H, et al. A comparison of the effect of free access to reduced fat products or their full fat equivalents on food intake, body weight, blood lipids and fat-soluble antioxidants levels and haemostasis variables. Eur J Clin Nutr 1998; 52:389–395.

71. Stefanick ML, Mackey S, Sheehan M, Ellsworth N, Haskell WL, Wood PD. Effects of diet and exercise in men and postmenopausal women with low levels of HDL cholesterol and high levels of LDL cholesterol. N Engl J Med 1998; 339:12–20.

72. Thuesen L, Henriksen LB, Engby B. One-year experience with a low-fat, low-cholesterol diet in patients with coronary heart disease. Am J Clin Nutr 1986; 44:212–219.

73. Knopp RH, Walden CE, Retzlaff BM, et al. Long-term cholesterol-lowering effects of 4 fat-restricted diets in hypercholesterolemic and combined hyperlipidemic men. The Dietary Alternatives Study. JAMA 1997; 278:1509–1515.

74. Simon MS, Heilbrun LK, Boomer A, et al. A randomized trial of a low-fat dietary intervention in women at high risk for breast cancer. Nutr Cancer 1997; 27:136–142.

75. Toubro S, Astrup A. Randomised comparison of diets for maintaining obese subjects' weight after major weight loss: ad lib, low fat, high carbohydrate diet v fixed energy intake. BMJ 1997; 314:29–34.

76. Buzzard IM, Asp EH, Chlebowski RT, et al. Diet intervention methods to reduce fat intake: nutrient and food group composition of self-selected low-fat diets. J Am Diet Assoc 1990; 90:42–50, 53.

77. Puska P, Iacono JM, Nissinen A, et al. Controlled, randomised trial of the effect of dietary fat on blood pressure. Lancet 1983; 1:1–5.

78. Hammer RL, Barrier CA, Roundy ES, Bradford JM, Fisher AG. Calorie-restricted low-fat diet and exercise in obese women. Am J Clin Nutr 1989; 49:77–85.

79. Rumpler WV, Seale JL, Miles CW, Bodwell CE. Energy-intake restriction and diet-composition effects on energy expenditure in men. Am J Clin Nutr 1991; 53:430–436.

80. Shintani TT, Hughes CK, Beckham S, O'Connor HK. Obesity and cardiovascular risk intervention through the ad libitum feeding of traditional Hawaiian diet. Am J Clin Nutr 1991; 53(6 Suppl): 1647S–1651S.

81. Schlundt DG, Hill JO, Pope-Cordle J, Arnold D, Virts KL, Katahn M. Randomized evaluation of a low fat ad libitum carbohydrate diet for weight reduction. Int J Obes Relat Metab Disord 1993; 17:623–629.

82. Powell JJ, Tucker L, Fisher AG, Wilcox K. The effects of different percentages of dietary fat intake, exercise, and calorie restriction on body composition and body weight in obese females. Am J Health Promot 1994; 8:442–448.

83. Harris JK, French SA, Jeffery RW, McGovern PG, Wing RR. Dietary and physical activity correlates of long-term weight loss. Obes Res 1994; 4:307–313.

84. Shah M, McGovern P, French S, Baxter J. Comparison of a low-fat, ad libitum complex-carbohydrate diet with a low-energy diet in moderately obese women. Am J Clin Nutr 1994; 59:980–984.

85. Jeffery RW, Hellerstedt WL, French SA, Baxter JE. A randomized trial of counseling for fat restriction versus calorie restriction in the treatment of obesity. Int J Obes Relat Metab Disord 1995; 19:132–137.

86. Pascale RW, Wing RR, Butler BA, Mullen M, Bononi P. Effects of a behavioral weight loss program stressing calorie restriction versus calorie plus fat restriction in obese individuals with NIDDM or a family history of diabetes. Diabetes Care 1995; 18:1241–1248.

87. Siggaard R, Raben A, Astrup A. Weight loss during 12 week's ad libitum carbohydrate-rich diet in overweight and normal-weight subjects at a Danish work site. Obes Res 1996; 4:347–356.

88. Harvey-Berino J. The efficacy of dietary fat vs. total energy restriction for weight loss. Obes Res 1998; 6:202–207.

89. Pritchard JE, Nowson CA, Wark JD. Bone loss accompanying diet-induced or exercise-induced weight loss: a randomised controlled study. Int J Obes Relat Metab Disord 1996; 20:513–520.

90. De Graaf C, Drijvers JJ, Zimmermanns NJ, et al. Energy and fat compensation during long-term consumption of reduced fat products. Appetite 1997; 29:305–323.

91. Banting W. Letter on Corpulence, Addressed to the Public. 2nd ed. Harrison and Sons, London, 1863.

92. Foster GD, Wyatt HR, Hill JO, et al. A randomized trial of a low-carbohydrate diet for obesity. N Engl J Med 2003; 348:2082–2090.

93. Samaha FF, Iqbal N, Seshadri P, et al. A low-carbohydrate as compared with a low-fat diet in severe obesity. N Engl J Med 2003; 348:2074–2081.

94. Brehm BJ, Seeley RJ, Daniels SR, D'Alessio DA. A randomized trial comparing a very low carbohydrate diet and a calorie-restricted low fat diet on body weight and cardiovascular risk factors in healthy women. J Clin Endocrinol Metab 2003; 88:1617–1623.

95. Stern L, Iqbal N, Seshadri P, et al. The effects of low-carbohydrate versus conventional weight loss diets in severely obese adults: one-year follow-up of a randomized trial. Ann Intern Med 2004; 140:778–785. Astrup A. Correspondence with author.

96. Pirozzo S, Summerbell C, Cameron C, Glasziou P. Should we recommend low-fat diets for obesity? Obes Rev 2003; 4:83–90.

97. Saris WH, Astrup A, Prentice AM, et al. Randomized controlled trial of changes in dietary carbohydrate/fat ratio and simple vs complex carbohydrates on body weight and blood lipids: the CARMEN study. The Carbohydrate Ratio Management in European National diets. Int J Obes Relat Metab Disord 2000; 24:1310–1318.

98. Rolls BJ, Pirraglia PA, Jones MB, Peters JC. Effects of olestra, a noncaloric fat substitute, on daily energy and fat intakes in lean men. Am J Clin Nutr 1992; 56:84–92.

99. Burley VJ, Blundell JE. Evaluation of the action of a non-absorbable fat on appetite and energy intake in lean healthy males. In: Ailhaud G, Guy-Grand B, Lafontan M, Ricquier D, eds. Obesity in Europe. John Libbey, London, 1992, pp. 63–65.

100. Cotton JR, Weststrate JA, Blundell JE. Replacement of dietary fat with sucrose polyester: effects on energy intake and appetite control in nonobese males. Am J Clin Nutr 1996; 63:891–896.

101. Bray G, Sparti A, Windhauser M, York DA. Effect of two weeks fat replacement of olestra on food intake and energy metabolism. FASEB J 1995; 9:A439.

102. Roy J, Lovejoy JC, Windhauser M, Bray G. Metabolic effects of fat substitution with olestra. FASEB J 1997; 11:A358.

103. Drewnowski A. Energy density, palatability, and satiety: implications for weight control. Nutr Rev 1998; 56:347–353.

104. Pi-Sunyer FX. Effect of the composition of the diet on energy intake. Nutr Rev 1990; 48:94–105; discussion 114–131.

105. Bell EA, Castellanos VH, Pelkman CL, Thorwart ML, Rolls BJ. Energy density of foods affects energy intake in normal-weight women. Am J Clin Nutr 1998; 67:412–420.

106. Paeratakul S, Ferdinand DP, Champagne CM, Ryan DH, Bray GA. Fast-food consumption among US adults and children: dietary and nutrient intake profile. J Am Diet Assoc 2003; 103:1332–1338.

14 Diets and Exercise Programs for Weight Loss

Lisa Sanders, Kathleen Page, Dena Bravata, and Marguerite Brainerd

KEY POINTS

- All diets work by reducing calorie consumption. Low-fat and low-carbohydrate diets use different strategies to reach the same end of calorie reduction.
- Both low-fat and low-carbohydrate diets can be safe and effective strategies for short-term weight loss.
- Given that greater weight loss is associated with greater adherence and longer duration of diet, and the lack of data on which diet works best, potential dieters should be encouraged to consider a variety of diet strategies and choose one that they can most easily integrate into their daily life for the long term.
- Exercise will modestly enhance weight loss and weight maintenance and, given its other demonstrated health benefits, should be recommended for everyone trying to lose weight.
- Exercise programs should be started gradually and work toward recommended goals of at least 30 min of daily moderate activity for overall health benefits and toward an ultimate goal of 60 min of daily physical activity for weight loss and weight maintenance.

1. INTRODUCTION

Fifty-eight million Americans are overweight or obese, and one in four say they are trying to lose that weight *(1)*. Mounting evidence suggests that losing even a portion of the extra weight will improve health and prolong life. A recent study published in the *Annals of Internal Medicine* found that although intentional weight loss was linked to the greatest increase in lifespan, simply trying to lose weight, independent of any real weight loss, was almost as beneficial *(2)*.

Potential dieters have plenty of choice. Hundreds of titles crowd the diet book nook of any bookstore. A search of a popular Internet book vender using the phrase "diet book" turned up more than 50,000 titles *(3)*. Yet, in this vast commercial array of books, scientific evidence mixes with pseudoscience. The books present a confusing variety of competing claims and promises that can baffle even the most sophisticated would-

From: *Nutritional Health: Strategies for Disease Prevention, Second Edition*
Edited by: N. J. Temple, T. Wilson, and D. R. Jacobs © Humana Press Inc., Totowa, NJ

be dieter. Should you choose "the delicious, doctor-designed foolproof plan" or the "ultimate weight solution"? Should you eliminate fat or carbohydrates? Will success come from the "power of protein," the "hormone connection," or the "fat flush plan"? All are available. And all promise the same thing: buyers will lose the weight they want easily, safely, and effectively.

Given that they all claim to do the same thing, does it matter which diet is chosen? Weight loss efforts are notorious for their poor success rate—one factor behind the proliferation of diet programs. There is no evidence that any single weight loss program works best; indeed, most research shows that almost any diet can produce modest weight loss in many and significant weight loss in a few. At present there are no data on which weight-loss program may be most effective for a given individual. However, choosing the wrong diet may cause adverse health effects.

In this chapter we will briefly review the evidence on the most popular diets to help guide clinicians and dieticians choose a diet that is most likely to be safe and effective for a given individual. We will also review the most recent data on the role of exercise in weight loss. Although the wealth of information can seem confusing, what is beginning to emerge is the idea that there are many options for those who wish to lose weight and a careful consideration of the options may improve the odds that the chosen diet will be successful.

2. ELEMENTS OF A SUCCESSFUL WEIGHT-LOSS PROGRAM

We reviewed a variety of diet and exercise studies and guidelines to isolate the elements of those successful weight-loss programs that have received widespread support. In general, these strategies fall into several broad categories: reducing caloric intake, increasing caloric expenditure, improving adherence to a dietary program, and identifying other behaviors associated with successful weight loss.

It is universally accepted that weight loss occurs when energy expenditure exceeds energy intake. An energy deficit of 500–1000 kcal/d will result in a loss of approx 1–2 lbs/wk and an average total weight loss of approx 8% after 6 mo (4). Although weight regain is common, two-thirds of the weight that is lost by dieting is maintained at 1 yr (5). The National Heart, Lung and Blood Institute Obesity Education Initiative Expert Panel recommends a low-calorie diet that supplies 1000–1200 kcals/d for women and 1200–1600 kcals/d for men (4). An alternative strategy is presented in Table 1.

However, simply restricting calories, using any type of diet, is difficult. Because of this, caloric restriction is usually combined with other strategies in an effort to improve adherence with the dietary program and resultant weight loss. Although all the components of a successful weight-loss support are not known, four characteristics associated with success have been described (4–6).

First, keeping track of what is eaten may enhance adherence to a reduced-calorie diet. The Weight Control Registry is a group of thousands of dieters with a documented weight loss of more than 30 lbs that has been maintained for more than 1 yr (7). Many of these dieters report that keeping track of what they ate was an important strategy for both weight loss and weight maintenance. Other research has shown that dieters have difficulty recalling what they eat over the course of a day, which can make keeping track of calories a challenge (8). Moreover, without a diary, eaters are most likely to have particular difficulty recalling foods that are high in fat and calorie dense (9).

Table 1
Alternative Approach for Estimating Energy Intake Goal of Initial Weight-Loss Diet

Initial body weight (pounds)[a]	Suggested goals for energy intake (kcal/d)
150–199	1000–1200
200–249	1200–1500
250–299	1500–1800
300–349	1800–2000
>350	2000

[a]Initial body weight refers to pre-diet weight, not target weight.
From ref. 5.

Second, regular eating patterns, whether it is three meals a day or multiple small meals—eaten in an established pattern—is associated with better odds of weight maintenance and weight loss *(10)*. In particular, eating breakfast regularly was a strategy used by successful dieters to lose weight and maintain weight loss *(11–13)*.

Third, exercise and increased activity increase caloric expenditures—the other half of the weight-loss equation. Although how much and which types of exercise are best is an ongoing debate, exercise remains a component of most weight loss and maintenance strategies *(4,5)*. Dieters need to find a form of exercise and activity that they consider pleasant and work to integrate these into a daily routine *(4,5,13)*.

Finally, inadequate sleep has been linked to weight gain *(14,15)*. So, those trying to lose weight should regularly get enough sleep.

Weight gain is the result of multiple factors of lifestyle and behaviors. Individuals trying to lose weight should identify behaviors linked to their own weight gain and work to change these habitual behaviors. Setting small and achievable weight and behavior goals allows dieters to experience success, and this can be used to motivate additional lifestyle alterations. Strategies, such as self-monitoring (daily records of food intake and physical activity), stimulus control (avoiding triggers that prompt eating), and problem solving (identifying barriers to successful change and developing techniques for coping), can support the change process *(16)*. Working with others who are experienced in the practices of successful weight loss can be useful to the dieter who must make dozens of choices each day that will affect the success of their endeavor *(4,5,16)*. Frequent patient-provider contact (every 1–2 wk) is associated with better long-term results *(4,5)*.

3. LOW-CARBOHYDRATE DIETS

Despite the concerns of numerous medical and dietary organizations, low-carbohydrate diets are currently extraordinarily popular. The top two low-carbohydrate diet books, *Dr. Atkins' Diet Revolution (17)*, and the more recent *South Beach Diet (18)* by fellow cardiologist Arthur Agatston, have sold more than 10 million copies in the past 2 yr. An estimated 30 million Americans have turned to low-carbohydrate diets to lose their excess weight *(19)*. This remarkable popularity has brought new research scrutiny into the safety and efficacy of short-term use of these diets. However, many questions remain unanswered.

A link between carbohydrates and obesity was postulated long before our own diet-obsessed time. In the 19th century, physician Anthelm Brillat-Savarin wrote in his seven-volume work, *The Physiology of Taste (20)*, that his "stout" patients ate diets rich in breads, rice, and potatoes. He attributed obesity to a natural predisposition combined with "floury and feculent substances which man makes the prime ingredients of his daily nourishment." Fifty years later, a cabinetmaker named William Banting went on a diet, which excluded all carbohydrate (except red wine) and lost 25% of his 202 lb over the course of 1 yr. He extolled the virtues of this diet in a best-selling pamphlet, remarking that "the great charms and comfort of the system are that its effects are palpable within a week of trial and creates a natural stimulus to persevere for a few weeks more" *(21)*. Banting also noted that he lost this weight without feeling hungry. Those qualities—a diet made exclusively of the richest of foods, allowing many dieters to lose weight quickly and without hunger—have made low-carbohydrate diets one of the most profitable mines in the modern diet industry.

Dr. Atkins' Diet Revolution was first published in 1972, with several editions and updates in the intervening decades. In it, Atkins recommends eliminating virtually all carbohydrates in the first 2 wk of the diet. Dieters may consume up to 20 g/d of carbohydrate—the equivalent of one slice of bread per day—if you were allowed to eat bread. (*See* Table 2 for a more complete nutritional picture of the induction diet.) The way the diet does this is by allowing the consumption of unlimited fat and protein but limiting carbohydrate choices to vegetables alone, and, at least initially, only those vegetables with the lowest carbohydrate content. Most fruits, and all pastas, breads, and sweets, are banished. The purpose of this phase of the diet is to use up all the glycogen stores in the body and induce the body to use fat rather than carbohydrates for fuel. In doing this, the dieter will become mildly ketotic—a state that Atkins dubs "benign dietary ketosis."

After the initial induction phase, dieters move on to the ongoing diet in which they can add back some carbohydrates—principally some fruits and a few more vegetables. The author recommends limiting carbohydrates to less than 60 g/d as long as dieters wish to continue losing weight. The goal is to add back as many nonstarchy carbohydrates as possible while remaining ketotic. Dieters stay in this phase of the diet until the goal weight is achieved. At that point dieters can increase their carbohydrate intake again, although carbohydrates will still make up less one-quarter of their total calorie intake. Breads, pastas, and starches along with most sweets are banished forever.

In comparison, the *South Beach Diet* is a relative newcomer to the marketplace. Published in 2002, its success has surpassed even Dr. Atkins'. Like its rival, the South Beach diet gets rid of practically all carbohydrates initially, then slowly adds back what author Agatston calls "good" carbohydrates—complex carbohydrates containing lots of fiber. (*See* Table 2 for a nutritional analysis of the diet.) The book also emphasizes choosing "good fats," namely monounsaturated and polyunsaturated fatty acids over "bad fats," that is, saturated and trans fats.

Despite their commercial success, the strategy employed by these diets—replacing most carbohydrates with fats and protein—runs counter to the traditional high-carbohydrate, low-fat fare usually recommended for weight loss. A few recent studies, however, have shown that these diets can be both safe and effective in the short run. Long-term effects—on weight loss and health—are still to be examined *(22)*.

Table 2
Nutritional Analysis of Popular Diets

Nutrient	Food guide pyramid (recommended)	Atkins introduction phase	The South Beach diet	The Zone diet	Weight Watchers diet	Eat More, Weigh Less
Total calories	1593	1487	1552	1385	1647	1220
Carbohydrates in grams (% cals)	237 (60)	27 (7)	50 (13)	105 (29)	238 (56)	241 (78)
Protein in grams (% cals)	92 (23)	156 (43)	140 (36)	109 (31)	82 (19)	47 (15)
Fat in grams (% cals)	37 (21)	80 (50)	86 (36)	61 (39)	46 (24)	10 (7)
Saturated fat in grams (% cals)	9 (5)	29 (18)	24 (14)	25 (16)	11 (6)	1 (0.7)
Cholesterol (mg)	82	1175	290	235	69	4
Sodium (mg)	1920	2506	3540	3349	3324	1214
β-Carotene (μg)	557	166	405	407	3488	602
Vitamin C (mg)	170	166	149	277	198	401
Calcium (mg)	978	493	654	1120	1197	800
Iron (mg)	15	21	10	10	29	20
Vitamin E (mg)	6	9	19	10	29	7
Folate (μg)	410	341	194	380	654	389
Fiber (g)	32	15	12	23	32	41

3.1. Efficacy and Safety of the Low-Carbohydrate Diet

The research done to date suggests that low-carbohydrate diets are effective in producing short-term weight loss. In a meta-analysis of more than 100 studies of low-carbohydrate diets, Bravata et al. found that these diets did produce short-term weight loss (22). However, this weight loss was a result of calorie restriction—not carbohydrate restriction. In other words, successful low-carbohydrate dieters were eating not just fewer carbohydrates, but fewer calories as well.

Several randomized, controlled trials have compared low-carbohydrate diets with their conventional low-fat, low-calorie counterparts (23–27). These are summarized in Table 3. In a randomized, controlled trial of 53 obese, healthy women, Brehm et al. (23) reported a mean weight loss of 8.5 (±1) kg in 6 mo for the women in the low-carbohydrate diet arm vs 3.9 (±1) kg in dieters following a more conventional diet. The most dramatic weight loss came in the first few weeks of the diet, with those in the low-carbohydrate diet arm losing 7.6 kg in the first 3 mo compared with 4.2 kg in the low-fat arm. Yancy et al. (24) saw an even greater weight loss in a 6-mo study of 120 overweight men and women with high cholesterol levels. In that randomized, controlled trial, the low-carbohydrate group lost almost twice as much as the low-fat/low-calorie arm: 12 kg vs 6.5 kg.

However, obesity is a chronic disease and treatment needs to provide a long-term solution. And in this arena, the evidence suggests that low-carbohydrate diets are no better than other diets at producing durable weight loss. When low-carbohydrate dieters and low-fat dieters are followed for 1 yr, the difference between the two diets disappears. Samaha et al. evaluated a group of 132 severely obese subjects with a high rate of diabetes and metabolic syndrome, who were randomized to either a low-carbohydrate or a low-fat diet (25). Again, weight loss at 6 mo was greater for the low-carbohydrate group, who lost on average 5.8 kg, compared with the low-fat group, who lost a modest 1.9 kg. In a follow-up study by Stern et al. (26), the low-carbohydrate dieters had maintained most of their weight loss (5.1 kg) at 1 yr but the low-fat dieters had continued their slow reduction, with a mean weight loss of 3.1 kg, and the difference between the groups had become statistically insignificant.

As a group, the studies had significant limitations. First, several studies did not report the number of calories consumed—a key limitation because weight loss is clearly associated with caloric intake. Second, all studies have reported a high drop-out rate, ranging from 21% (6-mo study by Brehm et al. [23]) to 41% in the year-long study by Stern et al. (26). Only one study showed a difference in drop-out rates between groups: Yancy et al. (24) reported a 24% drop-out rate in the low-carbohydrate group compared with a 43% rate in the low-fat diet. Finally, the different studies had different degrees of intervention: participants in the study conducted by Foster et al. (27) met with a dietitian only once to discuss the diet, whereas in the trial by Yancy et al. subjects met regularly with counselors to review diet and adherence issues. Despite these limitations, these studies suggest that low-carbohydrate diets are as effective in producing short-term weight loss as the more traditional low-fat, low-calorie diet.

Safety has been a significant concern with the growing popularity of the low-carbohydrate diet. The American Heart Association, the American Dietetic Association, and other groups have cautioned against the use of these diets primarily because of concerns over their effect on lipids (28–30). Each of the recent studies evaluated the change in lipids in dieters on the low-carbohydrate and low-fat diets. Somewhat surprisingly, all

Table 3
Randomized Trials Comparing Low-Carbohydrate and Low-Fat/Low-Calorie Diets

Author	Cohort	Duration (mo)	Weight loss (kg)		Change in blood lipids
			Low-carbohydrate group	Low-fat/low-calorie group	
Foster et al. (27)	Obese healthy	6	7	3.2	HDL-C increased in the low-carbohydrate group
		12	4.4	2.5	HDL-C increased and TG decreased more in low-carbohydrate group
Samaha et al. (25)	Severely obese healthy	6	5.8	1.9	Low-carbohydrate dieters had greater decreases in TG
Stern et al. (26)	Severely obese healthy (same cohort as Samaha et al.)	12	5.1	3.1	TG decreased more and HDL-C decreased less in low-carbohydrate group
Brehm et al. (23)	Obese healthy women	6	8.5	3.9	No difference between groups
Yancy et al. (24)	Obese, hypercholesterolemia	6	12	6.5	HDL-C increased and TG decreased more in low-carbohydrate group

HDL-C, high-density lipoprotein-cholesterol; TG, triglycerides.

showed that lipid profiles improved in both diets (*see* Table 3). Because weight loss is known to produce improvements in cholesterol, it may be that the improvements in cholesterol resulted from the weight loss rather than from a specific change in diet. The effect of the low-carbohydrate diets on lipids in the absence of weight loss is unknown. In all five randomized, controlled trials, total cholesterol and low-density lipoprotein-cholesterol (LDL-C) were equally reduced on both diets. In three of the five studies, triglyceride levels and high-density lipoprotein-cholesterol (HDL-C) levels were better in the low-carbohydrate diet arms—changes associated with lower risk of cardiovascular disease. However, the long-term effects of low-carbohydrate diets on lipids remain poorly characterized.

Yancy et al. specifically evaluated patients with hyperlipidemia to characterize the potential cholesterol-raising effects of low-carbohydrate diets in this high-risk population. Even among this group, the change in cholesterol between the low-fat and the low-carbohydrate group was not statistically significant. However, two participants in the low-carbohydrate diet dropped out because of elevations in LDL-C measured at 3 mo (from 4.8 to 7.4 mmol/L in one patient; 4.7 to 5.7 mmol/L in the other). And although mean LDL-C was unchanged in the low-carbohydrate group by the end of the study, 13 of the remaining 44 participants (30%) in the low-carbohydrate arm experienced a greater than 10% increase in LDL-C compared with five of the 31 (16%) in the low-fat arm. This difference was not statistically significant ($p > 0.2$), perhaps because of the size of the study. Nevertheless, in each of these studies, most low-carbohydrate dieters had an improvement in overall lipid profile with a stable LDL-C and improved HDL-C and triglycerides.

Taken together, these studies suggest that for those individuals who lose weight on low-carbohydrate diets, the benefits of weight loss on cholesterol may outweigh the short-term harm thought to be associated with consuming a diet that provides more saturated fats and fewer carbohydrates than have traditionally been recommended for patients with elevated lipids. Long-term effects on lipids and cardiovascular health are still unknown and some individuals will experience an increase in LDL-C and total cholesterol. At this time, there is no way to distinguish between those who will respond adversely and those who will not. Given this, anyone starting on this type of diet should have their lipid profile checked regularly.

Although serum cholesterol has received the most attention, there are other health concerns about low-carbohydrate diets, including increased risk of gout, kidney stones, dehydration, and constipation. Some low-carbohydrate diets (The Protein Power Diet or The Zone) recommend replacing carbohydrates with protein rather than fat. High-protein diets are linked with renal injury in those with chronic renal disease and there is some concern that a diet high in protein can injure healthy kidneys as well. In a recent study based on the Nurses' Health Study data, a diet high in protein was associated with more rapid decline of renal function in women with existing renal disease, although women with normal kidneys showed no change in renal function when followed for 11 yr *(33)*. However, this was an observational cohort study and although somewhat reassuring, does not completely answer the question of the safety of high-protein diets.

Ketosis is also associated with greater calcium loss in the urine. There is concern that this persistent leaching of calcium from bones will promote osteoporosis. However, there have been no long-term studies that specifically evaluate this outcome. Overall, it is clear that there are still many concerns about diets that promote ketosis. The safety of low-carbohydrate diets will be an important area of research as there have been no long-term follow-up studies on their safety beyond 1 or 2 yr.

3.2. The Physiology of Low-Carbohydrate Diets

Why did these diets work at all? The utility of a strategy of replacing low-calorie carbohydrates with higher-calorie fats or isocaloric proteins to promote weight loss is completely counterintuitive. Atkins and other advocates of low-carbohydrate diets maintain that a diet low in carbohydrates confers some "metabolic advantage." Although Atkins never defined this advantage directly, he did suggest two possible mechanisms. First, metabolizing proteins takes more energy than that required to dispose of either fats or carbohydrates. However, even at the most restrictive phase of the Atkins diet, proteins comprise 35% of the calories consumed (34) and although that is more than twice the protein recommended in the recommended dietary allowance (RDA), it seems unlikely to consume the number of calories involved in the weight loss seen in these diets.

Atkins also claimed that on his diet you can "flush fat away" (35) and, in fact, dieters who are ketotic will lose ketones in stool and urine. However, Brehm et al. and Samaha et al. found no link between ketosis and weight loss in their randomized, controlled trials (23,25). And in a meta-analysis done by Bravata et al. (22) dieters consuming 20 g of carbohydrates or less—who were therefore ketotic—lost no more weight than those on low-carbohydrate diets that allowed higher levels of carbohydrate intake.

Skeptics have focused on the loss of water weight associated with depleting glycogen stores in the liver as a possible cause of the rapid weight loss (36). However, Brehm et al. note that in the first 2 wk of their study, dieters in the low-fat and low-carbohydrate groups lost the same amount of weight on average, suggesting that diuresis alone does not account for the greater weight loss. Moreover, in that study, body composition after dieting for 6 mo was not significantly different in the two groups, making changes in total body water an unlikely cause of the difference in weight loss.

Advocates of low-carbohydrate diets downplay the role of calories in promoting the weight loss seen in these diets, and in fact Atkins originally subtitled his book "the high calorie way to stay thin forever." However, there is good evidence that calorie restriction remains the most important factor in weight loss even in this diet. In the four randomized, controlled trials that measured calories (23–26), all found that on average the low-carbohydrate group reduced their calorie intake to the same extent as those on an explicitly low-calorie, low-fat diet. This was observed even though those on the low-carbohydrate diet were not instructed to reduce their calories or to count calories. Although some researchers see this as essentially debunking the low-carbohydrate diet myth by removing the promise of losing weight without restricting calories, others see this as an advantage: if you can get dieters to eat less, without even trying, then weight loss will be easier and transient weight loss has a better chance of becoming permanent.

Why would dieters following a low-carbohydrate diet eat a low calorie diet? Some researchers point to the loss of appetite caused by ketosis as a reason for the decreased intake of calories. However, as noted previously, in the most recent studies, weight loss in those who were ketotic was no greater than in those who were not (22,23,25). Restricting the variety of foods available for consumption is a well-established technique in weight loss and undoubtedly plays an important role here. But is there another factor as well? In a low-carbohydrate diet, eaters are choosing from some of the most filling foods available. By eating a diet high in protein and the most filling types of carbohydrates, low-carbohydrate eaters are able to consume fewer calories because the foods they do eat allow them to feel full with fewer calories.

Studies dating back three decades have suggested that protein, in particular, promotes the feeling of satiety, primarily through the release of cholecystokinin triggered by its consumption. Cholecystokinin works locally, by inhibiting gastric emptying and thereby promoting gastric distention. In addition, it acts as a central nervous system messenger signaling satiety through the hypothalamus *(37,38)*. Increasing the amount of protein in a meal can increase satiety and reduce overall food, and caloric, intake. In an analysis of meals on the low-carbohydrate diet done by Freedman et al., protein made up 35% of the Atkins diet plan *(34)*, much higher than the quantity recommended in the RDA. In an analysis of meal composition of those who had been following a low-carbohydrate diet for one year, Stern et al. found that dieters ate less protein than Atkins recommended (20% of total caloric intake) but still considerably more than their low-fat counterparts and the amount suggested in the United States Department of Agriculture's RDA.

The evidence of the sating effects of fats is less clear. Although some studies suggest that dietary fat increases the intervals between meals, certainly one measure of satiety, many others suggest that high-fat foods will increase the amount eaten at a meal. The Atkins diet provides 59% of daily calories in fat *(34)*, far in excess of the upper limit of the adequate macronutrient distribution range. Fat consumption remained high after one year *(26)*. Despite the high fat content of these meals, total calorie consumption in the low-carbohydrate group was no different from those in the arm with explicit calorie limitations. Although the specific contribution of fats in the Atkins diet remains uncertain, what is clear in this diet with higher than recommended consumption of protein and fat, is that overall intake is frequently reduced enough to cause weight loss.

3.3. Glycemic Index: Good and Bad Carbohydrates

The specific types of carbohydrates allowed in most low-carbohydrate diets may also contribute to the increased satiety noted by dieters. Although commonly portrayed as eliminating all carbohydrates from the diet, even the strictest popular low-carbohydrate diets eliminate only certain types of carbohydrates. More permissive low-carbohydrate diets, such as the Zone diet, restrict carbohydrates to 40% of daily calories *(32)*. Sugar Busters *(39)*, which eliminates all foods containing flour or sugar, allows far more carbohydrates than Atkins or Agatston, but again only certain types of carbohydrates. All these diets completely ban highly processed carbohydrates and those containing sugar, while allowing varying degrees of access to most vegetables, fruits, and unrefined grains. In general, the carbohydrates that are allowed are those that are most filling—those that contain high levels of fiber, the lowest amount of carbohydrate and, perhaps not coincidentally, the fewest calories.

The rationale for distinguishing between types of carbohydrates is based on the observation, made decades ago, that some carbohydrates have a much greater effect on blood glucose than others. Twenty-five years ago Jenkins et al. introduced a system of classifying these differences,` which they dubbed the glycemic index (GI) *(40)*. The GI compares the change in blood glucose prompted by the consumption of a set amount of carbohydrate in any given food to that caused by the consumption of a standard amount of either white bread or, in earlier tables, glucose *(41)*. The greater the change in blood glucose, the higher the GI of the test food.

Essentially everything that affects the rate at which the carbohydrate is broken down into its component sugars will affect the GI of a food. Thus, the structure of the carbohydrate itself, the degree of refinement and processing, and the presence of fats and fiber will each contribute to the final GI of a food.

One characteristic not taken into consideration by the GI is the amount of carbohydrate in a given food. This means that the GI overestimates the effect of certain foods that are high in fiber and starch, such as carrots or cantaloupe. The carbohydrate contained in cantaloupe has a very high GI—65, about the same as that of many sugary foods, such as Fruit Loops®, a popular sweetened cereal (GI 69). Cantaloupe, however, contains only a small amount of this carbohydrate—6 g per half-cup serving—whereas Fruit Loops are almost all carbohydrate, containing 13 g of carbohydrate for the same half-cup serving. So, although the GI is almost the same for both foods, serving for serving, the glycemic effect of the carbohydrate will be much greater for the Fruit Loops than for the cantaloupe. Because of this discrepancy, the concept of glycemic load was developed.

Glycemic load takes into consideration both the GI of the food, as well as the amount of the carbohydrate it contains *(42)*. Thus, although cantaloupe and Fruit Loops have the same GI, their glycemic load is quite different—4 for cantaloupe vs 18 for the Fruit Loops. The concept of glycemic load is slowly replacing GI in the nutrition literature; however, much of the research done to date on the effects of carbohydrates on weight gain and loss was based on GI.

Does glycemic response to food as measured by either the GI or glycemic load contribute to weight gain or loss? There is evidence that it does. A recent paper by Harvard pediatrician David Ludwig in the *Journal of the American Medical Association* argues that the hyperglycemia caused by foods with a high GI exaggerates the normal anabolic responses to eating *(41)*. The rapid increase in blood glucose caused by high-GI foods triggers a compensatory surge in blood insulin. This, in turn, enhances the uptake of nutrients by insulin-responsive tissues, stimulates glycogenesis and lipogenesis, and suppresses gluconeogenesis and lipolysis. The hyperinsulinemia also causes a dramatic drop in blood glucose concentration, and this relative hypoglycemia has been associated with hunger and initiation of feeding in rats and humans. Moreover, insulin-induced hypoglycemia appears to provoke prolonged overeating, persisting well after restoration of normal blood glucose levels *(41)*.

Low-carbohydrate-diet advocates cite insulin's anabolic role in the body as a cause of obesity by promoting fat storage and inhibition of lipolysis. And indeed, there is research to suggest that high-GI foods can promote obesity, at least in lab animals *(41)*. Rats fed amylopectin, a high-GI starch, for up to 8 mo became morbidly obese *(41)*. Whether this is an important cause of obesity in humans has yet to be determined.

Additionally, there are studies that suggest a low-GI diet can promote weight loss. In one study, cited by Ludwig, obese teenage boys who ate a low-GI breakfast were less hungry and consumed fewer calories during the rest of the day than those fed a high-GI breakfast. In another study, young men given a low-GI diet for 9 d ate less, and expended more calories, than those fed a high-GI diet *(41)*. In a third study, obese women were placed on a low-calorie diet containing either low-GI or high-GI foods. Those on the low-GI diet lost more weight and were found to have lower fasting insulin levels *(42)*. Other studies have not shown significant weight loss when high-GI foods were replaced with low-GI foods and therefore the contribution of GI manipulation to weight loss is still controversial (43). Nevertheless, many researchers believe that low-GI foods promote greater satiety and lower insulin response than do high-GI foods and may be useful in weight loss.

Low-carbohydrate diets may work, then, by emphasizing the consumption of highly sating foods—primarily proteins and low-GI carbohydrates—and that, in turn, allows dieters to experience less hunger and consume fewer calories. Thus, a successful low-carbohydrate diet will also be a low-calorie diet.

Another mechanism may be at work in dieters who choose low-GI foods. There is good evidence that successful weight loss causes a drop in resting energy expenditure. Some researchers theorize that this reduction in calorie expenditure contributes to decreasing weight loss (the plateau phenomenon) and subsequent weight gain. A recent study by Pereira et al. (43b) suggests that a low-GI diet may defend dieters from some, though not all, of this decrease in resting energy expenditure. In that study, researchers assigned 22 adults to either a low glycemic load (and lower carbohydrate) diet or a traditional low-fat, high-carbohydrate, and high glycemic load diet and measured resting energy expenditure before and after they had lost 10% of their baseline weight. Subjects who had lost weight using a low glycemic load diet had only half the reduction in resting energy expenditure of that seen in those on the high glycemic load diet (5.9 vs 10.6%). Further study will be needed to determine if this difference is sustained and if it aids in better weight loss and maintenance. Nevertheless, the study suggests that perhaps with some foods, a calorie is not just a calorie, and that some calories are better for weight loss and maintenance than others.

4. LOW-FAT DIETS

4.1. Dietary Fat and Obesity

Dietary fat has long been blamed for much of the obesity in the US population. This is discussed in Chapter 13. Several mechanisms have been proposed to explain why a diet high in fat should lead to greater body fat. First, fat is the most energy-dense macronutrient, providing 9 kcals/g compared to just 4 kcals/g for carbohydrates and protein. Also, fats make food more flavorful and palatable, qualities that promote greater consumption. Fats also take less energy to metabolize than either carbohydrates or proteins, reducing the thermic effect of food—a small, but potentially significant, energy expenditure (44).

Epidemiological evidence also links high-fat diets to obesity. Cultures that consume low-fat diets have much less obesity than that found in cultures that consume high-fat diets. Moreover, when populations move from a low fat consuming environment to a more Western environment where high levels of dietary fat are the norm, the rates of obesity skyrocket (45).

4.2. Low-Fat Diets for Weight Loss

Because of these links between fat consumption and obesity, reducing dietary fat has been a favored strategy for weight loss starting in the 1980s. Advocates of low-fat diets suggest that replacing dietary fat with carbohydrates will allow dieters to eat the same volume of food and yet consume few calories and thereby lose weight. But do they work?

Although there is evidence that a reduced-fat diet can promote modest weight loss, restricting calories, as well as fats, is far more effective method for weight loss than restricting dietary fat alone.

The effectiveness of low-fat diets has been evaluated extensively. In a recent meta-analysis, Pirozzo et al. looked at nearly 600 subjects, mostly women, randomized in six studies to either a low-fat or a low-calorie diet *(46)*. The diets were found to be equally effective. At 6 mo, those on the low-fat diet had lost 5.8 kg compared with the low-calorie group who lost 6.5 kg. At 12 mo, both groups had regained some of their weight with the low-fat group maintaining a weight loss of 2.3 kg and the low-calorie group 3.4 kg. At 18 mo the low-fat group had regained most of their weight, whereas those on a low-calorie diet were still an average of 2.3 kg below their baseline weight. However, there was no statistically significant difference between the two groups at any point in the study.

Most reviews of the literature suggest that combining a low-fat diet with a low-calorie diet works better than either strategy alone. In a meta-analysis of 18 studies following just over 1100 dieters assigned to either a low-fat regimen, a low-calorie regimen, or a combination of both, Bray et al. *(47)* found that dieters combining a low-calorie with a low-fat diet lost more weight than those on either diet alone. Likewise, a meta-analysis of low-fat diets published in the Clinical Guidelines on the Identification, Evaluation and Treatment of Overweight and Obesity in Adults, published by the National Heart, Lung and Blood Institute in 1998, found that diets that restrict fat without specifically restricting calories are effective, but not nearly as effective as diets that restrict both *(4)*. Another long-time low-fat diet promoter, the National Cholesterol Education Program, now recommends combining a moderate fat diet (30–35% fat) with a low-calorie diet to reduce obesity and improve blood lipids *(48)*.

Why is calorie restriction needed? The theory behind a low-fat diet is that if you remove the foods containing high-calories fats, what you would be left with should be foods that are lower in calories. That may have been the case at one time but the marketplace has provided us with a large variety of foods that are low in fat yet high in calories. Many of the "reduced fat" foods—designed for dieters trying to lose weight by restricting fat—contain the same number of calories as their full fat counterparts. Some have even more. The original message—to eat less meat, milk, and butter and consume more fruits and vegetables—has been drowned in the roar of a million lower-fat foods arriving on supermarket shelves. Obesity researcher David Katz *(49)* has dubbed this "the Snackwell® effect" after the popular low-fat cookie company whose success led the way for other low-fat, high-calorie foods. This relatively new phenomenon has prompted most experts to abandon the low-fat diet and replace it with a diet that limits both fat and calories.

4.3. Safety of Low-Fat Diets

It may seem odd to discuss the safety of a low-fat diet but studies assessing the effect of these diets on blood lipids show that the effects are not universally beneficial. A diet low in fat has been shown to lower total cholesterol and LDL-C. However, HDL-C also drops when dietary fat is reduced. The Framingham Risk score relies on HDL-C as well as total cholesterol. Using this widely accepted algorithm, reducing HDL-C as well as total cholesterol will result in a higher cardiovascular risk score *(50)*. The effects of diet on blood lipids are reviewed in Chapter 6.

In addition, a low-fat diet will be a diet high in carbohydrates. Such a diet can cause an increase in triglycerides in many populations. In a recent review, Parks and Hellerstein *(51)* noted that this effect was greatest in those who were overweight and those with insulin resistance, the very group most likely to be started on a low-fat, high-carbohydrate diet. This effect was mitigated to some extent by the consumption of fiber-rich foods and weight loss. In addition, there is some evidence that carbohydrate-induced hypertriglyceridemia may resolve over time, at least in some individuals.

In summary, a low-fat diet can be an effective method for weight loss primarily when coupled with a low-calorie diet. Most low-fat diets restrict fat intake to around 30% of calories, combined with a deficit of 500–1000 kcal/d, resulting in a weight loss of 1–2 lbs/wk. These diets are safe for most overweight and obese patients, especially when they are high in fiber. Low-fat diets will reduce the HDL-C levels in many dieters. In addition, very obese dieters and those with insulin resistance are at risk of developing an increase in triglycerides and thus a worsening of their lipid profile on a low-fat diet and so may not be ideal candidates.

5. LOW-CALORIE DIETS

In essence, as argued under Heading 4, all effective diets are low-calorie diets because decreasing energy intake is still the most powerful and effective method for weight loss available. There are approx 3500 kcals stored in every pound of fat, defining the deficit needed to produce a single pound of weight loss. Proponents of low-fat or low-carbohydrate diets have argued over the past decades that the success of their diets lies not in calorie restriction but in the specific restriction they advocate. But at this point most experts agree that the primary method for losing weight in all these diets is calorie restriction *(4,5,34)*. Reducing dietary fat or eliminating high-GI carbohydrates may enhance the weight loss that is stimulated by an energy deficit, but these are garnishes on a main dish of calorie restriction.

Despite near universal agreement among experts that calorie restriction is the cornerstone of weight loss, it is news to many dieters. According to a recent poll, less than half of overweight and obese adults (42%) try to limit their intake of calories, although nearly two-thirds say they are trying to limit fat intake *(52)*. The current focus on macronutrient content (low carbohydrate vs low fat) has distracted the overweight public from the principle consideration: calories. Refocusing attention back to calorie content should be an important component in weight loss and weight maintenance strategies. For this reason, a low-calorie diet is an essential tool in weight loss counseling.

The goal of a low-calorie diet should be to provide the greatest range of food choices to the consumer to allow for nutritional adequacy and compliance, while still resulting in a slow but steady rate of weight loss. Unlike low-fat or low-carbohydrate diets, which limit food choice, a good low-calorie diet offers a wide variety of foods but restricts portion size. Low-calorie diets have been studied extensively. In the National Heart, Lung and Blood Institute Guideline, a systematic review of the literature, showed that a low-calorie diet (1000–1200 kcal/d) produces, on average, an 8% decrease in weight when followed for 6 mo–1 yr *(4)*. In that review a handful of studies followed dieters for up to 4 yr and found that despite some weight gain, mean weight loss averaged 4% even after several years. The more recent systematic review in the US Preventive Health Task Force recommendations came to the same conclusion *(5)*.

There are a variety of low-calorie diets in the marketplace. For the most part they focus their calorie-restricting strategies by restricting either fat or high-GI carbohydrates, although most end up limiting intake of both. Examples of low-calorie/moderate-fat diets include Weight Watchers, Jenny Craig, and diets that focus on energy density, such as Volumetrics *(53)*. Examples of low-calorie/moderate-carbohydrate diets include The Zone, Sugar Busters, and diets that focus on reducing GI or glycemic load, such as The New Glucose Revolution *(54)*. In each of these diets, reducing daily calories is an explicit goal. (For nutritional analysis and menus of sample diets, *see* Tables 2 and 4.)

The strength of these diets is that they allow a wide variety of foods to be consumed. One of the reasons dieters frequently give for nonadherence to a particular diet is the lack of variety in the foods they are allowed to eat. The low-calorie diets also allow eaters to choose foods that will provide the greatest satiety. In low-fat diets, the limitation on fats often results in a limitation on protein. Proteins promote a feeling of fullness. When these are dramatically restricted, dieters frequently complain of hunger. Low-carbohydrate diets frequently restrict intake of complex carbohydrates and provide a smaller volume of food for per meal. Volume is also associated with the sensation of satiety *(55)*. Low-calorie diets, by contrast, are more likely to draw on all forms of foods so as to provide a meal that is more filling and satisfying.

In summary, there are many diets available to those interested in weight loss. Current research shows that each of the strategies outlined above can be used successfully to aid not only in weight loss but in lifelong weight maintenance, the real goal of any informed dieter. Those interested in losing weight should be encouraged to experiment with different options and to focus on finding ways to eat those foods that they can adhere to for the long run, rather than seeking the elusive "simple rapid weight loss solution."

6. EXERCISE AND WEIGHT LOSS

There is clear and convincing evidence that exercise has many health benefits including dramatic reductions in the risk of developing chronic diseases such as diabetes, hypertension, and coronary artery disease. The evidence for the use of exercise in weight loss and weight maintenance is less convincing. Exercise should result in weight loss by increasing energy expenditure and by increasing the rate at which calories are metabolized. Whereas physics and common sense tell us that exercise should also play an important role in weight loss, most studies suggest that exercise has not lived up to that expectation. Systematic reviews assessing the effect of exercise on weight loss and maintenance, either alone or when paired with diet, have shown only very modest gains when compared to diet alone *(4)*. Thirty minutes of moderate-intensity activity at least 5 d/wk has been shown to provide the basic health benefit and has been the usual recommendation for the promotion of weight loss and weight maintenance *(4,56)*. Recent studies suggest that this amount of physical activity is not sufficient to promote weight loss or even prevent weight gain *(57–59)*, and several advisory bodies, including the Institute of Medicine and the American College of Sports Medicine, have recently recommended 1 h/d of exercise, 5–7 d/wk, when this activity is being used to aid in weight loss or weight maintenance—twice the amount recommended for disease prevention *(57,58)*.

Table 4
Comparison of Sample Menus From Popular Diets

Meal	Food guide pyramid	Atkins' induction	South Beach phase 1	The Zone	Weight Watchers	Eat More, Weigh Less
Breakfast	3/4 c orange juice, 1/2 c oatmeal, 1 slice white toast with 1 tsp margarine, 1 tsp jelly, 1/2 c skim milk	2 scrambled eggs, 2 strips bacon, coffee	6 oz vegetable juice, 1/2 c egg substitute, 1/2 c skim milk, 2 slices Canadian bacon, coffee or tea with skim milk	1 c grapes, 1 tortilla stuffed with 2 oz low-fat cheese, 2 slices Canadian bacon, scallions, peppers, tomato, 2 T guacamole	1 oz Total cereal, 1/2 c skim milk, 1 slice whole wheat bread, 1 pat margarine, orange	1/2 grapefruit, 1 package oatmeal, 1 oz raisins, 1 c skim milk, tea
Snack	6 oz apple juice		2 oz turkey, scallions, red pepper with 2 T low-fat mayonnaise rolled in 2 lettuce leaves			
Lunch	1 c split pea soup, tuna and sprouts sandwich, mixed green salad with 1 T low-calorie dressing, chocolate mint pie	Bacon (1 slice) cheese-burger (4 oz hamburger, 1 oz cheese, no bun), small salad, seltzerwater	6 oz tuna, with 1/3 c each: cucumber, tomato, celery radishes, avocado, low-calorie vinegrette, sugar-free gelatin	1 slice bread, 2 oz Canadian bacon, lettuce, tomato, dill pickle, 1 oz low-fat cheese, 1/2 c plain low-fat yogurt, 1/3 c canned peaches	2 oz roast beef on rye bread, carrots, tossed green salad, low-calorie dressing, 1 c skim milk, 10 grapes	1 corn tortilla, 2 tsp salsa, 1/2 c black beans, 1/2 c canned tomatoes, onions, 1/4 c green peas, 1 c salad, 1/4 cantaloupe
Snack	10 saltine crackers, 6 oz V-8		Celery stuffed with a wedge of Laughing Cow cheese		1 oz almonds, 1 fig bar	
Dinner	3 oz sirloin steak, 1/2 c corn and zucchini combo, lettuce and tomato salad with 1 T low-calorie dressing, Yogurt strawberry parfait	Clear consumme, 11/2 c shrimp salad, 4 oz steak, salad with dressing, 1 c sugarless Jello with tsp sugarfree whipped toping	Baked chicken breast, eggplant sliced, baked with pepper, onion, 1 tsp olive oil, 1/2 c part skim ricotta cheese, 1/2 tsp unsweetened cocoa powder	4 oz pork chop sauted with 2 tsp white wine, 1 c steamed broccoli, 1 c large tossed salad with 4 tsp olive oil and vinegar dressing	1 c beef boullion soup, 2 saltines, 2.5 oz salmon broiled, 3/4 c zucchini, 1/2 baked potato	1 c brown rice with 1/4 c tofu, stir fry vegetables (broccoli, cabbage, scallions, bean sprouts, peppers, snow peas, carrots) teriyaki sauce, 2 oz wine, 1/4 c pineapple, 1 c salad 1 orange
Snack	3 graham crackers, 1 c skim milk				1/2 c chocolate ice cream, 1/2 c skim milk	1/2 c strawberries

6.1. Exercise Alone for Weight Loss

Exercise alone as a strategy for weight loss has been well studied over the past two decades. Two recent systematic reviews conclude that the use of exercise, without a calorie-reducing diet, can produce modest weight loss. Garrow and Summerbell *(60)* found a mean 3-kg weight loss in men and 1.4 kg in women when compared with nonexercising controls. Similarly, a National Institutes of Health (NIH) review of 12 randomized, control trials of exercise in the absence of diet calculated a mean weight loss of 2.4 kg *(4)*.

In the studies reviewed by the NIH, the intensity of physical activity was described as "moderate." The frequency of physical activity was between three and seven sessions per week and the duration of each session ranged from 30 to 60 min. Almost all exercise programs in these studies used aerobic exercise—most commonly, brisk walking. Although these studies did not estimate the number of calories expended in exercise, an approximation can be calculated using estimates of calorie expenditure: brisk walking consumes between 5 and 8 kcal/min depending on the weight of the walker. Using these approximations, a 30-min walk done 5 d/wk will consume between 150 and 240 kcal/d— the equivalent of 750–1200 kcal/wk. If caloric intake remains stable, exercisers should be able to lose about one pound per month. The mean weight loss of 2.4–3 kg for 4–6 mo found in their meta-analyses is consistent with these approximations.

There is some evidence that exercise can be as effective in weight loss as diet, but only if the amount of exercise is increased so that the net calorie deficit achieved is as much as that achieved through calorie restriction. In two recent studies by Ross et al. *(62,63)* obese men and women were randomized to use either exercise or diet in order to produce a net calorie deficit of 500 (women) to 700 (men) kcal/d. Half maintained a constant caloric intake and exercised to expend 500–700 kcal/d, whereas the other half reduced their calorie intake by this amount while maintaining the same level of activity. Exercisers had supervised daily exercise sessions in which they walked or jogged on a motorized treadmill at approx 80% maximum heart rate for an average of 60 min. After 3 mo there was no difference in weight loss between the two groups (men lost 7.6 kg through exercise, 7.4 kg through diet *(62)*; women lost 6.1 kg through exercise, 5.2 kg through diet *(63)*. Reduction in body fat was significantly greater in the exercise group than in the diet group in both sexes. This study suggests that exercise can be used as a method for weight loss even in the absence of diet, but that the amount of exercise needed to achieve this end is greater than the 30 min/d for 5 d/wk that is frequently recommended.

6.2. Exercise in Addition to Diet for Weight Loss

The addition of exercise to diet may modestly improve weight loss; greater intensity and duration is associated with greater weight loss *(4,59,64,65)*. Based on a systematic review of 15 randomized, controlled studies the NIH Expert Panel recommends that dieters should combine exercise with diet for weight loss. Twelve of the fifteen showed a greater weight loss in the groups combining exercise with diet over the diet only group. Overall, the mean difference was 1.9 kg *(4)*.

The NIH group noted that the subjects in the diet plus exercise groups usually participated in supervised exercise sessions lasting between 30 and 60 min done three times a week at an intensity of 60–80% of maximum heart rate. A randomized trial of diet and exercise in overweight women by Jakicic et al. *(64)* showed that greater duration of exercise—an average 280 min/wk—was associated with significantly greater weight loss than the usually recommended 150–180 min/wk.

6.3. Exercise in Weight Loss Maintenance

Physical activity is considered an important component of weight loss maintenance, and several observational studies have shown a strong inverse relationship between physical activity and long-term weight gain *(4,66,67)*. In a systematic review of observational studies, Anderson et al. *(67)* found that in the six studies assessing the effects of exercise on weight loss maintenance, groups with higher amounts of exercise were significantly more successful in maintaining weight loss than groups with lower amounts of physical activity.

Most randomized, controlled trials have shown only small differences between those who did and those who did not use exercise for weight maintenance. In a systematic review evaluating the effects of physical activity, only three of the eight included studies showed a statistically significant difference in weight gain when exercise plus diet was used to maintain weight loss *(66)*. When study results were combined, those who exercised during weight maintenance regained a mean 1.8 kg less during a 20-mo follow-up.

Again, the amount of exercise may be key to its success in weight maintenance. Studies of successful dieters suggest that 1500–2800 kcal/wk of physical activity is associated with weight maintenance *(66–68)*.

Based in part on this evidence, the Institute of Medicine and the American College of Sports Medicine have recently issued guidelines that greatly increase the amount of exercise recommended for weight loss and weight maintenance. These guidelines recommend 60 min/d of exercise, 4–6 d/wk for an average energy expenditure of 2000 kcal/wk *(58,59)*. Moderate intensity exercise is generally recommended but organizations would not discourage most individuals from engaging in more vigorous activity as well, recognizing that calories are burned more quickly with more vigorous activity than with moderate activity.

In many studies, brisk walking was the preferred type of exercise. Data from the National Weight Control Registry suggests that walking is the type of exercise most used by people who have lost and maintained their weight loss *(70)*. Given this, many experts in the field recommend walking as the exercise type of choice. Recently, pedometers have become popular as a tool to both monitor and motivate exercise *(70)*. There is evidence that just by wearing a pedometer people increase the amount that they walk *(71)*. At this point there are still no data that pedometers enhance weight loss, but that may be because most studies are too short (8–12 wk) to allow for significant weight loss *(72)*. Current goals of 10,000 steps per day can more than double the walking done by many Americans.

Although most studies have looked at the effects of aerobic exercise on weight loss, resistance exercise in promoting weight loss has also been evaluated. In theory, strength-building exercise should improve weight loss by increasing muscle tone and by preserving fat free mass and resting metabolic rate, which tend to decline with weight loss. However, in a review of the literature Jakicic *(58)* found that resistance exercise combined with diet has no clear weight loss benefit over diet alone. Studies comparing resistance training plus diet to either aerobic training plus diet or to diet alone have found no difference in weight loss or resting metabolic rate, although there have been differing results regarding changes in fat free mass *(73–77)*. Although studies on effects of resistance exercise on weight loss have been small and of short duration, current evidence suggests that, when combined with diet, the addition of strength building exercise offers no advantage over aerobic exercise in achieving weight loss.

7. SUMMARY

Current evidence suggests that all weight loss diets work primarily through calorie restriction. Greater weight loss is associated with greater adherence and longer duration of diet. Those seeking to lose weight should be encouraged to find a diet that is lower in calories, as well as palatable and enjoyable to promote long-term adherence. Low-fat and low-carbohydrate diets use different strategies to reach the same end of calorie reduction. Both will improve lipids for most, though not all, dieters. Long-term health consequences of the low-carbohydrate diet are as yet unknown, but the benefits of intentional long-term weight reduction are clear.

Exercise will modestly enhance weight loss and weight maintenance and, given its other demonstrated health benefits, should be recommended for everyone trying to lose weight. Efficacy may be greater when exercise duration is longer or intensity higher. When tailoring exercise programs for individuals, it is important to keep in mind that many factors play a role in the effectiveness of physical activity for weight management, including gender, age, genetics, adherence to exercise programs, and existing medical conditions. Current evidence suggests that all exercise programs should be started gradually and work toward recommended goals of at least 30 min of daily moderate activity for overall health benefits and progress toward higher amounts of exercise with a goal of 60 min daily physical activity for weight loss and weight maintenance.

REFERENCES

1. Available at website: http://www.shapeup.org/media/surveys/x-factor.html. Last accessed May 17, 2004.
2. Gregg EW, Gerzoff RB, Thompson TJ, Williamson DF. Intentional weight loss and death in overweight and obese US adults 35 years of age and older. Ann Intern Med 2003; 138:383–389.
3. Available at website: http://www.amazon.com/exec/obidos/search-handle-form/103-1974694-7791865. Last accessed July 2, 2004.
4. NIH/NHLBI Clinical guidelines on the identification, evaluation and treatment of overweight and obesity in adults National Institutes of Health, 1998.
5. Klein S, Sheard NF, Pi-Sunyer X, et al. Weight management through lifestyle modification for the prevention and management of type 2 diabetes: rationale and strategies. A statement of the American Diabetes Association, the North American Association for the Study of Obesity and the American Society for Clinical Nutrition. Am J Clin Nutr 2004; 80;257–263.
6. McTigue KM, Harris R, Hemphill B, et al. Screening and intervention for obesity in adults: summary of the evidence for the U.S. Preventive Services Task Force. Ann Intern Med 2003; 139:933–949.
7. Wyatt HR, Grunwald GK, Mosca CL, et al. Long-term weight loss and breakfast in subjects in the National Weight Control Registry. Obes Res 2002; 10:78–82.
8. Lichtman SW, Pisarska K, Berman ER, Discrepancy between self reported and actual caloric intake and exercise in obese subjects, N Engl J Med 1992; 327:1893–1898.
9. Heitmann BL, Lissner L. Dietary underreporting by obese individuals—is it specific or non-specific? BMJ 1995; 311:986–989.
10. Jenkins DJ, Wolever TM, Vuksan V, et al. Nibbling versus gorging: metabolic advantages of increased meal frequency. N Engl J Med 1989; 321:929–934.

11. Wyatt HR, Grunwald GK, Mosca CL, Klem ML, Wing RR, Hill JO. Long-term weight loss and breakfast in subjects in the National Weight Control Registry. Obes Res 2002; 10:78–1082.

12. Schlundt DG, Hill JO, Sbrocco T, Pope-Cordle J, Sharp T. The role of breakfast in the treatment of obesity: a randomized clinical trial. Am J Clin Nutr 1992; 55:645–651.

13. Wing, RR, Hill JO. Successful weight loss maintenance. Annu Rev Nutr 2001; 21:323–341.

14. Ayas NT, White DP, Al-Delaimy WK, et al. A prospective study of self reported sleep duration and incident diabetes in women. Diabetes Care 2003; 26:380–384.

15. Geliebter A, Gluck ME, Tanowitz M, Aronoff NJ, Zammit GK. Work shift period and weight change. Nutrition 2000; 16:27–29.

16. Farquhar JW. The American Way of Life Need not be Hazardous to your Health. Perseus Publishing, New York, 1987.

17. Atkins RC. Dr. Atkins' Diet Revolution: The High Calorie Way to Stay Thin Forever. David McKay Company Inc, New York, 1972.

18. Agatston A. The South Beach Diet. Random House, New York, 2003.

19. Gotinez V. Catering to low carb dieters. Dallas Morning News, 1/10/2004.

20. Brillat Savarin A, Fisher MFK. The physiology of taste. Counterpoint Press, Washington, DC, 2000.

21. Banting W. Letter on Corpulence, Addressed to the Public. 2nd ed. Harrison and Sons, London, England, 1863.

22. Bravata DM, Sanders L, Huang J, Krumholz HM, Olkin I, Gardner CD. Efficacy and safety of low-carbohydrate diets: a systematic review. JAMA 2003; 289:1837–1850.

23. Brehm BJ, Seeley RJ, Daniels SR, D'Alessio DA. A randomized trial comparing a very low carbohydrate diet and a calorie-restricted low fat diet on body weight and cardiovascular risk factors in healthy women. J Clin Endo Metab 2003; 88:1617–1623.

24. Yancy WS, Olsen MK, Guyton JR, Bakst RP, Westman EC. A low-carbohydrate, ketogenic diet versus a low-fat diet to treat obesity and hyperlipidemia. Ann Intern Med 2004; 140:769–777.

25. Samaha FF, Iqbal N, Seshadri P, et al. A low-carbohydrate as compared with a low-fat diet in severe obesity. N Engl J Med 2003; 348:2074–2081.

26. Stern L, Iqbal N, Seshadri P, et al. The effects of low-carbohydrate versus conventional weight loss diets in severely obese adults: one-year follow-up of a randomized trial. Ann Intern Med 2004; 140:778–785.

27. Foster GD, Wyatt HR, Hill JO, et al, A randomized trial of a low-carbohydrate diet for obesity. N Engl J Med 2003; 348:2082–2090.

28. Available at website http://www.americanheart.org/presenter.jhtml?identifier=11234. Last accessed March 6, 2003.

29. St Jeor ST, Howard BV, Prewitt TE, Bovee V, Bazarre T, Eckel PH. Dietary protein and weight reduction: a statement for healthcare professionals from the nutrition committee of the Council on Nutrition, Physical Activity and Metabolism of the American Heart Association. Circulation 2001; 104:1869–1874.

30. Stein K. High protein low carbohydrate diets: do they work? J Am Diet Assoc 2000; 100:760–761.

31. Eades MR. Protein Power: The High Protein/Low Carbohydrate Way to Lose Weight, Feel Fit and Boost your Health—In Just Weeks! Bantam Books, New York, 1996.

32. Sears B, Lawson B. The Zone: A Dietary Roadmap to Lose Weight Permanently: Reset Your Genetic Code: Prevent Disease: Achieve Maximum Physical Performance. Harper Collins, New York, 1995.

33. Knight EL, Stampler MJ, Hankinson SE, Spiegelman D, Curhan GC. The impact of protein intake on renal function decline in women with normal renal function or mild renal insufficiency. Ann Intern Med 2003; 138:460–467.

34. Freedman MR, King J, Kennedy E. Popular diets: a scientific review. Obes Res 2001; 9:5S–17S.

35. Atkins RC. Dr. Atkins' New Diet Revolution: The Amazing No-Hunger Weight-Loss Plan that has Helped Millions Lose Weight and Keep it off. Avon Books, New York, 1992.

36. Denke M. Metabolic effects of high-protein, low-carbohydrate diets. Am J Cardiology 2001; 88:56–61.

37. Gutzwiller JP, Drewe J, Ketterer S, Hildebrand P, Krautheim A, Beglinger C. Interaction between CCK and a preload on reduction of food intake is mediated by CCK-A receptors in humans. Am J Physiol Regul Integr Comp Physiol 2000; 279:R189–R195.

38. Stacher G . Satiety effects of cholecystokinin and ceruletide in lean and obese men. Ann NY Acad Sci 1985; 448:431–436.

39. Stewart HL, Bethea MC, Andrews SS, Balart LA. The New Sugar Busters: Cut Sugar to Lose Weight. Ballantine Books, New York, 2003.
40. Jenkins DJA, Wolever TMS, Taylor RH, Barker H, Fielden H, Baldwin JM. Glycemic index of foods: a physiological basis for carbohydrate exchange. Am J Clin Nutr 1981; 34:362–366.
41. Ludwig D. The glycemic index: physiological mechanisms relating to obesity, diabetes and cardiovascular disease. JAMA 2002; 287:2414–2423.
42. Brand-Miller JC, Holt SHA, Pawlak DB, McMillan J. Glycemic index and obesity. Am J Clin Nutr 2002; 76(suppl):281S–28S.
43. Sloth B, Krog-Mikkelsen I, Flint A, et al. No difference in body weight decrease between a low-glycemic-index and a high-glycemic-index diet but reduced LDL cholesterol after 10-wk ad libitum intake of the low-glycemic-index diet. Am J Clin Nutr 2004; 80:337–347.
43b. Pereira MA, Swain J, Goldfine AB, Rifai N, Ludwig DS. Effects of a low-glycemic load diet on resting energy expenditure and heart disease risk factors during weight loss. JAMA 2004; 292:2482–2490.
44. Willett W. Is dietary fat a major determinant of body fat? Am J Clin Nutr 1998; 67(suppl)556S–562S.
45. Kato H, Tillotson J, Nichaman MZ, Rhoads GG, Hamilton HB. Epidemiologic studies of coronary heart disease and stroke in Japanese men living in Japan, Hawaii and California. Am J Epidemiol 1973; 97:37–385.
46. Pirozzo S, Summerbellc, Cameron C, Glasziou P. Advice on low-fat diets for obesity. The Cochrane Database of Systematic Reviews 2004.
47. Bray GA, Popkin B. Dietary fat intake does affect obesity! Am J Clin Nutr 1998; 68:1157–1173.
48. Available at website: http://www.nhlbi.nih.gov/cgi-bin/chd/step2intro.cgi. Last accessed March 10, 2004.
49. Katz D. Special Diets In Weight Management: Do They Work? Roundtable discussion; American College of Preventive Medicine annual conferene, 2004.
50. Third Report of the National Cholesterol Education Program (NCEP) Expert Panel on Detection, Evaluation, and Treatment of High Blood Cholesterol in Adults (Adult Treatment Panel III) Final Report. Circulation 2002; 106:3143–3421.
51. Parks EJ, Hellerstein MK. Carbohydrate induced hypertriglyceridemia: historical perspective and biological mechanisms. Am J Clin Nutr 2000; 71:412–433.
52. Available at http://www.shapeup.org/media/surveys/x-factor.htm. Last accessed January 5, 2004.
53. Rolls B, Barnett RA. The Volumetrics Weight-Control Plan. Harper Collins, New York, 2000.
54. Brand-Miller J, Wolever TMS, Foster-Powell K, et al. The New Glucose Revolution: The Authoritive Guide to The Glycemic Index. Marlowe and Company, New York, 2002.
55. Rolls BJ, Castellanos VH, Halford JC. Volume of food consumed affects satiety in men. Am J Clin Nutr 1998; 67:1170–1177.
56. US Department of Health and Human Services. Physical Activity and Health: A Report of the Surgeon General. US Department of Health and Human Services, Washington, DC, 1996.
57. Institute of Medicine. Dietary Reference Intakes for Energy, Carbohydrates, Fiber, Fat, Protein, and Amino Acids (Macronutrients). National Academy of Sciences, Institute of Medicine, Washington, DC, 2002.
58. Jakicic JM, Clark K, Coleman E, et al. American College of Sports Medicine position stand. Appropriate intervention strategies for weight loss and prevention of weight regain for adults. Med Sci Sports Exerc 2001; 33:2145–2156.
59. Saris WHM, Blair SN, van Baak MA, et al. How much physical activity is enough to prevent unhealthy weight gain? Outcome of the IASO 1st Stock Conference and consensus statement. Obes Rev 2003; 4:101–114.
60. Garrow JS, Summerbell CD. Meta-analysis: effect of exercise, with or without dieting, on the body composition of overweight subjects. Eur J Clin Nutr 1995; 49:1–10.
61. Wing RR. Physical activity in the treatment of the adulthood overweight and obesity: Current evidence and research issues. Med Sci Sports Exerc 1999; 31:S547–S552.
62. Ross R, Dagnone D, Jones PJH, et al. Reduction in obesity and related comorbid conditions after diet-induced weight loss or exercise-induced weight loss in men. Ann Intern Med 2000; 133:92–103.
63. Ross R, Janssen I, Dawson J, et al. Exercise-induced reduction in obesity and insulin resistance in women: a randomized controlled trial. Obesity Res 2004; 12:789–798.

64. Jakicic JM, Marcus BH, Gallagher K, Napolitano M, Lang W. Effects of exercise duration and intensity on weight loss in overweight, sedentary women. JAMA 2003; 290:1323–1330.

65. Miller WC, Koceja DM, Hamilton EJ. A meta-analysis of the past 25 years of weight loss research using diet, exercise, or diet plus exercise intervention. Int J Obesity 1997; 21:941–947.

66. Fogelholm M, Kukkonen-Harjula K. Does physical activity prevent weight gain - A systematic review. Obes Rev 2000; 1:95–111.

67. Anderson JW, Konz EC, Frederich RC, Wood CL. Long-term weight-loss maintenance: a meta-analysis of US studies. Am J Clin Nutr 2001; 74:579–584.

68. Klem ML, Wing RR, McGuire MT, Seagle HM, Hill JO. A descriptive study of individuals successful at long-term maintenance of substantial weight loss. Am J Clin Nutr 1997; 66:239–246.

69. Schoeller DA, Shay K, Kushner RF. How much physical activity is needed to minimize weight gain in previously obese women? Am J Clin Nutr 1997; 66:551–556.

70. Tudor-Locke C, Bassett DR, Jr. How many steps/day are enough? Preliminary pedometer indices for public health. Sports Med 2004; 34(1):1–8.

71. Swartz AM, Strath SJ, Bassett DR, et al. Increasing daily walking improves glucose tolerance in overweight women. Prev Med 2003; 37:356–362.

72. Tudor-Locke C, Ainsworth BE, Whitt MC, et al. The relationship between pedometer-determined ambulatory activity and body composition variables. Int J Obes Relat Metab Disord 2001; 25:1571–1578.

73. Wadden TA, Vogt RA, Anderson, RE, et al. Exercise in the treatment of obesity: effects of four interventions on body composition, resting energy expenditure, appetite, and mood. J Consult Clin Psychol 1997; 65:296–277.

74. Ballor DL, Harvey-Berion JR, Ades PA, Cryan J, Calles-Escandon J. Contrasting effects of resistance and aerobic training on body composition and metabolism after diet-induced weight loss. Metabolism 1996; 45:179–183.

75. Geliebter A, Maher MM, Gerace L, Gutin B, Heymsfield SB, Hashim SA. Effects of strength or aerobic training on body composition, resting metabolic rate, and peak oxygen consumption in obese dieting subjects. Am J Clin Nutr 1997; 66:557–563.

76. Kraemer WJ, Volek JS, Clark KL, et al. Influence of exercise training on physiological and performance change with weight loss in men. Med Sci Sports Exerc 1999; 31:1320–1329.

77. Kraemer WJ, Volek JS, Clark KL, et al. Physiological adaptations to a weight-loss dietary regimen and exercise programs in women. J Appl Physiol 1997; 93:270–279.

15 The Developmental Origins of Chronic Disease in Adult Life

David J.P. Barker

KEY POINTS

- Low birth-weight, as a result of slow fetal growth, is associated with increased rates of coronary heart disease and the related disorders, stroke, hypertension, and type 2 diabetes; these associations extend across the normal range of birth-weight.
- They are thought to be consequences of developmental plasticity, the phenomenon by which one genotype can give rise to a range of different physiological or morphological states in response to environmental conditions during development.
- People who were small at birth may be vulnerable to later disease because they have reduced functional capacity in key organs, such as the kidney, altered settings of hormones and metabolism, or altered responses to adverse influences in the postnatal environment.
- Slow growth in infancy and rapid weight gain after the age of 2 yr further increase the risk of later disease.
- Slow fetal growth is the product of the mother's body composition and diet before and during pregnancy, together with her metabolism.

1. DEVELOPMENTAL ORIGINS

The recent discovery that people who develop coronary heart disease (CHD) grew differently to other people during fetal life and childhood has led to a new "developmental" model for the disease *(1,2)*. The model proposes that nutrition during fetal life, infancy, and early childhood establishes functional capacity, metabolic competence, and responses to the later environment by changing gene expression *(3)*. There is now clear evidence that the pace and pathway of early growth is a major risk factor for the development of chronic disease in adult life.

To explore the developmental origins of chronic disease required studies of a kind that had not hitherto been carried out. It was necessary to identify groups of men and women now in middle or late life, whose size at birth had been recorded at the time. Their birth-weight could thereby be related to the later occurrence of CHD. In Hertfordshire, UK, from 1911 onward, when women had their babies they were attended by a midwife, who recorded the birth-weight. A health visitor went to the baby's home at intervals through-

From: *Nutritional Health: Strategies for Disease Prevention, Second Edition*
Edited by: N. J. Temple, T. Wilson, and D. R. Jacobs © Humana Press Inc., Totowa, NJ

out infancy, and the weight at 1 yr was recorded. Table 1 shows the findings in 10,636 men born between 1911 and 1930 *(1,4)*. Hazard ratios for CHD fell with increasing birth-weight. There were stronger trends with weight at 1 yr. A subsequent study confirmed a similar trend with birth-weight among women, but no trend with weight at 1 yr *(4)*. Table 2 shows findings for the first sample of men to have glucose tolerance tests *(5)*. The percentage with impaired glucose tolerance or type 2 diabetes fell steeply with increasing birth-weight, and with weight at 1 yr. There were similar trends with birth-weight among women.

The association between low birth-weight and CHD has now been replicated among men and women in Europe, North America, and India *(6–12)*. The association between low weight gain in infancy and CHD in men has been confirmed in Helsinki *(13)*. Low birth-weight has been shown to predict altered glucose tolerance in studies around the world *(14–18)*.

2. CONFOUNDING VARIABLES

These findings suggest that influences linked to early growth have an important effect on the risk of CHD and type 2 diabetes. It has been argued, however, that people whose growth was impaired *in utero* and during infancy may continue to be exposed to an adverse environment in childhood and adult life, and it is this later environment that produces the effects attributed to intrauterine influences. There is now strong evidence that this argument cannot be sustained.

In a number of studies data on lifestyle, including smoking habits, employment, alcohol consumption, and exercise, were collected. In the Nurses' Health Study in the United States allowance for these influences had little effect on the association between birth-weight and CHD *(8)*. Similar results came from Sweden and the United Kingdom *(6,10)*. In studies of type 2 diabetes and blood pressure the associations with size at birth are again independent of social class, cigarette smoking, and alcohol consumption. Adult lifestyle, however, adds to the effects of early life: for example, the prevalence of impaired glucose tolerance is highest in people who had low birth-weight but became obese as adults *(5,14–18)*. As described under Heading 4, slow fetal growth may also alter the body's response to socioeconomic influences in later life. Associations between low birth-weight and altered glucose tolerance and raised blood pressure have been found in numerous studies of children, which is a further argument against these associations being the product of confounding variables in adult life.

3. BIOLOGICAL BASIS

Like other living creatures in their early life, human beings are "plastic" and able to adapt to their environment. The development of the sweat glands provides a simple example of this. All humans have similar numbers of sweat glands at birth, but none of them function. In the first 3 yr after birth a proportion of the glands become functional, depending on the temperature to which the child is exposed. The hotter the conditions, the greater the number of sweat glands that are programmed to function. After 3 yr the process is complete and the number of sweat glands is fixed. Thereafter, the child who has experienced hot conditions will be better equipped to adapt to similar conditions in later life, because people with more functioning sweat glands cool down faster.

Table 1
Hazard Ratios (95% Confidence Intervals) for Death From CHD According
to Weight at Birth and at Age 1 Yr in 10,636 Men in Hertfordshire

		Death from CHD	
Weight (lb)		Before 65 yr	All ages
At birth			
	≤5.5	1.50 (0.98–2.31)	1.37 (1.00–1.86)
	–6.5	1.27 (0.89–1.83)	1.29 (1.01–1.66)
	–7.5	1.17 (0.84–1.63)	1.14 (0.91–1.44)
	–8.5	1.07 (0.77–1.49)	1.12 (0.89–1.40)
	–9.5	0.96 (0.66–1.39)	0.97 (0.75–1.25)
	>79.5	1.00	1.00
p for trend		0.001	0.005
Age 1 yr			
	≤18	2.22 (1.33–3.73)	1.89 (1.34–2.66)
	–20	1.80 (1.11–2.93)	1.58 (1.15–2.16)
	–22	1.96 (1.23–3.12)	1.66 (1.23–2.25)
	–24	1.52 (0.95–2.45)	1.36 (1.00–1.85)
	–26	1.36 (0.82–2.26)	1.29 (0.93–1.78)
	≥27	1.00	1.00
p for trend		<0.001	<0.001

This brief description encapsulates the essence of developmental plasticity: a critical period when a system is plastic and sensitive to the environment, followed by loss of plasticity and a fixed functional capacity. For most organs and systems the critical period occurs *in utero*. There are good reasons why it may be advantageous, in evolutionary terms, for the body to remain plastic during development. It enables the production of phenotypes that are better matched to their environment than would be possible if the same phenotype was produced in all environments. Developmental plasticity is defined as the phenomenon by which one genotype can give rise to a range of different physiological or morphological states in response to different environmental conditions during development *(19)*. Plasticity during intrauterine life enables animals, and humans, to receive a "weather forecast" from their mothers that prepares them for the type of world in which they will have to live *(20)*. If the mother is poorly nourished, she signals to her unborn baby that the environment it is about to enter is likely to be harsh. The baby responds to these signals by adaptations, such as reduced body size and altered metabolism, which help it to survive a shortage of food after birth. In this way plasticity gives a species the ability to make short-term adaptations, within one generation, in addition to the long-term genetic adaptations that come from natural selection. Because, as Mellanby noted long ago, the ability of a human mother to nourish her baby is partly determined when she herself is *in utero*, and by her childhood growth, the human fetus is receiving a weather forecast based not only on conditions at the time of the pregnancy, but on conditions a number of decades before *(3,21)*. This may be advantageous in populations that experience periodic food shortages.

Table 2
Percentage of Men Aged 64 Yr With Impaired Glucose Tolerance or Diabetes
According to Weight at Birth and at Age 1 Yr in 370 Men in Hertfordshire

Weight (lb)		% of men with 2-h glucose of ≥7.8 mmol/L	Odds ratio (95% CI)[a]
At birth			
	≤5.5	40	6.6 (1.5–28)
	–6.5	34	4.8 (1.3–17)
	–7.5	31	4.6 (1.4–16)
	–8.5	22	2.6 (0.8–8.9)
	–9.5	13	1.4 (0.3–5.6)
	>9.5	14	1.0
p for trend	<0.001		
Age 1 yr			
	≤18	43	8.2 (1.8–38)
	–20	32	4.8 (1.2–19)
	–22	30	4.2 (1.1–16)
	–24	18	2.1 (0.5–7.9)
	–26	19	2.1 (0.5–9.0)
	≥27	13	1.0
p for trend	<0.001		

[a]Adjusted for body mass index.

Until recently, we have overlooked a growing body of evidence that systems of the body that are closely related to adult disease, such as the regulation of blood pressure, are also plastic during early development. In animals it is surprisingly easy to produce life-long changes in the blood pressure and metabolism of a fetus by minor modifications to the diet of the mother before and during pregnancy (22,23).

The different size of newborn human babies exemplifies plasticity. The growth of babies has to be constrained by the size of the mother, otherwise normal birth could not occur. Small women have small babies: in pregnancies after ovum donation they have small babies even if the woman donating the egg is large (24). Babies may be small because their growth is constrained in this way or because they lack the nutrients for growth. As McCance wrote, "The size attained in utero depends on the services which the mother is able to supply. These are mainly food and accommodation" (25). Because the mother's height or pelvic dimensions are generally not found to be important predictors of the baby's long-term health, research into the developmental origins of disease has focused on the nutrient supply to the baby, while recognizing that other influences, such as hypoxia and stress, also influence fetal growth. This focus on fetal nutrition was endorsed in a recent review (26). The availability of nutrients to the fetus is influenced by the mother's nutrient stores and metabolism, as well as by her diet during pregnancy. In developing countries many babies are undernourished because their mothers are chronically malnourished. Despite current levels of nutrition in Western countries the nutrition of many fetuses and infants remains suboptimal because the nutrients available are unbalanced or because their delivery is constrained by maternal metabolism. Globally, size at birth in relation to gestational age is a marker of fetal nutrition *(26)*.

4. DEVELOPMENTAL ORIGINS HYPOTHESIS

The developmental origins hypothesis proposes that CHD, type 2 diabetes, stroke, and hypertension originate in developmental plasticity, in response to undernutrition during fetal life and infancy *(2,27)*. Why should fetal responses to undernutrition lead to disease in later life? The general answer is clear: "life history theory," which embraces all living things, states that, during development, increased allocation of energy to one trait, such as brain growth, necessarily reduces allocation to one or more other traits, such as tissue repair processes. Smaller babies, who have had a lesser allocation of energy, must incur higher costs and these, it seems, include disease in later life. A more specific answer to the question is that people who were small at birth are vulnerable to later disease through three kinds of process. First, they have less functional capacity in key organs, such as the kidney. One theory holds that hypertension is initiated by the reduced number of glomeruli found in people who were small at birth *(28)*. A reduced number necessarily leads to increased blood flow through each glomerulus. Over time, this hyperfiltration is thought to lead to the development of glomerulo-sclerosis which, combined with the loss of glomeruli that accompanies normal aging, leads to accelerated age-related loss of glomeruli, and a self-perpetuating cycle of rising blood pressure and glomerular loss.

A second process by which slow fetal growth may be linked to later disease is in the setting of hormones and metabolism. An undernourished baby may establish a "thrifty" way of handling food. Insulin resistance, which is associated with low birth-weight, may be viewed as persistence of a fetal response by which blood glucose concentrations were maintained for the benefit of the brain, but at the expense of glucose transport into the muscles and muscle growth *(29)*.

A third link between low birth-weight and later disease is that people who were small at birth are more vulnerable to adverse environmental influences in later life. Observations on animals show that the environment during development permanently changes not only the body's structure and function but also its responses to environmental influences encountered in later life *(20)*. Table 3 shows the effect of low income in adult life on CHD among men in Helsinki *(30)*. As expected, men who had a low taxable income had higher rates of the disease. There is no agreed explanation for this, but the association between poverty and CHD is a major component of the social inequalities in health in many western countries. Among the men in Helsinki the association was confined to men who had slow fetal growth and were thin at birth, defined by a ponderal index (birth-weight/length^3) of less than 26 kg/m^3 (*see* Table 3). Men who were not thin at birth showed no association of CHD with income, which implies that they were resilient to the effects of low income.

One explanation for these findings emphasizes the psychosocial consequences of a low position in the social hierarchy, as indicated by low income and social class, and suggests that perceptions of low social status and lack of success lead to changes in neuroendocrine pathways and hence to disease *(31)*. The findings in Helsinki seem consistent with this. People who were small at birth are known to have persisting alter-

Table 3
Hazard Ratios (95% CI) for CHD in 3629 Men in Helsinki According
to Ponderal Index at Birth (Birth-Weight/Length^3) and Taxable Income in Adult Life

Household income in pounds sterling/yr	Hazard ratios	
	Ponderal index ≤ 26.0 kg/m3 (n = 1475)	Ponderal index >26.0 kg/m3 (n = 2154)
<15,700	1.00	1.19 (0.65–2.19)
15,700	1.54 (0.83–2.87)	1.42 (0.78–2.57)
12,400	1.07 (0.51–2.22)	1.66 (0.90–3.07)
10,700	2.07 (1.13–3.79)	1.44 (0.79–2.62)
≤8400	2.58 (1.45–4.60)	1.37 (0.75–2.51)
p for trend	<0.001	0.75

ations in responses to stress, including raised serum cortisol concentrations (32). It is suggested that persisting small elevations of cortisol concentrations for many years may have effects similar to those seen when tumors lead to more sudden, large increases in glucocorticoid concentrations. People with Cushing's syndrome, the result of overactivity of the adrenal cortex, are insulin-resistant and have raised blood pressure, both of which predispose to CHD.

5. CHILDHOOD GROWTH AND CORONARY HEART DISEASE

Figure 1 shows the growth of 357 men who were either admitted to hospital with CHD or died from it (13). They belong to a cohort of 4630 men who were born in Helsinki, and their growth is expressed as Z-scores. The Z-score for the cohort is set at zero, and a boy maintaining a steady position as large or small in relation to other boys would follow a horizontal path on the figure. Boys who later developed CHD, however, were small at birth, remained small in infancy, but had accelerated gain in weight and body mass index (BMI) thereafter. In contrast, their heights remained below average. Table 4 shows that, as in Hertfordshire, the hazard ratios for CHD fell with increasing weight at 1 yr. Whereas in Hertfordshire measurements at 1 yr were restricted to weight, in Helsinki length was also recorded. Table 4 shows that hazard ratios for CHD fell with increasing length and, more strongly, with BMI. Small size at this age predicted CHD independently of size at birth. There may therefore be at least two pathways of development that lead to CHD among men in this cohort. One begins with slow growth *in utero*, and low birth-weight and thinness at birth, thought to be a consequence of fetal undernutrition. The other begins with poor weight gain during infancy, which is associated with two markers of poor living conditions, namely low parental socioeconomic status and overcrowding in the home. The effect of rapid weight gain after infancy, shown in Fig. 1, is confined to men on the first pathway. Rapid weight gain has no effect on the risk of disease among men following the second pathway (13).

Among the 4130 girls in the same birth cohort, the 87 who later developed CHD showed a broadly similar pattern of growth to the boys (12). They were, however, short

Table 4
Hazard Ratios for CHD According to Body Size
at Age 1 Yr in 4630 Men in Helsinki

Body Size	Hazard ratio (95% CI)
Weight (kg)	
≤9	1.82 (1.25–2.64)
–10	1.17 (0.80–1.71)
–11	1.12 (0.77–1.64)
–12	0.94 (0.62–1.44)
>12	1.00
p for trend	<0.0001
Height (cm)	
≤73	1.55 (1.11–2.18)
–75	0.90 (0.63–1.27)
–77	0.94 (0.68–1.31)
–79	0.83 (0.58–1.18)
>79	1.00
p for trend	0.007
BMI	
≤16	1.83 (1.28–2.60)
–17	1.61 (1.15–2.25)
–18	1.29 (0.91–1.81)
–19	1.12 (0.77–1.62)
>19	1.00
p for trend	0.0004

at birth rather than thin. They had rapid height growth in infancy, but became thin. This persisted up to the age of 4 yr, after which they gained weight rapidly. In both sexes disease risk was related to the tempo of weight gain rather than to body size at any particular age.

Table 5 shows hazard ratios for CHD according to birth-weight and fourths of BMI at age 11 yr among 13,517 men and women in Helsinki representing the combined older and younger birth cohorts, born between 1924 and 1933 and 1934 and 1944 (27). The risks of disease fell with increasing birth-weight and rose with increasing BMI at age 11 yr. The pattern was similar in the two sexes.

6. TYPE 2 DIABETES AND HYPERTENSION

People who were small at birth remain biologically different from people who were larger, and these differences include an increased susceptibility to type 2 diabetes and hypertension. Table 6 is based on the same cohort of men and women shown in Table 5,

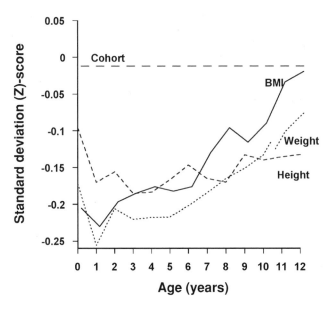

Fig. 1. Mean Z-scores for height, weight, and body mass index during childhood in 357 boys who later developed coronary heart disease within a cohort of 4630 boys. At any age, the mean Z-score for the cohort is set a 0, whereas the standard deviation is set at 1.

Table 5
Hazard Ratios for CHD According to Birth-Weight and BMI
at Age 11 Yr Among 13,517 Men and Women in Helsinki

Birth-weight (kg)	BMI at age 11 yr			
	<15.7	–16.6	–17.6	>17.6
Hospital admissions and deaths (1235 cases)				
<3.0	1.4 (991)	1.6 (719)	1.8 (581)	2.1 (560)
–3.5	1.3 (1394)	1.5 (1422)	1.5 (1264)	1.6 (1246)
–4.0	1.3 (827)	1.4 (984)	1.3 (1122)	1.4 (1110)
>4.0	1.0 (167)	1.2 (254)	1.1 (413)	1.0 (463)
Deaths (480 cases)				
<3.0	1.4	1.8	2.1	3.0
–3.5	1.4	1.9	2.2	2.7
–4.0	1.9	1.8	1.7	1.6
>4.0	1.0	1.4	1.6	1.3

Figures in parentheses are numbers of subjects.

and again shows odds ratios according to birthweight and fourths of BMI at age 11 yr. The two disorders are associated with the same general pattern of growth as CHD *(27)*. Risk of disease falls with increasing birth-weight and rises with increasing BMI.

Associations between low birth-weight and type 2 diabetes, shown in Table 2, have been found in other studies *(5,14–18)*. The association with hypertension has also been

Table 6
Odds Ratios (95% CI) for Type 2 Diabetes and Hypertension According
to Birth-Weight and BMI at Age 11 Yr Among 13,517 Men and Women in Helsinki

Birth-weight (kg)	BMI at age 11			
	<15.7	–16.6	–17.6	>17.6
Type 2 diabetes (698 cases)				
<3.0	1.3 (0.6–2.8)	1.3 (0.6–2.8)	1.5 (0.7–3.4)	2.5 (1.2–5.5)
–3.5	1.0 (0.5–2.1)	1.0 (0.5–2.1)	1.5 (0.7–3.2)	1.7 (0.8–3.5)
–4.0	1.0 (0.5–2.2)	0.9 (0.4–1.9)	0.9 (0.4–2.0)	1.7 (0.8–3.6)
>4.0	1.0	1.1 (0.4–2.7)	0.7 (0.3–1.7)	1.2 (0.5–2.7)
Hypertension (2997 cases)				
<3.0	2.0 (1.3–3.2)	1.9 (1.2–3.1)	1.9 (1.2–3.0)	2.3 (1.5–3.8)
–3.5	1.7 (1.1–2.6)	1.9 (1.2–2.9)	1.9 (1.2–3.0)	2.2 (1.4–3.4)
–4.0	1.7 (1.0–2.6)	1.7 (1.1–2.6)	1.5 (1.0–2.4)	1.9 (1.2–2.9)
>4.0	1.0	1.9 (1.1–3.1)	1.0 (0.6–1.7)	1.7 (1.1–2.8)

found elsewhere *(33)*. There is a substantial literature showing that birth-weight is associated with differences in blood pressure and insulin sensitivity within the normal range *(5,14,18,34)*. These differences are found in children and adults but they tend to be small. A 1-kg difference in birth-weight is associated with around 3-mmHg difference in systolic pressure. The contrast between this small effect and the large effect on hypertension (*see* Table 6) suggests that lesions that accompany poor fetal growth and that tend to elevate blood pressure, and which may include a reduced number of glomeruli, have a small influence on blood pressure within the normal range because counter-regulatory mechanisms maintain normal blood pressure levels. As the lesions progress through, for example, hyperfiltration of the reduced number of glomeruli and consequent glomerulosclerosis, these mechanisms are no longer able to maintain homeostasis and, as a result, blood pressure rises. This may initiate a cycle of rise in blood pressure resulting in further progression of the lesions and further rise in blood pressure *(28,35)*. Direct evidence in support of this has come from a study of the kidneys of people killed in road accidents. Those being treated for hypertension had fewer, but larger, glomeruli *(36)*. Evidence to support the development of self-perpetuating cycles comes from a study of elderly people in Helsinki among whom the effect of birth-weight on blood pressure was confined to those being treated for hypertension *(37)*. Despite their treatment the blood pressures of those who had low birth-weight were markedly higher, whereas among the normotensive subjects birth-weight was unrelated to blood pressure. Whether measured in the clinic or by ambulatory methods, there was a more than 20-mmHg difference in systolic pressure between those who weighed 2500 g (5.5 lb) or less at birth and those who weighed 4000 g (8.8 lb) or more. An inference is that by the time they reached old age most of the people with lesions acquired *in utero* had developed clinical hypertension. Studies in South Carolina bear on this issue. They show that among 3236 hypertensive patients, the blood

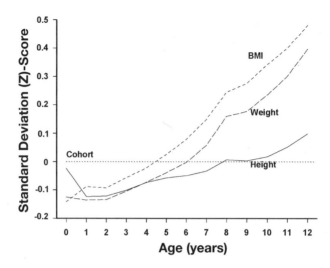

Fig. 2. Mean Z-scores for height, weight, and body mass index during childhood in 290 boys and girls who later developed type 2 diabetes within a cohort of 8760 children. At any age, the mean Z-score for the cohort is set at 0, whereas the standard deviation is set at 1.

pressures of those with low birth-weight tended to be more difficult to control with medication *(38)*.

Figure 2 shows the growth of boys and girls, in the younger Helsinki cohort, who later developed type 2 diabetes. They had below average body size at birth and at 1 yr, after which their weight and BMI rose progressively to exceed the average *(39)*. Table 7 shows the relation between age at "adiposity rebound" and later type 2 diabetes. After the age of 2 yr the degree of obesity of young children, as measured by BMI, decreases to a minimum around 6 yr of age before increasing again—the so-called adiposity rebound. The age at adiposity rebound ranges from around 3 to 8 yr or more. Table 7 shows that early adiposity rebound is strongly related to a high BMI in later childhood, as has previously been shown *(40)*. It also predicts an increased incidence of type 2 diabetes in later life. This new observation has now been replicated in a longitudinal study in Delhi, India *(41)*. In both studies an early adiposity rebound was found to be associated with thinness at birth and at 1 yr *(39,41)*. It is not, therefore, the young child who is overweight who is at greatest risk of type 2 diabetes but the one who is thin but subsequently gains weight rapidly.

7. COMPENSATORY GROWTH

When undernutrition during early development is followed by improved nutrition, many animals and plants stage accelerated or "compensatory" growth *(27)*. Compensatory growth has costs, however, which in animals include reduced life-span *(42)*. There are a number of processes by which, in humans, undernutrition and small size at birth followed by rapid childhood growth could lead to cardiovascular disease and type 2 diabetes in later life *(13,16)*. Rapid growth may be associated with persisting hormonal and metabolic changes. Larger body size may increase the functional demand on functional capacity that has been reduced by slow early growth—fewer glomeruli

Table 7
BMI at Age 11 Yr and Cumulative Incidence of Type 2 Diabetes
According to Age at Adiposity Rebound in 8760 Men and Women in Helsinki

Age at adiposity rebound (yr)	Mean BMI at age 11 yr	Cumulative incidence of diabetes % (n)		
	All	Men	Women	All
≤4	19.7	8.1 (86)	8.9 (112)	8.6 (198)
5	17.6	6.2 (904)	2.5 (864)	4.4 (1768)
6	17.0	3.7 (1861)	2.5 (1456)	3.2 (3317)
7	16.8	2.4 (249)	2.1 (243)	2.2 (492)
≥8	16.7	3.0 (135)	0.7 (150)	1.8 (285)
p for trend	<0.001	<0.001	0.002	<0.001

for example. Rapid weight gain may lead to an unfavorable body composition. Babies that are small and thin at birth lack muscle, a deficiency that will persist as the critical period for muscle growth occurs *in utero* and there is little cell replication after birth *(43)*. If they develop a high body mass during later childhood, they may have a disproportionately high fat mass in relation to lean body mass, which will lead to insulin resistance *(44)*.

8. PATHWAYS TO DISEASE

New studies, especially the Helsinki studies with their detailed information on child growth and socioeconomic circumstances, increasingly suggest that the pathogenesis of CHD and the disorders related to it depend on a series of interactions occurring at different stages of development. To begin with, the effects of the genes acquired at conception may be conditioned by the early environment. Table 8 is based on a study of 476 elderly people in Helsinki *(45)*. It shows mean fasting plasma insulin concentrations according to which of two polymorphisms of the peroxisome proliferator-activated receptor *(PPAR)*-γ gene was present. The Pro12Pro polymorphism is known to be associated with insulin resistance, indicated by elevated fasting plasma insulin concentrations. Table 8 shows, however, that this effect occurs only among men and women who had low birth-weight. Conversely, low birth-weight has been consistently linked to later insulin resistance *(18)*, but Table 8 shows that this effect occurs only among people with the Pro12Pro polymorphism. As birth-weight serves as a marker of fetal nutrition *(26)*, this gene–birth-weight interaction may reflect a gene–nutrient interaction during development.

The effects of the intrauterine environment on later disease are conditioned not only by events at conception but also by events after birth. Tables 5 and 6 show how the effects are conditioned by childhood weight gain. Table 3 shows that the effects of low ponderal index at birth are conditioned by living conditions in adult life. Table 9 shows how the effects of low birth-weight on later hypertension are conditioned by living conditions in childhood, indicated by the occupational status of the father *(46)*. Among all the men and women low birth-weight was associated with an increased incidence of hypertension, as has been shown before *(33)*. This association, however, was present only among those who were born into families where the father was a laborer or of lower middle class.

Table 8

Mean Fasting Insulin Concentrations in 426 Elderly People
in Helsinki According to *PPAR-γ* Gene Polymorphism and Birth-Weight

| | Birth-weight (g) | | | |
	<3000	*3000–3500*	*>3500*	p *for trend*
Pro12Pro	84 (56)[a]	71 (161)	65 (107)	0.003
Pro12Ala/Ala12Ala	60 (37)	60 (67)	65 (48)	0.31
p for difference	0.008	0.02	0.99	

[a]Fasting insulin (pmol/L) (*n*).

Table 9

Cumulative Incidence (%) of Hypertension According to Birth-Weight
and Father's Social Class in 8760 Men and Women in Helsinki

| | Father's social class | | | |
Birth-weight (g)	*Laborer*	*Lower middle class*	*Upper middle class*	p *for trend*
<3000	22.2	20.2	10.5	0.002
–3500	18.8	15.2	10.6	<0.001
–4000	14.5	12.5	10.3	0.04
>4000	11.1	15.6	15.7	0.11
p for trend	<0.001	0.05	0.79	

It seems that the pathogenesis of cardiovascular disease and type 2 diabetes cannot be understood within a model in which risks associated with adverse influences at different stages of life add to each other *(47)*. Rather, disease is the product of branching paths of development. The environment triggers the branchings. The pathways determine vulnerability of each individual to what lies ahead. The pathway to CHD can originate either in slow fetal growth as a consequence of undernutrition, or in poor infant growth as a consequence of poor living conditions.

The effects of slow fetal growth and low birth-weight, and the effects of postnatal development, depend on environmental influences and paths of development that precede and follow them. Low birth-weight or any other single influence, does not have "an" effect that is best estimated by a pooled estimate from all published studies. A recent pooled estimate led to the conclusion that because the effects of birth-weight on blood pressure within the normal range are small, the effects on disease are also small *(48)*. Such a conclusion is biologically fallacious for the reasons already described under "developmental origins hypothesis." It is also statistically fallacious because it discounts interactions of the kind described. As René Dubos *(49)* wrote: "The effects of the physical and social environments cannot be understood without knowledge of individual history." Unravelling disease causation, and hence the way to prevent it, will therefore require an understanding of heterogeneity.

9. STRENGTH OF EFFECTS

Low birth-weight, though a convenient marker in epidemiological studies, is an inadequate description of the phenotypic characteristics of a baby that determine its long-term health. The wartime famine in the Netherlands produced lifelong insulin resistance in babies who were *in utero* at the time, but with little alteration in birth-weight *(50)*. In babies, as in children, slowing of growth is a response to a poor environment, especially undernutrition, but body size at birth does not adequately describe the long-term morphological and physiological consequences of undernutrition. The same birth-weight can be attained by many different paths of fetal growth, and each is likely to be accompanied by different gene–environment interactions *(26)*. Nevertheless, birth-weight provides a basis for estimating the magnitude of the effects of the fetal phase of development on later disease, although it is likely to underestimate them.

Because the risk of cardiovascular disease is influenced both by small body size at birth and during infancy and by rapid weight gain in childhood, estimation of the risk of disease attributable to early development requires data on fetal, infant, and childhood growth. Currently, the Helsinki studies are the main source of information *(27)*. Table 5 shows that men and women who had birth-weights higher than 4 kg (8.8 lb) and whose prepubertal BMI was in the lowest fourth had around half the risk of CHD when compared with people who had birth-weights lower than 3 kg (6.6 lb), but whose BMI was in the highest fourth. The hazard ratios for admissions and deaths were 0.80 (95% CI 0.72–0.90) for each kilogram increase in birth-weight and 1.06 (1.03–1.10) for each kilogram per meter^2 increase in BMI at age 11 yr. The hazard ratios for deaths alone were 0.83 (0.69–0.99) and 1.10 (1.04–1.16), respectively.

Table 10 is based on the younger Helsinki cohort, born between 1934 and 1944. Subjects were divided according to thirds of body size at birth and whether their standard deviation score for BMI decreased or increased between ages 3 and 11 yr. Among men, ponderal index at birth was more strongly related to CHD than birth-weight, whereas among women, length at birth was stronger. If each man in the cohort had been in the highest third of ponderal index at birth, and each woman in the highest third of birth length, and if each man or woman had lowered their BMI score between ages 3 and 11 yr, the incidence of CHD would have been reduced by 25% in men and 63% in women *(27)*.

Table 6 showed that men and women who had birth-weights higher than 4 kg and whose prepubertal BMI was in the lowest fourth had around half the risk of type 2 diabetes and hypertension when compared with people who had birth-weights lower than 3 kg but whose BMI was in the highest fourth. The odds ratio for type 2 diabetes was 0.67 (95% CI 0.58–0.79) for each kilogram increase in birth-weight and 1.18 (95% CI 1.13–1.23) for each kilogram per meter^2 increase in BMI at age 11 yr. The corresponding figures for hypertension were 0.77 (95% CI 0.71–0.84) and 1.07 (95% CI 1.04–1.09).

In Table 11 subjects are again divided into six groups according to thirds of birth-weight and whether their standard deviation score for BMI decreased or increased between ages 3 and 11 yr. For both type 2 diabetes and hypertension there were independent effects of birth-weight and change in BMI score. The patterns of odds ratios and incidence shown in Tables 6 and 11 were similar in the two sexes. If each individual in

Table 10
Cumulative Incidence (%) of CHD According to Body Size
at Birth and Change in Standard Deviation Score for BMI
Between Ages 3 and 11 Yr Among 6345 Men and Women in Helsinki

Birth size	Change in standard deviation score for BMI between ages 3 and 11	
	Decrease	Increase
Men		
Birth-weight (kg)		
<3.2	8.8 (512)[a]	9.0 (476)[a]
−3.6	6.9 (662)	11.3 (512)
>3.6	5.9 (740)	8.6 (521)
Ponderal index (kg/m3)		
<25	8.0 (411)	11.7 (394)
−27	7.6 (649)	10.8 (556)
>27	6.2 (838)	7.2 (539)
Women		
Birth-weight (kg)		
<3.2	1.6 (563)	3.8 (604)
−3.6	1.5 (612)	2.5 (438)
>3.6	0.7 (450)	3.6 (334)
Birth length (cm)		
<49	1.5 (543)	4.2 (520)
−50	1.5 (452)	3.3 (338)
>50	0.8 (609)	2.6 (496)

[a]Cumulative incidence, % (n) of coronary heart disease (hospital admissions and deaths). There were 279 cases in men and 66 in women.

the cohort had been in the highest third of birth-weight and had lowered their standard deviation score for BMI between ages 3 and 11 yr, the incidence of type 2 diabetes would have been reduced by 52% and the incidence of hypertension by 25% (27).

10. MATERNAL INFLUENCES ON FETAL NUTRITION

Size at birth is the product of the fetus's trajectory of growth, which is set at an early stage in development, and the materno-placental capacity to supply sufficient nutrients to maintain that trajectory. In Western communities, randomized, controlled trials of maternal macronutrient supplementation have indicated relatively small effects on birth-weight (51). This has led to the view that regulatory mechanisms in the maternal and placental systems act to ensure that human fetal growth and development is little influenced by normal variations in maternal nutrient intake, and that there is a simple relationship between a woman's body composition and the growth of her fetus. Recent experimental studies in animals and observational data in humans challenge these concepts (52). They suggest that a mother's own fetal growth and her dietary intakes and body composition can exert major effects on the balance between the fetal demand for

Table 11
Cumulative Incidence, %(n) of Type 2 Diabetes and Hypertension
According to Birth-Weight and Change in Standard Deviation Score for BMI
Between Ages 3 and 11 Yr Among 6424 Men and Women in Helsinki

Birth-weight (kg)	Change in standard deviation score for BMI between ages 3 and 11	
	Decrease	Increase
Type 2 diabetes (227 cases)		
<3.2	3.1 (1075)	5.5 (1080)
–3.6	2.4 (1274)	4.3 (950)
>3.6	1.5 (1190)	5.4 (855)
Hypertension (1036 cases)		
<3.2	15.9 (1075)	21.3 (1080)
–3.6	14.8 (1274)	19.4 (950)
>3.6	12.0 (1190)	13.9 (855)

nutrients and the materno-placental capacity to meet that demand. Specific issues that have not yet been adequately addressed include: (1) maternal effects on the trajectory of fetal growth; (2) intergenerational effects; (3) paradoxical effects on placental growth; and (4) the importance of the mother's body composition and the balance of macronutrients in her diet.

10.1. The Fetal Growth Trajectory

A rapid trajectory of growth increases the fetus's demand for nutrients. Though this demand is greatest late in pregnancy, its magnitude is thought to be primarily determined by genetic and environmental effects on the trajectory of fetal growth, which is set at an early stage in development. Experimental studies of pregnant ewes have shown that, although a fast growth trajectory is generally associated with larger fetal size and improved neonatal survival, it renders the fetus more vulnerable to a reduced materno-placental supply of nutrients in late gestation. Thus, maternal undernutrition during the last trimester adversely affects the development of rapidly growing fetuses with high requirements, while having little effect on those growing more slowly (53). Rapidly growing fetuses were found to make a series of adaptations in order to survive, including fetal wasting and placental oxidation of fetal amino acids to maintain lactate output to the fetus (52). Experiments in animals have shown that alterations in the maternal diet around the time of conception can change the fetal growth trajectory. In a recent study, rats were fed a 9% casein low-protein diet in the periconceptional period. This led to structural changes at the blastocyst stage of embryonic development, reduced fetal growth rates, small size at birth, and raised blood pressure in the offspring during adult life (23). The sensitivity of the human embryo to its environment is being increasingly recognized with the development of assisted reproductive technology (54). The trajectory of fetal growth is thought to increase with improvements in periconceptional nutrition, and is faster in male fetuses. The consequent greater vulnerability of male fetuses to undernutrition may contribute to the higher death rates from CHD among men.

10.2. Intergenerational Effects

Experimental studies in animals have shown that undernutrition can have effects on reproductive performance which may persist for several generations. Among rats fed a protein-deficient diet over 12 generations, there was a progressive fall in fetal growth rates. When restored to a normal diet, it took three generations before growth and development were normalized *(55)*.

Strong evidence for major intergenerational effects in humans has come from studies showing that a woman's birth-weight influences the birth-weight of her offspring *(56)*. A study in the United Kingdom showed that whereas low-birth-weight mothers tended to have thin infants with a low ponderal index, the father's birth-weight was unrelated to ponderal index at birth *(57)*. The effect of maternal birth-weight on thinness at birth is consistent with the hypothesis that in low-birth-weight mothers the fetal supply line is compromised and unable to meet fetal nutrient demand. Potential mechanisms underlying this effect include alterations in the uterine or systemic vasculature, changes in maternal metabolism, or impaired placentation.

10.3. Placental Size and Transfer Capabilities

Although the size of the placenta gives only an indirect measure of its capacity to transfer nutrients to the fetus, it is nonetheless strongly associated with fetal size at birth. Experiments in sheep have shown that maternal nutrition in early pregnancy can exert major effects on the growth of the placenta and thereby alter fetal development *(58)*. The effects produced depend on the nutritional status of the ewe in the periconceptional period. In ewes that were poorly nourished around the time of conception, low nutrient intakes in early pregnancy reduced the size of the placenta. Conversely, in ewes well nourished around the time of conception, low intakes in early pregnancy resulted in increased placental size *(58)*. Placental expansion may be an adaptation by the fetus to extract more nutrients from the mother, but apparently it can only occur in previously well-nourished ewes. Although this seems paradoxical, in sheep farming it is common practice for ewes to be put on rich pasture prior to mating and then on poor pasture for a period in early pregnancy, in order to increase the size of the lambs at birth.

There is evidence of a similar suppressive effect of high dietary intakes on placental growth in humans *(59)*. Among 538 women who delivered at term in Southampton, UK, those with high dietary intakes in early pregnancy, especially of carbohydrate, had smaller placentas, particularly if this was combined with low intakes of dairy protein in late pregnancy. These effects were independent of the mother's body size, social class, and smoking, and resulted in alterations in the ratio of placental weight to birth-weight (placental ratio). Further evidence that maternal diet can alter placental growth has come from analyses of the Dutch famine, in which famine exposure in early pregnancy increased placental weight *(60)*.

The U-shaped relation between the placental ratio and later CHD and raised blood pressure indicates that effects on placental growth may be of long-term importance *(61,62)*. Babies with a disproportionately small placenta may suffer as a consequence of an impaired placental supply capacity; those with a disproportionately large placenta may become catabolic and waste in order to supply amino acids for placental consumption *(63)*.

10.4. Maternal Diet and Body Composition

Evidence supporting a long-term effect of levels of maternal nutrient intake during pregnancy has come from a follow-up study of children whose mothers took part in a randomized, controlled trial of calcium supplementation in pregnancy in Argentina *(64)*. Supplementation was associated with lowering of the offspring's blood pressure in childhood, although it was not associated with any change in birth-weight. Follow-up studies after the Dutch famine of 1944–1945 found that severe maternal caloric restriction at different stages of pregnancy was variously associated with obesity, dyslipidemia, and insulin resistance in the offspring, and there is preliminary evidence of an increased risk of CHD *(50,65,66)*. Again, these effects were largely independent of size at birth.

In the Dutch studies, famine exposure per se was not associated with raised blood pressure in the offspring, but there was an effect of macronutrient balance. Maternal rations with a low protein density were associated with raised blood pressure in the adult offspring *(67)*. This adds to the findings of studies in Aberdeen, UK, which showed that maternal diets with either a low or a high ratio of animal protein to carbohydrate were associated with raised blood pressure in the offspring during adult life *(68)*.

In the Aberdeen study, maternal diets with a high protein density were not only associated with raised blood pressure in the offspring but also with insulin deficiency and impaired glucose tolerance *(69)*. Although it may seem counter-intuitive that a high-protein diet should have adverse effects, these findings are consistent with the results of controlled trials of protein supplementation in pregnancy, which show that high protein intakes are associated with reduced birth-weight *(70)*. The Aberdeen findings have recently been replicated in a follow-up study of men and women in Motherwell, UK, whose mothers were advised to eat a diet high in meat protein and low in carbohydrate during pregnancy *(71)*. Those whose mothers had high intakes of meat and fish in late pregnancy, but low intakes of carbohydrate, had raised blood pressure, particularly if the mother also had a low intake of green vegetables. Although raised blood pressure was also related to low birth-weight, taking account of birth-weight had little effect on the relation between the maternal diet and the offspring's blood pressure. One possibility is that the effect on blood pressure may be a consequence of the metabolic stress imposed on the mother by an unbalanced diet in which high intakes of essential amino acids are not accompanied by the micronutrients required to use them. These high intakes create an excess that is potentially toxic unless they are degraded and oxidized. The degradation of essential amino acids consumes nonessential amino acids, which are synthesized by the body. Their synthesis requires cofactors, especially folate and other B vitamins *(3)*. Direct evidence of metabolic stress in the offspring comes from analysis of their fasting plasma cortisol concentrations *(72)*. Men and women whose mothers had high intakes of meat and fish and low intakes of green vegetables had raised cortisol concentrations.

The fetus does not live on the mother's diet alone: that would be too dangerous a strategy. It also lives off stored nutrients and the turnover of protein and fat in the mother's tissues *(73)*. Maternal size and body composition account for up to 20% of the variability in birth-weight *(74)*. Gestational diabetes is known to be associated with adverse long-term outcomes in the offspring *(75)*. More recently, studies in Europe and India have shown that high maternal weight and adiposity are associated with adult development of insulin deficiency, type 2 diabetes, and CHD in the offspring *(9,16,76)*. Of great importance is an increasing body of consistent evidence showing strong links between low maternal weight or BMI and insulin resistance in the adult offspring *(50,69,77)*. Table 12 shows plasma glucose and insulin concentrations in Chinese men and women aged around 45 yr following a standard oral glucose challenge. Low maternal BMI at 38 wk of pregnancy was associated with raised plasma glucose and insulin concentrations *(77)*. Results for maternal BMI in early pregnancy, around 15 wk, were stronger. In contrast to these associations between maternal BMI and insulin resistance, thin maternal skinfold thicknesses and low pregnancy weight gain have been consistently associated with raised blood pressure in the offspring *(78–81)*. One of the metabolic links between maternal body composition and birth size is protein synthesis. Women with a greater lean body mass have higher rates of protein synthesis in pregnancy *(82)*. Variation in rates of maternal protein synthesis explains a quarter of the variability in birth length.

The list of chronic diseases whose origins lie in early development now extends beyond cardiovascular disease and type 2 diabetes. There is strong evidence that osteoporosis is another of the body's "memories" of undernutrition at a critical early stage of development *(83)*. This is perhaps unsurprising given that rickets has served as a longstanding example of the persisting structural changes induced by early undernutrition. More surprising is suggestive evidence linking early development with depression *(84)*. There is also clear evidence that schizophrenia originates through developmental abnormalities of the fetal brain in response to an adverse intrauterine environment *(85)*.

11. RESEARCH CHALLENGES

Further research has to address two overarching questions.

11.1. Environmental Influences

What are the environmental influences that, acting through the mother, or directly on the infant and young child, alter gene expression and thereby permanently change the body's structure and function? Research on maternal influences will need to address: (1) effects on the fetal growth trajectory; (2) effects on placental growth; and (3) intergenerational effects.

11.2. Pathogenesis

How do gene–environment interactions during development translate into chronic disease? Through a combination of clinical and experimental studies, progress is being made in understanding the developmental origins of altered glucose–insulin and lipid metabolism, stress responses, blood pressure, and renal function.

12. DISEASE PREVENTION

The evidence presented in this chapter indicates that prevention of a substantial proportion of chronic diseases, including cardiovascular disease, type 2 diabetes, and osteoporosis, may depend on interventions at a number of stages of development. Strategies that target infants and young children may give the most immediate benefit but improving the intrauterine environment is an important long-term goal. There is sufficient knowledge to implement preventive programs now. More research is needed, however, to increase the effectiveness of these programs.

Table 12
Mean 2-h Plasma Glucose and Insulin Concentrations
According to Maternal BMI in Late Pregnancy in 584 Chinese Men and Women

	Maternal BMI				
	≤ 23	−24.5	−26	>26	*p* for trend
2-h glucose (mmol/L)	7.6	6.6	6.7	5.7	0.003
2-h insulin (pmol/L)	304	277	282	177	0.007

MOTHER

- An optimal diet begins before pregnancy. In developing countries micronutrients in the diet may be limiting factors in fetal growth, whereas in Western countries macronutrient balance, especially between protein and carbohydrate, seems likely to be important.
- Women require an optimal body composition before pregnancy, with avoidance of excessive thinness or overweight.
- It is not known whether the greatest benefits for the next generation will come from improving the nutrition of adult women, adolescent girls, or girl children. Any rational policy needs to address all three.

INFANT

- The growth in weight and length during the first year after birth needs to be protected by good infant feeding practices and avoidance of recurrent infections.

CHILD

- Young children who were small or thin at birth should not gain weight rapidly after the age of 2 yr, so that their BMIs increase in relation to those of other children.

ADULT

- People who were small at birth are more vulnerable to adverse influences acting in adult life. At present these are known to include obesity and aspects of psychosocial stress.

13. CONCLUSIONS

Low birth-weight is now known to be associated with increased rates of CHD and the related disorders stroke, hypertension, and type 2 diabetes. These associations have been extensively replicated in studies in different countries and are not the result of confounding variables. They extend across the normal range of birth-weight and depend on lower birth-weights in relation to the duration of gestation rather than the effects of premature birth. The associations are thought to be consequences of developmental plasticity, the phenomenon by which one genotype can give rise to a range of different physiological or morphological states in response to different environmental conditions during development. Recent observations have shown that impaired growth in infancy and rapid childhood weight gain exacerbate the effects of impaired prenatal growth. CHD and the disorders related to it arise through a series of interactions between environmental influences and the pathways of development that preceded them. These diseases are the product of branching pathways of development in which the branchings are triggered by the environment before and after birth.

The demonstration that normal variations in fetal size and thinness at birth have implications for health throughout life has prompted a re-evaluation of the regulation of fetal development. Impetus has been added to this re-evaluation by recent findings showing that a woman's dietary balance and body composition in pregnancy are related to levels of cardiovascular risk factors and the risk of CHD in her offspring in adult life without necessarily affecting size at birth. These observations challenge the view that the fetus is little affected by changes in maternal nutrition, except in circumstances of famine. There is an increasing body of evidence that a woman's own fetal growth, and her diet and body composition before pregnancy, play a major role in determining the future health of her children. A new vision of optimal early human development is emerging which takes account of both short- and long-term outcome.

REFERENCES

1. Barker DJP, Osmond C, Winter PD, Margetts B, Simmonds SJ. Weight in infancy and death from ischaemic heart disease. Lancet 1989; 2:577–580.
2. Barker DJP. Fetal origins of coronary heart disease. BMJ 1995; 311:171–174.
3. Jackson A.A. All that glitters. British Nutrition Foundation Nutrition Bulletin 2000; 25:11–24.
4. Osmond C, Barker DJP, Winter PD, Fall CHD, Simmonds SJ. Early growth and death from cardiovascular disease in women. BMJ 1993; 307:1519–1524.
5. Hales CN, Barker DJP, Clark PMS, et al. Fetal and infant growth and impaired glucose tolerance at age 64. BMJ 1991; 303:1019–1022.
6. Frankel S, Elwood P, Sweetnam P, Yarnell J, Davey Smith G. Birthweight, body mass index in middle age, and incident coronary heart disease. Lancet 1996; 348:1478–1480.
7. Stein CE, Fall CHD, Kumaran K, Osmond C, Cox V, Barker DJP. Fetal growth and coronary heart disease in South India. Lancet 1996; 348:1269–1273.
8. Rich-Edwards JW, Stampfer MJ, Manson JE, et al. Birth weight and risk of cardiovascular disease in a cohort of women followed up since 1976. BMJ 1997; 315:396–400.
9. Forsén T, Eriksson JG, Tuomilehto J, Teramo K, Osmond C, Barker DJP. Mother's weight in pregnancy and coronary heart disease in a cohort of Finnish men: follow up study. BMJ 1997; 315:837–840.
10. Leon DA, Lithell HO, Vagero D, et al. Reduced fetal growth rate and increased risk of death from ischaemic heart disease: cohort study of 15,000 Swedish men and women born 1915–29. BMJ 1998; 317:241–245.
11. Forsen T, Eriksson JG, Tuomilehto J, Osmond C, Barker DJP. Growth in utero and during childhood among women who develop coronary heart disease: longitudinal study. BMJ 1999; 319:1403–1407.
12. Forsen T, Osmond C, Eriksson JG, Barker DJP. Growth of girls who later develop coronary heart disease. Heart 2004; 90:20–24.
13. Eriksson JG, Forsen T, Tuomilehto J, Osmond C, Barker DJP. Early growth and coronary heart disease in later life: longitudinal study. BMJ 2001; 322:949–953.
14. Lithell HO, McKeigue PM, Berglund L, Mohsen R, Lithell UB, Leon DA. Relation of size at birth to non-insulin dependent diabetes and insulin concentrations in men aged 50–60 years. BMJ 1996; 312:406–410.
15. McCance DR, Pettitt DJ, Hanson RL, Jacobsson LTH, Knowler WC, Bennett PH. Birth weight and non-insulin dependent diabetes: thrifty genotype, thrifty phenotype, or surviving small baby genotype? BMJ 1994; 308:942–945.
16. Forsén T, Eriksson J, Tuomilehto J, Reunanen A, Osmond C, Barker D. The fetal and childhood growth of persons who develop type 2 diabetes. Ann Intern Med 2000; 133:176–182.
17. Rich-Edwards JW, Colditz GA, Stampfer MJ, et al. Birthweight and the risk for type 2 diabetes mellitus in adult women. Ann Intern Med 1999; 130:278–284.
18. Newsome CA, Shiell AW, Fall CHD, Phillips DIW, Shier R, Law CM. Is birthweight related to later glucose and insulin metabolism—a systematic review. Diabet Med 20:339–348.

19. West-Eberhard MJ. Phenotypic plasticity and the origins of diversity. Ann Rev Ecolo System 1989; 20:249.
20. Bateson P, Martin P. Design for a Life: How Behaviour Develops. Jonathan Cape, London, 1999.
21. Mellanby E. Nutrition and child-bearing. Lancet 1933; 2:1131–1137.
22. Widdowson EM, McCance RA. The effect of finite periods of undernutrition at different ages on the composition and subsequent development of the rat. Proc R Soc Lond B 1963; 158:329–342.
23. Kwong WY, Wild A, Roberts P, Willis AC, Fleming TP. Maternal undernutrition during the pre-implantation period of rat development causes blastocyst abnormalities and programming of postnatal hypertension. Development 2000; 127:4195–4202.
24. Brooks AA, Johnson MR, Steer PJ, Pawson ME, Abdalla HI. Birth weight: nature or nurture? Early Hum Dev 1995; 42:29–35.
25. McCance RA. Food, growth and time. Lancet 1962; 621–626.
26. Harding JE. The nutritional basis of the fetal origins of adult disease. Int J Epidemiol 2001; 30:15–23.
27. Barker DJP, Eriksson JG, Forsén T, Osmond C. Fetal origins of adult disease: strength of effects and biological basis. Int J Epidemiology 2002; 31:1235–1239.
28. Brenner BM, Chertow GM. Congenital oligonephropathy: an inborn cause of adult hypertension and progressive renal injury? Curr Opin Nephrol Hypertens 1993; 2:691–695.
29. Phillips DIW. Insulin resistance as a programmed response to fetal undernutrition. Diabetologia 1996; 39:1119–1122.
30. Barker DJP, Forsén T, Uutela A, Osmond C, Eriksson JG. Size at birth and resilience to the effects of poor living conditions in adult life: longitudinal study. BMJ 2001; 323:1273–1276.
31. Marmot M, Wilkinson RG. Psychosocial and material pathways in the relation between income and health: a response to Lynch et al. BMJ 2001; 322:1233–1236.
32. Phillips DIW, Walker BR, Reynolds RM, et al. Low birth weight predicts elevated plasma cortisol concentrations in adults from 3 populations. Hypertension 2000; 35:1301–1306.
33. Curhan GC, Chertow GM, Willett WC, et al. Birth weight and adult hypertension and obesity in women. Circulation 1996; 94:1310–1315.
34. Huxley RR, Shiell AW, Law CM. The role of size at birth and postnatal catch-up growth in determining systolic blood pressure: a systematic review of the literature. J Hypertens 2000; 18:815–831.
35. Ingelfinger JR. Is microanatomy destiny? N Eng J Med 2003; 348:99,100.
36. Keller G, Zimmer G, Mall G, Ritz E, Amann K. Nephron Number in Patients with Primary Hypertension. N Eng J Med 2003; 348:101–108.
37. Ylihärsilä H, Eriksson JG, Forsén T, Kajantie E, Osmond C, Barker DJP. Self-perpetuating effects of birth size on blood pressure levels in elderly people. Hypertension 2003; 41:446–450.
38. Lackland DT, Egan BM, Syddall HE, Barker DJP. Associations between birthweight and antihypertensive medication in black and white Americans. Hypertension 2002; 39:179–183.
39. Eriksson JG, Forsen T, Tuomilehto J, Osmond C, Barker DJP. Early adiposity rebound in childhood and risk of type 2 diabetes in adult life. Diabetologia 2003; 46:190–194.
40. Rolland-Cachera MF, Deheeger M, Guilloud-Bataille M, Avons P, Patois E, Sempe M. Tracking the development of adiposity from one month of age to adulthood. Ann Hum Biol 1987; 14:219–229.
41. Bhargava SK, Sachdev HS, Fall CHD, et al. Relation of serial changes in childhood body mass index to impaired glucose tolerance in young adulthood. N Eng J Med 2004; 350:865–875.
42. Metcalfe NB, Monaghan P. Compensation for a bad start: grow now, pay later? Trends Ecol Evol 2001; 16:254–260.
43. Widdowson EM, Crabb DE, Milner RDG. Cellular development of some human organs before birth. Arch Dis Child 1972; 47:652–655.
44. Eriksson JG, Forsen T, Jaddoe VWV, Osmond C, Barker DJP. Effects of size at birth and childhood growth on the insulin resistance syndrome in elderly individuals. Diabetologia 2002; 45:342–348.
45. Eriksson JG, Lindi V, Uusitupa M, et al. The effects of the Pro12Ala polymorphism of the peroxisome proliferator-activated receptor-γ2 gene on insulin sensitivity and insulin metabolism interact with size at birth. Diabetes 2002; 51:2321–2324.
46. Barker DJP, Forsén T, Eriksson JG, Osmond C. Growth and living conditions in childhood and hypertension in adult life: longitudinal study. J Hypertens 2002; 20:1951–1956.

47. Kuh D, Ben-Shlomo Y. A Life-Course Approach to Chronic Disease Epidemiology. Oxford University Press, Oxford, 1997.

48. Huxley R, Neil A, Collins R. Unravelling the fetal origins hypothesis. Lancet 2002; 360:2074, 2075.

49. Dubos R. Mirage of Health. Allen and Unwin, London, 1960.

50. Ravelli ACJ, van der Meulen JHP, Michels RPJ, et al. Glucose tolerance in adults after prenatal exposure to famine. Lancet 1998; 351:173–177.

51. Kramer MS. Effects of energy and protein intakes on pregnancy outcome: an overview of the research evidence from controlled clinical trials. Am J Clin Nutr 1993; 58:627–635.

52. Barker DJP. Mothers, Babies and Health in Later Life. Churchill Livingstone, Edinburgh, 1998.

53. Harding JE, Liu L, Evans P, Oliver M, Gluckman P. Intrauterine feeding of the growth-retarded fetus: can we help? Early Hum Dev 1992; 29:193–197.

54. Walker SK, Hartwick KM, Robinson JS. Long-term effects on offspring of exposure of oocytes and embryos to chemical and physical agents. Hum Reprod Update 2000; 6:564–567.

55. Stewart RJC, Sheppard H, Preece R, Waterlow JC. The effect of rehabilitation at different stages of development of rats marginally malnourished for ten to twelve generations. Br J Nutr 1980; 43:403–412.

56. Emanuel I, Filakti H, Alberman E, Evans SJW. Intergenerational studies of human birthweight from the 1958 birth cohort. I. Evidence for a multigenerational effect. Br J Obstet Gynaecol 1992; 99:67–74.

57. Godfrey KM, Barker DJP, Robinson S, Osmond C. Maternal birthweight and diet in pregnancy in relation to the infant's thinness at birth. Br J Obstet Gynaecol 1997; 104:663–667.

58. Robinson JS, Owens JA, de Barro T, et al. Maternal nutrition and fetal growth. In: Ward RHT, Smith SK, Donnai D, eds. Early fetal growth and development. Royal College of Obstetricians and Gynaecologists, London, 1994, pp. 317–334.

59. Godfrey K, Robinson S, Barker DJP, Osmond C, Cox V. Maternal nutrition in early and late pregnancy in relation to placental and fetal growth. BMJ 1996; 312:410–414.

60. Lumey LH. Compensatory placental growth after restricted maternal nutrition in early pregnancy. Placenta 1998; 19:105–111.

61. Martyn CN, Barker DJP, Osmond C. Mothers' pelvic size, fetal growth, and death from stroke and coronary heart disease in men in the UK. Lancet 1996; 348:1264–1268.

62. Barker DJP, Bull AR, Osmond C, Simmonds SJ. Fetal and placental size and risk of hypertension in adult life. BMJ 1990; 301:259–262.

63. Robinson JS, Chidzanja S, Kind K, Lok F, Owens P, Owens JA. Placental control of fetal growth. Reprod Fertil Dev 1995; 7:333–344.

64. Belizan JM, Villar J, Bergel E, et al. Long term effect of calcium supplementation during pregnancy on the blood pressure of offspring: follow up of a randomised controlled trial. BMJ 1997; 315:281–285.

65. Roseboom TJ, van der Meulen JH, Osmond C, Barker DJ, Ravelli AC, Bleker OP. Plasma lipid profiles in adults after prenatal exposure to the Dutch famine. Am J Clin Nutr 2000; 72:1101–1106.

66. Roseboom TJ, van der Meulen JH, Osmond C, et al. Coronary heart disease after prenatal exposure to the Dutch famine, 1944-45. Heart 2000; 84:595–598.

67. Roseboom TJ, van der Meulen JH, van Montfrans GA, et al. Maternal nutrition during gestation and blood pressure in later life. J Hypertens 2001; 19:29–34.

68. Campbell DM, Hall MH, Barker DJP, Cross J, Shiell AW, Godfrey KM. Diet in pregnancy and the offspring's blood pressure 40 years later. Br J Obstet Gynaecol 1996; 103:273–280.

69. Shiell AW, Campbell DM, Hall MH, Barker DJ. Diet in late pregnancy and glucose-insulin metabolism of the offspring 40 years later. Br J Obstet Gynaecol 2000; 107:890–895.

70. Rush D. Effects of changes in maternal energy and protein intake during pregnancy, with special reference to fetal growth. In: Sharp F, Fraser RB, Milner RDG, eds. Fetal Growth. Royal College of Obstetricians and Gynaecologists, London, 1989, pp. 203–233.

71. Shiell AW, Campbell-Brown M, Haselden S, Robinson S, Godfrey KM, Barker DJP. A high meat, low carbohydrate diet in pregnancy: relation to adult blood pressure in the offspring. Hypertension 2001; 38:1282–1288.

72. Herrick K, Phillips DIW, Haselden S, Shiell AW, Campbell-Brown M, Godfrey KM. Maternal consumption of a high-meat, low-carbohydrate diet in late pregnancy: relation to adult cortisol concentrations in the offspring. J Clin Endocrin Metab 2003; 88:3554–3560.

73. James WPT. Long-term fetal programming of body composition and longevity. Nutr Rev 1997; 55:S41–S43.

74. Catalano PM. Husten LP, Thomas AJ, Fung CM. Effect of maternal metabolism on fetal growth and body composition. Diabetes Care 1998; 21:B85–B90.

75. Silverman BL, Purdy LP, Metzger BE. The intrauterine environment: implications for the offspring of diabetic mothers. Diabetes Reviews 1996; 4:21–35.

76. Fall CHD, Stein CE, Kumaran K, et al. Size at birth, maternal weight, and type 2 diabetes in South India. Diabet Med 1998; 15:220–227.

77. Mi J, Law C, Zhang K-L, Osmond C, Stein C, Barker DJP. Effects of infant birthweight and maternal body mass index in pregnancy on components of the insulin resistance syndrome in China. Ann Intern Med 2000; 132:253–260.

78. Margetts BM, Rowland MGM, Foord FA, Cruddas AM, Cole TJ, Barker DJP. The relation of maternal weight to the blood pressures of Gambian children. Int J Epidemiol 1991; 20:938–943.

79. Godfrey KM, Forrester T, Barker DJP, et al. Maternal nutritional status in pregnancy and blood pressure in childhood. Br J Obstet Gynaecol 1994; 101:398–403.

80. Clark PM, Atton C, Law CM, Shiell A, Godfrey K, Barker DJP. Weight gain in pregnancy, triceps skinfold thickness and blood pressure in the offspring. Obstet Gynaecol 1998; 91:103–107.

81. Adair LS, Kuzawa CW, Borja J. Maternal energy stores and diet composition during pregnancy program adolescent blood pressure. Circulation 2001; 104:1034–1039.

82. Duggleby SL, Jackson AA. Relationship of maternal protein turnover and lean body mass during pregnancy and birth length. Clin Sc 2001; 101:65–72.

83. Cooper C, Javaid MK, Taylor P, Walker-Bone K, Dennison E, Arden N. The fetal origins of osteoporotic fracture. Calcif Tissue Int 2002; 70:391–394.

84. Thompson CH, Syddall HE, Rodin I, Osmond C, Barker DJP. Birth weight and the risk of depressive disorder in late life. Br J Psychiatry 2001; 179:450–455.

85. Jones P, Rodgers B, Murray R, Marmot M. Child developmental risk factors for adult schizophrenia in the British 1946 birth cohort. Lancet 1994; 344:1398–1402.

16 Trends in Dietary Guidelines Around the Global Village

Jayne V. Woodside, Geraldine Cuskelly, and Norman J. Temple

KEY POINTS

- Numerous countries have published food guides that provide advice on the overall diet for the general public. One example is the American Food Guide Pyramid.
- Other dietary recommendations published in different countries are those focused on reducing the risk of chronic disease; they are usually intended for health professionals.
- A third type of dietary recommendations concern nutrient intake. An example is the recommended dietary allowance used in the United States and Canada. These are intended for health professionals and play an important role in food labels.
- There is evidence suggesting that certain dietary supplements may be beneficial, especially folate, selenium, chromium, calcium, vitamin D, and fish oil.

1. INTRODUCTION

The ultimate goal of nutritional research is the provision of healthier foods. To allow people to make healthier food choices, research findings have to be translated into information that the majority of the general population can understand and accept. An educating process is required; governments attempt such education by using a set of nutritional recommendations or dietary guidelines that are evidence-based, authoritative, and comprehensible. This chapter examines the various attempts that have been made in a number of countries to formulate such recommendations. Various types of messages are transmitted from a consensus of nutritional scientists to both the general population and to health professionals.

Different sets of recommendations and dietary guidelines, have emerged since the late 1960s. They advise on how to make food choices that will give the best chance of long-term health. These guidelines are of two general types: one is based on foods ("eat five servings a day of fruit and vegetables") and is intended for the general public, whereas the other is based on particular food components, especially fat, sugar, dietary fiber, salt, and alcohol ("no more than 30% of energy from fat") and is directed mainly at health professionals. Unfortunately, conflicts can arise between the recommendations of, on the

From: *Nutritional Health: Strategies for Disease Prevention, Second Edition*
Edited by: N. J. Temple, T. Wilson, and D. R. Jacobs © Humana Press Inc., Totowa, NJ

one hand, nutritional scientists who formulate dietary guidelines and, on the other hand, the wishes of parts of the food industry who may see their profits threatened if the proposed guidelines are published and widely followed. This can result in dietary guidelines being watered down because of pressure from industry lobby groups.

The other type of dietary recommendations concern the quantities of essential nutrients that people should consume. For example, the American version has for many years been the recommended dietary allowances (RDAs). These technical numbers can then be converted into informational devices, for example, for use on food labels. In underdeveloped countries and communities, nutritional policy has been focused on attempts to reach the RDA (or an equivalent set of recommendations concerning essential nutrients) for as many people and nutrients as possible. In contrast, in affluent countries and communities, intakes near the RDA can be assumed for most nutrients for most people and the RDA may serve as an alert in rare cases of undernutrition.

These various types of public health nutrition recommendations are examined in this chapter. Finally, we discuss the merits of using supplements.

2. FOOD GUIDES

Numerous countries have published food guides that provide advice on the overall diet for the general public. Several of these have been reviewed by Painter and colleagues (1). The underlying idea is that dietary guidelines need to be expressed in terms of foods and in ordinary language. Food guides tend to center on a colored diagram or poster. Several examples are described in the following Subheadings.

2.1. United States

The food guide used in the United States is the Food Guide Pyramid (Fig. 1), developed by the US Department of Agriculture and first published in 1991. Its structure emphasizes the message that the bulk of the diet should comprise food from the grain (bread and cereal) group and, to a slightly lesser extent, from the vegetable and fruit groups. As we move up the pyramid, recommended consumption drops: from the milk and cheese group and from the meat, poultry, and fish group. At the top, consumption is least from fats, oils, and sweets. The pyramid is presently undergoing a major revision.

Nestle (2) has detailed the considerable controversy that accompanied the development of this document. This reflects the fact that official advice on diet is at least as much about appeasing special interest groups, especially the meat lobby, as it is about providing the best advice for improvement of the national health. A major source of the problem is that the government department given the job of producing the food guide was the US Department of Agriculture, whose *raison d'etre* is protection of the agriculture industry rather than national health.

Perhaps the biggest flaw in the pyramid is that it gives little guidance within each food group on the tremendous variation in nutritional quality of the different foods. For instance, within the grain group, there is no distinction between white bread and whole-grain bread. Similarly, fatty meats are lumped together with lean ones, and whole milk with skim.

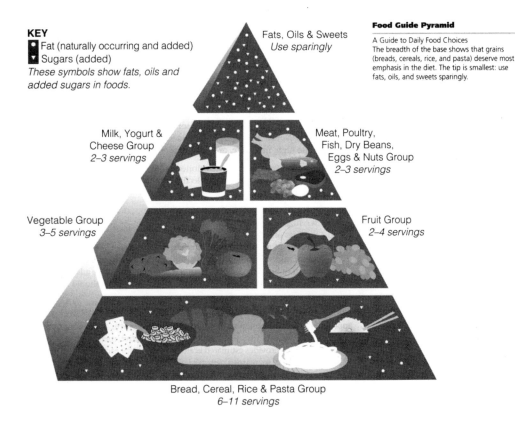

KEY
- Fat (naturally occurring and added)
- Sugars (added)

These symbols show fats, oils and added sugars in foods.

Fats, Oils & Sweets
Use sparingly

Food Guide Pyramid

A Guide to Daily Food Choices
The breadth of the base shows that grains (breads, cereals, rice, and pasta) deserve most emphasis in the diet. The tip is smallest: use fats, oils, and sweets sparingly.

Milk, Yogurt & Cheese Group
2–3 servings

Meat, Poultry, Fish, Dry Beans, Eggs & Nuts Group
2–3 servings

Vegetable Group
3–5 servings

Fruit Group
2–4 servings

Bread, Cereal, Rice & Pasta Group
6–11 servings

Fig. 1. Food Guide Pyramid. (Produced by the US Department of Agriculture. For the full color image and more useful information, *see* www.nal.usda.gov/fnic/Fpyr/pyramid.html.)

2.2. Canada

The food guide used in Canada is Canada's Food Guide to Healthy Eating (Fig. 2). This has three key differences from the American pyramid: (1) the food groups are portrayed as a rainbow (but with similar relative proportions of the different food groups); (2) fruit and vegetables are combined into one group; and (3) foods, such as fats and sweets (as well as alcoholic beverages and water), are not depicted on the actual rainbow drawing but are treated separately in a group called "Other Foods."

The guide states three times that foods lower in fat should be chosen more often. However, it is unclear what impact such advice is likely to have. The guide has similar inadequacies as those noted with respect to the American pyramid. The following words are written alongside the grain group: "Choose whole grain and enriched products more often." However, "enriched" usually means refined cereals that are depleted in fiber and numerous nutrients.

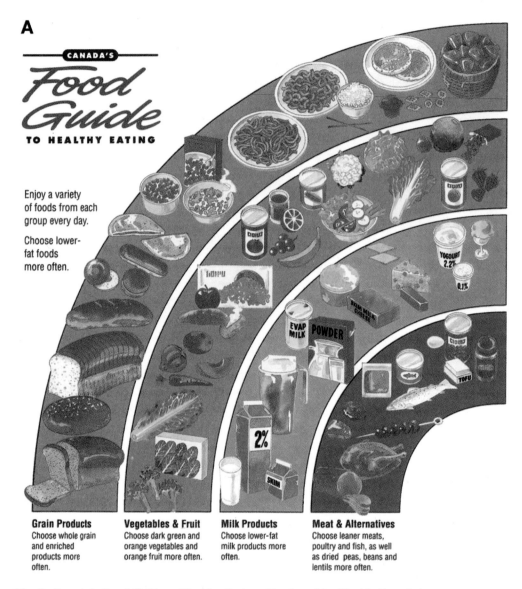

A

Enjoy a variety
of foods from each
group every day.

Choose lower-
fat foods
more often.

Grain Products	**Vegetables & Fruit**	**Milk Products**	**Meat & Alternatives**
Choose whole grain and enriched products more often.	Choose dark green and orange vegetables and orange fruit more often.	Choose lower-fat milk products more often.	Choose leaner meats, poultry and fish, as well as dried peas, beans and lentils more often.

Fig. 2. Canada's Food Guide to Healthy Eating. (Produced by Health Canada.)

2.3. United Kingdom

The Balance of Good Health is a pictorial food guide produced by the Food Standards Agency showing the proportion and types of foods that are needed to make up a healthy balanced diet. The food guide is depicted as a plate with food sectors. It resembles the Canadian guide in that fruit and vegetables are combined into one group, and the US guide in that fatty and sugary foods are included in the pictorial representation.

The Balance of Good Health is based on the UK government's Eight Guidelines for a Healthy Diet, which are:

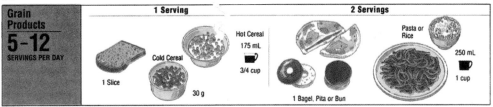

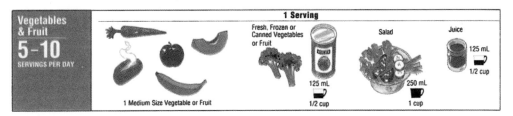

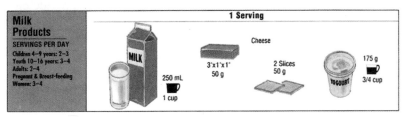

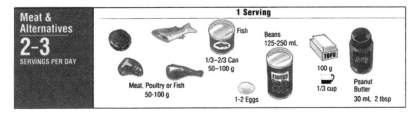

Fig. 2. *(continued from opposite page)*

1. Enjoy your food.
2. Eat a variety of different foods.
3. Eat the right amount to be a healthy weight.
4. Eat plenty of foods rich in starch and fiber.
5. Eat plenty of fruit and vegetables.
6. Do not eat too many foods that contain a lot of fat.
7. Do not have sugary foods and drinks too often.
8. If you drink alcohol, drink sensibly.

2.4. Other Countries

The Swedish guide is plate-shaped, similar to the UK guide, but has one distinct feature: written prominently across it are the words: "Choose fiber-rich and low-fat products." The guide used in China and Korea is a pagoda that resembles the American pyramid. The Australian food guide predates the US guide and is similar to it.

2.5. Comment

Some food guides are limited by not including foods representative of diverse cultures. To address this in the United States, the Food Guide Pyramid has been adapted to include additional foods so that it can be used by other cultures, such as people from Southeast Asia *(3)*.

These various food guides all convey essentially the same message. If followed, then the diet will almost certainly provide all nutrients in amounts that meet RDA recommendations. The guides encourage consumption of at least five servings of fruit and vegetables daily and also encourage a diet that is rich in starch but modest in protein. However, those guides, such as the American pyramid, that do not emphasize high-fiber choices can easily result in a diet low in fiber. For example, six servings of refined cereals, three servings of whole fruit or vegetables, and two servings of fruit or vegetable juice will provide only about 15 g of fiber. Similarly, the guide does not emphasize low-fat choices. This is a more complex issue. First, it can result in a diet high in fat. Second, although people do strive to reduce their fat intake, the diet may still be unbalanced in that low-fat foods often have their fat replaced by refined carbohydrates (sugar and starch). Third, there is little guidance regarding the type of fats to cut down on. As a result, the diet can still be high in saturated fat (and trans fats) but low in polyunsaturated fats, especially n-3 fats.

Several differences between the food guides are noteworthy. An important difference concerns the use of quantitative recommendations. This is done in the United States, Canada, Australia, United Kingdom, China, and Korea but not in Portugal, Mexico, and Sweden. Specifying the recommended numbers of servings might be expected to assist consumers in selecting a healthier diet. However, to what extent individuals pay attention to the recommended amounts is not known. As with several other aspects of the construction of these food guides, this is an area that deserves investigation.

Fruits and vegetables are grouped together in some guides (Canada, United Kingdom, China, Korea, Portugal, and Mexico) but are in separate groups in others (Germany, United States, Sweden, and Australia). In the United States and Canada, potatoes go with other vegetables; in Sweden potatoes and root vegetables are given their own group distinct from other vegetables. Several countries—Korea, the United Kingdom, Portugal, Germany, and Mexico—include potatoes with grains. Keeping potatoes separate from other vegetables is probably sensible, as potatoes are poor in phytochemicals, have a high glycemic index, and are often consumed as fries (and may therefore have a high content of oxidized fat).

Another inconsistency is in the placement of legumes. The American pyramid places soybeans and "legumes" with vegetables but "dry beans" with meat, poultry, and fish. In Canada, beans are included with meat, hence the name of that food group: "meat and alternatives." This schism in the placement of legumes reflects the fact that legumes are a low-fat, protein-rich alternative to meat but are also a good source of fiber and various nutrients, such as folate.

One problem with the food guides is that manufactured products often contain mixtures of diverse foods or their derivatives, along with several additives. Accordingly, placing manufactured foods in the pyramid is often difficult. How does a shopper perceive a label on, for example, "Breakfast Apple Crisp"? Is this food a valuable means to obtain fruit or is it a significant source of fat and sugar?

3. FOOD COMPONENT GUIDELINES
TO COUNTER CHRONIC DISEASE

Globally, different agencies publish sets of dietary recommendations that are aimed at reducing the impact of chronic disease and are usually intended for health professionals. The clear intention of these guides is that the advice filters down to the general population.

3.1. United States

Several professional bodies in the United States publish dietary recommendations. Among the most well-known are those from the American Heart Association *(4)* which, not surprisingly, focus on the prevention of cardiovascular disease. Their recommendations include:

- Limit total fat intake to lower than 30% of energy.
- Limit intake of saturated fat and trans-fatty acids to less than 10% of energy.
- Limit cholesterol to less than 300 mg/d.
- Limit salt to less than 6 g/d.
- Limit alcohol consumption (no more than two drinks per day for men or one drink per day for women).
- Emphasize low-fat and fat-free dairy products.
- Maintain a healthy body weight.

3.2. Canada

Canada also has a set of guidelines formulated with the goal of reducing the impact of chronic disease. These are Nutrition Recommendations for Canadians. They are broadly similar to the above guidelines from the American Heart Association. However, they make no mention of cholesterol but do provide advice on fluoride and caffeine. These guidelines are currently being revised.

3.3. World Health Organization

The 1990 dietary guidelines from the World Health Organization (WHO) *(5)* are also broadly similar to the American ones. Whereas the Canadian guidelines recommend that carbohydrate should contribute 55% of energy, WHO recommends a figure of 55–75%. This likely reflects the fact that the target populations for WHO include millions of the world's poor who, out of necessity, consume a high-carbohydrate diet, often centered on polished rice. WHO also recommends a fiber intake of 27–40 g/d, protein of 10–15% of energy, and refined sugars of less than 10% of energy.

These guidelines were modified in 2003 *(6)*. The noteworthy changes were as follows. Specific goals were set for n-6 polyunsaturated fats (5–8% of energy), n-3 fats (1–2%), and trans-fatty acids (<1%). The maximum recommended salt intake was lowered to 5 g/d. There is no longer a specific recommendation for dietary fiber but rather a general recommendation for fruit, vegetables, and whole-grain foods.

3.4. United Kingdom

The Committee on Medical Aspects of Food and Nutrition Policy (COMA) consists of independent experts drawn from research, academia, clinical medicine, and public health. The committee also has members with a background in the food industry and others who represent consumers. Its reports provide the UK government with advice on matters relating to nutrition, diet, and health. In 1991 the committee published quantitative population goals for fats and carbohydrates as part of a report on dietary reference values (7). Of the population's average percentage of total energy (including alcohol), total fat should average 33%, of which saturated fat should be 10%, polyunsaturated fat 6% (not more than 10%), and trans-fatty acids not more than 2%. Nonstarch polysaccharides should be 18–24 g/d (corresponding to around 30–35 g/d dietary fiber) and nonmilk extrinsic sugars should not exceed 60 g/d or 10% of total dietary energy.

COMA was disbanded in March 2000. A new committee, The Scientific Advisory Committee on Nutrition, has been set up, which continues to advise the UK Health Department and the Food Standards Agency on nutrition.

4. RECOMMENDATIONS FOR NUTRIENT INTAKE

The other major set of dietary recommendations concerns the intake of nutrients. As before, numerous countries produce their own sets of standards, and, again, they are intended primarily for health professionals. The information they provide reaches the public in different ways. In particular, they also play an important role in food labels.

4.1. United States and Canada

The RDA reflects the average daily amount of a nutrient considered necessary to meet the needs of most healthy people. The RDA has been in use in the United States for several decades, longer in fact than the type of dietary guidelines described above. In the late 1990s a new set of recommendations were formulated: the dietary reference intakes (DRIs). DRIs were developed by the Institute of Medicine of the National Academy of Sciences together with Health Canada and are used in both the United States and Canada. The RDA is now part of the DRI. For those nutrients where there is insufficient information to establish a RDA, estimates are made, known as adequate intakes (AI). Values of RDA and AI are given for 14 vitamins and 12 minerals. Values are also given for energy, carbohydrates, essential (n-3 and n-6) fatty acids, protein, and dietary fiber. Tables are broken down by age and sex. DRI includes two other tables. The estimated average requirement (EAR) is the mean requirement of a group for a particular nutrient. The EAR for a nutrient will meet the nutrient need of half the population within that age and gender group. The other table within the DRI gives tolerable upper intake levels (UL). This is the maximum amount of potentially toxic nutrients that appears safe for most healthy people to consume on a regular basis. Whereas RDA and AI are targets to aim for, UL provides a warning against overconsumption of nutrients, especially from supplements.

The Canadian equivalent of RDA was for many years the Recommended Nutrient Intakes (RNI). However, as noted in the previous paragraph, Canada collaborated with the United States in the development of DRI. At the time of writing (2005) the RNI are being phased out and DRI phased in. The logic behind this move is to help harmonize food labels across the world's largest trading border. The most notable differences between

RNI and RDA are that the latter have significantly higher values for calcium, folate, and vitamins C, D, and E.

4.2. United Kingdom

Early COMA reports based their recommendations on recommended daily intake and RDA. These were set deliberately high (compared with average requirements) to minimize the risk of undernutrition. The intention was to apply recommended daily intake and RDA to groups of people rather than to individuals.

New values, called dietary reference values (DRV), were set in a 1991 report *(7)*. This report improved the scientific basis for making practical dietary guidelines in a number of ways. It looked at the concept of health, not merely the avoidance of deficiency diseases. It also took a new approach by defining more than one figure for each nutrient, thus recognizing the broad range of requirements of individuals within a population. Finally, although the criteria to determine the values were not always backed by strong evidence, it was judged to be the best possible and set a framework for amendments as new information from research becomes available.

The DRV are based on the assessment of the distribution of requirements for each nutrient, and aid interpretation of dietary information on both groups and individuals. They are estimates of requirements for a population, and are intended to provide guidance rather than make recommendations. Three values are defined. First, the EAR is the mean requirement of a group for a particular nutrient or for energy. About half will usually need more than the EAR, and half will need less. Second, the RNI is the amount of a nutrient (calculated as mean EAR + 2 SD) that is sufficient for almost all individuals in a group (about 97%). It therefore exceeds the requirement of most people and habitual intakes above RNI are almost certain to be adequate. Finally, the lower reference nutrient intake (LRNI) is the amount of a nutrient or energy (calculated as mean EAR – 2 SD) that is sufficient for only a few individuals in a group who have low needs. Habitual intakes below the LRNI by an individual will almost certainly be inadequate. The DRV has obvious similarities to the American DRI: EAR is essentially the same in both sets of guides, whereas the RNI (of the DRV) is equivalent to the RDA and AI (of the DRI).

DRV are scientifically more sound and comprehensive than in the preceding publications, as DRV were set for energy, protein, fats, sugars, starches, nonstarch polysaccharides, 13 vitamins, and 15 minerals. These guidelines for nutrient intake can be used as yardsticks for surveys (EAR), in guidance of dietary composition (RNI), for food labels (EAR), and to provide a general guide in assessing the adequacy of an individual's diet (LRNI/RNI).

5. THE MERITS OF SUPPLEMENTS

The conventional wisdom is that we can obtain adequate amounts of all nutrients from a normal diet. In other words, following the American pyramid will result in a diet that meets the RDA (and likewise for guides in other countries). Moreover, there is a dearth of hard evidence that supplements of most vitamins and minerals will have a favorable impact on health. But, on the other hand, for several nutrients (and fish oil) a case can be made for the merits of supplements. The evidence is most clear-cut among people whose diets are marginally deficient, and in such groups as pregnant women and the elderly. This evidence is reviewed here.

5.1. Folate

Folate provides perhaps the most compelling example that supplements of a nutrient may be warranted. Intervention trials have demonstrated that supplements of folic acid (the form of folate used in supplements) can prevent a substantial proportion of neural tube defects, such as spina bifida (8). In 1996, in response to this evidence, the Food and Drug Administration mandated that all grain foods in the United States be supplemented with folic acid. Quite likely folic acid supplements only achieve this benefit because so many women consume diets poor in the vitamin.

Several cohort studies have reported a strong protective association between blood level or dietary intake of folate and risk of coronary heart disease (CHD) (9–12). Subjects whose folate status is in the top quartile or quintile may have a risk of CHD that is 30% or more lower than those in the bottom group. This may be partly explained by the fact that folic acid is effective at lowering the level of blood homocysteine (13).

Evidence has also appeared in recent years indicating that folate may also be protective against some types of cancer, especially colorectal and pancreatic cancer (14–16). It may also be protective against breast cancer, especially in women with a relatively high alcohol intake (17).

5.2. Selenium

There is strong evidence that selenium exerts an anticarcinogenic action. This has been reported in numerous epidemiological studies and in one controlled trial. This is reviewed in Chapter 9.

5.3. Chromium

This mineral is reviewed in Chapter 5. It appears that a substantial fraction of the population may have a suboptimal intake of chromium. This apparently reduces insulin sensitivity and may thereby be a factor in the chain of events leading to type 2 diabetes. Chromium supplementation at a dose of 200–1000 μ/d, especially in the form of chromium picolinate, seems to help improve insulin sensitivity and glucose control.

5.4. Calcium

The RDA for calcium is 1200 mg for adults aged over 50 yr. This is equivalent to a liter of milk. There is no doubt that large numbers of people consume inadequate amounts of the mineral. This is especially the case in non-Caucasians, who frequently have lactose intolerance. A survey in Canada revealed that a quarter of women have a calcium intake of less than 500 mg/d (18).

There is good evidence that a long-term low intake of calcium plays an important role in the development of osteoporosis (19). The mineral may also be protective against hypertension (19).

5.5. Vitamin D

In the United States, Canada, and some other countries milk is fortified with this nutrient. But if milk consumption is low, then vitamin D status may be poor because there are few other dietary sources. This is especially the case for those living in northern latitudes, such as Canada and the northern states of the United States, because of lack of ultraviolet light from sunshine for much of the year. Vitamin D insufficiency is most common in the elderly. This may be a risk factor for osteoporosis *(20)*. The possibility that vitamin D is also protective against cancer is discussed in Chapter 9. Caution must be exercised when using vitamin D supplements as there is a risk of toxicity because of overdosing: the DRI states that the UL is only 5–10 times higher than the RDA.

5.6. Fish Oil

Impressive evidence has accumulated indicating that fish (especially fatty fish) and fish oil, and their active ingredient, long-chain n-3 fatty acids, have a protective action against the risk of CHD, sudden death, and stroke *(21)*. This is reviewed in Chapter 8. For a person who chooses not to eat fish regularly, fish oil may provide most or all of the benefit.

5.7. Antioxidant Vitamins

Epidemiological evidence has repeatedly suggested that supplements of antioxidant vitamins, vitamin E in particular, may protect against cardiovascular disease *(22)*. However, intervention trials with clinical end points have failed to show clear evidence of benefit with supplements of vitamin E or β-carotene *(22)*. In fact, in the case of β-carotene supplementation in smokers, there is some evidence that such supplementation may actually increase cancer risk *(23,24)*. These trials should act as a caution that solid evidence is required before jumping to conclusions that supplements may actually prevent disease.

5.8. Comment

It seems likely that in most cases where supplements appear to be beneficial, this is only because large numbers of people have an inadequate diet and may therefore be marginally deficient in various nutrients. For that reason our first priority should clearly be to encourage people to improve the overall quality of their diets, but at the same time, we need to be realistic and recognize that a substantial section of the population will continue to eat a far from ideal diet. Moreover, it may well be that for maximum effectiveness some of the supplements discussed here need to be consumed in amounts greater than is obtainable from a normal diet.

The conclusions reached here are generally consistent with those made by Willett and Stampfer *(25)*:

Given the greater likelihood of benefit than harm, and considering the low cost, we conclude that a daily multivitamin that does not exceed the RDA of its component vitamins makes sense for most adults. Substantial data suggest that higher intakes of folic acid, vitamin B_6, vitamin B_{12}, and vitamin D will benefit many people, and a multivitamin will ensure an adequate intake of other vitamins for which the evidence of benefit is indirect. A multivitamin is especially important for women who might become pregnant; for persons who regularly consume one or two alcoholic drinks per day; for the elderly, who tend to absorb vitamin B_{12} poorly and are often deficient in vitamin D; for vegans, who require supplemental vitamin B_{12}; and for poor urban residents, who may be unable to afford adequate intakes of fruit and vegetables.

The ideal supplement should be safe, effective, and cheap. Recent discoveries in nutrition have brought such a supplement several steps closer to becoming a reality.

There is considerable skepticism over the use of supplements within the nutrition community. This is readily understandable in light of the enormous dishonesty that accompanies the marketing of supplements, as documented in Chapter 17. It is therefore essential that recommendations for the use of supplements be based on solid evidence stemming from the results of well-conducted studies.

6. CONCLUSIONS

The various sets of recommendations described in this chapter are a work in progress. The three altogether different types of recommendations serve entirely distinct purposes. Food guides, such as the American pyramid, are directed at the general population and, for that reason, are meant to be easily understood and highly flexible, something that is far easier to aim for than to achieve. But as we have seen, the various guidelines often fail to put enough emphasis on a generous intake of fiber and on clear quantitative and qualitative advice concerning fat intake. There are also numerous differences between the guides in the placement of different foods. More research is clearly needed into how to optimize the presentation of the guides so that users are encouraged to consume the healthiest diet. As national diets around the world continue their rapid evolution, the food guides will also need to evolve.

The guidelines concerned with countering chronic disease are also a work in progress. As they are intended for health professionals, there is obviously far less of a challenge in grabbing the attention of the reader. However, the contrast in the various guidelines points to the debates that have taken place but have not yet been settled. Obviously, it is a question of focusing on the most important nutritional issues. But what are they? The apparent disagreement is reflected in the differences in the inclusion of such dietary components as salt, cholesterol, fiber, and caffeine.

The development of the DRI in the United States and Canada is dramatic in that one set of recommendations concerning intake of nutrients (the RDA) was replaced by several tables. Clearly, the committee that developed the DRI felt that the obvious loss in terms of simplicity was a necessary price to pay for giving health professionals a more complete set of tools, and a similar argument can be made for the introduction of DRV in the United Kingdom.

There are several challenges in developing recommendations concerning nutrient intake. One is differentiating between two distinct objectives: achieving a diet that is adequate in each nutrient so that there is *no risk of deficiency*, and achieving an *optimal intake for health*. Although not explicitly stated, the section on supplements focuses more on the latter than the former.

Clearly, guidelines must address the key nutritional issues of their target population. In developed countries, the focus will be primarily on the prevention of chronic diseases. But in less developed countries malnutrition is still a serious problem. However, such chronic diseases as obesity are becoming rapidly more prevalent in many less developed countries and food guides must stay abreast of these changes in population health.

One conclusion is inescapable: this entire field will be the scene of considerable debate, controversy, and research for years to come.

REFERENCES

1. Painter J, Rah JH, Lee YK. Comparison of international food guide pictorial representations. J Am Diet Assoc 2002; 102:483–489.
2. Nestle M. Food politics. How the Food Industry Influences Nutrition and Health. University of California Press, Berkeley, Calif, 2002.
3. Achterberg, C, McDonnell E, Bagby R. How to put the Food Guide Pyramid into practice. J Am Diet Assoc 1994; 94:1030–1035.
4. Krauss RM, Eckel RH, Howard B, Appel LJ, Daniels SR, Deckelbaum RJ, et al. AHA Dietary Guidelines: revision 2000: A statement for healthcare professionals from the Nutrition Committee of the American Heart Association. Circulation 2000; 102:2284–2299.
5. Report of a WHO study group. Diet, nutrition and the prevention of chronic diseases. Tech Rep Ser 797. World Health Organization, Geneva, 1990.
6. Report of a joint WHO/FAO expert consultation. Diet, nutrition and the prevention of chronic diseases. Tech Rep Ser 916. World Health Organization, Geneva, 2003.
7. Committee on Medical Aspects of Food Policy. Dietary Reference Values for Food Energy and Nutrients for the United Kingdom. HMSO, London, 1991.
8. MRC Vitamin Study Research Group. Prevention of neural tube defects: results of the Medical Research Council Vitamin Study. Lancet 1991; 338:131–137.
9. Voutilainen S, Rissanen TH, Virtanen J, Lakka TA, Salonen JT. Low dietary folate intake is associated with an excess incidence of acute coronary events: The Kuopio Ischemic Heart Disease Risk Factor Study. Circulation 2001; 103:2674–2680.
10. Chasan-Taber L, Selhub J, Rosenberg IH, et al. A prospective study of folate and vitamin B6 and risk of myocardial infarction in US physicians. J Am Coll Nutr 1996; 15:136–143.
11. Rimm EB, Willett WC, Hu FB, et al. Folate and vitamin B6 from diet and supplements in relation to risk of coronary heart disease among women. JAMA 1998; 279:359–364.
12. Folsom AR, Nieto FJ, McGovern PG, et al. Prospective study of coronary heart disease incidence in relation to fasting total homocysteine, related genetic polymorphisms, and B vitamins: the Atherosclerosis Risk in Communities (ARIC) study. Circulation 1998; 98:204–210.
13. Wald DS, Bishop L, Wald NJ, et al. Randomized trial of folic acid supplementation and serum homocysteine levels. Arch Intern Med 2001; 161:695–700.
14. Kim YI. Folate and carcinogenesis: evidence, mechanisms, and implications. J Nutr Biochem 1999; 10:66–88.
15. Kim YI. Folate and cancer prevention: a new medical application of folate beyond hyperhomocysteinemia and neural tube defects. Nutr Rev 1999; 57:314–321.
16. La Vecchia C, Negri E, Pelucchi C, Franceschi S. Dietary folate and colorectal cancer. Int J Cancer 2002; 102:545–547.
17. Rohan TE, Jain MG, Howe GR, Miller AB. Dietary folate consumption and breast cancer risk. J Natl Cancer Inst 2000; 92:266–269.
18. Gray-Donald K, Jacobs-Starkey L, Johnson-Down L. Food habits of Canadians: reduction in fat intake over a generation. Can J Public Health 2000; 91:381–385.
19. Heaney RP. Calcium intake and the prevention of chronic disease. From osteoporosis to premenstrual syndrome. In: Wilson T, Temple NJ, eds. Nutritional Health: Strategies for Disease Prevention. Humana Press, Totowa, NJ, 2001, pp. 31–50.
20. Gennari C. Calcium and vitamin D nutrition and bone disease of the elderly. Public Health Nutr 2001; 4:547–559.
21. Kris-Etherton PM, Harris WS, Appel LJ, for the Nutrition Committee. Fish consumption, fish oil, omega-3 fatty acids, and cardiovascular disease. Circulation 2002; 106:2747–2757.
22. Young IS, Woodside JV. Antioxidants in health and disease. J Clin Pathol 2001; 54:176–186.
23. Omenn GA, Goodman GE, Thornquist MD, et al. The effects of a combination of β-carotene and vitamin A on lung cancer and cardiovascular disease. N Engl J Med 1996; 334:1150–1155.
24. Albanes D, Heinonen OP, Huttunen JK, et al. Effects of α-tocopherol and β-carotene supplements on cancer incidence in the Alpha-Tocopherol Beta-Carotene Cancer Prevention Study. Am J Clin Nutr 1995; 62:1427S–1430S.
25. Willett WC, Stampfer MJ. Clinical practice. What vitamins should I be taking, doctor? N Engl J Med 2001; 345:1819–1824.

17 Marketing Dietary Supplements for Health and Profit

Norman J. Temple and Diane H. Morris

Hope springs eternal in the human breast.
—A. Pope, Essay on Man, Epistle i.

KEY POINTS

- Use of dietary supplements has increased rapidly in recent years and around half of people in North America now use supplements regularly.
- Supplements are marketed by a variety of different methods, including health food stores, infomercials, multilevel marketing, bulk mail, spam e-mails, and internet websites.
- A large part of the marketing of supplements involves giving information that is unreliable or dishonest.
- There is very little regulation of the marketing of supplements in the United States. However, Canada is now in the process of enforcing strict regulations.
- Advice is given for evaluating claims made for supplements and advice for the general public.

1. INTRODUCTION

Dietary supplements are defined in the United States as vitamins, minerals, amino acids, herbs, enzymes and extracts, metabolites, constituents, and/or concentrates derived from plants and animals. They are sold as liquids, tablets, capsules, powders, soft gels, and geltabs *(1)*. In Canada, dietary supplements are regulated as natural health products and include vitamins and minerals, herbal and homeopathic remedies, traditional medicines (e.g., Chinese), probiotics, essential fatty acids, amino acids, and other products *(2)*. These products are not conventional foods but are designed to supplement the diet.

Regulating the colossal and growing dietary supplement industry and protecting consumers from fraudulent and misleading products and health claims is a daunting enterprise. Clearly, dietary supplement manufacturers have succeeded in convincing consumers to buy their products, but an important question remains unanswered: What benefits do consumers receive from the billions of dollars they spend on supplements? Our aim in this chapter is to examine the main methods of marketing supplements,

From: *Nutritional Health: Strategies for Disease Prevention, Second Edition*
Edited by: N. J. Temple, T. Wilson, and D. R. Jacobs © Humana Press Inc., Totowa, NJ

provide examples of egregious marketing strategies and claims, review the current regulatory status of dietary supplements in Canada and the United States, and outline ways in which health professionals can help consumers protect themselves from unscrupulous or even dishonest supplement marketers. What is especially remarkable is the meager amount of peer-reviewed research that has investigated this area and the effect that this lack of research has on our ability to make recommendations regarding informed supplement use.

2. GROWTH OF THE DIETARY SUPPLEMENT INDUSTRY

In 2001 US consumers spent almost $18 billion on dietary supplements, including $4.2 billion for herbs and other botanical remedies *(3)*. In one 2002 survey, more than two-thirds (69%) of US adults reported taking supplements *(4)*. The median intake was one pill per day. However, other studies have found lower levels of supplement use. Findings from National Health and Nutrition Examination Survey (1999–2000) revealed that 52% of US adults reported using vitamin/mineral supplements in the previous month *(5)*. A survey carried out in 2000 found that 34% of Americans took a vitamin/mineral supplement every day and 39% took one every month *(6)*. The latter survey also reported that herbal supplements were taken by 6% of Americans daily and by 8% monthly. Canadian surveys revealed that 41% of adults questioned had taken a supplement on the day of the survey *(7)*, whereas 68% had taken a supplement in the previous month *(8)*.

The use of dietary supplements has increased sharply in recent years *(5,6)*; sales increased nearly 80% between 1994 and 2000 *(9)*. According to a Canadian survey conducted in 2000, the use of vitamins rose 10% during the previous 2 yr, whereas the use of herbal supplements jumped threefold in the previous 3 yr *(8)*.

The profile of people most likely to use dietary supplements are female, older, white, nonsmokers, regular exercisers, and better educated *(4–11)*. Supplement use tends to be higher among those with a higher income *(8,10)*, although this is not a consistent finding *(9)*. Two studies reported that supplement use is highest in those who are healthiest *(5,7)*, but one study indicated the reverse *(10)*.

3. MARKETING STRATEGIES USED BY MANUFACTURERS

Dietary supplements are among the hottest items sold in grocery stores, pharmacies, supermarkets, national discount chain stores, and health food stores, as well as through TV programs, the Internet, direct sales, and mail-order catalogs *(12)*. This section describes some marketing strategies used by manufacturers.

A few years ago a freshman at Eagle Rock Junior High won first prize at the Greater Idaho Falls Science Fair. He was attempting to show how conditioned we have become to alarmists practicing junk science and spreading fear of everything in our environment. In his project he urged people to sign a petition demanding strict control or total elimination of the chemical "dihydrogen monoxide." And for plenty of good reasons: it can cause excessive sweating and vomiting; it is a major component in acid rain; it can cause severe burns in its gaseous state; accidental inhalation can kill you; it contributes to erosion; it decreases the effectiveness of automobile brakes; and it has been found in tumors of terminal cancer patients.

He asked 50 people if they supported a ban on the chemical. Forty-three said yes, six were undecided, and only one knew that the chemical was water. This anecdote indicates the very poor level of scientific knowledge of the large majority of people in North America. This fact is exploited by the people engaged in the marketing of supplements.

3.1. Direct Contact With Consumers

Health food stores (HFS) are a popular source of dietary supplements *(12)*. That some HFS staff act in dishonest, uninformed, or unethical ways was demonstrated in a study conducted in Hawaii in 1998 *(13)*. A woman visited 40 HFS. In each one, she stated that her mother had advanced breast cancer and requested advice. In 36 (90%) of the HFS, one or more products were recommended. The most common ones recommended were shark cartilage (recommended in 17 HFS), followed by essiac (an herbal treatment), maitake mushroom, Coenzyme Q_{10}, and vitamin C. In all, 38 different products were recommended. No sales person mentioned potential adverse effects associated with taking the supplements. The cost of the supplements of shark cartilage, essiac, and maitake ranged from $300–$3400.

In a similar study conducted in Ontario, Canada, the investigator posed as a mother of a child with Crohn's disease *(14)*. Of the 32 HFS visited, 23 (72%) offered advice. The advice given was remarkably inconsistent, with 30 different herbs and nutritional supplements recommended. A third study was carried out in London *(15)*. Here, the UK researcher stated that she had been getting headaches lately. The researcher visited 29 HFS; of these, 25 (86%) recommended a specific product. As before, a wide variety of products were recommended. In addition, seven of the stores (24%) recommended diet or lifestyle change. One disturbing aspect of this study was that the researcher presented with what could be a serious disease, yet only seven of the HFS (24%) suggested a visit to a physician. By contrast, 18 of the HFS (62%) suggested a cause of the headaches.

Save-On-Foods is a supermarket chain in Canada. In one of their Edmonton stores, one of us (NT) talked with a salesperson in the health food section whose job was to provide advice for customers. When questioned, the clerk admitted that she had no relevant qualifications, was paid minimum wage, and had been instructed to refer customers to a book that recommended a wide variety of supplements.

The lack of staff training in science, nutrition, and clinical medicine, coupled with the economic incentives to sell products, places many consumers at risk. One fear is that this marketing environment may lead some consumers to choose unproven therapies over conventional medical treatment when they are seriously ill *(9)*.

3.2. Infomercials

Another form of distribution of many types of health-related products is by infomercials. These TV programs are produced and paid for by commercial companies. They resemble regular TV programs but are, in reality, a form of advertising. They typically last for 30 min and air during the night.

Here we describe an infomercial that was aired on Canadian TV many times during 2003. It consisted of an interview with Robert Barefoot, the author of a book on calcium (*The Calcium Factor: The Scientific Secret of Health and Youth*) *(16)* that appears to be popular, as indicated by its sales ranking at Amazon.com. In the infomercial, Barefoot made a series of claims for calcium that have no supporting evidence. He claimed that calcium can both reverse and prevent cancer; turn on DNA and thereby enhance youth; and prevent heart disease, a condition he states is unrelated to cholesterol. The infomercial directed potential customers to a toll-free number for placing orders from Today's Health, a company in Boston. The type of calcium being sold was supposedly coral calcium from Japan, costing 10 times more than regular calcium from a drug store.

Setting aside the ecologic and ethical issues of harvesting calcium from fragile, endangered coral environments, this infomercial made outrageous claims for effectiveness, contained bogus science, provided no scientific evidence for claims, although at the same time offering the product at a huge mark-up in price. Indeed, this infomercial resembled the classic snake oil sales pitch of a previous era. Fortunately for consumers, Barefoot's infomercial caught the eye of the US Federal Trade Commission (FTC), which took legal action in June 2003 against him, his business associates, and two companies for making false and unsubstantiated claims about their product's health benefits. The FTC is seeking to bar permanently the ads for Barefoot's coral calcium and obtain refunds for consumers who purchased it *(17,18)*.

3.3. Multilevel Marketing

Many products—from Avon cosmetics to Tupperware—are sold by direct marketing, a strategy in which company salespeople recruit other salespeople. The foot soldiers and everyone up the chain get a commission for their sales. This marketing strategy is popular among manufacturers of dietary supplements. Its focus is profit, not consumer health.

Body Wise International, for example, rewards so-called consultants for selling product and also for "sponsoring" other independent consultants. According to the company website, consultants can use this form of network marketing to generate "substantial incomes" *(19)*. The science behind some of the company's products is questionable, as evidenced in a public lecture given in 2002 in Edmonton by Tim Tierney. Although Tierney did not claim to be an expert, he was giving the views of Dr. Jesse Stoff, who was described in the advertising leaflet for the lecture as "the world's leading viroimmunologist." A check of MEDLINE, however, failed to produce a single publication by Stoff, though he has authored several populist nutrition books of dubious credibility.

Tierney made some rather strange statements in his lecture, including that milk causes osteoporosis. However, the real purpose of the lecture was the promotion of various products sold by Body Wise. Tierney claimed that several people had been cured of cancer by the products. Indeed, the products seem to cure pretty much everything. For evidence of its efficacy, the audience was given, not references to papers in journals, but statements by half a dozen people describing fantastic cures experienced by themselves or others. The products come with money back guarantees. The company website *(19)* refers to two unpublished research studies that examined immune function (number of natural-killer cells) rather than clinical end points.

3.4. Bulk Mail

Bulk mail ("junk mail") is a common form of advertising, especially for supplements that promise weight loss. A typical advertisement for apple cider vinegar capsules was mailed to residents of Edmonton, Alberta, in 2002. The advert stated:

You can even eat as much as you like and still lose weight! ....an intake of 4000 calories a day can actually help you to lose weight, each day you'll feel better, more energized and lose weight.....(the capsules) really do help to drain off your fat deposits and eliminate that extra weight once and for all.

Other egregious claims made for apple cider vinegar include "normalizing blood circulation" and "neutralizing the toxicity in the body" *(20)*. These terms may sound impressive to anxious consumers who fret about their health, but they have no meaning in the scientific community.

3.5. Spam E-Mails

Spam e-mails are a cheap and easy way for manufacturers to promote their dietary supplements to tens of thousands, if not millions, of people. As a result large numbers of products are being touted, most of them of highly dubious value. As an example, Sleep Away Thermogenesis Diet is a product that contains aloe and collagen. The e-mail gave no evidence to support the value of aloe but makes the following grandiose claim for collagen: "The body absorbs collagen protein while sleeping releasing stored brown fat to be used as energy" *(21)*. Neither ingredient has any recognized value in weight control.

3.6. Internet Websites

According to the FTC more than 90 million Americans use the Internet to find health information. The Internet is well suited to mass marketing as it provides low-cost access to a global market. Unfortunately, its easy accessibility and openness make it an ideal forum for selling questionable products.

An analysis was recently published of herbal products marketed on the Internet *(22)*. It was discovered that among 338 websites that sold herbal remedies, 273 (81%) made one or more health claims. Of these 273, more than half (55%) made a claim that a product could treat, prevent, diagnose, or cure a specific disease, and half of them failed to show the standard federal disclaimer related to health claims.

Some internet marketers have the computer savvy to extend their promotions beyond mere advertising—they enhance sales by embedding misleading metatags on their websites so as to increase the chances that consumers will see the website. The FTC does not condone this practice *(23)*.

The marketing of supplements that supposedly increase the body's production of human growth hormone (HGH) provides an example of how some companies attempt to mislead consumers using the Internet. HGH is a potent hormone that affects the metabolism of glucose, protein, and fat, and the growth and maturation of the skeleton. A paper in the *New England Journal of Medicine* reported that men aged 60 yr and older who were treated with HGH experienced a decrease in adipose tissue mass and an increase in both lean body mass and skin thickness *(24)*. These positive findings make HGH potentially marketable as an "anti-aging" formula. What the supplement websites do not tell consumers is that in clinical studies HGH was injected because its peptide structure would be digested if the hormone were taken orally, thus rendering it ineffective. This creates something of a problem for sellers of supplements.

One approach around the problem is a supplement called UltraMax HGH. The manufacturer, Ageless Foundation Laboratories, claims that its product stimulates the pituitary gland to produce more HGH. Among its many supposed benefits, UltraMax HGH is claimed to increase muscle tone, decrease body fat, restore hair color and thickness, reduce the appearance of wrinkles, normalize blood pressure, and improve memory and vision *(25)*. According to the company's website, the ingredients include niacin, several amino acids (arginine, lysine, tyrosine, glutamine, and pyroglutamic acid), anterior pituitary peptides, ornithine α-ketoglutarate, "glycoamino-acid complex," "somatotrophin mediating factors (free-form amino acid duplex glycine and γ-amino butyric acid)," "novel polyose complex (pharmaceutical glucose polymers)," and L-DOPA from broad bean. The product is described on the website *(25)* as being:

> *...100% natural. There are no drugs in the product. There are no synthetic ingredients or chemicals in the product either. It is composed of ... herbs such as broad bean, which is a very rare and expensive herb from the Amazonian rain forests that go into the body and stimulates the body's own natural production of human growth hormone.*

A similar product is Sunbright produced by Life Force. According to the company website *(26)*, the ingredients that stimulate release of HGH are arginine and ornithine. The preparation also contains 10 herbs and four other substances. Amongst the many benefits that will supposedly occur with regular use are: weight loss, strength and endurance, enhanced sexual function and desire; skin tone, texture, and appearance; restoration of hair color and luster; and greater resistance to illness.

Neither website provides supporting evidence that the supplements actually increase the body's production of HGH, and the only evidence for the claims of improved health comes in the form of testimonials. Instead of credible evidence, they refer to but do not specify the "clinical studies" showing that HGH has been tested on people for several decades. It is true that there has been extensive clinical research on HGH, but the product sold by these companies is not the same compound used in clinical studies. Furthermore, there is no evidence, based on a MEDLINE search, that the products sold by these companies have been tested in clinical trials. Some studies have suggested that ornithine α-ketoglutarate, an ingredient of UltraMax HGH, may increase HGH levels, but this effect was achieved at a dose many times greater than that supplied by UltraMax HGH *(27)*. Both websites claim that their products are free of side effects. It is highly implausible that the products can increase the body's production of a potent hormone that has multiple effects, yet poses no risk of side effects. Hormones carry the risk of serious side effects, as the research on the safety of hormone replacement therapy for menopausal women attests *(28)*.

4. REGULATIONS ON THE MARKETING OF SUPPLEMENTS

The explosive growth of the dietary supplement industry over the last decade has created many regulatory challenges for federal agencies. Refer to Table 1 for a list of agencies involved in regulating dietary supplements in the United States and Canada.

4.1. United States

The Nutrition Labeling and Education Act of 1990 gave the Food and Drug Administration (FDA) the authority to require the manufacturers of dietary supplements to furnish evidence that their products are safe *(29)*. The FDA was also empowered to approve the health claims for these products. However, enactment of the Dietary Supplement and Health Education Act (DSHEA) of 1994 freed dietary supplement manufactur-

Table 1
Agencies in the United States and Canada Involved in Regulating Dietary Supplements

United States

Food and Drug Administration
www.fda.gov
Center for Food Safety and Applied Nutrition (CFSAN)
www.cfsan.fda.gov
CFSAN's Office of Nutritional Products, Labeling, and Dietary Supplements
www.cfsan.fda.gov/~dms/onplds.html
Federal Trade Commission
www.ftc.gov

Canada

Health Canada
www.hc-sc.gc.ca
Health Products and Food Branch
www.hc-sc.gc.ca/hpfb-dgpsa/index_e.html
Natural Health Products Directorate
www.hc-sc.gc.ca/hpfb-dgpsa/nhpd-dpsn/index.html

ers from many FDA regulations *(29)*. Whereas manufacturers were required by the Nutrition Labeling and Education Act regulations to prove that a dietary supplement is *safe*, the FDA must prove under DSHEA regulations that a supplement is *unsafe*. This shift in regulatory policy places burdens on a federal agency with important public health responsibilities but limited resources. Moreover, manufacturers are now free to make health-related claims (structure/function claims). However, manufacturers are not permitted to state explicitly that the product will cure or prevent a disease, and they must state that the FDA has not evaluated the agent. In other words, a manufacturer may now claim that a supplement "boosts the immune system," "makes the body burn fat while you sleep," or "fights cholesterol," provided they stop short of saying that the supplement prevents infectious disease, cures obesity, or prevents heart disease. Needless to say, the distinction is lost on most consumers. Put bluntly, the 1994 law, together with the lack of resources at the FDA to enforce regulations, has given supplement manufacturers carte blanche to employ deceptive marketing that often looks and smells like fraud.

Dr. Marion Nestle, of New York University, traced the history of how the supplement industry succeeded in pressuring Congress to pass DSHEA, thereby allowing the supplement industry almost unlimited freedom to market supplements *(29)*:

Today, marketers of supplements are permitted to make practically any claim they want for the health benefits of their products; they may vary the ingredient contents of their products with impunity. They do not have to remove potentially harmful products from the market unless taken to court by the FDA, and they do not have to prove that their products bestow the benefits claimed for them. This remarkable situation is the result of the industry's persistence and skill in generating public pressure on Congress to restrict the FDA's regulatory mission.

The serious problems with the current regulatory climate was recently addressed by the editors of the Journal of the American Medical Association *(30)*:

> *If dietary supplements have or promote ... biological activity, they should be considered to be active drugs. On the other hand, if dietary supplements are claimed to be safe because they lack or have minimal biological activity, then their ability to cause physiologic changes to support "structure/function" claims should be challenged, and their sale and distribution as products to improve health should be curtailed. Manufacturers of dietary supplements are trying to have it both ways. They claim their products are powerfully beneficial, on the one hand, but harmless on the other. To claim both makes no sense, and to claim either without trails demonstrating efficacy and safety is deceptive. The public should wonder why dietary supplements have effectively been given a free ride. New legislation is needed for defining and regulating dietary supplements.*

A similar article was published in the *New England Journal of Medicine* with a focus on herbal supplements *(31)*.

4.2. Canada

The situation in Canada has for years been every bit as dishonest as that in the United States. However, in 1999 Health Canada created a new organization, the Natural Health Products Directorate, to regulate dietary supplements. The directorate's mission is to ensure that Canadians have access to natural health products (NHPs) that are safe, effective, and of high quality *(2)*. New regulations were published in June 2003 and took effect in January 2004, but with the actual implementation being done during a 6-yr period. Whereas previous products had been regulated as drugs or foods, the new regulations specify that NHPs are a subset of drugs with their own unique regulations. A key feature of the new regulations is that the requirements for safety and good manufacturing practices fall on the companies that manufacture, package, label, import, or distribute NHPs. By the end of the 6-yr transition period, all manufacturers, importers, packagers, and labelers of NHPs must have site licenses, and any new NHP must have a product license. The regulations require a premarket review of products to assure Canadians that label information is truthful and health claims are supported by appropriate types of scientific evidence. The effect of these new regulations should be that by 2006 or 2007 the outrageous marketing activities documented in this chapter will have largely disappeared from Canada.

5. HELPING CONSUMERS MAKE INFORMED CHOICES ABOUT DIETARY SUPPLEMENTS

A healthy dose of skepticism is a consumer's best protection against fraudulent and misleading claims, promotion, and products. Unfortunately, two surveys indicate that large sections of the American public have a poor understanding of the issues involved. In one study, 28% of adults believed the following statement to be true: "[herbal supplements] are safe because they are natural" *(32)*. The other survey reported that 61% of people believe that supplements are helpful for people with colds, 49% for influenza, and 16% for HIV/AIDS *(9)*. Clearly, consumers need help in two key areas: evaluating health claims and understanding basic science principles.

It is not only the general public who need more education on these issues. Dietitians, for instance, are not as knowledgeable about dietary supplements as they should be. A survey revealed that dietetic interns and program directors receive less than one hour of classroom instruction on herbal supplements, although 79% had been asked about these products *(33)*.

5.1. Evaluating Health Claims

Given the abundant and innovative forms of marketing of dietary supplements, consumers need help sorting through the health claims. Although each supplement and each form of marketing is unique, suspicious claims share several features, including *(23)*:

1. A reliance on anecdotal evidence, especially testimonials.
2. A lack of supporting evidence from papers published in peer-reviewed journals.
3. The use of unscientific and unsupported theories to rationalize the use of supplements (e.g., claims that a supplement boosts immunity or detoxifies the body).
4. Money-back guarantees.
5. The use of claims that the product represents a "scientific breakthrough" or an "ancient remedy."
6. The use of claims suggesting that the product is an effective cure for a broad range of ailments. For example, a list might include insomnia, HIV/AIDS, cancer, memory loss, and fibromyalgia; no one product can cure, prevent, or treat such an array of diseases or medical conditions.
7. The use of impressive-sounding medical terms. Legitimate manufacturers take the time to explain medical terms and ingredients so that consumers know what they are buying.

5.2. Understanding Basic Science

The science underlying reported health benefits of dietary supplements can be baffling to consumers as well as to health care providers. When working with the public, health professionals can offer the following simple rules to help consumers determine whether dietary supplement manufacturers offer reliable health and product information based on good science *(12)*:

1. If in doubt, obtain advice from a legitimate health professional, such as a doctor, dietitian, or pharmacist, before purchasing a supplement.
2. Take advice given by staff at health food stores with a grain of salt—many are motivated more by sales than by concern for a customer's health, and lack basic training in nutrition, biochemistry, and medicine.
3. Ignore heavily biased infomercials and websites of supplement manufacturers, and do not trust the advice given by people engaged in multilevel marketing.
4. Give little credence to evidence based on testimonials: people's health often improves *despite* the treatment rather than *because of it.*
5. Use common sense. Remember the fundamental rule: if things look too good to be true, they usually are.
6. Check with a local or national nonprofit health organization, such as the Canadian Diabetes Association, the American Heart Association, etc., to obtain information about diet and nutritional recommendations for managing a disease.
7. Check the health and dietary supplement websites of federal government agencies and legitimate medical organizations for information about dietary supplements. Some helpful websites are listed in Table 2. For example, a consumer newly diagnosed with cancer might consider taking a shark cartilage supplement based on claims made by a dietary

Table 2
Internet Resources on Dietary Supplements and Health Fraud

Dietary Supplements

Buying Medicines and Medical Products Online (Food and Drug Administration)
www.fda.gov/oc/buyonline/
Cancer.gov (National Cancer Institute)
www.cancer.gov
Dietary Supplements and Herbal Information (National Agricultural Library)
www.nal.usda.gov/fnic/etext/000015.html
Dietary Supplements—Warnings and Safety Information (Food and Drug Administration)
www.cfsan.fda.gov/~dms/ds-warn.html
Healthfinder
www.healthfinder.gov
Mayo Clinic
www.mayoclinic.com
MEDLINEplus Guide to Healthy Web Surfing
www.nlm.nih.gov/medlineplus/healthywebsurfing.html
Memorial Sloan-Kettering Cancer Center's About Herbs, Botanicals and Other Products
www.mskcc.org
National Center for Complementary and Alternative Medicine
www.nccam.nih.gov
Supplement Watch
www.supplementwatch.com.

Health Fraud

National Council Against Health Fraud
www.ncahf.org
Quackwatch
www.quackwatch.org
A highly informative website for exposing fraud in the sale of various supplements,
including herbs and weight-loss products, is www.dietfraud.com. Also check the Federal
Trade Commission's Operation Cure-All website at www.ftc.gov/bcp/conline/edcams/
cureall for information about false health claims and products. There are also several
books available*(39–41)*.

supplement manufacturer. But before making a decision, they can turn to the National
Cancer Institute's website for detailed information about this supposed cancer cure, its
history of use, evidence of anticancer components, and the findings of animal and clinical
trials, if any, and reports of adverse effects *(37)*. This information was not available to
consumers a few years ago.

Four science issues deserve elaboration. First, many consumers do not realize that
supplements may pose a risk of toxicity and "natural" does not mean "safe." For example,
thousands of people in the United States suffered significant harm from ephedra, a naturally occurring, adrenaline-like stimulant derived from the Chinese herbal Ma huang
(31,38). Safety concerns prompted Health Canada in January 2002 to issue a voluntary
recall of ephedra-containing dietary supplements and a warning to consumers to stop

using such products *(39)*. Its sale remained legal in the United States, although the Department of Health and Human Services issued an advisory in 2003 about ephedra's adverse effects, the FDA sent warning letters to companies marketing dietary supplements containing the compound, and the FTC took action against two direct marketers of weight-loss products formulated with ephedra *(38,40)*. Eventually, in December 2003, its sale was banned by the FDA. Another hazardous supplement is kava, which has been linked to several deaths, mainly from liver toxicity, in the United States and Europe *(41)*. Kava has been banned in the European Union, whereas in Canada, people have been advised not to consume it. Yet it is still sold in the United States.

Second, consumers do not realize that taking complex mixtures of herbs alongside prescription medicines for prolonged periods of time may result in serious side effects. This is especially true when a sick individual is taking medication whose action might be affected by an herb. For example, St. John's wort accelerates the metabolic degradation of many drugs and may cause a reduction in their effectiveness *(42)*. The seriousness of such drug interactions was apparent in February 2000 when the FDA issued a public health advisory, informing health professionals that a significant drug interaction between St. John's wort and indinavir, a protease inhibitor used to treat HIV/ AIDS, had been confirmed and asking them to check with their patients about the simultaneous use of the two products *(43)*.

Third, consumers may not be aware that, unlike prescription and over-the-counter drugs, herbal supplements generally lack standardization of active ingredients. For example, a wide variation in the concentration of active components in different samples of ginseng was reported in one study *(44)*. This finding probably reflects differences in such factors as the species of plant, the part of the plant used, and the processing method. Thus, an herb that was reportedly effective in one study may not be effective in others. In short, herbal treatments have few of the careful testing and quality controls seen with new drug development or the manufacturing practices required to produce drugs of consistent purity, quality, and content.

Finally, some consumers may think that adults and children alike can derive health benefits from dietary supplements, and some manufacturers are eager to promote this view. In truth, many—maybe most—dietary supplements have not been tested in children to determine their safety or effectiveness. The FTC noted an increase in advertising that promotes dietary supplements as cures or preventive agents for various childhood ailments, such as colds, ear infections, asthma, and attention deficit/hyperactivity disorder. Parents are advised to read ingredient labels and check with reliable medical authorities before giving their children dietary supplements beyond simple vitamin and mineral formulations *(45)*.

6. CONCLUSIONS

The marketing of dietary supplements provides a situation where ethics, honesty, and a sincere desire to improve the health of consumers take a backseat to maximizing sales and profit. Consumers have embraced the regular use of dietary supplements with zeal, but they have turned a blind eye to issues of safety and efficacy—to the delight of supplement manufacturers. Marketers of dietary supplements have rushed to fill consumer demand for health products, in many cases using scientific evidence the way a drunk uses a lamp post: more for support than illumination.

It is entirely possible that on balance the supplement industry actually does more harm than good to people's health. This is because many people are persuaded to take worthless—and possibly harmful—supplements for the prevention and treatment of a health condition and forgo a beneficial intervention. Why eat extra portions of fruit and vegetables every day in order to lower your risk of cancer when you can much more easily take shark cartilage tablets? Why get flu shots when the same protection can be achieved with echinacea? Why cut down on your intake of hamburgers when the saturated fat can be neutralized with garlic? The supplement industry has built an empire, but the emperor is almost naked.

Is there an answer to the question posed at the beginning of this chapter: What benefits do consumers receive from the billions they spend on dietary supplements? One answer is that, yes, consumers receive health benefits from some dietary supplements. Occasionally, a supplement taken by large numbers of people based on weak evidence turns out to be effective. For example, St. John's wort became popular for the treatment of mild to moderate depression, despite the meager quality of the supporting evidence. Nevertheless, it has stood up reasonably well to careful testing (46). But such cases are very much the exception. (See Chapter 11, which discusses the possible benefits of herbs.) In addition, given the ample evidence that some North Americans have diets of poor quality (47), many consumers would benefit from taking a limited group of nutrients in the form of a single nutrient or multivitamin-mineral supplement. (See Chapter 16)

Consumers may also derive other, less tangible, benefits from dietary supplements. Healthy consumers, empowered to take control of their health, may look to dietary supplements as a way to keep themselves out of doctors' offices. Consumers at the other end of the spectrum, faced with life-threatening conditions and searching desperately for medical cures, may derive some psychological benefits from taking dietary supplements they believe may ease their symptoms or prolong life.

Unfortunately, the positive side of dietary supplements is overshadowed by an industry that exploits consumers' lack of understanding of basic science, robs them of money for expensive but worthless supplements, and endangers their health when the use of unproven dietary supplements prevents them from obtaining standard medical treatment.

In the final analysis, an educated consumer is the best consumer when it comes to dietary supplements. And the need for education also applies to health professionals and the general public alike. In addition to general education, there is also a need for greater vigilance of the industry by government agencies. Finally, more research is needed that identifies the key constituents in herbs and other products, their mechanisms of action, drug interactions, and adverse reactions. And, most of all, carefully conducted clinical research is needed so as to clearly identify in what medical conditions and for what groups of persons these supplements can be justified.

REFERENCES

1. Food and Drug Administration, Center for Food Safety and Applied Nutrition. 2001. Overview of dietary supplements, available at www.cfsan.fda.gov/~dms/ds-oview.html. Last accessed August 29, 2003.
2. Health Canada, Natural Health Products Directorate. Natural health products regulations, available at www.hc-sc.gc.ca/hpfb-dgpsa/nhpd-dpsn/nhp_regs_e.html. Last accessed August 29, 2003.
3. Nutrition Business Journal's annual industry overview VII. Nutrition Business Journal. May/June 2002.

4. National Harris Interactive Survey. Released December 23, 2002. http://www.harrisinteractive.com/news/allnewsbydate.asp?NewsID=560. Last accessed April 7, 2003.

5. Radimer K, Bindewald B, Hughes J, Ervin B, Swanson C, Picciano MF. Dietary supplement use by US adults: data from the National Health and Nutrition Examination Survey, 1999–2000. Am J Epidemiol 2004; 160:339–349.

6. Millen AE, Dodd KW, Subar AF. Use of vitamin, mineral, nonvitamin, and nonmineral supplements in the United States: The 1987, 1992, and 2000 National Health Interview Survey results. J Am Diet Assoc 2004; 104:942–950.

7. Troppmann L, Johns T, Gray-Donald K. Natural health product use in Canada. Can J Public Health 2002; 93:426–430.

8. Angus Reid Study, released May 19, 2000. www.ipsos-reid.com/ca/. Accessed February 13, 2002.

9. Blendon RJ, DesRoches CM, Benson JM, Brodie M, Altman DE. Americans' views on the use and regulation of dietary supplements. Arch Intern Med 2001; 161:805–810.

10. Satia-Abouta J, Kristal AR, Patterson RE, Littman AJ, Stratton KL, White E. Dietary supplement use and medical conditions: the VITAL study. Am J Prev Med 2003; 24:43–51.

11. Gunther S, Patterson RE, Kristal AR, Stratton KL, White E. Demographic and health-related correlates of herbal and specialty supplement use. J Am Diet Assoc 2004; 104:27–34.

12. Food and Drug Administration. An FDA guide to dietary supplements. FDA Consumer 1999. Available at vm.cfsan.fda.gov/~dms/fdsupp.html. Last accessed August 29, 2003.

13. Gotay CC, Dumitriu D. Health food store recommendations for breast cancer patients. Arch Fam Med 2000; 9:692–699.

14. Calder J, Issenman R, Cawdron R. Health information provided by retail health food outlets. Can J Gastroenterol 2000; 14:767–771.

15. Vickers AJ, Rees RW, Robin A. Advice given by health food shops: is it clinically safe? J R Coll Physicians Lond 1998; 32:426–428.

16. Barefoot RR, Reich CM. The calcium factor: the scientific secret of health and youth. Bokar Consultants, Wickenburg, AZ, 2002.

17. Memorial Sloan-Kettering Cancer Center. June 16, 2003. FTC charges marketers of coral calcium supplement with making false claims and issues warnings to website operators. Available at www.mskcc.org/mskcc/html/14009.cfm. Last accessed August 29, 2003.

18. National Center for Complementary and Alternative Medicine. June 17, 2003. NCCAM consumer advisory on coral calcium. Available at nccam.nih.gov/health/alerts/coral/coral.htm. Last accessed August 29, 2003.

19. www.bodywise.com. Last accessed March 9, 2003. Formerly: www.healthywave.com.

20. BioActive Nutrients.com. Apple cider vinegar. Available at www.bioactivenutrients.com/AppleCider Vinegar.html. Last accessed Sept. 2, 2003.

21. http://AloeFormulas.com. Last accessed November 7, 2003.

22. Morris CA, Avorn J. Internet marketing of herbal products. JAMA 2003; 290:1505–1509.

23. Federal Trade Commission. June 2001. Health claims on the Internet: Buyer beware. Available at www.ftc.gov/bcp/conline/features/healthclaims.htm. Last accessed August 29, 2003.

24. Rudman D, Feller AG, Nagraj HS, Gergans GA, Lalitha PY, Goldberg AF, et al. Effects of human growth hormone in men over 60 years old. N Engl J Med 1990; 323:1–6.

25. www.ultramaxhgh.com. Last accessed March 29, 2003.

26. http://www.mgi-pages.com/colon/HGH.htm. Last accessed March 30, 2003.

27. Talbott SM. A guide to understanding dietary supplements. The Haworth Press, NY, 2003.

28. Women's Health Initiative Investigators. Risks and benefits of estrogen plus progestin in healthy post-menopausal women: principal results from the Women's Health Initiative randomized controlled trial. JAMA 2002; 288:321–333.

29. Nestle M. The Politics of Food. How the Food Industry Influences Nutrition and Health. University of California Press, Berkeley, 2002.

30. Fontanarosa PB, Rennie D, DeAngelis CD. The need for regulation of dietary supplements—lessons from ephedra. JAMA 2003; 289:1568–1570.

31. Marcus DM, Grollman AP. Botanical medicines—the need for new regulations. N Engl J Med 2002; 347:2073–2076.

32. Americans' food and nutrition attitudes and behaviors –American Dietetic Association's Nutrition and You: Trends 2000. Released January 3, 2000. www.eatright.org/pr/2000/010300a.html. Last accessed 9 April, 2003.

33. Box S, Creswell B, Hagan DW. Alternative health care education in dietetic training programs: a survey of perceived needs. J Am Diet Assoc 2001; 101:108–110.

34. Professional Guide to Complementary & Alternative Therapy. Springhouse, Springhouse, Pennsylvania, 2002.

35. Sarubin Fragakis A. The Health Professional's Guide to Popular Dietary Supplements, 2nd ed. American Dietetic Association, Chicago, 2003.

36. Fetrow CW, Avila JR, eds. Professionals' Handbook of Complementary & Alternative Medicine. Springhouse, Springhouse, Pennsylvania, 2001.

37. National Cancer Institute. Cancer.gov website: Cartilage (bovine and shark). Available at www.cancer.gov. Last accessed August 29, 2003.

38. Food and Drug Administration. Feb. 28, 2003. HHS acts to reduce potential risks of dietary supplements containing ephedra. FDA News. Available at www.fda.gov/bbs/topics/NEWS/2003/NEW00875.html. Last accessed Sept. 9, 2003.

39. Health Canada. Jan. 9, 2002. Advisory: Health Canada requests recall of certain products containing Ephedra/ephedrine. Available at www.hc-sc.gc.ca/English/protection/warnings/2002/2002_01e.htm. Last accessed Sept. 4, 2003.

40. Federal Trade Commission. July 1, 2003. FTC charges direct marketers of ephedra weight loss products with making deceptive efficacy and safety claims. Available at www.ftc.gov/opa/2003/07/ephedra.htm. Last accessed Sept. 2, 2003.

41. Health Canada. Jan. 16, 2002. Advisory: Health Canada is advising consumers not to use any products containing kava. Available at media.healthcanada.net/English/protection/warnings/2002/2002_02e.htm. Last accessed Sept. 4, 2003.

42. Moore LB, Goodwin B, Jones SA, Goodwin B, Jones SA, Wisely GB. St. John's wort induces hepatic drug metabolism through activation of the pregnane X receptor. Proc Natl Acad Sci USA 2000; 97:7500–7502.

43. Food and Drug Administration. Feb. 10, 2000. FDA Public Health Advisory: Risk of drug interactions with St. John's wort and indinavir and other drugs. Available at www.fda.gov/cder/drug/advisory/stjwort.htm. Last accessed Sept. 2, 2003.

44. Harkey MR, Henderson GL, Gershwin ME, Stern JS, Hackman RM. Variability in commercial ginseng products: an analysis of 25 preparations. Am J Clin Nutr 2002; 75:600,601.

45. Federal Trade Commission. May 2000. Promotions for kids' dietary supplements leave sour taste. FTC Consumer Feature. Available at www.ftc.gov. Last accessed August 29, 2003.

46. Memorial Sloan-Kettering Cancer Center website: About Herbs, Botanicals & Other Products: St. John's wort (*Hypericum perforatum*). Available at www.mskcc.org. Last accessed August 29, 2003.

47. Briefel RR, Johnson CL. Secular trends in dietary intake in the United States. Annu Rev Nutr 2004; 24:401–431.

18 Optimizing Nutrition for Exercise and Sports

Richard B. Kreider and Brian Leutholtz

KEY POINTS

1. General recommendations.
- Stress high-carbohydrate, nutrient-dense, isoenergetic diet designed to maintain weight.
- Take a low-dose daily multivitamin (with iron for women).
- Taper training intensity and carbohydrate load before competition.
- Consume a prepractice or preworkout carbohydrate/protein snack 30–60 min before exercise.
- Consume plenty of water and sports drinks during exercise (particularly in the heat).
- Consume a postpractice carbohydrate/protein snack within 30 min of exercise.
- If you have to train in the morning, ingest an evening snack before going to bed.
- Only consider sport-specific use of effective and legal ergogenic aids.

2. Potentially effective supplements for strength/power/sprint athletes.
- Water/sports drinks.
- Carbohydrate.
- Creatine.
- Bicarbonate loading.
- Sodium phosphate.
- Glycerol (to counteract dehydration).

3. Potentially effective supplements for endurance athletes.
- Water/sports drinks.
- Carbohydrate.
- Caffeine.
- Sodium phosphate.
- Glycerol (to counteract dehydration).
- Creatine.

From: *Nutritional Health: Strategies for Disease Prevention, Second Edition*
Edited by: N. J. Temple, T. Wilson, and D. R. Jacobs © Humana Press Inc., Totowa, NJ

Factors Affecting Peak Performance

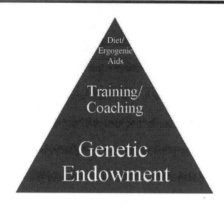

Fig. 1. Factors that affect performance.

4. Possible anticatabolic nutrients that may help athletes tolerate training.
- Sports drinks.
- Carbohydrate.
- Postexercise carbohydrate, protein, essential amino acids (EAA), and glutamine.
- Creatine.
- Metabolite β-hydroxy β-methylbutyrate monohydrate.

5. Possible nutrients to enhance the immune system.
- Postexercise carbohydrate, protein, and EAA.
- Vitamin C.
- Zinc.
- Glutamine.
- Echinacea.

1. INTRODUCTION

The primary factors that affect exercise performance capacity include an individual's genetic endowment, the quality of training, and effective coaching (*see* Fig. 1). Beyond these factors, nutrition plays a critical role in optimizing performance capacity. In order for athletes to perform well, their training and diet must be optimal. If athletes do not train enough or have an inadequate diet, their performance may be decreased *(1)*. On the other hand, if athletes train too much without a sufficient diet, they may be susceptible to becoming overtrained (*see* Fig. 2).

Because optimizing training and dietary practices are critical to peak performance, athletes have searched for various ways to improve exercise performance capacity through the use of *ergogenic aids*. An ergogenic aid is any training technique, mechanical device, nutritional practice, pharmacological method, or psychological technique that can improve exercise performance capacity and/or enhance training adaptations *(2)*. This includes aids that may help prepare an individual to exercise, improve the efficiency of exercise, and/or enhance recovery from exercise. Ergogenic aids may also allow an individual to tolerate heavy training to a greater degree by helping them recover

Training Stimulus

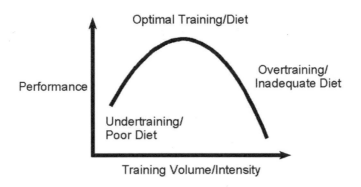

Fig. 2. Relationship of training volume/intensity to performance.

faster or helping them stay healthy during intense training. This chapter presents an overview of the role that nutrition has on optimizing sport performance; describes nutritional guidelines that athletes should employ to optimize training adaptations; and evaluates the potential ergogenic value of various nutrients that have been proposed to improve exercise capacity and/or training adaptations.

2. ENERGY DEMANDS FOR ACTIVE INDIVIDUALS

The first component in optimizing training and performance through nutrition is to ensure that the athlete is consuming enough calories to offset energy expenditure *(1,3,4)*. People who participate in a general fitness program (e.g., exercising 30–40 min/d, three times per week) can generally meet nutritional needs following a normal diet (e.g., 1800–2400 kcals/d or about 25–35 kcals/kg/d for a 50–80 kg individual) because their caloric demands from exercise are not too great (e.g., 200–400 kcals/session) *(5)*. However, athletes involved in moderate levels of intense training (e.g., 2–3 h/d of intense exercise performed five to six times per week) or high volume intense training (e.g., 3–6 h/d of intense training in one to two workouts for 5–6 d/wk) may expend 600–1200 kcals/h or more during exercise. For this reason, their caloric needs may approach 50–80 kcals/kg/d (2500–8000 kcals/d for a 50–100 kg athlete). For elite athletes, energy expenditure during heavy training or competition may be enormous. For example, energy expenditure for cyclists to compete in the Tour de France has been estimated as high as 12,000 kcals/d (150–200 kcals/kg/d for a 60–80 kg athlete) *(6–8)*. In addition, caloric needs for large athletes (i.e., 100–150 kg) may range between 6000 and 12,000 kcals/d depending on the volume and intensity of different training phases *(8)*.

Although some exercise physiologists and nutritionists argue that athletes can meet caloric needs simply by consuming a well-balanced diet, it is often very difficult for larger athletes and/or athletes engaged in high volume/intense training to be able to eat enough food to meet caloric needs. Maintaining an energy deficient diet during training often leads to significant weight loss (including muscle mass), illness, onset of physical and psychological symptoms of overtraining, and reductions in performance *(9)*. Nutritional

Table 1
Dietary Macronutrient Guidelines for Athletes

Nutrient	Proposed ergogenic value	Summary of research findings
Carbohydrate	Primary fuel used for anaerobic and high-intensity aerobic exercise. Increasing dietary availability proposed to increase glycogen content and increase exercise capacity.	Athletes engaged in heavy training need to consume a diet high in carbohydrate (55–65% of caloric intake). Ingesting 8–10 g/kg/d of carbohydrate during heavy training has been suggested as one strategy to maintain muscle and liver glycogen levels and reduce the incidence of overtraining.[a] However, recent evidence indicates that power athletes may only need to ingest 35–45% of caloric intake in the form of carbohydrate to maintain muscle glycogen levels.
Protein	Increasing dietary availability of protein has been suggested to be a means of maintaining nitrogen balance and enhancing gains in muscle mass.	Protein balance studies indicate that athletes involved in heavy training need to ingest 1.5–2.0 g/kg/d of protein in order to maintain nitrogen balance (about 1.5 times the RDA). Although most athletes consume enough protein in their diet, some athletes are susceptible to protein malnutrition (dancers, gymnasts, runners, swimmers, etc.). Studies indicate that supplementing the diet with protein above that necessary to maintain protein balance does not increase strength or muscle mass. However, ingesting protein and carbohydrate following exercise can improve glycogen and protein synthesis.
Fat	Primary fuel for moderate- to low-intensity exercise. Some have proposed that increasing fat and/or derivatives of fat may enhance endurance exercise performance. Others suggest that increasing fat content in the diet may help moderate insulin levels, thus promoting fat loss.	It is generally recommended that athletes consume less than 1 g/kg/d of fat in their diet (<30% of calories). Studies indicate that individuals who successfully maintain weight loss consume less than 40 g/d of fat. Studies generally do not indicate that fat supplementation enhances exercise performance, although supplements that increase fat use during exercise may enhance time to exhaustion.

[a] 1 kg = 2.2 lbs.
RDA, recommended daily allowance.

analyses of athletes' diets have revealed that many are susceptible to maintaining negative energy intakes during training. Susceptible populations include runners, cyclists, swimmers, triathletes, gymnasts, skaters, dancers, wrestlers, boxers, and athletes attempting to lose weight too quickly *(4)*. In addition, female athletes have been reported to have a high incidence of eating disorders *(4)*. Consequently, it is important for the exercise physiologist working with athletes to ensure that athletes are well-fed and consume enough calories to offset the increased energy demands of training and maintain body weight.

Although this sounds relatively simple, intense training often suppresses appetite and/or alters hunger patterns so that many athletes do not feel like eating *(4)*. Some athletes do not like to exercise within several hours after eating because of sensations of fullness and/or a predisposition to gastrointestinal distress. Further, travel and training schedules may limit food availability and/or the types of food that athletes are accustomed to eating. This means that care should be taken to plan meal times in concert with training, as well as to make sure that athletes have sufficient availability of nutrient-dense foods throughout the day for snacking between meals (e.g., drinks, fruit, carbohydrate/protein bars) *(9)*. For this reason, sport nutritionists often recommend that athletes consume four to six meals per day and snack in between meals to meet energy needs. Use of nutrient-dense energy bars and high-calorie carbohydrate/protein supplements often provide a convenient way for athletes to supplement their diet to maintain energy intake during training.

3. GENERAL MACRONUTRIENT GUIDELINES FOR ATHLETES

The second component to optimizing training and performance through nutrition is to ensure that athletes consume the proper amounts of carbohydrate, protein, and fat in their diet. Table 1 summarizes macronutrient guidelines for athletes. The following discussion provides additional insight on how to structure the diet of athletes to optimize performance. Individuals engaged in a general fitness program can typically meet macronutrient needs by consuming a normal diet (i.e., 55% carbohydrate [3–5 g/kg/d], 20% protein [0.8–1.0 g/kg/d], and 25% fat [0.5–1.5 g/kg/d]). However, athletes involved in moderate- and high-volume training need greater amounts of carbohydrate and protein in their diet to meet macronutrient needs.

3.1. Carbohydrate

Carbohydrates serve as the primary fuel for high-intensity intermittent or prolonged exercise. Carbohydrate is stored in the muscle (about 15 g/kg) and liver (about 80–100 g). Intense exercise significantly depletes muscle and liver glycogen stores. The depleted stores are replenished from dietary carbohydrate. Unfortunately, when significant amounts of carbohydrate are depleted, it may be difficult to fully replenish carbohydrate levels within 1 d. Consequently, when athletes train once or twice per day over a period of days, carbohydrate levels may gradually decline, leading to fatigue, poor performance, and/or overtraining.

Athletes involved in moderate amounts of intense training (e.g., 2–3 h/d of intense exercise performed five to six times per week) typically need to consume a diet consisting of 55–65% carbohydrate (i.e., 5–8 g/kg/d or 250–1200 g/d for 50–150-kg athletes) to maintain liver and muscle glycogen stores *(3)*. Research has also shown that athletes

Table 2
Proposed Nutritional Ergogenic Aids for Athletes: Carbohydrate and Carbohydrate Byproducts

Nutrient	Theoretical ergogenic value	Summary of research findings/recommendations
Colosolic acid	Colosolic acid activates the "shuttle" that attracts glucose molecules, which are then transported into cells for energy. The result would be a stabilizing of blood glucose levels.	A review of PubMed revealed only one research study identifying colosolic acid as a glucose transport activator in vitro (35).
Dihydroxy-acetone phosphate (DHAP)	Supplementation with DHAP has been suggested to enhance glycolytic and oxidative metabolism. In addition, DHAP and pyruvate supplementation have been suggested to promote fat loss and extend endurance exercise capacity by serving as a fuel during exercise.	Few well-controlled studies have evaluated the ergogenic value of DHAP. Several studies have reported that DHAP supplementation (16–75 g/d) improved maximal VO_2 and promoted fat loss in obese individuals on hypocaloric diets (36). However, more research is needed before definitive conclusions can be made.
Fructose 1,6-diphosphate (FDP)	FDP serves as an intermediate step in glycolysis after the energy requiring steps of converting glucose to glucose-6-phosphate. Theorized to increase blood adenosine triphosphate (ATP) and 2,3-diphosphoglycerate levels, enhance dissociation of oxygen from hemoglobin, and serve as an efficient source of carbohydrate to enhance exercise capacity.	Studies indicate that FDP supplementation (0.25 g/kg) can serve as an effective fuel source during exercise (37). Some studies indicate that exercise capacity may be improved in patients with peripheral vascular disease. However, recent studies in healthy subjects indicate that FDP supplementation has no advantage over other forms of carbohydrate.
Glucose/ electrolyte solution (GES) sport drinks	Ingesting sport drinks during prolonged exercise (e.g., 6–8 oz of 6–8% solution every 5–15 min) has been found to help maintain blood glucose availability to the muscle and improve time to exhaustion in moderately intense exercise bouts (e.g., 70% of VO_2 max) lasting 3–4 h.	Numerous studies indicate that ingesting GES drinks during exercise maintains blood glucose levels, helps promote fluid retention, and decreases dehydration (38). Recommended for exercise bouts lasting more than 60 min, particularly if exercising in hot/humid environments. Ingesting highly concentrated carbohydrate drinks (i.e., >15%) may slow gastric emptying and promote dehydration.
Pinitol	D-Pinitol or (3-O-methyl-chiroinositol) is a plant extract that has been reported to stimulate glucose uptake into L6 cells (39).	A recent study found that co-ingestion of low doses of D-pinitol with creatine monohydrate augmented whole body creatine retention (40).
Calcium D-glucarate (CDG) Calcium glucarate Glucaric acid	Supplementation with calcium D-glucarate, calcium glucarate, and glucaric acid have been purported to help enhance metabolism, recovery, and growth by helping the body eliminate toxins, waste products, and carcinogens. In addition, the theory suggests that since D-glucaric acid and CDG have been found to help eliminate excess estrogen, it may help bodybuilders improve androgen/estrogen blance (44)	D-Glucarate acid is an important nutrient that promote the removal of toxins, carcinogens, and excess estrogen from the body. Although there may be some potential health benefits of supplementing the diet with CDG, there is no evidence that CDG supplementation at the recommeneded doses would affect training adaptations, body composition, or help atheletes reduce excess estrogen levels (44).

(continued)

318

Polylactate (PL)	PL is a semisoluble amino acid/lactate salt that has been theorized to be easily converted to pyruvate for entrance into the tricarboxylic acid (TCA) cycle and thereby enhance carbohydrate availability during endurance exercise.	Few studies have evaluated the ergogenic value of PL supplementation. One study reported that in comparison to a placebo and maltodextrin trial, PL supplementation during exercise (7% GES solution) promoted higher pH and bicarbonate levels reported that addition with no differences in performance (42). Conversely, another study reported that addition of PL to a glucose polymer drink did not affect physiological responses to exercise or performance (43).
Pyruvate	Supplementation of pyruvate with DHAP has been suggested to enhance fat loss and extend endurance exercise capacity by serving as a fuel during exercise.	Studies indicate that calcium pyruvate (6–25 g/d) with or without DHAP (16–75 g/d) supplementation promoted significantly more fat loss in obese individuals on hypocaloric diets 44,45). However, (there are little data to support that the dosages currently marketed to promote fat loss (i.e., 0.5–2 g/d) affect body composition or exercise responses.
Ribose	Ribose is a naturally occurring five-carbon sugar (pentose) that is primarily found in the body as a constituent of riboflavin (vitamin B$_2$), nucleic acids, nucleotides, and nucleosides. Supplementation has been theorized to increase ATP availability and recovery during intense exercise.	Some medical studies indicate that ribose supplementation (10–60 g/d) can increase ATP availability in certain patient populations, blunt the ischemia threshold in heart patients, and enhance the predictive value of thallium exercise tests (46–48). Most recent studies show no ergogenic value in athletes (49,50).

Table 3
Proposed Nutritional Ergogenic Aids: Lipids and Lipid Byproducts

Nutrient	Proposed ergogenic value	Summary of research findings
Conjugated linoleic acids (CLA)	CLA are essential fatty acids found primarily in fat from whole dairy products. Animal studies indicate that adding CLA to dietary feed decreases body fat, increases bone mass, has anticarcinogenic properties, enhances immunity, and inhibits atherosclerotic progression (51). Consequently, CLA supplementation in humans has been suggested to help manage body composition, delay loss of bone, and provide health benefit.	Although animal studies are impressive (52,53) and some studies suggest benefits at some but not all dosages (54,55), most studies conducted on humans show little to no effect on body composition or muscle growth (56,57).
Glycerol	Glycerol has been reported to promote fluid retention by decreasing urine formation. Glycerol added to water may be beneficial to hyperhydrate athletes before exercise in an effort to prevent dehydration during exercise.	Although studies indicate that glycerol can significantly enhance body fluid, studies are mixed on whether it can improve exercise capacity (58–60).
L-Carnitine	Carnitine serves as a transporter of fatty acids from the cytosol into the mitochondria and helps modulate the metabolism of coenzyme-A. Studies indicate that fatty acid oxidation is regulated in part by the ability to shuttle fatty acids into the mitochondria for entrance into the TCA cycle. Consequently, L-carnitine supplementation has been theorized as a means of enhancing fat oxidation and sparing muscle glycogen during exercise as well as promoting fat loss.	Although there are some data showing that L-carnitine supplementation may be beneficial for some patient populations, most well controlled studies indicate that L-carnitine supplementation does not affect muscle carnitine content, fat metabolism, and/or weight loss in overweight or trained subjects (61,62). One study reported that L-carnitine supplementation during a period of intensified training helped athletes tolerate training to a better degree (63).
Medium chain triglycerides (MCT)	MCT are shorter chain fatty acids that can easily enter the mitochondria of the cell and be converted to energy through fat metabolism (64). Theoretically, MCT feedings should serve as an efficient fuel source for exercise possibly serving to enhance endurance capacity.	Studies are mixed regarding whether MCT can serve as an effective source of fat during exercise metabolism and/or improve exercise performance (64–67).
n-3 Fatty acids	n-3 Fatty acids have been reported to serve as antioxidants, enhance immunity, and to decrease acid risk of cardiovascular disease. Some have suggested that n-3 fatty acid supplementation in athletes would decrease muscle damage and help maintain immune function.	Although there is evidence that n-3 fatty supplementation (1–3 g/d) may affect lipid peroxidation and immune responses, most studies indicate no ergogenic benefit on aerobic or anaerobic power (68).

involved in high-volume intense training (e.g., 3–6 h/d of intense training in one to two workouts for 5–6 d/wk) may need to consume 8–10 g/kg/d of carbohydrate (i.e., 400–1500 g/d for 50–150-kg athletes) to maintain muscle glycogen levels. This would be equivalent to consuming 0.5–2.0 kg/d of spaghetti. Preferably, the majority of dietary carbohydrate should come from complex carbohydrates with a low to moderate glycemic index (e.g., grains, starches, and fruit). However, because it is physically difficult to consume that much carbohydrate per day when an athlete is involved in intense training, many nutritionists and exercise physiologists recommend that athletes consume concentrated carbohydrate juices/drinks and/or consume high-carbohydrate supplements to meet carbohydrate needs. Although this amount of carbohydrate is not necessary for the fitness-minded individual who only trains three to four times per week for 30–60 min, it is essential for competitive athletes engaged in intense moderate- to high-volume training.

3.2. Protein

There has been considerable debate regarding protein needs of athletes (10–13). Initially, it was recommended that athletes do not need to ingest more than the recommended daily allowance (RDA) for protein (i.e., 0.8–1.0 g/kg/d). However, research over the last decade has indicated that athletes engaged in intense training need to ingest about 1.5–2 times the RDA (i.e., 1.5–2.0 g/kg/d) to maintain protein balance. If an insufficient amount of protein is obtained from the diet, an athlete will maintain a negative nitrogen balance resulting in protein catabolism and slow recovery. Over time, this may lead to lean muscle wasting and training intolerance.

For people involved in a general fitness program, protein needs can generally be met by ingesting 0.8–1.0 g/kg/d of protein. It is generally recommended that athletes involved in moderate amounts of intense training consume 1–1.5 g/kg/d of protein (50–225 g/d for a 50–150-kg athlete), whereas athletes involved in high-volume intense training consume 1.5–2.0 g/kg/d of protein (75–300 g/d for a 50–150-kg athlete) (10). This protein need would be equivalent to ingesting 3–11 servings of chicken or fish per day for a 50–150-kg athlete. Although smaller athletes typically can ingest this amount of protein in their normal diet, larger athletes often have difficulty consuming this much dietary protein. In addition, a number of athletic populations have been reported to be susceptible to protein malnutrition (e.g., runners, cyclists, swimmers, triathletes, gymnasts, dancers, skaters, wrestlers, and boxers). Therefore, care should be taken to ensure that athletes consume a sufficient amount of quality protein in their diet to maintain nitrogen balance (e.g., 1.5–2 g/kg/d).

However, it should be noted that not all protein is the same. Proteins differ based on the source of the protein, the amino acid profile of the protein, and the methods of processing or isolating the protein (14). These differences influence availability of amino acids that have been reported to possess biological activity (e.g., α-lactalbumin, β-lactoglobulin, glycomacropeptides, immunoglobulins, lactoperoxidases, and lactoferrin), and the rate and metabolic activity of the protein (15). For example, different types of proteins (e.g., casein and whey) are digested at different rates, and this directly affects catabolism and anabolism (14–17). Therefore, care should be taken not only to make sure that the athlete consumes enough protein in their diet but also that the protein is high quality. The best dietary sources of low-fat and high-quality protein are light, skinless chicken, fish, egg whites, and skim milk (casein and whey) (14). The best sources of high-

Table 4
Proposed Nutritional Ergogenic Aids: Protein and Amino Acids

Nutrient	Proposed ergogenic value	Summary of research findings
α-Keto-glutarate (α-KG)	α-KG is an intermediate in the TCA cycle that is involved in aerobic energy metabolism. There is some clinical evidence that α-KG may serve as an anticatabolic nutrient after surgery (69,70).	It is unclear whether α-KG supplementation during training affects training adaptations.
α-Keto-isocaproate (KIC)	KIC is a branched-chain keto acid that is a metabolite of leucine. In a similar manner as metabolite β-hydroxy β-methylbutyrate monohydrate (HMB), leucine and metabolites of leucine are believed to possess anticatabolic properties (71). the effects of KIC supplementation during training on body composition.	There is some clinical evidence that KIC may spare protein degradation in clinical populations (72,73). However, we are not aware of any studies that have evaluated the effects of KIC supplementation dring training on bod composition.
Arginine, ornithine, lysine	Clinical studies indicate that supplementation of these amino acids may stimulate growth hormone release serving to preserve muscle mass during bed rest. In addition, some studies indicate that arginine supplementation improve immune status. Consequently, some have suggested that supplementation of these amino acids during training may increase muscle mass and strength gains.	Recent studies indicate that supplementation with arginine, ornithine, and/or lysine (10–25 g/d), does not enhance the effect of exercise stimulation or power in experienced weightlifters (74,75).
Aspartate, asparagine	These amino acids serve as precursors to oxaloacetate in the TCA cycle. Supplementation has been theorized to spare muscle glycogen use and enhance endurance performance capacity.	Some well-controlled studies support the ergogenic value of aspartate and arginine supplementation on sparring muscle glycogen use and improving exercise capacity (76–78). However, additional research is necessary.
Branched-chain amino acids (BCAA)	Exercise-induced decreases in BCAA levels has been suggested to contribute to central fatigue as well as muscle catabolism. Supplementation of BCAA with sports drinks may increase BCAA availability and decrease the ratio of free tryptophan/BCAA. Theoretically, this may minimize serotonin production in the brain and delay central fatigue. Additionally, BCAA supplementation has been reported to decrease exercise-induced protein degradation and/or muscle enzyme release (an indicator of muscle damage) possibly by promoting an anticatabolic hormonal profile (27,79). Theoretically, BCAA supplementation during intense training may help minimize protein degradation and thereby lead to greater gains in fat-free mass.	A number of studies have reported that BCAA supplementation (4–16 g) can affect physiological and psychological responses to exercise. However, it is unclear the degree to which these potentially beneficial effects may affect performance. In terms of training, there is some evidence to support contentions that BCAA supplementation may affect catabolism and body composition (80–82) particularly when training at altitude.

(continued)

322

Creatine	The availability of phosphocreatine (PC) stores in the muscle significantly affects the amount of energy generated during brief periods of high-intensity exercise. Creatine supplementation has been hypothesized to increase muscle creatine content, help maintain adensoine triphosphate (ATP) during and following high-intensity, short-duration exercise.	Numerous studies have indicated that creatine supplementation increases high-intensity exercise performance and muscle mass during training (83). Performance gains are typically 5–15% greater than controls while muscle mass gain are 2–5 pounds greater than controls during 4–12 wk of training (84,85). The gains in muscle mass appear to be a result of an improved ability to perform high-intensity exercise enabling an athlete to train harder and thereby promote greater training adaptations and muscle hypertrophy (89–91).
Essential amino acids (EAA)	Recent studies have indicated that ingesting 3–6 g of EAA before (89,90) and or following exercise stimulates protein synthesis (91–95). Theoretically, this may enhance gains in muscle mass during training.	Recent research indicates that ingesting EAA with carbohydrate immediately following resistance exercise in elderly subjects promoted significantly greater training adaptations as compared to waiting until 2 h after exercise to consume the supplement (96). Although more data are needed, there is strong theoretical rationale and some supportive evidence that EAA supplementation may enhance protein synthesis and training adaptations.
Glutamine	Glutamine has been reported to increase cell volume and stimulate protein (97,98) and glycogen synthesis (99). Glutamine availability also directly affects lymphocytic function. Theoretically, glutamine supplementation prior to and/or following exercise (e.g., 6-10) may help to optimize cell hydration, protein synthesis, and maintain immune function leading to greater training adaptations.	A recent study found that subjects who supplemented their diet with glutamine (5 g) and BCAA (3 g) enriched whey protein during training promoted about a 2-lb greater gain in muscle mass and greater gains in strength than ingesting whey protein alone (100). Although more data are needed, there appears to be a strong scientific rationale and some preliminary evidence to indicate that glutamine may help build muscle.
β-hydroxy β-methylbutyrate (HMB)	Leucine and metabolites of leucine such a α-ketoisocaproate (KIC) have been reported to inhibit protein degradation. The anticatabolic effects have been suggested to be regulated by the leucine metabolite HMB. Adding HMB to dietary feed improved carcass quality in sows and steers. It has been hypothesized that supplementing the diet with leucine and/or HMB may inhibit protein degradation during resistance training.	Supplementing the diet with 1.5 to 3 g/d of calcium HMB has been reported to increase muscle mass and strength particularly among untrained subjects initiating training (101–104) and the elderly (105). Gains in muscle mass are typically 0.5 to 1 kg greater than controls during 3–6 wk of training. There is also recent evidence that HMB may lessen the catabolic effects of prolonged exercise (106) and that there may be additive effects of co-ingesting HMB with creatine (107,108).

(continued)

Table 4 (*continued*)
Proposed Nutritional Ergogenic Aids—Protein and Amino Acids

Nutrient	Proposed ergogenic value	Summary of research findings
Ornithine-α-ketoglutarate (OKG).	OKG is believed to possess anabolic/catabolic effects. Animal and clinical studies have suggested that patients administered OKG experienced improved protein balance. Theoretically, OKG may provide some value for athletes engaged in intense training.	A recent study reported that OKG supplementation (10 g/d) during 6 wk of resistance training promoted greater gains in bench press (*109*). However, no significant differences were observed in squat strength, training volume, or gains in muscle mass.
Tryptophan	Tryptophan is an amino acid that increases during prolonged exercise as fatty acids are mobilized for fat oxidation. Increases in brain concentrations of tryptophan have been reported to contribute to fatigue as well as increase endogenous opioid production. Tryptophan supplementation has been theorized to help athletes tolerate pain and enhance endurance exercise capacity.	Most studies indicate that increases in tryptophan in the blood and brain contributes to central fatigue. Although an initial study suggested that L-tryptophan supplementation improved endurance exercise performance whereas exercising at 80% of maximal exercise capacity (*110*), another study indicated that L-tryptophan had no effect or promoted an ergolytic effect on performance (*111*).

TCA, tricarboxylic acid cycle.

quality protein found in nutritional supplements are whey, casein, milk proteins, soy, and egg protein (14,18).

3.3. Fat

The dietary recommendations of fat intake for athletes are similar to or slightly greater than those recommended for nonathletes to promote health. Maintenance of energy balance, replenishment of intramuscular triacylglycerol stores, and adequate consumption of essential fatty acids are of greater importance among athletes and allow for somewhat increased intake (19). This depends on the athlete's training state and goals. For example, higher-fat diets appear to maintain circulating testosterone concentrations better than low-fat diets (20,21). This may have relevance to the documented suppression of testosterone that may occur during volume-type overtraining (22). Generally, it is recommended that athletes consume a moderate amount of fat (approx 30% of their daily caloric intake), whereas increases up to 50% of energy can be safely ingested by athletes during regular high-volume training (19). For athletes attempting to decrease body fat, however, it has been recommended that they consume 0.5–1 g/kg/d of fat. This is because some weight loss studies indicate that people who are most successful in losing weight and maintaining the weight loss are those who ingest less than 40 g/d of fat in their diet (23). Certainly, the type of dietary fat (e.g., n-6 vs n-3; saturation state) is a factor in such research and could play an important role in any discrepancies (24,25). Strategies to help athletes manage dietary fat intake include teaching them which foods contain various types of fat so they can make better food choices and how to how to count fat grams.

3.4. Nutrient Timing

In addition to the general nutritional guidelines described above, research has also demonstrated that the timing and composition of meals consumed may play a role in optimizing performance, training adaptations, and preventing overtraining. In this regard, it takes about 3–4 h for carbohydrate to be digested and begin to be stored as muscle and liver glycogen. Consequently, pre-exercise meals should be consumed about 3–4 h before exercise (3). This means that if an athlete trains in the afternoon, breakfast is the most important meal to top off muscle and liver glycogen levels. Research has also indicated that ingesting a light carbohydrate and protein snack 30–60 min before exercise (e.g., 50 g of carbohydrate and 5–10 g of protein) serves to increase carbohydrate availability toward the end of an intense exercise bout, increase availability of amino acids during exercise, maintain insulin levels, and decrease exercise-induced catabolism (10,26,27).

When exercise lasts more than 1 h, athletes should ingest glucose/electrolyte solution (GES) drinks to maintain blood glucose levels, help prevent dehydration, and reduce the immunosuppressive effects of intense exercise (28–31). Within 30 min following intense exercise, athletes should consume carbohydrate and protein (e.g., 1 g/kg of carbohydrate and 0.5 g/kg of protein), as well as consume a high-carbohydrate meal within 2 h of the exercise (32,33). This nutritional strategy has been found to accelerate glycogen resynthesis, as well as promote a more anabolic hormonal profile that may hasten recovery (32–34). Finally, for 2–3 d before competition, athletes should taper training by 30–50% and consume 200–300 g/d of *extra* carbohydrate in their diet.

Table 5
Proposed Nutritional Ergogenic Aids—Vitamins

Nutrient	Recommended dietary allowance	Proposed ergogenic value	Summary of research findings
Vitamin A	Males 900 μg/d Females 700 μg/d	Constituent of rhodopsin (visual pigment) and is involved in night vision. Some suggest that vitamin A supplementation may improve sport vision.	No studies have shown that vitamin A supplementation improves exercise performance (112).
Vitamin D	5 μg/d (age <51)	Promotes bone growth and mineralization. Enhances calcium absorption. Supplementation with calcium may help prevent bone loss in osteoperotic populations.	Co-supplementation with calcium may help prevent bone loss in athletes susceptible to osteoporosis (113). However, vitamin D supplementation does not enhance exercise performance (112).
Vitamin E	15 mg/d	As an antioxidant, it has been shown to help prevent the formation of free radicals during intense exercise and prevent the destruction of red blood cells, improving or maintaining oxygen delivery to the muscles during exercise. Some evidence suggests that it may reduce risk to heart disease or decrease incidence of recurring heart attack.	Numerous studies show that vitamin E supplementation can decrease exercise-induced oxidative stress (114–116). However, most studies show no effects on performance at sea level. At high altitudes, vitamin E may improve exercise performance (117). Additional research is necessary to determine whether long-term supplementation may help athletes better tolerate training.
Vitamin K	Males 120 μg/d Females 90 μg/d	Important in blood clotting. There is also some evidence that it may affect bone metabolism in postmenopausal women.	Vitamin K supplementation (10 mg/d) in elite female athletes has been reported to increase calcium-binding capacity of osteocalcin and promoted a 15–20% increase in bone formation markers and a 20–25% decrease in bone resorption markers suggesting an improved balance between bone formation and resorption (118).
Thiamin (B$_1$)	Males 1.2 mg/d Females 1.1 mg/d	Coenzyme (thiamin pyrophosphate) in the removal of CO_2 from decarboxylic reactions from pyruvate to acetyl coenzyme A (CoA) and in TCA cycle. Supplementation is theorized to improve anaerobic threshold and CO_2 transport.Deficiencies may decrease efficiency of energy systems.	Dietary availability of thiamin does not appear to affect exercise capacity when athletes have a normal intake (119).

(continued)

326

Riboflavin (B$_2$)	Males 1.3 mg/d Females 1.7 mg/d	Constituent of flavin nucleotide coenzymes involved in energy metabolism. Theorized to enhance energy availability during oxidative metabolism.	Dietary availability of riboflavin does not appear to affect exercise capacity when athletes have a normal intake (119).
Niacin (B$_3$)	Males 16 mg/d Females 14 mg/d	Constituent of coenzymes involved in energy metabolism. Theorized to blunt increases in fatty acids during exercise, reduce cholesterol, enhance thermoregulation, and improve energy availability improve energy availability during oxidative metabolism.	Studies indicate that niacin supplementation (100–500 mg/d) can help decrease blood lipid levels and increase homocysteine levels in hypercholesteremic patients (120,121). However, niacin supplementation (280 mg) during exercise has been reported to decrease exercise capacity blunting the mobilization of fatty acids (122).
Pyridoxine (B$_6$)	1.3 mg/d (age <51)	Has been marketed as a supplement that will improve muscle mass, strength, and aerobic power in the lactic acid and oxygen systems. It also may have a calming effect that has been linked to an improved mental strength.	In well-nourished athletes, pyridoxine failed to improve aerobic capacity, or lactic acid accumulation (119). However, when combined with vitamins B$_1$ and B$_{12}$, it may increase serotonin levels and improve fine motor skills that may be necessary in sports like pistol shooting and archery (123,124).
Cyano-cobalamin (B$_{12}$)	2.4 mg/d	A coenzyme involved in the production of DNA and serotonin. DNA is important in protein and red blood cell synthesis. Theoretically, it would increase muscle mass, the oxygen-carrying capacity of blood, and decrease anxiety.	In well-nourished athletes, no ergogenic effect has been reported. However, when combined with vitamins B$_1$ and B$_6$, cyanocobalamin has been shown to improve performance in pistol shooting (124). This may be caused by increased levels of serotonin, a neurotransmitter in the brain, which may reduce anxiety.

(continued)

Table 5 (*continued*)
Proposed Nutritional Ergogenic Aids—Vitamins

Nutrient	Recommended dietary allowance	Proposed ergogenic value	Summary of research findings
Folic acid (folate)	400 mg/d	Functions as a coenzyme in the formation of DNA and red blood cells. An increase in red blood cells could improve oxygen delivery to the muscles during exercise. Believed to be important to help prevent birth defects and may help decrease homocysteine levels.	Studies suggest that increasing dietary availability of folic acid during pregnancy can lower the incidence of birth defects (125). In addition, it may decrease homocysteine levels (a risk factor for heart disease) (126). In well-nourished and folate deficient-athletes, folic acid did not improve exercise performance (127).
Pantothenic acid	5 mg/d	Acts as a coenzyme for acetyl CoA. This may benefit aerobic or oxygen energy systems.	Research has reported no improvements in aerobic performance with acetyl CoA supplementation. However, one study reported a decrease in lactic acid accumulation, without an improvement in performance (128).
β-Carotene	None	Serves as an antioxidant. Theorized to help minimize exercise-induced lipid peroxidation and muscle damage.	Research indicates that β-carotene supplementation with or without other antioxidants can help decrease exercise-induced peroxidation. Over time, this may help athletes tolerate training. However, it is unclear whether antioxidant supplementation affects exercise performance (115).
Vitamin C	Males 90 mg/d Females 75 mg/d	Used in a number of different metabolic processes in the body. It is involved in the synthesis of epinephrine, iron absorption, and is an antioxidant. Theoretically, it could benefit exercise performance by improving metabolism during exercise. There is also evidence that vitamin C may enhance immunity.	In well-nourished athletes, vitamin C supplementation does not appear to improve physical performance (129,130). However, there is some evidence that vitamin C supplementation (e.g., 500 mg/d) following intense exercise may the incidence of upper respiratory tract infections (131–133).

Recommended dietary allowances based on the 2002 Food and Nutrition Board, National Academy of Sciences National Research Council recommendations.

This *carbohydrate loading* technique has been shown to supersaturate carbohydrate stores before competition and improve endurance exercise capacity *(3)*. Thus, the type of meal and timing of eating are important factors in maintaining carbohydrate availability during training and potentially decreasing the incidence of overtraining.

4. PROPOSED NUTRITIONAL ERGOGENIC AIDS

Nutritional ergogenic aids include alterations in the composition of the diet, timing of eating, and/or supplementation of various macro- and micronutrients that may enhance performance. Nutritional strategies that improve the preparation for exercise, the efficiency of exercise, performance capacity, and/or enhance the recovery from exercise may be viewed as ergogenic. Consequently, the final nutritional strategy for enhancing training and/or performance capacity in athletes is the appropriate use of effective, safe, and legal nutritional ergogenic aids. Although research has demonstrated that some nutritional strategies and nutrients may affect exercise training and/or performance capacity, the majority of nutritional ergogenic aids marketed to athletes do not affect performance. The following reviews macro- and micronutrients that have been proposed to improve exercise capacity.

4.1. Carbohydrate and Carbohydrate Byproducts

As stated previously, dietary carbohydrate availability can significantly affect muscle and liver carbohydrate stores and performance capacity. For this reason, in addition to the dietary guidelines described above, a significant amount of research has been conducted on determining ways to optimize carbohydrate availability during exercise and/or spare muscle glycogen use during exercise. Generally, increasing availability of any form of carbohydrate has the potential to improve exercise capacity by serving as an exogenous fuel source. Table 2 describes the proposed ergogenic value and summary of research findings for several forms of carbohydrate and carbohydrate byproducts that have been proposed to enhance exercise performance. Of the nutrients reviewed, GES sport drinks possess the greatest potential to improve exercise capacity. Although some clinical and/ or exercise benefits have been reported from colosolic acid, calcium D-glucarate, dihydroxyacetone phosphate, fructose 1,6-diphosphate, polylactate, pyruvate, and ribose supplementation, it is our view that additional research is necessary to determine the efficacy of these nutrients before they are recommended for athletes.

4.2. Lipids and Lipid Byproducts

Because fat can serve as a primary fuel source during low- to moderate-intensity exercise and most people have a considerable amount of fat stored as potential energy. Therefore, researchers have also investigated the effects of lipids and lipid byproducts on exercise capacity and training. The basic rationale is that if fat oxidation can be increased during exercise, carbohydrate stores can be spared, exercise capacity can be improved, and/or a greater amount of fat can be burned during exercise. Table 3 presents research findings for selected lipids and lipid byproducts that have been proposed to affect exercise performance. Of the nutrients presented, glycerol supplementation used as a means to hyperhydrate athletes susceptible to dehydration appears to possess the most ergogenic potential. Although basic research is promising, more research is needed in humans to determine whether conjugated linoleic acids supplementation affects body composition

Table 6
Proposed Nutritional Ergogenic Aids—Minerals

Nutrient	Recommended dietary allowance	Proposed ergogenic value	Summary of research findings
Boron	None	Boron has been marketed to athletes as a dietary supplement that may promote muscle growth during resistance training. The rationale was primarily based on an initial report that boron supplementation (3 mg/d) significantly increased β-estradiol and testosterone levels in postmenopausal women consuming a diet low in boron.	Studies, which have investigated the effects of 7 wk of boron supplementation (2.5 mg/d) during resistance training on testosterone levels, body composition, and strength, have reported no ergogenic value (136,137). There is no evidence at this time that boron supplementation during resistance-training promotes muscle growth.
Calcium	1000 mg/d (age 19–50 yr)	Involved in bone and tooth formation, blood clotting, and nerve transmission. Stimulates fat metabolism. Diet should contain sufficient amounts, especially in growing children/adolescents (139), female athletes, and postmenopausal women. Vitamin D needed to assist absorption.	Calcium supplementation may be beneficial in populations susceptible to osteoporosis (138). Additionally, calcium supplementation has been shown to promote fat metabolism and help manage body composition (139,140). Calcium supplementation provides no ergogenic effect on exercise performance.
Chromium	Males 35 mg/d Females 25 mg/d (age 19–50 yr)	Chromium, commonly sold as chromium picolinate, has been marketed with claims that the supplement will increase lean body mass and decrease body fat levels.	Animal research indicates that chromium supplementation increases lean body mass and reduces body fat. Early research on humans reported similar results (141), however, more recent well-controlled studies reported that chromium supplementation (200 to 800 mcg/d) does not improve lean body mass or reduce body fat (142,143).
Iron	Males 8 mg/d Females 18 mg/d (age 19–50)	Iron supplements are used to increase aerobic performance in sports that use the oxygen system. Iron is a component of hemoglobin in the red blood cell, which is a carrier of oxygen.	Most research shows that iron supplements do not appear to improve aerobic performance unless the athlete is iron-depleted and/or has anemia (144).
Magnesium	Males 420 Females 320	Activates enzymes involved in protein synthesis. Involved in adenosine triphosphate (ATP) reactions. Serum levels decrease with exercise. Some suggest that magnesium supplementation may improve energy metabolism/ATP	Most well-controlled research indicates that magnesium supplementation (500 mg/d) does not affect exercise performance in athletes unless there is a deficiency (145,146).

(continued)

330

Nutrient	RDA	Description	Research findings
Phosphorus (phosphate salts)	700 mg/d	Phosphate has been studied for its ability to improve all three energy systems, primarily the oxygen system or aerobic capacity.	Recent well-controlled research studies reported that sodium phosphate supplementation (4 g/d for 3 d) improved the oxygen energy system in endurance tasks (147,149). There appears to be little ergogenic value of other forms of phosphate (i.e., calcium phosphate, potassium phosphate). More research is needed to determine the mechanism for improvement.
Potassium	2000 mg/da	An electrolyte that helps regulate fluid balance, nerve transmission, and acid–base balance. Some suggest excessive increases or decreases in potassium may predispose athletes to cramping.	Although potassium loss during intense exercise in the heat has been anecdotally associated with muscle cramping, the etiology of cramping is unknown (150,151). It is unclear whether potassium supplementation in athletes decreases the incidence of muscle cramping (152). No ergogenic effects reported.
Selenium	55 µg/d	Marketed as a supplement to increase aerobic exercise performance. Working closely with vitamin E and glutathione peroxidase (an antioxidant), selenium may destroy destructive free radical production of lipids during aerobic exercise.	Although selenium may reduce lipid peroxidation during aerobic exercise, improvements in aerobic capacity have not been demonstrated (153,154).
Sodium	500 mg/da	An electrolyte that helps regulate fluid balance and nerve transmission.	During the first several days of intense training in the heat, a greater amount of sodium is lost in sweat. In addition, prolonged ultraendurance exercise may decrease sodium levels leading to hyponatremia. Increasing salt availability during heavy training in the heat has been shown to help maintain fluid balance and prevent hyponatremia (152,155).
Vanadyl sulfate (vanadium)	None	Vanadium may be involved in reactions in the body that produce insulin-like effects on protein and glucose metabolism. Owing to the anabolic of insulin, this has brought attention to vanadium as a supplement to increase muscle mass, enhance	Limited research has shown that type 2 diabetics may improve their glucose control; however, there is no proof that vanadyl sulfate has any effect on muscle mass, strength, or power (156,157).
Zinc	Males 11 mg/d Females 8 mg/d	Constituent of enzymes involved in digestion. Associated with immunity. Theorized to reduce incidence of upper respiratory tract infections in athletes involved in heavy training.	Studies indicate that zinc supplementation (25 mg/d) during training minimized exercise-induced changes in immune function (31,158–160).

Recommended dietary allowances based on the 2002 Food and Nutrition Board, National Academy of Sciences National Research Council recommendations.

[a]Estimated minimum requirement

Table 7
Proposed Nutritional Ergogenic Aids—Miscellaneous Nutrients

Nutrient	Proposed ergogenic value	Summary of research findings
Alcohol	It has been studied for its use as a psychological stress reducer in precision sports, such as riflery, archery, and dart throwing. It also has been investigated as an energy source.	Some limited research supports an ergogenic effect in precision sports like riflery when about one drink of alcohol is consumed (a blood alcohol of 0.02), 30–60 min before competition (162). However, its use is illegal in these sports and not recommended.
Alkaline salts (bicarbonate)	Sodium bicarbonate has been researched for its effect on improving power in sports that are of a short duration and use the lactic acid energy system.	Bicarbonate loading (e.g., 0.3 g/kg taken 60–90 min before exercise or 5 g taken 2 times/d for 5 d) has been shown to be an effective way to buffer acidity during high-intensity exercise lasting 1–3 min (163,164). This can improve exercise capacity in events like the 400–800-m run or 100–200-m swim (165).
Caffeine	Caffeine is a naturally derived stimulant found in many nutritional supplements, such as Gaurana, Bissey Nut, or Kola. Caffeine is also found in coffee, tea, soft drinks, energy drinks, and chocolate.	Studies indicate that ingestion of caffeine (e.g., 3–9 mg/kg taken 30–90 min before exercise) can spare carbohydrate use during exercise and thereby improve endurance (166,167).
Choline (lecithin)	Choline is considered an essential nutrient that is needed for cell membrane integrity and to facilitate the movement of fats in and out of cells. It is also a component of the neurotransmitter acetylcholine and is needed for normal brain functioning, particularly in infants. For this reason, phosphatidyl choline (PC) has been purported as a potentially effective supplement to promote fat loss as well as improve neuromuscular function.	There is some data from animal studies that support the potential value of PC as a weight-loss supplement (168). However, it is currently unclear whether PC supplementation affects body composition in humans. Studies have reported no apparent effects of PC supplementation during endurance exercise on performance (169,170).
Coenzyme Q10	It is found in the mitochondria and is involved in oxygen transport and adenosine triphosphate production. It is also an antioxidant that may help destroy free radicals during intense aerobic exercise.	Coenzyme Q10 has been found to improve heart function, aerobic capacity, and exercise performance in patients with heart disease, but not in healthy athletes (171,172).
Growth hormone releasing peptides (GHRP) and secretogues	Research has indicated that GHRP and other nonpeptide compounds (secretagogues) appear to help regulate growth hormone (GH) release (173,174). These observations have served as the basis for development of nutritionally-based GH stimulators (e.g., amino acids, pituitary peptides, "pituitary substances," macuna pruriens, broad bean, α-GPC).	Although there is clinical evidence that pharmaceutical grade GHRPs and some nonpeptide secretagogues can increase GH and insulin-like growth factor (IGF)-1 levels at rest and in response to exercise, it is currently unknown whether any of these nutritional alternatives would increase GH and/or affect training adaptations.

Inosine	Inosine is a building block for DNA and RNA that is found in muscle. It has a number of potentially important roles that may enhance training and/or exercise performance (175).	Although there is some theoretical rationale, available studies indicate that inosine supplementation has no apparent affect on exercise performance capacity (176–178).
Isoflavones	These are naturally occurring nonsteroidal phytoestrogens that have a similar chemical structure as the ipriflavone (a synthetic flavonoid drug used in the treatment of osteoporosis) (179). For this reason, soy protein (which is an excellent source of isoflavone) and isoflavone extracts have been investigated in the possible treatment of osteoporosis. More recently, the isoflavone extracts 7-isopropoxyisoflavone (ipriflavone) and 5-methyl-7-methoxy-isoflavone (methoxyisoflavone) have been marketed as "powerful anabolic" substances.	Although there may be some beneficial role of isoflavones in maintenance of bone mass in women, there is currently no peer-reviewed data indicating that ipriflavone or methoxyisoflavone supplementation affects exercise, body composition, or training adaptations.
Zinc-magnesium aspartate (ZMA)	Zinc and magnesium deficiency have been reported to reduce the production of testosterone and IGF-1. Athletes have been reported to have lower zinc and magnesium status. ZMA supplementation has been theorized to increase testosterone and IGF-1 leading to greater recovery, anabolism, and strength during training.	One study reported that a zinc-magnesium formulation increased testosterone and IGF-1 (two anabolic hormones) leading to greater gains in strength in football players participating in spring training (180). However, a recent study conducted in our lab was unable to reproduce these findings. More research is needed to evaluate the role of ZMA on body composition and strength during training before conclusions can be drawn.

during training and/or may possess health benefits. Based on current data, there appears to be limited ergogenic value of ʟ-carnitine and medium chain triglyceride supplementation. Finally, although there may be some health benefits from diets high in n-3 fatty acids, there is no evidence that supplementation with them affects exercise performance.

4.3. Protein and Amino Acids

Amino acids are the foundation of protein in the body and are essential for the synthesis of tissue-specific proteins, hormones, enzymes, and neurotransmitters *(10)*. Amino acids are also involved in the synthesis of energy through gluconeogenesis and regulation of numerous metabolic pathways. Consequently, it has been suggested that athletes may require additional protein in their diet to enhance muscle and tissue growth, the synthesis of hormones and enzymes necessary for energy metabolism, or serve as a potential energy substrate during exercise.

Table 4 describes the potential ergogenic value of amino acids, which have been purported to affect exercise capacity and/or promote training adaptations. Of the amino acids reviewed, creatine appears to be one of most effective and safe nutritional supplements to enhance anaerobic exercise capacity, strength, and gains in muscle mass during training. Studies have indicated that aspartate, branched-chain amino acids (leucine, isoleucine, and valine), essential amino acids (EAA), glutamine, and β-hydroxy β-methylbutyrate may affect exercise capacity, enhance recovery, and/or promote greater training adaptations. However, not all studies report the ergogenic value of the supplement and additional research is needed. Although there may be some clinical applications, there appears to be little ergogenic value of arginine, ornithine, lysine, and tryptophan supplementation for athletes.

4.4. Vitamins

Vitamins are essential organic compounds that serve to regulate metabolic processes, energy synthesis, neurological processes, and prevent destruction of cells. There are two primary classifications of vitamins: fat and water soluble. The fat-soluble vitamins include vitamins A, D, E, and K. The body stores fat-soluble vitamins and therefore excessive intake may result in toxicity. Water-soluble vitamins are the B vitamins and vitamin C; their water solubility reduces their risk of systemic toxicity caused by their improved ease of excretion in the urine.

Table 5 describes the RDA, proposed ergogenic benefit, and summary of research findings for fat- and water-soluble vitamins. Research has demonstrated that specific vitamins may possess some health benefit (e.g., vitamins C and E, niacin, and folic acid), although only a few have been reported to directly provide ergogenic value for athletes. However, some vitamins may help athletes tolerate training to a better degree by reducing oxidative damage (vitamins E and C) and/or help to maintain a healthy immune system during heavy training (vitamin C). However, dietary analyses of athletes have found deficiencies in caloric and vitamin intake, many sport nutritionists recommend that athletes consume a low-dose, one-a-day multivitamin and/or a vitamin-enriched postworkout carbohydrate/protein supplement during periods of heavy training. The American Medical Association also recently evaluated the available medical literature and recommended that Americans consume a one-a-day, low-dose multivitamin to promote general health and well-being *(134,135)*.

4.5. Minerals

Minerals are essential inorganic elements necessary for a host of metabolic processes. Minerals serve as structure for tissue, important components of enzymes and hormones, and regulators of metabolic and neural control. Some minerals have been found to be deficient in athletes or become deficient in response to training and/or prolonged exercise. When mineral status is inadequate, exercise capacity may be reduced. Dietary supplementation of minerals in deficient athletes has generally been found to improve exercise capacity. In addition, supplementation of specific minerals in nondeficient athletes has also been reported to affect exercise capacity.

Table 6 describes minerals that have been purported to affect exercise capacity in athletes. Of the minerals reviewed, several appear to possess health and/or ergogenic value for athletes under certain conditions. For example, calcium supplementation in athletes susceptible to premature osteoporosis may help maintain bone mass. There is also recent evidence that dietary calcium may help manage body composition. Iron supplementation in athletes prone to iron deficiency and/or anemia has been reported to improve exercise capacity. Sodium phosphate loading has been reported to increase maximal oxygen uptake, anaerobic threshold, and improve endurance exercise capacity by 8–10%. Increasing dietary availability of salt (sodium chloride) during the initial days of exercise training in the heat has been reported to help maintain fluid balance and prevent dehydration. Finally, zinc supplementation during training has been reported to decrease exercise-induced changes in immune function. Consequently, somewhat in contrast to vitamins, there appear to be several minerals that may enhance exercise capacity and/or training adaptations for athletes under certain conditions. However, although ergogenic value has been purported for the remaining minerals, there is little evidence that boron, chromium, magnesium, or vanadium affect exercise capacity or training adaptations in healthy individuals eating a normal diet.

4.6. Water

The most important nutritional ergogenic aid for athletes is water. Exercise performance can be significantly impaired when 2% or more of body weight is lost through sweat. For example, when a 70-kg athlete loses more than 1.4 kg of body weight during exercise (2%), performance capacity is often significantly decreased. Loss of more than 4% of body weight during exercise may lead to heat illness, heat exhaustion, heat stroke, and possibly death (161). For this reason, it is critical that athletes consume a sufficient amount of water and/or GES sports drinks during exercise to prevent excessive dehydration.

The normal sweat rate of individuals engaged in exercise ranges from 0.5–2.0 L/h depending on temperature, humidity, exercise intensity, and their sweat response to exercise (161). This means that to maintain fluid balance and prevent dehydration, athletes need to ingest 0.5–2 L/h of fluid to offset weight loss. This requires frequent ingestion of 6–8 oz of cold water or a GES sports drink every 5–15 min during exercise (161). Athletes should not depend on thirst to prompt them to drink because people do not typically get thirsty until they have lost a significant amount of fluid through sweat. In addition, athletes should weigh themselves before and following exercise training to ensure that they maintain proper hydration (161). The athlete should consume three cups of water for every pound lost during exercise to adequately rehydrate themselves after

Table 8
Categorization of the Ergogenic Value of Performance Enhancement, Muscle-Building, and Weight-Loss Supplements

Category	Muscle-building supplements	Weight-loss supplements	Performance enhancement
I. Apparently effective and generally safe	• Weight gain powders • Creatine • HMB (untrained individuals initiating training)	• Low-calorie foods, MRPs and RTDs that help individuals maintain a hypocaloric diet • Ephedra-, caffeine-, and salicin-containing thermogenic supplements taken at recommended doses in appropriate populations (ephedra is now banned by the FDA)	• Water and sports drinks • Carbohydrate • Creatine • Sodium phosphate • Sodium bicarbonate • Caffeine
II. Possibly effective	• Postexercise carbohydrate and protein • BCAA • Essential amino acids • Glutamine • Protein • HMB (trained subjects)	• High-fiber diets • Calcium • Phosphate • Green tea extract • Pyruvate/DHAP (at high doses)	• Postexercise CHO/PRO • Glutamine • EAA • BCAA • HMB (trained subjects) • Glycerol • Low doses of ephedrine/caffeine ephedrine is now banned by FDA)

(continued)

336

III. Too early to tell

- α-Ketoglutarate
- α-Ketoisocaproate
- Ecdysterones
- Growth hormone releasing peptides (GHRP) and secretogues
- HMB (trained athletes)
- Isoflavones
- Sulfo-polysaccharides (myostatin inhibitors)
- Zinc/magnesium aspartate

- Appetite suppressants and fat blockers (*Gymnema sylvestre*, chitosan)
- Thermogenics (synephrine, thyroid stimulators, cayenne pepper, black pepper, ginger root)
- Lipolytic nutrients (phosphatidyl choline, betaine, *Coleus forskohlii*, 7-keto DHEA)
- Psychotropic nutrients/herbs
- Chromium (nondiabetics)
- CLA
- HCA
- L-Carnitine
- Pyruvate (at low doses)
- Herbal diuretics
- High doses of ephedrine/caffeine

- Medium chain triglycerides
- Ribose

IV. Apparently not effective and/or dangerous

- Boron
- Chromium
- Conjugated linoleic acids (CLA)
- γ-Oryzanol (ferulic acid)
- Prohormones
- *Tribulus terrestris*
- Vanadyl sulfate (vanadium)
- Yohimbe (Yohimbine)

- Inosine
- High doses of ephedrine/caffeine

HMB, metabolite b-hydroxy b-methylbutyrate monohydrate; MRPs, meal replacement powders; FDA, Food and Drug Administration; CHO, charbohydrate; PRO, protein; BCAA, branched-chain amino acids; DHAP, dihydroxyacetone phosphate; DHEA, dihydroxy epiandrosterone; CLA, conjugated linoleic acids; HCA, hydroxycitic acid.

exercise *(161)*. Athletes should also train themselves to tolerate drinking greater amounts of water during training and make sure that they consume more fluid in hotter or humid environments. Preventing dehydration during exercise is one of the most effective ways to maintain exercise capacity. Finally, inappropriate and excessive weight loss techniques (e.g., cutting weight in saunas, wearing rubber suits, severe dieting, vomiting, and using diuretics) are extremely dangerous and should be prohibited.

4.7. Miscellaneous Substances

Table 7 shows various ergogenic substances not previously described. Of the nutrients described, sodium bicarbonate, caffeine, and echinacea appear to have the greatest potential to affect exercise performance and/or training adaptations. Sodium bicarbonate-loading (0.3 g/kg of baking soda) before exercise has been consistently reported to enhance bouts of high-intensity exercise lasting from 1 to 3 min in duration (e.g., a 400–800 m run). Although some athletes may experience gastrointestinal distress, bicarbonate loading appears to be a highly effective ergogenic aid for athletes as long as they can tolerate the supplementation protocol.

Caffeine is a naturally occurring stimulant found in many foods consumed in the normal diet (e.g., coffee, tea, and chocolate). Caffeine ingestion (3–9 mg/kg) before exercise has been reported to increase fat oxidation, spare muscle glycogen use, and enhance endurance exercise performance. The ergogenic effects of caffeine appear to be more pronounced in nonhabitual caffeine users and in habitual users who abstain from consuming caffeine for about 1 wk before competition. Although some athletic governing bodies have banned excessive intake of caffeine as an ergogenic aid, studies show that even when taken within the limits allowed by athletic governing bodies, caffeine may provide ergogenic benefit. Doses should be limited to 7 mg/kg or less to avoid a positive drug test for excess caffeine use. Because caffeine serves as a mild diuretic, there has been some concern whether caffeine intake before exercise may hasten dehydration. However, recent studies indicate that caffeine does not appear to influence hydration status in active individuals who follow normal fluid intake guidelines.

A more complete review of the general usefulness of herbal supplements can be found in Chapter 11. Echinacea is an herb that has been reported to enhance immune function and decrease the severity, duration, and incidence of colds and upper respiratory tract infections. Because intense training may compromise immune function in athletes, some have suggested that echinacea supplementation during heavy training may decrease the incidence of colds and infections, particularly when combined with vitamin C and/or zinc. Although there are data to support the immuno-enhancing effects of echinacea, we are aware of no studies that have determined whether use of echinacea in athletes helps maintain immune function during intense training.

5. SUMMARY

Dietary and nutritional practices of athletes can significantly affect exercise performance capacity. To optimize performance, athletes should: (1) eat enough calories to offset energy expenditure (typically 60–80 kcal/kg/d); (2) consume the proper amount of carbohydrate (5–10 g/kg/d), protein (1.5–2.0 g/kg/d), and fat (0.5–1.5 g/kg/d); (3) ingest meals and snacks at appropriate time intervals before, during, and/or following exercise to provide energy for exercise, as well as promote recovery following exercise; and (4) only consider using nutritional supplements that have been found to be an effective and safe means to improve performance capacity.

Table 8 categorizes supplements into those that we consider to be effective, those that are possibly effective, those where it is "too early to tell" but needing more research before any definitive conclusions can be drawn, and those that are apparently ineffective or potentially dangerous. The foundation for good performance begins with a good diet and intelligent training. For strength/power athletes, research has indicated that water, carbohydrate, postexercise carbohydrate/protein intake, creatine, sodium phosphate, and possibly sodium bicarbonate may have the greatest impact on optimizing performance and/or training adaptations. For endurance athletes, research suggests that carbohydrate loading, water/GES sports drinks, caffeine, sodium phosphate loading, and possibly, use of glycerol in an attempt to hyperhydrate before exercise may offer some ergogenic value. Sports drinks, carbohydrate, postexercise carbohydrate with protein or EAA, creatine, and metabolite b-hydroxy b-methylbutyrate monohydrate have been reported to help athletes tolerate exercise and training. In addition, postexercise carbohydrate, protein, EAA, and glutamine, as well as vitamin C, zinc, and echinacea, may help athletes maintain a healthy immune system during training. Use of these strategies can help optimize performance and/or help athletes tolerate intense periods of training.

REFERENCES

1. Kreider RB, Fry AC, O'Toole ML. Overtraining in Sport. Human Kinetics Publishers, Champaign, IL, 1998.
2. Williams MH. Nutrition for Health, Fitness, and Sport. ACB/McGraw-Hill, Dubuque, IA, 1999.
3. Sherman WM, Jacobs KA, Leenders N. Carbohydrate metabolism during endurance exercise. In: Kreider RB, Fry AC, O'Toole ML, eds. Overtraining in Sport. Human Kinetics Publishers, Champaign, Il, 1998, pp. 289–308.
4. Berning JR. Energy intake, diet, and muscle wasting. In: Kreider RB, Fry AC, O'Toole ML, eds. Overtraining in Sport. Human Kinetics, Champaign, IL, 1998, pp. 275–288.
5. Leutholtz B, Kreider R. Exercise and sport nutrition. In: Wilson T, Temple N, eds. Nutritional Health. Humana Press, Totowa, NJ, 2001, pp. 207–239.
6. Brouns F, Saris WH, Beckers E, et al. Metabolic changes induced by sustained exhaustive cycling and diet manipulation. Int J Sports Med 1989; 10(Suppl 1):S49–S62.
7. Brouns F, Saris WH, Stroecken J, et al. Eating, drinking, and cycling. A controlled Tour de France simulation study, Part II. Effect of diet manipulation. Int J Sports Med 1989; 10 Suppl 1:S41–S48.
8. Kreider RB. Physiological considerations of ultraendurance performance. Int J Sport Nutr 1991; 1:3–27.
9. Kreider RB. Nutritional considerations of overtraining. In: Stout JR, Antonio J, eds. Sport Supplements: A Complete Guide to Physique and Athletic Enhancement. Lippincott, Williams & Wilkins, Baltimore, MD, 2001, pp. 199–208.
10. Kreider RB. Dietary supplements and the promotion of muscle growth with resistance exercise. Sports Med 1999; 27:97–110.
11. Lemon PW, Tarnopolsky MA, MacDougall JD, Atkinson SA. Protein requirements and muscle mass/strength changes during intensive training in novice bodybuilders. J Appl Physiol 1992; 73:767–775.
12. Tarnopolsky MA, Atkinson SA, MacDougall JD, Chesley A, Phillips S, Schwarcz HP. Evaluation of protein requirements for trained strength athletes. J Appl Physiol 1992; 73:1986–1995.
13. Tarnopolsky MA, MacDougall JD, Atkinson SA. Influence of protein intake and training status on nitrogen balance and lean body mass. J Appl Physiol 1988; 64:187–193.
14. Bucci L, Unlu L. Proteins and amino acid supplements in exercise and sport. In: Driskell J, Wolinsky I, eds. Energy-Yielding Macronutrients and Energy Metabolism in Sports Nutrition. CRC Press, Boca Raton, FL, 2000, pp. 191–212.

15. Boirie Y, Dangin M, Gachon P, Vasson MP, Maubois JL, Beaufrere B. Slow and fast dietary proteins differently modulate postprandial protein accretion. Proc Natl Acad Sci USA 1997; 94:14930–14935.

16. Boirie Y, Gachon P, Corny S, Fauquant J, Maubois JL, Beaufrere B. Acute postprandial changes in leucine metabolism as assessed with an intrinsically labeled milk protein. Am J Physiol 1996; 271: E1083–E1091.

17. Dangin M, Boirie Y, Garcia-Rodenas C, et al. The digestion rate of protein is an independent regulating factor of postprandial protein retention. Am J Physiol Endocrinol Metab 2001; 280:E340–E348.

18. Kreider RB, Kleiner SM. Protein supplements for athletes: need vs. convenience. Your Patient & Fitness 2000; 14:12–18.

19. Venkatraman JT, Leddy J, Pendergast D. Dietary fats and immune status in athletes: clinical implications. Med Sci Sports Exerc 2000; 32:S389–S395.

20. Dorgan JF, Judd JT, Longcope C, et al. Effects of dietary fat and fiber on plasma and urine androgens and estrogens in men: a controlled feeding study. Am J Clin Nutr 1996; 64:850–855.

21. Hamalainen EK, Adlercreutz H, Puska P, Pietinen P. Decrease of serum total and free testosterone during a low-fat high-fibre diet. J Steroid Biochem 1983; 18:369,370.

22. Fry AC, Kraemer WJ, Ramsey LT. Pituitary-adrenal-gonadal responses to high-intensity resistance exercise overtraining. J Appl Physiol 1998; 85:2352–2359.

23. Pirozzo S, Summerbell C, Cameron C, Glasziou P. Should we recommend low-fat diets for obesity? Obes Rev 2003; 4:83–90.

24. Hu FB, Manson JE, Willett WC. Types of dietary fat and risk of coronary heart disease: a critical review. J Am Coll Nutr 2001; 20:5–19.

25. Vessby B. Dietary fat, fatty acid composition in plasma and the metabolic syndrome. Curr Opin Lipidol 2003; 14:15–19.

26. Cade JR, Reese RH, Privette RM, Hommen NM, Rogers JL, Fregly MJ. Dietary intervention and training in swimmers. Eur J Appl Physiol Occup Physiol 1991; 63:210–215.

27. Carli G, Bonifazi M, Lodi L, Lupo C, Martelli G, Viti A. Changes in the exercise-induced hormone response to branched chain amino acid administration. Eur J Appl Physiol Occup Physiol 1992; 64:272–277.

28. Burke LM. Nutrition for post-exercise recovery. Aust J Sci Med Sport 1997; 29:3–10.

29. Burke LM. Nutritional needs for exercise in the heat. Comp Biochem Physiol A Mol Integr Physiol 2001; 128:735–748.

30. Nieman DC, Fagoaga OR, Butterworth DE, et al. Carbohydrate supplementation affects blood granulocyte and monocyte trafficking but not function after 2.5 h or running. Am J Clin Nutr 1997; 66:153–159.

31. Nieman DC. Nutrition, exercise, and immune system function. Clin Sports Med 1999; 18:537–548.

32. Zawadzki KM, Yaspelkis BB, 3rd, Ivy JL. Carbohydrate-protein complex increases the rate of muscle glycogen storage after exercise. J Appl Physiol 1992; 72:1854–1859.

33. Tarnopolsky MA, Bosman M, Macdonald JR, Vandeputte D, Martin J, Roy BD. Postexercise protein-carbohydrate and carbohydrate supplements increase muscle glycogen in men and women. J Appl Physiol 1997; 83:1877–1883.

34. Kraemer WJ, Volek JS, Bush JA, Putukian M, Sebastianelli WJ. Hormonal responses to consecutive days of heavy-resistance exercise with or without nutritional supplementation. J Appl Physiol 1998; 85:1544–1555.

35. Murakami C, Myoga K, Kasai R, et al. Screening of plant constituents for effect on glucose transport activity in Ehrlich ascites tumour cells. Chem Pharm Bull (Tokyo) 1993; 41:2129–2131.

36. Stanko RT, Robertson RJ, Galbreath RW, Reilly JJ, Jr., Greenawalt KD, Goss FL. Enhanced leg exercise endurance with a high-carbohydrate diet and dihydroxyacetone and pyruvate. J Appl Physiol 1990; 69:1651–1656.

37. Myers J, Atwood JE, Forbes S, Evans B, Froelicher V. Effect of fructose 1,6-diphosphate on exercise capacity in patients with peripheral vascular disease. Int J Sports Med 1990; 11:259–262.

38. Convertino VA, Armstrong LE, Coyle EF, et al. American College of Sports Medicine position stand. Exercise and fluid replacement. Med Sci Sports Exerc 1996; 28:i–vii.

39. Bates SH, Jones RB, Bailey CJ. Insulin-like effect of pinitol. Br J Pharmacol 2000; 130:1944–1948.

40. Greenwood M, Kreider RB, Rasmussen C, Almada AL, Earnest CP. D-Pinitol augments whole body creatine retention in man. J Exerc Physiol Online 2001. Available: http://www.css.edu/users/tboone2/asep/GreenwoodNOVEMBER2001.pdf; 4:41–47.

41. Walaszek Z, Szemraj J, Narog M, et al. Metabolism, uptake, and excretion of a D-glucaric acid salt and its potential use in cancer prevention. Cancer Detect Prev 1997; 21:178–190.

42. Fahey T. The effects of ingesting polylactate or glucose polymer drinks during prolonged exercise. Int J Sport Nutr 1991; 1:49–56.

43. Swensen T, Crater G, Bassett DR, Jr., Howley ET. Adding polylactate to a glucose polymer solution does not improve endurance. Int J Sports Med 1994; 15:430–434.

44. Kalman D, Colker CM, Wilets I, Roufs JB, Antonio J. The effects of pyruvate supplementation on body composition in overweight individuals. Nutrition 1999; 15:337–340.

45. Stanko RT, Arch JE. Inhibition of regain in body weight and fat with addition of 3-carbon compounds to the diet with hyperenergetic refeeding after weight reduction. Int J Obes Relat Metab Disord 1996; 20:925–930.

46. Gross M, Kormann B, Zollner N. Ribose administration during exercise: effects on substrates and products of energy metabolism in healthy subjects and a patient with myoadenylate deaminase deficiency. Klin Wochenschr 1991; 69:151–155.

47. Hegewald MG, Palac RT, Angello DA, Perlmutter NS, Wilson RA. Ribose infusion accelerates thallium redistribution with early imaging compared with late 24-hour imaging without ribose. J Am Coll Cardiol 1991; 18:1671–1681.

48. Wagner DR, Gresser U, Kamilli I, Gross M, Zollner N. Effects of oral ribose on muscle metabolism during bicycle ergometer in patients with AMP-deaminase-deficiency. Adv Exp Med Biol 1991; 309B:383–385.

49. Op 't Eijnde B, Van Leemputte M, Brouns F, et al. No effects of oral ribose supplementation on repeated maximal exercise and de novo ATP resynthesis. J Appl Physiol 2001; 91:2275–2281.

50. Kreider RB, Melton C, Greenwood M, et al. Effects of oral d-ribose supplementation on anaerobic capacity and selected metabolic markers in healthy males. Int J Sport Nutr Exerc Metab 2003; 13:87–96.

51. Pariza MW, Park Y, Cook ME. The biologically active isomers of conjugated linoleic acid. Prog Lipid Res 2001; 40:283–298.

52. Park Y, Albright KJ, Liu W, Storkson JM, Cook ME, Pariza MW. Effect of conjugated linoleic acid on body composition in mice. Lipids 1997; 32:853–858.

53. DeLany JP, West DB. Changes in body composition with conjugated linoleic acid. J Am Coll Nutr 2000; 19:487S–493S.

54. Blankson H, Stakkestad JA, Fagertun H, Thom E, Wadstein J, Gudmundsen O. Conjugated linoleic acid reduces body fat mass in overweight and obese humans. J Nutr 2000; 130:2943–2948.

55. Gaullier JM, Berven G, Blankson H, Gudmundsen O. Clinical trial results support a preference for using CLA preparations enriched with two isomers rather than four isomers in human studies. Lipids 2002; 37:1019–1025.

56. Kreider RB, Ferreira MP, Greenwood M, Wilson M, Almada AL. Effects of conjugated linoleic acid supplementation during resistance training on body composition, bone density, strength, and selected hematological markers. J Strength Cond Res 2002; 16:325–334.

57. Zambell KL, Keim NL, Van Loan MD, et al. Conjugated linoleic acid supplementation in humans: effects on body composition and energy expenditure. Lipids 2000; 35:777–782.

58. Inder WJ, Swanney MP, Donald RA, Prickett TC, Hellemans J. The effect of glycerol and desmopressin on exercise performance and hydration in triathletes. Med Sci Sports Exerc 1998; 30:1263–1269.

59. Meyer LG, Horrigan DJ, Jr, Lotz WG. Effects of three hydration beverages on exercise performance during 60 hours of heat exposure. Aviat Space Environ Med 1995; 66:1052–1057.

60. Magal M, Webster MJ, Sistrunk LE, Whitehead MT, Evans RK, Boyd JC. Comparison of glycerol and water hydration regimens on tennis-related performance. Med Sci Sports Exerc 2003; 35:150–156.

61. Brass EP, Hiatt WR. Carnitine metabolism during exercise. Life Sci 1994; 54:1383–1393.

62. Villani RG, Gannon J, Self M, Rich PA. L-Carnitine supplementation combined with aerobic training does not promote weight loss in moderately obese women. Int J Sport Nutr Exerc Metab 2000; 10:199–207.

63. Volek JS, Kraemer WJ, Rubin MR, Gomez AL, Ratamess NA, Gaynor P. L-Carnitine L-tartrate supplementation favorably affects markers of recovery from exercise stress. Am J Physiol Endocrinol Metab 2002; 282:E474–E482.

64. Jeukendrup AE, Thielen JJ, Wagenmakers AJ, Brouns F, Saris WH. Effect of medium-chain triacylglycerol and carbohydrate ingestion during exercise on substrate utilization and subsequent cycling performance. Am J Clin Nutr 1998; 67:397–404.

65. Goedecke JH, Elmer-English R, Dennis SC, Schloss I, Noakes TD, Lambert EV. Effects of medium-chain triaclyglycerol ingested with carbohydrate on metabolism and exercise performance. Int J Sport Nutr 1999; 9:35–47.

66. Calabrese C, Myer S, Munson S, Turet P, Birdsall TC. A cross-over study of the effect of a single oral feeding of medium chain triglyceride oil vs. canola oil on post-ingestion plasma triglyceride levels in healthy men. Altern Med Rev 1999; 4:23–28.

67. Angus DJ, Hargreaves M, Dancey J, Febbraio MA. Effect of carbohydrate or carbohydrate plus medium-chain triglyceride ingestion on cycling time trial performance. J Appl Physiol 2000; 88:113–119.

68. Brilla LR, Landerholm TE. Effect of fish oil supplementation and exercise on serum lipids and aerobic fitness. J Sports Med Phys Fitness 1990; 30:173–180.

69. Hammarqvist F, Wernerman J, Ali R, Vinnars E. Effects of an amino acid solution enriched with either branched chain amino acids or ornithine-alpha-ketoglutarate on the postoperative intracellular amino acid concentration of skeletal muscle. Br J Surg 1990; 77:214–218.

70. Wernerman J, Hammarqvist F, Vinnars E. Alpha-ketoglutarate and postoperative muscle catabolism. Lancet 1990; 335:701–703.

71. Antonio J, Stout JR. Sport Supplements. Lippincott, Williams and Wilkins, Philadelphia, PA, 2001, pp. 118–120.

72. Mitch WE, Walser M, Sapir DG. Nitrogen sparing induced by leucine compared with that induced by its keto analogue, alpha-ketoisocaproate, in fasting obese man. J Clin Invest 1981; 67:553–562.

73. Van Koevering M, Nissen S. Oxidation of leucine and alpha-ketoisocaproate to beta-hydroxy-beta-methylbutyrate in vivo. Am J Physiol 1992; 262:E27–E31.

74. Procopio M, Maccario M, Savio P, et al. GH response to GHRH combined with pyridostigmine or arginine in different conditions of low somatotrope secretion in adulthood: obesity and Cushing's syndrome in comparison with hypopituitarism. Panminerva Med 1998; 40:13–17.

75. Wu G, Meininger CJ. Arginine nutrition and cardiovascular function. J Nutr 2000; 130:2626–2629.

76. Colombani PC, Bitzi R, Frey-Rindova P, et al. Chronic arginine aspartate supplementation in runners reduces total plasma amino acid level at rest and during a marathon run. Eur J Nutr 1999; 38:263–270.

77. Colombani P, Wenk C, Kunz I, et al. Effects of L-carnitine supplementation on physical performance and energy metabolism of endurance-trained athletes: a double-blind crossover field study. Eur J Appl Physiol Occup Physiol 1996; 73:434–439.

78. Tuttle JL, Potteiger JA, Evans BW, Ozmun JC. Effect of acute potassium-magnesium aspartate supplementation on ammonia concentrations during and after resistance training. Int J Sport Nutr 1995; 5:102–109.

79. Coombes JS, McNaughton LR. Effects of branched-chain amino acid supplementation on serum creatine kinase and lactate dehydrogenase after prolonged exercise. J Sports Med Phys Fitness 2000; 40:240–246.

80. Bigard AX, Lavier P, Ullmann L, Legrand H, Douce P, Guezennec CY. Branched-chain amino acid supplementation during repeated prolonged skiing exercises at altitude. Int J Sport Nutr 1996; 6:295–306.

81. Candeloro N, Bertini I, Melchiorri G, De Lorenzo A. [Effects of prolonged administration of branched-chain amino acids on body composition and physical fitness]. Minerva Endocrinol 1995; 20:217–223.

82. Schena F, Guerrini F, Tregnaghi P, Kayser B. Branched-chain amino acid supplementation during trekking at high altitude. The effects on loss of body mass, body composition, and muscle power. Eur J Appl Physiol Occup Physiol 1992; 65:394–398.

83. Williams MH. Facts and fallacies of purported ergogenic amino acid supplements. Clin Sports Med 1999; 18:633–649.

84. Kreider RB, Melton C, Rasmussen CJ, et al. Long-term creatine supplementation does not significantly affect clinical markers of health in athletes. Mol Cell Biochem 2003; 244:95–104.

85. Kreider RB. Effects of creatine supplementation on performance and training adaptations. Mol Cell Biochem 2003; 244:89–94.

86. Willoughby DS, Rosene JM. Effects of oral creatine and resistance training on myogenic regulatory factor expression. Med Sci Sports Exerc 2003; 35:923–929.

87. Willoughby DS, Rosene J. Effects of oral creatine and resistance training on myosin heavy chain expression. Med Sci Sports Exerc 2001; 33:1674–1681.

88. Volek JS, Duncan ND, Mazzetti SA, et al. Performance and muscle fiber adaptations to creatine supplementation and heavy resistance training. Med Sci Sports Exerc 1999; 31:1147–1156.

89. Tipton KD, Borsheim E, Wolf SE, Sanford AP, Wolfe RR. Acute response of net muscle protein balance reflects 24-h balance after exercise and amino acid ingestion. Am J Physiol Endocrinol Metab 2003; 284:E76–E89.

90. Wolfe RR. Regulation of muscle protein by amino acids. J Nutr 2002; 132:3219S–3224S.

91. Rasmussen BB, Wolfe RR, Volpi E. Oral and intravenously administered amino acids produce similar effects on muscle protein synthesis in the elderly. J Nutr Health Aging 2002; 6:358–362.

92. Tipton KD, Rasmussen BB, Miller SL, et al. Timing of amino acid-carbohydrate ingestion alters anabolic response of muscle to resistance exercise. Am J Physiol Endocrinol Metab 2001; 281:E197–E206.

93. Rasmussen BB, Tipton KD, Miller SL, Wolf SE, Wolfe RR. An oral essential amino acid-carbohydrate supplement enhances muscle protein anabolism after resistance exercise. J Appl Physiol 2000; 88:386–392.

94. Miller SL, Tipton KD, Chinkes DL, Wolf SE, Wolfe RR. Independent and combined effects of amino acids and glucose after resistance exercise. Med Sci Sports Exerc 2003; 35:449–455.

95. Biolo G, Williams BD, Fleming RY, Wolfe RR. Insulin action on muscle protein kinetics and amino acid transport during recovery after resistance exercise. Diabetes 1999; 48:949–957.

96. Esmarck B, Andersen JL, Olsen S, Richter EA, Mizuno M, Kjaer M. Timing of postexercise protein intake is important for muscle hypertrophy with resistance training in elderly humans. J Physiol 2001; 535:301–311.

97. Low SY, Taylor PM, Rennie MJ. Responses of glutamine transport in cultured rat skeletal muscle to osmotically induced changes in cell volume. J Physiol 1996; 492(Pt 3):877–885.

98. Rennie MJ, Ahmed A, Khogali SE, Low SY, Hundal HS, Taylor PM. Glutamine metabolism and transport in skeletal muscle and heart and their clinical relevance. J Nutr 1996; 126:1142S–1149S.

99. Varnier M, Leese GP, Thompson J, Rennie MJ. Stimulatory effect of glutamine on glycogen accumulation in human skeletal muscle. Am J Physiol 1995; 269:E309–E315.

100. Colker CM. Effects of supplemental protein on body composition and muscular strength in healthy athletic male adults. Curr Ther Res 2000; 61:19–28.

101. Gallagher PM, Carrithers JA, Godard MP, Schulze KE, Trappe SW. Beta-hydroxy-beta-methylbutyrate ingestion, part II: effects on hematology, hepatic and renal function. Med Sci Sports Exerc 2000; 32:2116–2119.

102. Gallagher PM, Carrithers JA, Godard MP, Schulze KE, Trappe SW. Beta-hydroxy-beta-methylbutyrate ingestion, Part I: effects on strength and fat free mass. Med Sci Sports Exerc 2000; 32:2109–2115.

103. Nissen S, Sharp R, Ray M, et al. Effect of leucine metabolite beta-hydroxy-beta-methylbutyrate on muscle metabolism during resistance-exercise training. J Appl Physiol 1996; 81:2095–2104.

104. Panton LB, Rathmacher JA, Baier S, Nissen S. Nutritional supplementation of the leucine metabolite beta-hydroxy-beta- methylbutyrate (hmb) during resistance training. Nutrition 2000; 16:734–739.

105 Vukovich MD, Stubbs NB, Bohlken RM. Body composition in 70-year-old adults responds to dietary beta-hydroxy-beta-methylbutyrate similarly to that of young adults. J Nutr 2001; 131:2049–2052.

106. Knitter AE, Panton L, Rathmacher JA, Petersen A, Sharp R. Effects of beta-hydroxy-beta-methylbutyrate on muscle damage after a prolonged run. J Appl Physiol 2000; 89:1340–1344.

107. Jowko E, Ostaszewski P, Jank M, et al. Creatine and beta-hydroxy-beta-methylbutyrate (HMB) additively increase lean body mass and muscle strength during a weight-training program. Nutrition 2001; 17:558–566.

108. O'Connor DM, Crowe MJ. Effects of beta-hydroxy-beta-methylbutyrate and creatine monohydrate supplementation on the aerobic and anaerobic capacity of highly trained athletes. J Sports Med Phys Fitness 2003; 43:64–68.

109. Chetlin RD, Yeater RA, Ullrich IH, Hornsby WG, Malanga CJ, Byrner RW. The effect of ornithine alpha-ketoglutarate (OKG) on healthy, weight trained men. J Exerc Physiol Online 2000; 3:Available at: www.css.edu/users/tboone2/asep/ChetlinV2.pdf.

110. Segura R, Ventura JL. Effect of L-tryptophan supplementation on exercise performance. Int J Sports Med 1988; 9:301–305.

111. Stensrud T, Ingjer F, Holm H, Stromme SB. L-tryptophan supplementation does not improve running performance. Int J Sports Med 1992; 13:481–485.

112 Williams MH. Vitamin supplementation and athletic performance. Int J Vitam Nutr Res Suppl 1989; 30.

113. Reid IR. Therapy of osteoporosis: calcium, vitamin D, and exercise. Am J Med Sci 1996; 312:278–286.

114. Goldfarb AH. Antioxidants: role of supplementation to prevent exercise-induced oxidative stress. Med Sci Sports Exerc 1993; 25:232–236.

115. Goldfarb AH. Nutritional antioxidants as therapeutic and preventive modalities in exercise-induced muscle damage. Can J Appl Physiol 1999; 24:249–266.

116. Appell HJ, Duarte JA, Soares JM. Supplementation of vitamin E may attenuate skeletal muscle immobilization atrophy. Int J Sports Med 1997; 18:157–160.

117. Tiidus PM, Houston ME. Vitamin E status and response to exercise training. Sports Med 1995; 20:12–23.

118. Craciun AM, Wolf J, Knapen MH, Brouns F, Vermeer C. Improved bone metabolism in female elite athletes after vitamin K supplementation. Int J Sports Med 1998; 19:479–484.

119. Fogelholm M, Ruokonen I, Laakso JT, Vuorimaa T, Himberg JJ. Lack of association between indices of vitamin B1, B2, and B6 status and exercise-induced blood lactate in young adults. Int J Sport Nutr 1993; 3:165–176.

120 Garg R, Malinow M, Pettinger M, Upson B, Hunninghake D. Niacin treatment increases plasma homocyst(e)ine levels. Am Heart J 1999; 138:1082–1087.

121. Alaswad K, O'Keefe JH, Jr, Moe RM. Combination drug therapy for dyslipidemia. Curr Atheroscler Rep 1999; 1:44–49.

122. Murray R, Bartoli WP, Eddy DE, Horn MK. Physiological and performance responses to nicotinic-acid ingestion during exercise. Med Sci Sports Exerc 1995; 27:1057–1062.

123. Bonke D. Influence of vitamin B1, B6, and B12 on the control of fine motoric movements. Bibl Nutr Dieta 1986:104–109.

124. Bonke D, Nickel B. Improvement of fine motoric movement control by elevated dosages of vitamin B1, B6, and B12 in target shooting. Int J Vitam Nutr Res Suppl 1989; 30:198–204.

125. Van Dyke DC, Stumbo PJ, Mary JB, Niebyl JR. Folic acid and prevention of birth defects. Dev Med Child Neurol 2002; 44:426–429.

126. Mattson MP, Kruman, II, Duan W. Folic acid and homocysteine in age-related disease. Ageing Res Rev 2002; 1:95–111.

127. Weston PM, King RF, Goode AW, Williams NS. Diet-induced thermogenesis in patients with gastrointestinal cancer cachexia. Clin Sci (Lond) 1989; 77:133–138.

128. Webster MJ. Physiological and performance responses to supplementation with thiamin and pantothenic acid derivatives. Eur J Appl Physiol Occup Physiol 1998; 77:486–491.

129. van der Beek EJ, Lowik MR, Hulshof KF, Kistemaker C. Combinations of low thiamin, riboflavin, vitamin B6 and vitamin C intake among Dutch adults. (Dutch Nutrition Surveillance System). J Am Coll Nutr 1994; 13:383–391.

130. van der Beek EJ. Vitamin supplementation and physical exercise performance. J Sports Sci 1991; 9 Spec No:77–90.

131. Pedersen BK, Bruunsgaard H, Jensen M, Krzywkowski K, Ostrowski K. Exercise and immune function: effect of ageing and nutrition. Proc Nutr Soc 1999; 58:733–742.

132. Petersen EW, Ostrowski K, Ibfelt T, et al. Effect of vitamin supplementation on cytokine response and on muscle damage after strenuous exercise. Am J Physiol Cell Physiol 2001; 280:C1570–C1575.

133. Nieman DC. Exercise immunology: nutritional countermeasures. Can J Appl Physiol 2001; 26:S45–S55.

134. Fletcher RH, Fairfield KM. Vitamins for chronic disease prevention in adults: clinical applications. JAMA 2002; 287:3127–3129.

135. Fairfield KM, Fletcher RH. Vitamins for chronic disease prevention in adults: scientific review. JAMA 2002; 287:3116–3126.

136. Green NR, Ferrando AA. Plasma boron and the effects of boron supplementation in males. Environ Health Perspect 1994; 102 Suppl 7:73–77.

137. Ferrando AA, Green NR. The effect of boron supplementation on lean body mass, plasma testosterone levels, and strength in male bodybuilders. Int J Sport Nutr 1993; 3:140–149.

138. Grados F, Brazier M, Kamel S, et al. Effects on bone mineral density of calcium and vitamin D supplementation in elderly women with vitamin D deficiency. Joint Bone Spine 2003; 70:203–208.

139. Zemel MB. Role of dietary calcium and dairy products in modulating adiposity. Lipids 2003; 38:139–146.

140. Zemel MB. Mechanisms of dairy modulation of adiposity. J Nutr 2003; 133:252S–256S.

141. Hasten DL, Rome EP, Franks BD, Hegsted M. Effects of chromium picolinate on beginning weight training students. Int J Sport Nutr 1992; 2:343–350.

142. Campbell WW, Joseph LJ, Anderson RA, Davey SL, Hinton J, Evans WJ. Effects of resistive training and chromium picolinate on body composition and skeletal muscle size in older women. Int J Sport Nutr Exerc Metab 2002; 12:125–135.

143. Volpe SL, Huang HW, Larpadisorn K, Lesser, II. Effect of chromium supplementation and exercise on body composition, resting metabolic rate and selected biochemical parameters in moderately obese women following an exercise program. J Am Coll Nutr 2001; 20:293–306.

144. Brutsaert TD, Hernandez-Cordero S, Rivera J, Viola T, Hughes G, Haas JD. Iron supplementation improves progressive fatigue resistance during dynamic knee extensor exercise in iron-depleted, nonanemic women. Am J Clin Nutr 2003; 77:441–448.

145. Bohl CH, Volpe SL. Magnesium and exercise. Crit Rev Food Sci Nutr 2002; 42:533–563.

146. Lukaski HC. Magnesium, zinc, and chromium nutrition and athletic performance. Can J Appl Physiol 2001; 26(Suppl):S13–S22.

147. Kreider RB, Miller GW, Williams MH, Somma CT, Nasser TA. Effects of phosphate loading on oxygen uptake, ventilatory anaerobic threshold, and run performance. Med Sci Sports Exerc 1990; 22:250–256.

148. Cade R, Conte M, Zauner C, et al. Effects of phosphate loading on 2,3 diphosphoglycerate and maximal oxygen uptake. Med Sci Sports Exerc 1984; 16:263–268.

149. Kreider RB, Miller GW, Schenck D, et al. Effects of phosphate loading on metabolic and myocardial responses to maximal and endurance exercise. Int J Sport Nutr 1992; 2:20–47.

150. Morton DP, Callister R. Characteristics and etiology of exercise-related transient abdominal pain. Med Sci Sports Exerc 2000; 32:432–438.

151. Noakes TD. Fluid and electrolyte disturbances in heat illness. Int J Sports Med 1998; 19(Suppl 2):S146–S149.

152. Sawka MN, Montain SJ. Fluid and electrolyte supplementation for exercise heat stress. Am J Clin Nutr 2000; 72:564S–572S.

153. Margaritis I, Tessier F, Prou E, Marconnet P, Marini JF. Effects of endurance training on skeletal muscle oxidative capacities with and without selenium supplementation. J Trace Elem Med Biol 1997; 11:37–43.

154. Tessier F, Margaritis I, Richard MJ, Moynot C, Marconnet P. Selenium and training effects on the glutathione system and aerobic performance. Med Sci Sports Exerc 1995; 27:390–396.

155. McCutcheon LJ, Geor RJ. Sweating. Fluid and ion losses and replacement. Vet Clin North Am Equine Pract 1998; 14:75–95.

156. Fawcett JP, Farquhar SJ, Walker RJ, Thou T, Lowe G, Goulding A. The effect of oral vanadyl sulfate on body composition and performance in weight-training athletes. Int J Sport Nutr 1996; 6:382–390.

157. Fawcett JP, Farquhar SJ, Thou T, Shand BI. Oral vanadyl sulphate does not affect blood cells, viscosity or biochemistry in humans. Pharmacol Toxicol 1997; 80:202–206.

158. Gibson RS, Heath AL, Ferguson EL. Risk of suboptimal iron and zinc nutriture among adolescent girls in Australia and New Zealand: causes, consequences, and solutions. Asia Pac J Clin Nutr 2002; 11 (Suppl 3):S543–S552.

159. Gleeson M, Bishop NC. Elite athlete immunology: importance of nutrition. Int J Sports Med 2000; 21(Suppl 1):S44–S50.

160. Singh A, Failla ML, Deuster PA. Exercise-induced changes in immune function: effects of zinc supplementation. J Appl Physiol 1994; 76:2298–2303.

161. Maughan RJ, Noakes TD. Fluid replacement and exercise stress. A brief review of studies on fluid replacement and some guidelines for the athlete. Sports Med 1991; 12:16–31.

162. Williams MH. Ergogenic and ergolytic substances. Med Sci Sports Exerc 1992; 24:S344–S348.

163. McNaughton L, Backx K, Palmer G, Strange N. Effects of chronic bicarbonate ingestion on the performance of high- intensity work. Eur J Appl Physiol Occup Physiol 1999; 80:333–336.

164. Kraemer WJ, Gordon SE, Lynch JM, Pop ME, Clark KL. Effects of multibuffer supplementation on acid-base balance and 2,3-diphosphoglycerate following repetitive anaerobic exercise. Int J Sport Nutr 1995; 5:300–314.

165. Matson LG, Tran ZV. Effects of sodium bicarbonate ingestion on anaerobic performance: a meta-analytic review. Int J Sport Nutr 1993; 3:2–28.

166. Graham TE. Caffeine and exercise: metabolism, endurance and performance. Sports Med 2001; 31: 785–807.

167. Applegate E. Effective nutritional ergogenic aids. Int J Sport Nutr 1999; 9:229–239.

168. Rama Rao SV, Sunder GS, Reddy MR, Praharaj NK, Raju MV, Panda AK. Effect of supplementary choline on the performance of broiler breeders fed on different energy sources. Br Poult Sci 2001; 42:362–367.

169. Buchman AL, Jenden D, Roch M. Plasma free, phospholipid-bound and urinary free choline all decrease during a marathon run and may be associated with impaired performance. J Am Coll Nutr 1999; 18:598–601.

170. Buchman AL, Awal M, Jenden D, Roch M, Kang SH. The effect of lecithin supplementation on plasma choline concentrations during a marathon. J Am Coll Nutr 2000; 19:768–770.

171. Svensson M, Malm C, Tonkonogi M, Ekblom B, Sjodin B, Sahlin K. Effect of Q10 supplementation on tissue Q10 levels and adenine nucleotide catabolism during high-intensity exercise. Int J Sport Nutr 1999; 9:166–180.

172. Kaikkonen J, Kosonen L, Nyyssonen K, et al. Effect of combined coenzyme Q10 and d-alpha-tocopheryl acetate supplementation on exercise-induced lipid peroxidation and muscular damage: a placebo-controlled double-blind study in marathon runners. Free Radic Res 1998; 29:85–92.

173. Bowers CY. Growth hormone-releasing peptide (GHRP). Cell Mol Life Sci 1998; 54:1316–1329.

174. Camanni F, Ghigo E, Arvat E. Growth hormone-releasing peptides and their analogs. Front Neuroendocrinol 1998; 19:47–72.

175. Hargreaves M, McKenna MJ, Jenkins DG, et al. Muscle metabolites and performance during high-intensity, intermittent exercise. J Appl Physiol 1998; 84:1687–1691.

176. Starling RD, Trappe TA, Short KR, et al. Effect of inosine supplementation on aerobic and anaerobic cycling performance. Med Sci Sports Exerc 1996; 28:1193–1198.

177. Williams MH, Kreider RB, Hunter DW, et al. Effect of inosine supplementation on 3-mile treadmill run performance and VO2 peak. Med Sci Sports Exerc 1990; 22:517–522.

178. McNaughton L, Dalton B, Tarr J. Inosine supplementation has no effect on aerobic or anaerobic cycling performance. Int J Sport Nutr 1999; 9:333–344.

179. Messina M, Messina V. Soyfoods, soybean isoflavones, and bone health: a brief overview. J Ren Nutr 2000; 10:63–68.

180. Brilla LR, Conte V. Effects of a novel zing-magnesium formulation on hormones and strength. J Exerc Physiol Online 2000;3: Available at: www.css.edu/users/tboone2/asep/BrillaV2.pdf.

19 Novel Foods

Today's Functional Foods Marketplace

Jill K. Rippe

KEY POINTS

- This chapter discusses various food trends including foods with a reduced content of sodium, cholesterol, fat, and carbohydrates (low carb), and foods containing nutraceuticals (food supplements).
- Food trends are discussed in relation to food labeling and health claims, popular diets, such as Atkins, and health issues, such as obesity and diabetes.
- Food trends have stimulated technological advancement in food ingredients and processing to meet consumer demands.
- Food supplements discussed include those providing protein (soy and dairy), and those that are intended to improve cardiovascular health (stanol esters, β-glucan, bioactive peptides, and n-3 fatty acids), bone and joint health (calcium, glucosamine, and chondroitin), eye health (lutein), the immune system (milk micronutrients, lactoferrin, lactoperoxidase, and colostrum), gut health (probiotics and prebiotics), body fitness (conjugated linoleic acid, amino acids, and glycomacropeptide), energy level, and for beauty.

1. INTRODUCTION

By definition, novel is "of a new kind or nature, strange, previously unknown," and food is "a nutritious substance that can be taken into an animal or a plant to maintain life and growth" *(1)*. This chapter is therefore an exploration of new, strange, and previously unknown kinds of nutrition. Humans are driven to create food availability out of need, but the form that it takes is in response to its relative abundance or scarcity, the technology available, the economic outlook, and the demands of trends present in any given culture.

New products are being introduced into food markets at a fast pace. ProductScan Online monitors consumer packaged food introductions from around the world and reported that there were 33,678 new products introduced in 2003, and a separate report finds that 50–75% of new products will fail and be off the market within 2 yr *(2)*. What is novel in food today may become obsolete tomorrow if there is no demand for it. However, an initially novel food may become commonplace if its attributes meet an ongoing need and it is made widely available.

From: *Nutritional Health: Strategies for Disease Prevention, Second Edition*
Edited by: N. J. Temple, T. Wilson, and D. R. Jacobs © Humana Press Inc., Totowa, NJ

Presented here is a snapshot of novel foods at the dawn of the 21st century. These foods are summarized in two categories that relate food and health: reduction of nutrients viewed as unhealthy and supplementation of nutrients viewed as healthy. Identification of product and ingredient examples are given (*see* Tables 1 and 2 for websites) to complete the picture of what has been and is available in the marketplace and how it came about.

2. REDUCTION OF NUTRIENTS VIEWED AS UNHEALTHY

Since the 1980s there have been a series of high-visibility issues in the United States relating food and health. One arena has been the demand to reduce components in foods that are viewed as harmful, such as excess sodium, cholesterol, fat, and carbohydrates.

2.1. Reduction of Sodium in Foods

Sodium content in foods became a hot topic when health studies linked high sodium intake and hypertension, leading to an Food and Drug Administration (FDA)-approved health claim that "diets low in sodium may reduce the risk of high blood pressure" *(3)*. Introduction of reduced-sodium foods peaked in the 1990s *(4)*. Table salt was criticized as a "bad" food. The alternatives created are still available, including Morton Lite Salt® as a blend of sodium and potassium chloride, and Nu-Salt® (Cumberland Packaging), AlsoSalt® (Also Salt), and Cardia Salt Alternative® (AMBI) as various blends of potassium chloride without sodium chloride. Sodium reduction in traditionally salt-preserved foods, such as cheese and some meats, is technically feasible, but products with less or no sodium chloride taste bland and "flat" to those unaccustomed to it. Those not on special diets appear loath to give up real salt flavor.

2.2. Reduction of Cholesterol in Foods

Two FDA-approved health claims addressed fat reduction: one saying "diets low in fat may reduce the risk of some cancers" *(5)* and the other saying "diets low in saturated fat and cholesterol may reduce the risk of heart disease" *(6)*. As cholesterol is associated with animal fat, a number of whole foods came under attack: eggs, red meat, bacon, cheese, and other dairy products with fat. Initial efforts were to employ new high technology, such as supercritical fluid extraction *(7)* and steam stripping *(8)*, to remove cholesterol from foods. These processes, although effective, proved too costly and the emphasis moved to reducing the fat that carried the cholesterol.

One clever innovation that has survived from this period is extended shelf life pasteurized liquid egg white in a carton, where the cholesterol-rich egg yolk has been removed. Examples of this include ConAgra Foods Egg Beaters®, Papetti Foods All Whites®, and Morning Star Scramblers®. No need to crack eggs: the convenience, flavor, and health aspects have outweighed the added cost.

2.3. Reduction of Fat in Foods

A trend that has had a lasting impact on foods is fat reduction. It started by trying to remove fat completely. For many high-fat foods, maintaining a desirable taste and texture as a "fat free" product was a considerable challenge. During the 1990s a tremendous effort went into the development of fat-replacement ingredients. Many of these were digestible carbohydrates, so the calorie load of foods using these could still be decep-

Table 1
Product Websites

Salt replacers	Soy foods	Oat foods	Probiotics
www.alsosalt.com	www.8thcontinent.com	www.americanoats.com	www.actimel.com
www.drugtopics.com	www.deanfoods.com	www.bioferme.fi	www.biogaia.se
www.mortonsalt.com	www.drsoy.com	www.graindrops.com	www.everybody.ie
www.nusalt.com	www.genisoy.com	www.oatly.com	www.lanimoo.com
Liquid egg white	www.hansens.com	*n-3 Fatty acids*	www.skanedairy.com
www.conagrafoods.com	www.imaginefoods.com	www.eggland.com	www.stonyfield.com
www.kelloggs.com	www.kraft.com	www.georgewestonfoods.com.au	www.valio.com
www.michaelfoods.com	www.lunabar.com	www.mbegg.mb.ca/nutrtion3.html	www.yakult.com.au
Reduced fat	www.snappleaday.com	www.smartbalance.com	*CLA*
www.kraft.com	www.stonyfield.com	*Bone and joint health*	www.cytodyne.com
www.olean.com	www.tofutti.com	www.1stvitality.co.uk/logic/juice4joints.htm	www.eas.com
Low carb	www.turtlemountain.com	www.jointjuice.com	*Amino acids*
www.atkins.com	www.vitasoy-usa.com	www.motionpotion.net	www.4-womenshealth.com
www.atlastfoods.com	www.westsoy.biz	www.myvitanet.com/johepodrmix.html	www.bsnonline.net
www.carboptions.com	www.wholesoycom.com	www.petitsfilous.co.uk	www.powerbar.com
www.fritolay.com	*Dairy related*	*Lutein*	www.prolab.com
www.generalmills.com	www.balance.com	www.glucerna.com	*GMP*
www.hphood.com	www.coldfusionfoods.com	www.hainpurefoods.com	www.hungeroff.com
www.kraft.com	www.eas.com	www.organicfoods-inc.com	www.prycerna-weight-loss.com
www.michelob.com	www.lactaid.com	www.ross.com	*Energy beverages*
www.saralee.com	www.metrx.com	www.sunsweet.com	www.adirondackpure.com
www.tropicana.com	www.nuvim.com	*Lactoferrin*	www.bevnet.com
Sweeteners	www.powerbar.com	www.morinagamilk.co.jp	www.hansens.com
www.equal.com	www.snickersmarathon.com	www2.maeil.com	www.upstatefarmscoop.com
www.sooolite.com	www.urbanbiologics.com	*Colostrum*	*Beauty foods*
www.splenda.com	www.valio.fi	www.bomba.at	www.eccobella.com
www.sweetnlow.com	*Stanol esters*	www.lifeway.net	www.nestle.com
www.sweetone.com	www.benecol.com	www.newlifefoods.net	www.skincola.com
Protein—other	www.minutemaid.com		
www.quorn.com	www.takecontrol.com		

CLA, conjugated linoleic acid; GMP, glycomacropeptide.

Table 2
Ingredient Websites

Carbohydrate fibers	*Sweeteners—nontraditional*
www.avebe.com	www.biospherics.com
www.benefiber.com	www.chinanaturalproduct.com
www.cargillhft.com	www.hollandsweetener.com
www.cpkelco.com	www.magnasweet.com
www.dansico.com	www.neotame.com
www.dow.com	www.overseal.co.uk
www.fmcbiopolymer.com	www.sooolite.com
www.futureceuticals.com	*Dairy related*
www.ifcfiber.com	www.americancasein.com
www.imperialsensus.com	www.arlafoodsingredients.com
www.larex.com	www.armor-proteines.com
www.matsutani.com	www.daviscofoods.com
www.midwestgrain.com	www.dmv-international.com
www.opta-food.com	www.glanbiaingredients.com
www.orafti.com	www.idb.ie
www.pizzeys.com	www.ingredia.fr
Fat replacers	www.lactalis.fr/bba
www.ars.usda.gov	www.mainstreetingredients.com
www.avebe.com	www.nzmp.com
www.cargillhft.com	www.proliantinc.com
www.cosucra.com	www.protient.com
www.cpkelco.com	www.spipolyols.com
www.dansico.com	www.tateandlyle.com
www.dow.com	*Protein—soy*
www.fmcbiopolymer.com	www.admworld.com
www.foodstarch.com	www.cargillsoyprotein.com
www.futureceuticals.com	www.nutriant.com
www.grainprocessing.com	www.solae.com
www.ifcfiber.com	www.solbar.com
www.imperialsensus.com	*Protein—other*
www.kraftfoodingredinets.com	www.cosucra.com
www.olean.com	www.mainstreetingredients.com
www.opta-food.com	www.manildra.com
www.orafti.com	www.midwestgrain.com
www.parmalat-ingredients.com	www.norbencompnay.com
www.primerafoods.com	www.quorn.com
www.tateandlyle.com	*Supplements—other*
	www.cargillhft.com
	www.clarinol.com
	www.kemin.com

tively high despite a "fat free" label. These fat replacers included ingredients, such as starches and maltodextrins from corn, tapioca, and potato; fibers from oat, corn, rice, and peas; and stabilizers, such as pectin and microcrystalline cellulose. Only a few specially processed, protein-based fat replacers appeared. Ingredient suppliers were looking for the "magic bullet" that could transform fat-laden foods into "fat free" without obvious changes in flavor or texture.

2.3.1. FAT AND DAIRY FOODS

Manufacturers of high-fat dairy foods felt threatened, so they countered with intense research efforts and a resulting host of new products. Skim milk was relabeled as "fat free" and gained popularity over 3–4% fat whole milk. But many other dairy products had to be reformulated in dramatic ways. Exemplifying the effort, Kraft Foods introduced lines of reduced-fat and "fat-free" dairy products that included cream cheese, processed cheese, and natural cheese. Consumer interest in many "fat-free" products declined as most products fell short in flavor and texture. However, reduced-fat dairy products have prevailed.

2.3.2. FAT AND SNACK FOODS

Looking at the huge snack food market in the United States, Proctor & Gamble developed Olestra®: "the no-fat cooking oil with the full-fat flavor." A fat unlike any other, it is a nonabsorbable, noncaloric fat substitute that was approved for use in the United States in 1996. But it was not without criticism; pundits pointed out that Olestra leached nutrients from the body in addition to having gastrointestinal side effects (9). Despite this, in the late 1990s it was introduced into Frito-Lay's WOW® line of chips, as well as in RJR Nabisco's Wheat Thins® and Ritz® crackers. Only three chip products remain on the market today. Despite the technological achievement of a functional noncaloric fat, the product has had limited appeal within the United States and has not been approved for use elsewhere. The magic bullet for fat free has been elusive.

2.4. Reduction of Digestible Carbohydrates: "Low-Carb" Foods

In 2002, dietary attention in America became fixated on reduction of high levels of digestible carbohydrate in foods (10). This was bolstered by dual national health alarms of rising levels of adult type 2 diabetes, as well as obesity in adults and children (11,12). The low-carb concept gained attention in 1972 with the bestseller, Dr. Atkins Diet Revolution, promoting a high-protein, low-carbohydrate diet for weight loss and improved health (13). Additional bestseller diets have supported versions of the controlled carbohydrate intake message: the Zone Diet (14), Sugar Busters (15), and the South Beach Diet (16). In 1999, ProductScan reported that there were only 47 products introduced as low-carb in the United States, but by 2003 they reported more than 600 (17), and in 2004 it continued to escalate.

2.4.1. ATKINS FOODS

Tied to the success of the Atkins diet has been the introduction of a family of more than 100 high-protein, low-carb products currently marketed in seven lines under the Atkins name: Advantage® nutritional bars, shake mixes, and ready-to-drink beverages; Endulge® candy bars, ice cream, and cheesecake treats; Nutritional Approach® bakery products;

Crunchers® snack foods; kitchen syrups and condiments; Morning Start® cereals and breakfast bars; and Quick Cuisine® bake mixes and pasta sides. Other Atkins-endorsed products have appeared, including a low-carb refrigerated dairy drink, Carb Countdown®, as well as restaurant menu items. The major food companies have jumped on the bandwagon and have introduced products low in net carbs, such as General Mills Total® Protein Cereal, Sarah Lee Delightful® White and Wheat breads, Frito-Lays Edge® taco chips, Michelob Ultra® beer, Tropicana's Light n' Healthy® orange juice, Unilever's Carb Options®, and Kraft's CarbWell® line of foods. Low-carb food sections are appearing in American grocery stores as manufacturers are rethinking how to take digestible carbohydrates out of everything, especially staple items, such as bread, pasta, rice, and potatoes.

2.4.2. REDUCING DIGESTIBLE CARBOHYDRATES

Carbohydrate reduction in food is achieved through a combination of means. Elimination of digestible sugars and replacement with nonnutritive intense sweeteners and/or sugar alcohols provides sweetness and reduction of carbohydrate calories. Replacement of a portion of any remaining carbohydrates with soluble and insoluble fibers provides further reduction of carbohydrate calories. And last, addition of higher protein and/or fat allows greater reduction in total carbohydrates while providing alternative nutritional energy sources.

2.4.2.1. Use of Intense Sweeteners

Tabletop substitute sweeteners have proved more popular than substitute salt. Products, such as Sweet N'Low® (saccharin; Cumberland Packaging), Equal® (aspartame; also known as Canderel® in Europe; Merisant), Splenda® (sucralose; McNeil Nutritionals), Sweet One® (acesulfame K; Stadt Holdings), and cyclamate are in common use worldwide where approved. The newest options for artificial sweeteners include Twinsweet® (aspartame and acesulfame; Holland Sweetner) and Neotame® (The Nutrasweet Co.) Alternatives to these artificial sweeteners are addition of the natural botanical extracts of licorice root (glycyrrhizin), stevia plant leaves (stevioside), thaumatin (Talin®; Palatinit MGBH), and Lo Han Kuo fruit that have intense sweetening properties.

2.4.2.2. Use of Sugar Alcohols

Sugar alcohols are less sweet than sucrose but they are synergistic with the noncaloric sweeteners, and they serve to provide bulk to replace the sugar removed. They include sorbitol, maltitol, isomaltitol, mannitol, lactitol, xylitol, erythritol, and glycerol. Sugar alcohols are not all similar in their blood sugar response or digestibility, including variable laxation effects *(18)*. The use of sugar alcohols has been critical to product functionality in development of low-carb ice creams, sweetened baked goods, chocolates, and sugar-free gums.

2.4.2.3. Use of Dietary Fibers

Many low-carb formulated foods use dietary fiber. Soluble and insoluble fibers from many sources are available with variable fiber concentration. A number of these are cross-functional as carbohydrate-based fat replacers (a fortunate technology transfer). Additional fibers include resistant maltodextrins and starches. Gums are also soluble fibers; particularly useful are lower viscosity products, such as larch gum (aribinogalactan), low-viscosity guar gum, and gum arabic. Still important are the more traditional fibers found in various grains, cereals, fruits, vegetables, seeds, and nuts (e.g., wheat, soy, oat, rice, apple, orange, tomato, sugar beet, pea, cottonseed, flax, and almond) that can be concentrated and prepared to very fine mesh powders.

2.5. Low Glycemic Foods

Approaches along the lines of the Atkins diet are not the only new ideas on controlled carbohydrates. Glycemic index (GI) was first introduced in 1981 by Jenkins et al. *(19)* and subsequently popularized in Australia and New Zealand in 1996 by Brand-Miller et al. with publication of *The GI Factor (20)*. In essence, this is a measure of the rate at which a food substance raises the blood sugar after ingestion. Foods can be registered for a GI rating label in Australia, New Zealand, and South Africa, whereas Sweden permits a "balance your blood sugar claim" *(21)*. In this context, a new natural low-calorie bulk sweetener called tagatose is attractive for having almost no glycemic response *(22)*. Tagatose can be found in the United States in Pasco Brands' Light and Tasty® frozen juices, whereas the Kellogg Company has patents on the use of tagatose in ready-to-eat cereals and Pepsi has patents in its use in diet soda formulations. Alternative approaches to low GI are exemplified by the CarboLite sugarless candy bar At Last® with erythritol and inulin.

3. SUPPLEMENTATION OF NUTRIENTS VIEWED AS HEALTHY: NUTRACEUTICALS

So far improvements to the health value of food by removal of components viewed as "unhealthy" have been discussed. An alternative strategy is the supplementation of food with healthful components in the form of proteins, vitamins, minerals, probiotics, prebiotics/fiber, botanicals, and bioactive proteins. In 1989, nutraceuticals were defined as "any substance that is a food or part of a food that provides medical and/or health benefits, including prevention and treatment of disease" *(23)*. There is no legal definition of such substances in the United States, but in Japan, "one of the world's most important and developed markets for functional foods," there is a legal category of "foods of specified health uses" that address this concept *(24)*. The concept of functional foods is discussed in Chapter 20.

3.1. Protein Supplementation

Traditionally, concentrated protein has come from meat, poultry, fish, egg, and dairy in the form of whole foods. Plant-based forms of whole food protein tend to be less concentrated and come from legumes, such as soybeans, chick peas, and lentils, that are amino acid-complemented with cereal grains, such as corn, rice, or wheat. Isolating proteins from their sources is feasible with such technologies as membrane filtration that allows large-scale protein purification. Table 3 compares protein composition from traditional vs concentrated sources. Protein supplementation with a variety of these concentrated proteins has allowed the production of new foods with specific functionalities, health benefits, and nutritional profiles.

Table 3
Comparison of Concentrated Protein Sources

Protein source	Type	Protein "as is" %
Beef *(25)*	Composite raw lean cuts	21
Poultry *(25)*	Composite raw meat only	20
Fish (tuna) *(25)*	Composite raw	23
Egg *(25)*	Whole raw	13
Dairy *(25;* Table 2)	Fluid whole milk	3.3
	Nonfat dry milk	35
	Milk protein concentrate	40–80
	Milk protein isolate	85–90
	Total milk protein	90
	Caseinate	90
	Micellar casein dry	90
	Fluid whey	0.9
	Dry whey	12
	Whey protein concentrate	34–80
	Whey protein isolate	85–90
Soy *(25,* Table 2)	Soy flour	35–50
	Soy protein concentrate	55–70
	Soy protein isolate	80–90
Wheat *(25,* Table 2)	Wheat flour	6–14
	Vital wheat gluten	75
	Wheat protein isolate	80–90
Rice *(25,* Table 2)	Rice flour	7–11
	Rice protein concentrate	40–70
	Rice protein isolate	75–80
Pea (Table 2)	Pea protein concentrate	40–60
	Pea protein isolate	80
Quorn (Table 1)	Quorn nuggets	25

3.1.1. SOY

The FDA approved the following health claim for soy: "Diets low in saturated fat and cholesterol and that include soy protein may reduce the risk of heart disease" *(26)*. In addition, the natural presence of isoflavones, such as genistein and daidzein, in many soy protein foods are of interest to women's health as sources of phytoestrogens to relieve menopausal symptoms *(27)*. Soy beverages, like Silk®, 8th Continent®, SoyDream®, and Vitasoy®, are recent additions to refrigerated dairy cases as mainstream alternatives to milk. Shelf-stable, aseptic boxes of soy milk are found worldwide. Making use of the isolated soy proteins are nutritional beverages, such as Westsoy ready-to-drink SmartPlus®, meal replacements, such as the single-serve, shelf-stable juice/soy Snapple-A-Day®, smoothie juice/soy beverages, such as Hansen's Protein Smoothie®, and cultured soy drinks Silk aLive! ® and WholeSoy Cultured Soy®. Nutritional bars with more than 6.25 g of soy protein per serving, such as GeniSoy®, Dr. Soy®, and Clif Luna®, are another popular category. Other soy products mimic dairy counterparts. Examples include the Tofutti® line with soy alternatives to cream cheese, sour cream, processed cheeses, and ice cream, and also Turtle Mountain soy frozen desserts, such as the low-carb product Carb Escapes®. Soy yogurts with live cultures are found in products, such as Silk®, Wholesoy®, and Stonyfield Farm's O'Soy®. Textured soy protein is a meat analog made by an extruded process that adds texture to the protein fiber *(28)*; it is found in products such as Kraft's soy Boca Burgers®.

3.1.2. Dairy: Milk Protein, Whey, and Casein

Dairy protein is no longer just milk and cheese. Numerous nutritional bars and beverages can now be found with a high content of dairy protein. Combinations of fast-acting (digesting) whey proteins and slow-acting caseins are critical in such products as MET-Rx® meal replacement powder beverage. Designed for athletes as balanced nutrition before and after workouts, the MRP concept has proved so convenient that it moved mainstream into single-serve, shelf-stable beverages, such as EAS Myoplex®, and nutritional bars, such as Balance Bar®, that contain dairy and soy protein. Ironically, the success of nutritional bars has brought protein supplementation full circle to the "original" high-energy bar: the candy bar. Masterfoods' popular Snickers® candy bar now has a companion higher protein Marathon® bar. A novel treat made from whey protein isolate is Crystal Pro® or Muscle Candy™ (Urban Biologics), a sucralose sweet and sour granulated protein that fizzes in your mouth as it dissolves. On the frozen end, high-protein, low-carb frozen desserts, such as Atkins Endulge® and extruded the frozen stick novelty, Cold Fusion's Protein Juice Bars®, represent the range of functionality achievable with isolated dairy proteins.

Concentration of milk, casein, or whey to a 90% protein powder reduces carbohydrates to the 1% range. As the carbohydrate is lactose, this allows concentrated dairy protein to be used in applications where further dilution reduces the lactose content of the product to less than 0.5 g/serving. Fluid milks must use lactase enzymes to break down lactose in products, such as Lactaid® lactose-free fluid milk.

3.1.3. Nontraditional Food Proteins

As an alternative source of protein to meat, Quorn® was developed based on mycoprotein, a plant related to edible fungi. It looks and tastes similar to chicken and is made into nuggets, noodle shapes, and "grounds." It originated in the United Kingdom and has become available in at least six other European countries and the United States.

3.2. Food Supplementation for Cardiovascular Health

3.2.1. Stanol Esters

Numerous clinical trials have shown that plant sterols can lower blood cholesterol *(29)*. The FDA allows a claim that "associates diets that include plant sterol/stanol esters with reduced risk of heart disease" *(30)*. First introduced in Finland, Benecol® was the first margarine-type spread to contain stanol esters and is now available in Spain as a fluid milk, Kaiku Benecol®, and in the United Kingdom as Benecol Yogurt Drink®. Unilever's Take Control® is another margarine-type spread. Introduced in 2003, Heart Wise® orange juice from Minute Maid has been supplemented with plant stanol esters and carries the claim "proven to help reduce cholesterol."

3.2.2. β-GLUCAN

Another FDA-approved health claim addresses soluble fiber, including β-glucan from whole oats: "Oat fibers may reduce the risk of heart disease" *(31)*. In the United States, a frozen dessert based on oats called OatScream® is available. A popular oat-based beverage, Oatly Oat Drink®, is manufactured in Sweden by Ceba Foods. In Finland, two products made by Bioferme, Ltd., are an oat beverage and a probiotic yogurt-type product called Yosa®. A Norwegian introduction is Graindrops® by BioSophia. Featuring oat, rice, and spelt drinks, these cereal beverages are made by the Japanese Koji fermentation process creating organic "bio-dynamic" milk alternatives.

3.2.3. BIOACTIVE PEPTIDES

Bioactive peptides that have been shown to control blood pressure can be made by hydrolysis of milk proteins by various lactic acid bacteria *(32)*. A new beverage based on patented Evolus® fermented milk technology, developed by Finland's Valio, promotes reduced blood pressure. A hydrolyzed whey protein isolate, BioZate®, manufactured by Davisco Foods, is also designed for reduction of blood pressure.

3.2.4. n-3 FATTY ACIDS

The major n-3 fatty acids are eicosapentanoic acid and docosahexanoic acid, both primarily sourced from fish oil, and α-linolenic acid, found in vegetable oils, such as flax, canola, and walnut *(33)*. Interest in n-3 fatty acids includes an FDA limited claim on their association with reduction in risk of coronary heart disease *(34)*. Special chicken feed produces eggs enhanced with n-3 fatty acids. They are available in Canada and as Eggland's Best Eggs® in the United States. In Australia, George Weston Foods and Clover Corp. joined forces to create Tip Top Up®, a white bread fortified with encapsulated fish oil docosahexanoic acid. A patented margarine product, Smartbalance® from GFA Foods, combines canola, soy, and olive oil with balanced n-6 and n-3 fatty acids for heart health.

3.3. Food Supplementation for Bone and Joint Health

3.3.1. CALCIUM

Calcium is important in multiple health concerns. An FDA health claim relates the intake of calcium with a reduced risk of osteoporosis *(35)*. Emerging research is also finding that "dietary calcium plays a key role in the regulation of energy metabolism and obesity risk" and that dairy sources of calcium have a greater effect in decreasing body fat *(36)*. An ingredient innovation taking advantage of high-calcium byproducts from dairy protein concentration has resulted in a natural, highly bioavailable calcium source called "milk minerals." It can be found in products, such as Yoplait's Petits Filous® yogurt for infants and toddlers. Although milk, yogurt, and cheese may have been traditional sources of dietary calcium, there are now calcium-fortified juices, cereals, breads, frozen desserts, soy products, and more. Calcium-fortified orange juice, which was introduced in the early 1990s by Tropicana, was the first high-calcium beverage to rival milk.

3.3.2. CHONDROITIN AND GLUCOSAMINE

Glucosamine and chondroitin are often used together to slow cartilage damage and alleviate arthritis *(37)*. Joint health beverages are becoming a popular vehicle to deliver glucosamine in a readily absorbed form. Product examples include Joint Juice®, Nutravail Technologies Drink UP™ Good-for-you-beverages, and BioEssentials' Motion Potion®. Other beverages contain both glucosamine and chondroitin: Logic's Juice4Joints® and Amerifit's FlexAble® orange drink. A Dutch company, Yagua, manufactures a drink called Free Move® with collagen hydrolysate and glucosamine to promote flexibility and relieve repetitive strain injury.

3.4. Food Supplementation for Eye Health

Lutein, a carotenoid pigment, is an antioxidant that has mostly been associated with decreasing the risk of eye disease, such as age-related macular degeneration *(38)*. It can be found in Ross Product's Ensure® balanced nutrition and Glucerna® diabetic weight-control meal replacement beverages, Sunsweet's Prune Juice +®, Hain Celestial's veggie and carrot juices, and Whole Grain Crunch® cereal. It may soon be found in egg substitutes, fermented milks, and yogurt products.

3.5. Food Supplementation for Boosting the Immune System

3.5.1. MILK MICRONUTRIENTS

NuVim® is a unique milk-juice beverage supplemented with two patented micronutrients isolated from milk: LactoMune® assists the human immune system and LactoActin® promotes muscle flexibility and sturdy joints. These components are from the milk of select cows in New Zealand that are raised under a program that stimulates their immune system by using feeding and husbandry techniques. The overall impact of drinking NuVim is described as the maintenance of good health, more energy, and faster recovery times from physical activity.

3.5.2. LACTOFERRIN AND LACTOPEROXIDASE

Lactoferrin, an iron-binding bioactive protein, and lactoperoxidase, an enzyme that is part of a natural antimicrobial defense system in animals, can both be isolated from milk *(39)*. Morinaga Milk in Japan has a "biotics" yogurt called Lactoferrin Yogurt®, whereas in South Korea Maeil Dairy adds lactoferrin to Absolute Masterpiece® baby food. Aside from their bioactivity as food supplements, both lactoperoxidase and lactoferrin have application as natural preservatives in foods. Lactoferrin has been approved in the United States for use in meat as a natural antimicrobial and its application in beef is forthcoming *(40)*.

3.5.3. COLOSTRUM

Colostrum, a serum rich in immunoglobulin G that comes from the first milk of mammals, is commercially isolated from cow's milk *(41)*. Used as a boost to the immune system, it has been a popular supplement in Scandinavia, Saudi Arabia, and Asia. Beverages containing colostrums include a kefir beverage from Lifeway called Basics Plus®, a juice drink from Bomba in Austria called Sol(e)ution®, and NewLife Colostrum® from Australia.

3.6. Food Supplementation for Gut Health: Probiotics and Prebiotics

Probiotic is defined as a "microbial culture beneficial to health by restoring balance to the intestinal flora" and prebiotics are "nondigestible oligosaccharides that support the growth of colonies of certain bacteria in the colon…so changing and possibly improving the colonic flora" *(42)*. Together, they are referred to as synbiotics. Probiotics for gut health are one of the functional food success stories, particularly in Europe *(43)*. A Japanese fermented skimmed milk, Yakult®, was introduced into Europe in 1995 and has been successful there, as well as in Japan. In France, Danone's probiotic beverage Actimel® (recently introduced in America as DanActive®) had been introduced into 15 countries as of 2003, whereas Yoplait has introduced the skim milk probiotic beverage Everybody® in Ireland. In the United States, all of Stonyfield Farms' line of yogurts and smoothie beverages contain six live cultures, and the smoothies contain inulin, a polyfructose (oligosaccharide) that functions as a prebiotic fiber and promotes beneficial microflora in the intestine. Meadow Gold Dairies in Hawaii launched iS® (short for Immuno-Stimulation) in 2002, a prebiotic juice and milk blend. The Swedish firm Probi has licensed probiotic cultures to Skanemejerier that are found in fruit juice products under the name ProViva®. And in Finland, Valio was the first to gain worldwide license to Lactobacillus GG in 1987 and had their first probiotics products launched in 1990. Their most recent introduction in Belgium under the Valio Gefilus® label is a probiotic Emmantel-type cheese.

Aseptic shelf-stable processing inactivates cultures, thereby losing probiotic functionality. However, an innovative solution was developed between aseptic process developer Tetra Pak and BioGaia AB in the creation of LifeTop® straws. The straw, internally coated with beneficial lactic acid bacterium, is wrapped and attached to the outside of beverage cartons. Upon consumption, the probiotic is released into the beverage. Two products are in European markets: Orchard Maid® organic drinkable yogurt by Farm Produce Marketing in the United Kingdom and Addera® nutritional beverage by Semper in Sweden.

3.7. Food Supplementation for Body Fitness

3.7.1. CONJUGATED LINOLEIC ACID

Conjugated linoleic acid, a natural ingredient in dairy, beef, poultry, and eggs, is reported to decrease body fat and increase muscle mass *(44)*. It has transitioned from capsules to foods and can be found in sports nutrition bars, such as Xenadrine®, and beverages, such as EAS Myoplex Deluxe®.

3.7.2. AMINO ACIDS

Some of the substances discussed here are reviewed in Chapter 18. Amino acids, such as L-creatine, L-glutamine, L-carnitine, L-taurine, and branched chain amino acids (L-leucene, L-valine, L-isoleucene), have become popular supplements in endurance, muscle building, and recovery sports products. Creatine is reported to increase lean muscle mass and have an "ergogenic effect" by storing energy in muscle. It is available in nutrition bars, such as ProLab's Lean Mass Creatine Bar®. Glutamine, reported to stimulate muscle growth and recovery, is added as glutamine peptides in products, such as BSN's anabolic sustained-release, muscle-building Lean Dessert Protein®. In Power Bar Energy Bites®, branched chain amino acids are added to the energy formulation, and a product by 4-Women's Health designed for female athletes is Somnabol-PM® for extended muscle protein synthesis during sleep.

3.7.3. GLYCOMACROPEPTIDE

Glycomacropeptide is a fragment of casein protein left after cheese making that can be concentrated from whey (isolated) or concentrated in whey. It is one of the only known phenylalanine-free natural proteins and offers a new protein option for children with phenylketonuria *(45)*. Alternatively, it is associated with appetite suppression and is used as a component of weight-loss formulations, such as the beverages Satietrol® by Pacific Health and Prycena® from Immunotec Research.

3.8. Food Supplementation for Energy

The launch of the Austrian product Red Bull in 1987 initiated a category of energy beverages that now numbers more than 150 products worldwide *(46)*. Ingredients, such as caffeine, taurine, glucoronolactone, inositol, guarana, L-carnitine, creatine, ginseng, and ginkgo biloba, along with vitamins and minerals, are combined in formulations to energize and stimulate. Milk has gotten energized as well, with caffeinated, flavored drinks, such as Nutra Java®, Schroeder's Hyper Cow®, and Upstate Farm's Intense Mocha Java Caffeine Kick®. Even water has been stimulated: Adirondack Pure's WOW® ("whacked out water") is sugar-free with the addition of caffeine from natural sources (yerba mate, guarana, and kola nut) and flavor, whereas Hansen's Energy Water® is fruit-flavored with glucose, ginseng, taurine, B vitamins, and electrolytes.

3.9. Food Supplementation for Skin Health: "Beauty Foods"

Popular in Japan and taking hold in Europe is the concept of "beauty foods" or "cosmeceutical foods" that promote healthy appearance, especially of the skin. Exemplified by the 2002 joint venture between French cosmetics firm L'Oreal and Swiss food giant Nestle to create the company Laboratoires Inneov, their objective is cosmetic nutritional supplements. The first food product from this venture has been Inneov Firmness®, containing Lacto-Lycopene, vitamin C, and soy isoflavones, "targeted at women over 40 concerned with loss of cutaneous firmness." From Swiss cosmetics firm Ecco Bella is Health by Chocolate®, "the delicious way to look beautiful," with cranberry seed oil, n-3 fatty acids, blueberry extract, lutein, lycopene, astaxanthin, and fiber. And an American product introduced in 2003 to New York was SkinCola®, a beverage to hydrate the skin, being a flavorless, noncarbonated purified water with "activated oxygen," zinc, and vitamins.

4. CONCLUSIONS

That food can first be envisioned and then designed to specific nutritional profiles, functionalities, and appearance is a novel concept for our time. The design process can entail both removal of what are viewed as unhealthy food components and supplementation or adding together healthy food components. As you read this, new food trends are in the making. What is known about the impact of our diet on health will change. Our lifestyles will change. Our food will change.

REFERENCES

1. Oxford American Dictionary and Thesaurus, American edition. Oxford University Press, NY, 2003, pp. 118,568.
2. Industry Watch Product Alert. Stagnito's New Product Magazine 2004; 1:8.
3. FDA. Code of Federal Regulations. 21CFR101.74 2002; 2:127–129.
4. Neff J. Is low sodium label worth its salt? Food Processing 1999;6. www.foodpro- cessing.com. Last accessed April 1, 2004.
5. FDA. Code of Federal Regulations. 21CFR101.73 2002; 2:126,127.
6. FDA. Code of Federal Regulations. 21CFR101.75 2002; 2:129–131.
7. Hegenbart SL. It's a gas: gas extraction in food processing. Food Product Design 1997(April). www.foodproductdesign.com. Last accessed April 1, 2004.
8. Kuntz LA. Fat facts for cookies and cakes. Food Product Design 1996(August). www.foodproduct design.com. Last accessed April 1, 2004.
9. Canadian food regulators give Olestra a thumbs down. Food & Drink Weekly 2000 (July 3). www.findarticles.com. Last accessed April 1, 2004.
10. Wilshire G. Low-carb going mainstream. Food Product Design 2004: 13(11):39–57.
11. FDA. Calories count: report of the working group on obesity. 2004(March). www.cfsan. fda.gov/~dms/owg-toc.html. Last accessed April 1, 2004.
12. The Centers for Disease Control. Obesity, diabetes on the increase in US. 2003. www.usgovinfo.about.com/library/weekly/aa010803a.htm. Last accessed April 1, 2004.
13. Atkins RC. Dr. Atkins Diet Revolution: The High Calorie Way to Stay Thin Forever. David McKay, NY, 1972.
14. Sears B. The Zone: A Revolutionary Life Plan to Put Your Body in Total Balance for Permanent Weight Loss, Higher Energy, a Happier State of Mind, a Healthier Heart. Harper Collins, NY, 1995.
15. Stewart L. Sugar Busters! Cut Sugar to Trim Fat. Ballantine, NY, 1998.
16. Agatston A. The South Beach Diet: the Delicious, Doctor Designed, Foolproof Plan for Fast and Healthy Weight Loss. Rodale Press, NY, 2003.
17. Neff J. Belt-tightening and the diet aisle: low-carb products are having an impact on many other aisles as well. Food Processing 2003: 64(10):34–40.
18. Sugar alcohols. Reduced calorie sweeteners: polyols. www.caloriecontrol.org. Last accessed April 1, 2004.
19. Jenkins DJ, Wolever TM, Taylor RH, et al. Glycemic index of foods: a physiological basis for carbohydrate change. Am J Clin Nutr 1981; 34:362–366.
20. Brand-Miller J, Foster-Powell K, Colagiuri S. The GI Factor: The Glycaemic Index Solution. Hodder & Stoughton, Sydney, 1997.
21. Glycemic Index. www.caloriecontrol.org/pr_glycemicindex.html. Last accessed April 1, 2004.
22. Bertelsen H, Hansen SJ, Laursen RS, et al. Tagatose. In: Nabors LO, ed. Alternative Sweeteners, 3rd ed. Marcel Dekker, NY, 2001, pp. 105–127.
23. DeFelice S. Foundation for Innovation in Medicine. www.fimdefelice.org. Last accessed April 1, 2004.
24. Nakajima K. Global dispatches Japan: regulation nation. Functional Foods & Nutraceuticals 2004(Jan): 16–18.
25. USDA Food Tables. www.nal.usda.gov/fnic/foodcomp. Last accessed April 1, 2004.
26. FDA. Code of Federal Regulations. 21CFR101.82 2002; 2:144–146.
27. Han KK, Soares JM Jr, Haidar MA, et al. Benefits of soy isoflavone therapeutic regimen on menopausal symptoms. Obset Gynecol 2002; 99:389–394.
28. Liu K. The second generation of soyfoods. In: Liu K, ed. Soybeans: Chemistry, Technology and Utilization. Aspen Publishers, Frederick, MD, 1999:412–441.
29. Institute of Food Science and Technology (UK). Phytosterol Esters. www.ifst.org/hottopic29.htm. Last accessed April 1, 2001.

30. FDA. Code of Federal Regulations. 21CFR101.83 2002; 2:146–149.
31. FDA. Code of Federal Regulations. 21CFR101.81 2002; 2:141–144.
32. Gedes SK, Harper WJ, Miller G. Bioactive components of whey and cardiovascular health. U.S. Dairy Export Council, 2001. www.wheyoflife.org/news/cardiohealth.pdf. Last accessed April 1, 2004.
33. Rudra, PK, Nair SSD, Leitch JW, Garg ML. Omega-3 polyunsaturated fatty acids and cardiac arrhythmias. In: Wildman EC, ed. Handbook of Nutraceuticals and Functional Foods. CRC Press, Boca Raton, FL, 2001, pp. 331–332.
34. FDA. Summary of qualified health claims permitted. vm.cfsan.fda.gov/~dms/ghc-sum.html. Last accessed April 1, 2004.
35. FDA. Code of Federal Regulations. 21CFR101.72 2002; 2:124–126.
36. Zemel MB, Miller SL. Dietary calcium and dairy modulation of adiposity and obesity risk. Nutr Rev 2004: 62:125–131.
37. American Arthritis Foundation. www.arthritis.org/condition/alttherapies/glucosamine.asp. Last accessed April 1, 2004.
38. National Eye Institute. Lutein and its role in eye disease prevention. July 2002. www.nei.nih.gov/news/statements/lutein.asp. Last accessed April 1, 2004.
39. Archibald A. Protein Power. Nutra Solutions 2004(March 1). www.nutrasolutions.com. Last accessed May 1, 2004.
40. Farmland National Beef. www.nationalbeef.com. Last accessed May 1, 2004.
41. Center for Nutritional Research. www.bovinecolostrum.com. Last accessed April 1, 2004.
42. Bender DA, Bender AE. In: Benders Dictionary of Nutrition and Food Technology, 7th ed. CRC Press, London, 1999, pp. 325,326.
43. Sloan AE. Up and coming markets. Nutraceuticals World 2003; 6(10):32–41.
44. Gaullier JM, Halse J, Hoye K, et al. Conjugated linoleic acid supplementation for 1 y reduces body fat mass in healthy overweight humans. Am J Clin Nutr 2004; 79:1118–1125.
45. DMI. Glycomacropeptide offers new option for people with PKU. 2003 www.doitwithdairy.com/presscover/pku.htm. Last accessed April 1, 2004.
46. Bev Reviews. www.bevnet.com. Last accessed April 1, 2004.

20 Functional Foods

A Critical Appraisal

Ted Wilson and David R. Jacobs, Jr.

KEY POINTS

- There is no universally agreed definition of functional foods. One operational definition is those foods whose consumption is associated with beneficial physiological changes that are outside of basic nutrition. Foods that qualify for a health claim may also be regarded as functional. Other foods may bear structure/function claims that have borne little scrutiny by unbiased experts. If the concept of functional food is to be helpful in marketing a healthful diet, the definition of a functional food should include those that improve and enhance health, including basic nutrition.
- The US Food and Drug Administration (FDA) has approved a series of legal "claims" that can appear on specified food labels. Other countries have taken diverse strategies to health claims.
- Functional foods reach the consumer in many, conceptually distinct forms. Of particular importance is the distinction between foods with special properties that depend on synergy of their natural constituents and foods that have been supplemented with purified compounds.
- The consumer learns about functional foods from marketing and government sources, whose motives may not be the same. Consumer health could be improved and government health care costs could be reduced with proper education. It remains to be seen whether the concept of functional foods is helpful in this regard. The promotion of functional foods does not come without perceived and real risks to the consumer. There is a need for legislation that will sort out which health claims are appropriate (based on evidence) and ban those that are not.

1. WHAT IS A FUNCTIONAL FOOD?

To a greater or lesser degree, all foods have nutritional functions and effects. We often desire protein-rich foods when our bodies are growing or when we build/replace muscle after a workout; we look for diets rich in carbohydrates to provide energy for the demands

From: *Nutritional Health: Strategies for Disease Prevention, Second Edition*
Edited by: N. J. Temple, T. Wilson, and D. R. Jacobs © Humana Press Inc., Totowa, NJ

of physical labor; we choose foods rich in fat to maintain the insulation provided by the skin's hypodermis; and finally we drink water to maintain fluidity and lubrication. We also need specific foods in our diet to provide micronutrients, such as animal products for vitamin B_{12} and citrus fruits for vitamin C. The foods selected are all functional in the sense that they provide energy and the required macronutrients and micronutrients. We also consume foods that contain substances whose presence in our diet, although not essential, will permit us to maintain an enhanced level of health. The foods containing such special substances might be called "functional foods," but according to Katan and De Roos [1], citing Baily [2], "Even in Japan, where functional foods originated, the term itself was not adopted because it was agreed that all foods are already functional."

Several definitions have been suggested for "functional food." Roberfroid and Slavin proposed it is "a food ingredient which affects physiological function(s) of the body in a targeted way so as to have positive effect(s) which may, in due course, justify health claims" [3]. The General Accounting Office of the US government has described a functional food as one with a "claim to have health benefits beyond basic nutrition" [4]. Palou et al. [5] assert, "Functional foods have at least one component, whether it be a nutrient or not, that affects the target functions of the organism in a specific, positive way and produces a physiological effect beyond its traditional nutritional value." They virtually equate functional foods with "novel foods," citing European legislation [6] that includes "transgenic foods; foods and ingredients that have a new molecular structure; those derived from micro-organisms, fungi, and algae; those from animals and plants that are reproduced from nontraditional methods; and those obtained with new production processes involving significant changes in the composition or structure of the foods or ingredients that affect their nutritional value, metabolism, or levels of nondesirable substances." Katan and De Roos [1] discuss definitions at length. They eschew the term "beyond basic nutrition," pointing out that even tap water could be seen as functional in helping to prevent "cystitis, kidney, and bladder stones, and possibly bladder cancer." Because all foods have some functionality, they assert that acknowledgement of market forces and the needs of the food industry should be part of the definition. Thus they state: "A functional food is a branded food which claims explicitly or implicitly to improve health or well-being" [1].

For the most part, therefore, functional foods typically contain one or more ingredients whose concentration has been manipulated to allow a manufacturer to make a health claim. This perspective is in sharp contrast to the view that functionality depends on the synergistic effects of foods as a whole [7,8], a point of view also discussed in this book in Chapter 10. For example, putting marketing aside, suppose the goal to be achieved by eating a functional food is to increase soluble fiber to reduce the blood cholesterol level. Many whole plant foods can be considered functional for this purpose: an apple (solid state) or apple sauce (semifluid state) could both be considered functional foods. In this particular case apple juice in its fluid state has little fiber and would not be considered functional. However, as noted by Katan and De Roos [1], these examples, although clearly satisfying the health aspect of functionality, do less well in satisfying marketing requisites. Another example is a breakfast cereal that is processed for improved palatability to increase our consumption of whole grains, nuts, and dried fruit, or to increase the fiber content (added bran) of the packaged product. Such a food could be considered a functional food; this example is a closer marriage of health and marketing requisites.

The General Accounting Office *(4)*, as well as Katan and De Roos *(1)*, find the distinction between functional foods and supplements to be blurred. The reason for this is as follows: purified compounds taken as a pill or powder are clearly supplements. This is because if a substance is extracted from a food and delivered in a pill, then it is not part of the food matrix and, in our opinion, is best thought of as a pharmaceutical (or nutraceutical). But if the same substance is purified, then added to a food, it is often called a functional food. Examples of this include foods that have been fortified with one or more substances, such as iron, calcium, or β-sitostanol, with the intent of affecting a physiological process; in these examples combating anemia, enhancing bone density, or lowering blood cholesterol, respectively. We find this distinction to be arbitrary and not helpful for consumers. Based on this reasoning, our consideration of functional foods does not include herbal supplements, which are discussed in Chapter 11. As stated previously, a more detailed description of the functionality of purified compounds, or their synergistic effects, is included in Chapter 10.

Given that all foods are functional, it is clear that the term "functional foods" arises essentially in a marketing or social policy context, highlighting only functions that go beyond basic nutrition *(9)*. We find a lack of clarity in the term "basic nutrition." We also find a tendency, spurred by a profit motive, to denigrate simple and inexpensive but highly nutritious foods. Thus, we suggest that from a purely health perspective, the most functional foods are whole grains, fruits, vegetables, nuts, legumes, and herbs, simply prepared in a manner consistent with making them palatable and convenient and their nutrient content bioavailable. We think that consumers, attracted by the term "functional food," might be surprised to learn that these healthful foods are generally not labeled "functional."

Whatever their merits, functional foods have received the attention and interest of regulatory bodies in Japan and the United States, and also of the World Health Organization. The Japanese government has led the way in providing officially designated health claims that apply to specific foods. The Foods for Specified Health Uses act of 1991 approved food labels that contain specific health claims. Foods for Specified Health Uses are those that contain a specific ingredient for a specific physiological purpose *(10)*. The act was revised in 2001 to permit foods rich in 14 different nutrients with proven physiological functions to be labeled with a health claim by the manufacturer.

In the United States, special functionality for a food often implies a food label that claims functionality. Such claims are of two distinct types. On the one hand, structure/function claims are weakly regulated, as described in Chapter 17. In contrast, health claims are tightly regulated by the Food and Drug Administration (FDA) as part of the Federal Food, Drug, and Cosmetic Act. Surprisingly, the FDA has not provided functional foods with a legal definition. As noted above, the General Accounting Office has defined a functional food as one that has a "claim to have health benefits beyond basic nutrition" *(11)*. Manufacturers seeking to provide a health claim on the food label must adhere to stringent regulations. The food-health claims approved by the FDA are listed under Heading 5 of this chapter.

Permitted food-health claims and their degree of regulation differ between countries; a description is provided in a recent WHO publication *(12)*. An excellent source of information concerning regulations on health claims for functional food in different countries around the world can be found at the website of Australia's National Centre of Excellence in Functional Foods Regulatory Affairs *(13)*.

To reiterate, the primary use of the term "functional food" has been in the arena of food marketing and consumer education. The term and the concepts surrounding it are intended to help sort out which food products should have a health claim and which should not, although the exact boundaries of the term are not well defined and, to the extent that they are defined, may not always make good sense. We can see the value for the consumer of well-placed health claims, whether for functionality or another health aspect of food. However, we also see possible problems associated with claims that stretch a point or that are made purely to increase sales, without due consideration for health consequences. We agree with Katan and De Roos *(1)* that there is a need for legislation that will sort out which health claims are appropriate (based on evidence) and ban those that are not. The rest of this chapter discusses functional foods from this perspective, along with associated health claims.

2. FUNCTIONAL FOODS: RAW, PROCESSED, AND SUPPLEMENTED

From a consumer perspective certain raw foods would be the classic functional foods; an example would be an apple. The hallmark of such foods is that they are eaten in their natural state or simply prepared. It is an advantage to the consumer that they can learn what is in the food based on tables of macro- and micronutrient content and can be further aware that plant foods, such as apples, also contain myriad apparently healthful phytochemicals that are either unidentified or untabulated *(14)*.

These foods are often processed by such methods as freezing, pasteurization, dehydrating, canning, and irradiating *(15)*. This can overcome problems of seasonal availability, limited shelf life, and may, to some extent, increase bioavailability of some nutrients. But processing can potentially affect the functionality of a food in several ways. The food's chemical nature can change. An orange, for example, is rich in fiber, vitamins, and various flavonoid compounds, whereas orange juice may be depleted in some of these constituents, especially the fiber. Oxidative injury, which is incurred during processing and as the product sits on a shelf, reduces its nutritional quality and, presumably, its functional food value. Much of the original ascorbate is degraded and continues to degrade *(16)*. Presumably the antioxidant flavones, such as hesperidin and naringenin, may also degrade. Note, however, that processing can also improve the quality of a functional food by adding materials that were destroyed during processing or were never present in the original food in significant quantities (for instance, supplementation of fruit juices with vitamin C and minerals); or by cooking to increase accessibility of cell contents, as in the case of lycopene, which is more bioavailable in cooked than in raw tomatoes *(17)*.

Foods are often supplemented with purified food components, vitamins, or minerals, in an attempt to enhance functionality or qualify the food as functional (permitting the food label to carry an FDA-approved "Health Claim." Soy protein is the classic example. It is often used as a filler to raise the protein content of a food. Such foods may also carry a health claim stating "Prevents Heart Disease." In many cases, a supplement labeled "soy protein" will actually be an extract of whole soybean rather than of purified soy protein. With such a food extract, some of the food matrix will be retained, a situation that we consider desirable. The advantage of the soy extract might be in the mix of isoflavones *(18)* or might be in the complex mix of constituents in any food matrix *(7,8)*. However, foods may also be supplemented with purified substances; although no health claim is allowed for such a formulation, the manufacturer may make a structure/function claim, and this is less tightly regulated than a health claim. Thus, vitamin C is often added at or above the amount originally found in a food to allow a packaging statement, such as "contains extra antioxidants."

Whether addition of purified substances to a food actually enhances its health value is often presumptive rather than having solid supporting evidence. There may be an evidence-based case for making a purified protein, vitamin, or mineral available in a dietary supplement. But why add such a substance to food and then call the food "functional"? This may make little sense from a health perspective but much sense from a marketing one. Indeed, based on recent evidence about antioxidants, such as β-carotene, for example, long-term consumption of a purified compound may even be harmful *(19–21)*. Yet before the large clinical trials of purified β-carotene, it met the paradigm that functional foods enthusiasts ask to be accepted as evidence: it was known to have antioxidant properties, it was associated with improved biomarkers in the short term, and it was associated with lower long-term risk in observational cohort studies.

Basing health claims only on short-term evidence may be a trap for industry, in that long-term outcomes may not jibe with short-term results; this might even result in long-term financial losses. The innovations in food marketing most likely to be of greatest health value to the population are those that increase consumption of simply prepared whole foods (or lightly processed whole foods that still contain most of their constituents), or that make available to the public nutritious foods that are not commonly eaten.

3. WHY HAS THE PUBLIC BECOME INTERESTED IN FUNCTIONAL FOODS?

A serious concern is how the public receives information about the relationship between diet and health. Publication and media coverage of medical studies of dietary components have helped educate the public about diet–disease interactions, at the same time increasing public interest in and awareness of the issues. Yet, not surprisingly given ambiguities inherent in the scientific process, this information flow is often vague and contradictory. Given space limitations and media attempts at simplification, information may be less than fully accurate; indeed, more complex presentations may be confusing to everyone except nutrition professionals. The average person is inundated with a plethora of information in the news about possible diet-food–health discoveries. These are born out of "press releases" that are sometimes based on the release of peer-reviewed publications, but are just as likely based on unpublished "research results" that never survive peer review.

One factor guiding the food purchase choices of consumers is the desire to improve their health. A recent survey indicated that 71% of the public believe that diet plays "a great role" in determining their health, a role perceived as being greater than the effects of exercise or family history *(22)*. Furthermore, 63% of Americans are eating at least one specific food just because it is supposed to have a health benefit. This is having a significant impact on how our food dollars are spent: $15 billion was spent on functional foods in 2001, which is 3% of all food spending of $503 billion *(23)*, and the popularity of this food niche has only grown since that time. We can also look at recent changes in the content of food labels and of the choices now available at fast food restaurants. These trends indicate that the functional foods concept is driving a change in consumer options by affecting consumer education and demand. As an example of increasing demand for new and healthier foods, consider McDonald's: it has become the world's largest seller of salads *(24)*.

4. GOVERNMENT INTEREST IN FUNCTIONAL FOODS

The rate of deaths from cancer in the United States could be lowered by one third if people altered their diet to include more protective foods *(25)*. The National Heart, Lung, and Blood Institute estimated that 2003 costs of cardiovascular disease to be $352 billion and an additional $190 billion for cancer *(26)*. Clearly, functional foods, to the extent that they coincide with protective foods, could have an immense ability to reduce the cost of health care. Governments are therefore in a position to promote their use, a possibility consistent with the views expressed in Chapter 23. In this context, we need to emphasize the importance of simply prepared whole foods, especially those of plant origin, which have great functionality, even if they are not especially profitable from a commercial perspective.

To help promote the consumption of functional foods that improve health, the FDA has a set of food–health claims that can be placed on food labels and used in advertising. Farm commodity and trade groups have also begun to use these dietary health claims in their advertising. This synergy among government, industry, and consumers is intended to save governments money and improve consumption of these health-enhancing products.

5. HEALTH CLAIMS THAT ARE CURRENTLY PERMITTED ON FOOD LABELING BY THE FDA

Although there is no universal list of which foods are agreed upon as being functional, one set of foods that could be considered to be functional are those marketed in the United States with specialized health claims on their labels. In the United States the content of such label claims are closely regulated by the FDA's Center for Food Safety and Applied Nutrition (CFSAN). These health claims are probably valuable to the general public in identifying certain functional foods *(27)*. A description of some of the new foods that carry these approved labels or make structure/function claims can be found in Chapter 19.

5.1. CFSAN Suggested or Required Labeling for Food–Health Claims

The following is a list of "model claim statements" *(27)*:

- "Regular exercise and a healthy diet with enough calcium helps teens and young adult white and Asian women maintain good bone health and may reduce their high risk of osteoporosis later in life."
- "Healthful diets with adequate folate may reduce a woman's risk of having a child with a brain or spinal cord defect."
- "Diets low in sodium may reduce the risk of high blood pressure, a disease associated with many factors."
- "Diets containing foods that are a good source of potassium and that are low in sodium may reduce the risk of high blood pressure and stroke."
- "Development of cancer depends on many factors. A diet low in total fat may reduce the risk of some cancers."

- "Low fat diets rich in fiber-containing grain products, fruits, and vegetables may reduce the risk of some types of cancer, a disease associated with many factors."
- "Low fat diets rich in fruits and vegetables (foods that are low in fat and may contain dietary fiber, vitamin A, or vitamin C) may reduce the risk of some types of cancer, a disease associated with many factors. Broccoli is high in vitamins A and C, and it is a good source of dietary fiber."
- "Diets low in saturated fat and cholesterol and rich in fruits, vegetables, and grain products that contain some types of dietary fiber, particularly soluble fiber, may reduce the risk of heart disease, a disease associated with many factors."
- "While many factors affect heart disease, diets low in saturated fat and cholesterol may reduce the risk of this disease."
- "Soluble fiber from foods such as [name of soluble fiber source, and, if desired, name of food product], as part of a diet low in saturated fat and cholesterol, may reduce the risk of heart disease. A serving of [name of food product] supplies ___ grams of the [necessary daily dietary intake for the benefit] soluble fiber from [name of soluble fiber source] necessary per day to have this effect."
- "25 grams of soy protein a day, as part of a diet low in saturated fat and cholesterol, may reduce the risk of heart disease. A serving of [name of food] supplies ___ grams of soy protein."
- "Foods containing at least 0.65 gram per serving of vegetable oil sterol esters, eaten twice a day with meals for a daily total intake of at least 1.3 grams, as part of a diet low in saturated fat and cholesterol, may reduce the risk of heart disease. A serving of [name of food] supplies ___ grams of vegetable oil sterol esters."
- "Diets rich in whole grain foods and other plant foods and low in total fat, saturated fat, and cholesterol may reduce the risk of heart disease and some cancers."
- "Supportive but not conclusive research shows that eating 1.5 ounces per day of walnuts, as part of a low saturated fat and low cholesterol diet and not resulting in increased caloric intake, may reduce the risk of coronary heart disease. See nutrition information for fat [and calorie] content."

5.2. Foods That May Qualify for "Health Claim Status" in the Future

Many foods are currently on the market that have not been endorsed by CFSAN for a health claim but may receive a health claim approval in the future and may then qualify for designation as a functional food. A brief description of some of the most popular potential associations is warranted. Red wine and grape juice provide polyphenolic compounds that may help decrease cardiovascular disease risk by providing antioxidants, improving intracoronary vasodilation, and preventing platelet aggregation *(28,29)*. Cranberry juice has been suggested to reduce urinary tract infections *(30)* and provide cardiovascular benefits in a manner similar to that associated with red wine *(31)*. Cold-water fish, such as cod and salmon, provide n-3 fatty acids that have been suggested to reduce the risk of cancer *(32)*, cardiovascular disease, and sudden cardiac arrest (*see* ref. *33*; *see also* Chapter 8). Organosulfur compounds in garlic have been suggested to provide beneficial effects on blood cholesterol levels that may protect against heart disease *(34)*. Green tea is rich in catechins that may be beneficial for reducing cancer *(35)* and cardiovascular disease *(36)*. Tomatoes are rich in lycopene and may be associated with reduction in prostate cancer risk *(37,38)*. Although much of the data collected in these studies are promising, many of the claims remain to be proven. Future studies may also determine that the apparent health protection associated with a food product may be owing to social or behavioral habits of the consumers of the product, and not caused by any specific functionality on the part of the product.

6. BENEFITS AND PROBLEMS ASSOCIATED WITH FUNCTIONAL FOOD HEALTH CLAIMS

Designating a food as functional by giving it a health claim can solve a consumer communication problem. For example, although many studies were published between 1978 and 1984 demonstrating that an "increased soluble fiber consumption may reduce risks of coronary heart disease," little change was observed in the fiber content of ready-to-eat cereals (during this time fiber content averaged 1.99 g/oz). However, after inclusion of FDA-approved health claims on the fiber content of high-fiber foods, cereals introduced between 1984 and 1987 averaged 3.59 g fiber/oz *(39,40)*. Furthermore, the knowledge of a beneficial link between fiber and coronary heart disease in persons with just a high school education increased from 1% in 1978 to 18% in 1986 *(40)*. Thus, if used judiciously, functionality can be an important tool in both marketing and consumer education.

Therefore, it seems that the use of packaging as a mode for nutrition information transfer has been helpful in educating the public about and promoting the consumption of healthful foods, including those that claim to be functional. However, there are potential problems for our overall nutritional quality. Consumption of functional foods could give the consumer a false sense of security and detract from a diet that enhances basic nutrition. Instead, the consumer may select packaged foods with a health claim that delivers a particular substance that may or may not be appropriate. In particular, because food package claims appear on food packaging and because many raw foods, apples for instance, generally have no actual packaging, an informational strategy that relies on package labels may actually lead consumers away from truly functional, simply prepared whole foods. It is also important that the public understands that a specific food-disease claim does not necessarily make the overall diet balanced and healthy.

Another potential problem is that some people may view functional foods as cures, rather than as preventive measures, and hence not seek medical attention in a timely manner. Functional foods taken in large amounts could interfere with the absorption, kinetics, or efficacy of prescription medications *(41)*. In general, there should be a concern, whether with supplements or with functional foods delivering purified compounds, that there may be interactions of various types: drug–supplement, drug–food, food–supplement, or food–food. In this regard it should be mentioned that the medical community remains poorly educated about the impact of basic nutrition on consumer health *(41)*, let alone the impact of functional foods.

The conflict between what the research community can support and what manufacturers want to market was highlighted at a recent meeting (November 2004) of the Korean Society of Food Science and Nutrition entitled, "The Current Prospects of Functional and Medicinal Food." At this meeting, research presentations were largely about functional properties of certain foods, based on studies of cells or short-term feeding, with findings extrapolated to long-term health. Exhibitors largely from the manufacturing side of functional foods, on the other hand, presented products that were closer to medicinal foods, in which certain substances had been manipulated for health-enhancing or marketing purposes. Many of these products should be treated in the same way as supplements or drugs.

7. CONCLUSIONS

There is no universal list of functional foods and the health claims associated with them, in part because there is so much debate regarding the appropriate definition of the term. The concept of functionality can be useful for explaining nutrition–disease associations to the public. The use of judicious health claims can provide the public with improved health and can potentially reduced health care costs. However, often a claim for functionality is made when a substance is delivered via a food outside of its natural food matrix. It may be more accurate to see such products as supplements in a food vehicle. If the concept of functionality is used primarily to obtain a marketing niche, it could damage the public health. A marketing program that promotes the consumption of one segment of our diet at the expense of others has the potential to create a diet that is neither balanced nor healthy. This problem becomes more serious when the marketing strategy is based on poor science.

REFERENCES

1. Katan MB, De Roos NM. Promises and problems of functional foods. Crit Rev Food Sci Nutr 2004; 44:369–377.
2. Baily R. Foods for Specified Health Use (FOSHU) as functional foods in Japan. Canadian Chemical News, May 18–19, 1999.
3. Roberfroid M, Slavin J. Nondigestible oligosaccharides. Crit Rev Food Sci Nutr 2000; 40:461–480.
4. Food Safety: Improvements Needed in Overseeing the Safety of Dietary Supplements and "Functional Foods." GAO/RCED-00-156. Washington, DC, July 11, 2000.
5. Palou A, Pico C, Bonet ML. Food safety and functional foods in the European Union: obesity as a paradigmatic example for novel food development. Nutr Rev 2004; 62(7 Pt 2):S169–S181.
6. Regulation on Novel Foods and Novel Foods Ingredients. Regulation-EC-258/97. 1997.
7. Jacobs DR, Steffen LM. Nutrients, foods, and dietary patterns as exposures in research: a framework for food synergy. Am J Clin Nutr 2003; 78(3 Suppl):508S–513S.
8. Liu RH. Health benefits of fruits and vegetables are from additive and synergistic combination of phytochemicals. Am J Clin Nutr 2003; 78:517S–520S.
9. IOM/NAS. Opportunities in the Nutrition and Food Sciences. Thomas PR, Earl R, eds. Institute of Medicine/National Academy of Sciences, National Academy Press, Washington, DC, 1994, p. 109.
10. Ohki K, Nakamura Y, Takano T. The Japanese nutritional health beverage market. In: Beverages in Nutrition and Health. Wilson T, Temple NJ, eds. Humana Press, Totowa, NJ, 2003, pp. 377–387.
11. Krasny LT. Labeling requirements for beverages in the United States. In: Beverages in Nutrition and Health. Wilson T, Temple NJ, eds. Humana Press, Totowa, NJ, 2003, pp. 389–401.
12. Hawkes C. Nutrition Labels and Health Claims: The Global Regulatory Environment. World Health Organization, Geneva, 2004, pp. 1–72.
13. Website of the National Centre of Excellence in Functional Foods Regulatory Affairs. www.nceff.com.au/regulatory/reg-news.htm. Last accessed January 5, 2005.
14. Eberhardt MV, Lee CY, Liu RH. Antioxidant activity of fresh apples. Nature 2000; 405:903, 904.
15. Slavin JL, Jacobs DR, Jr, Marquart L. Grain processing and nutrition. Crit Rev Food Sci Nutr 2000; 40:309–326.
16. Johnston CS. Orange juice: Are the health benefits of oranges lost during processing? In: Beverages in Nutrition and Health. Wilson T, Temple NJ, eds. Humana Press, Totowa, NJ, 2003, pp. 79–91.
17. Gartner C, Stahl W, Sies H. Lycopene is more bioavailable from tomato paste than from fresh tomatoes. Am J Clin Nutr 1997; 66:116–122.

18. Messina M, Messina V. Provisional recommended soy protein and isoflavone intakes for healthy adults: rationale. Nutr Today 2003; 38:100–109.

19. Clarke R, Armitage J. Antioxidant vitamins and risk of cardiovascular disease. Review of large-scale randomised trials. Cardiovasc Drugs Ther 2002; 16:411–415.

20. Lee DH, Folsom AR, Harnack L, Halliwell B, Jacobs DR Jr. Does supplemental vitamin C increase cardiovascular disease risk in women with diabetes? Am J Clin Nutr 2004; 80:1194–1200.

21. Miller ER, Pastor-Barriuso R, Dalal D, Riemersma RA, Appel LJ, Guallar E. Meta-analysis: high-dosage vitamin E supplementation may increase all-cause mortality. Ann Intern Med 2005; 142:37–46.

22. Anonymous. The consumer view on functional foods: yesterday and today. Food Insight May/June 2002.

23. Zawistowski J, Kitts DD. Functional foods—A new step in the evolution of food development. Clin Nutr Rounds 2004; 4(4).

24. Anonymous. The Economist. October 24, 2004.

25. Willett WC. Diet, nutrition, and avoidable cancer. Environ Health Perspect 1995; 103:165–170.

26. National Institute of Health. National Heart, Lung, and Blood Institute 2002 factbook. www.nhlbi.nih.gov/about/02factbk.pdf. Last accessed January 1, 2005.

27. US Food and Drug Administration Center for Food Safety and Applied Nutrition. Food Labeling Guide—Appendix C. Www.cfsan.fda.gov/~dms/flg-6c.html. Last accessed January 1, 2005.

28. Klatsky AL, Friedman GD, Armstrong MA, Kipp H. Wine, liquor, beer, and mortality. Am J Epidemiol 2003; 158:585–595.

29. Folts JD. Potential health benefits from the flavonoids in grape products on vascular disease. Adv Exp Med Biol 2002; 505:95–111.

30. Jepson RG, Mihaljevic L, Craig J. Cranberries for preventing urinary tract infections. Cochrane Database Syst Rev 2004; (2):CD001321.

31. Wilson T. Cranberry juice effects on health. In: Wilson T, Temple NJ, eds. Beverages in Nutrition and Health. Humana Press, Totowa, NJ, 2003, pp. 51–62.

32. Larsson SC, Kumlin M, Ingelman-Sundberg M, Wolk A. Dietary long-chain n-3 fatty acids for the prevention of cancer: a review of potential mechanisms. Am J Clin Nutr 2004; 79:935–945.

33. Lemaitre RN, King IB, Mozaffarian D, Kuller LH, Tracy RP, Siscovick DS. n-3 polyunsaturated fatty acids, fatal ischemic heart disease, and nonfatal myocardial infarction in older adults: the Cardiovascular Health Study. Am J Clin Nutr 2003; 77:319–325.

34. Banerjee SK, Maulik SK. Effect of garlic on cardiovascular disorders: a review. Nutr J 2002; 4:1–14.

35. Moyers SB, Kumar NB. Green tea polyphenols and cancer chemoprevention: multiple mechanisms and endpoints for phase II trials. Nutr Rev 2004; 62:204–211.

36. Imai K, Nakachi K. Cross sectional study of effects of drinking green tea on cardiovascular and liver diseases. BMJ 1995; 310:693–696.

37. Giovannucci E, Rimm EB, Liu Y, Stampfer MJ, Willett WC. A prospective study of tomato products, lycopene, and prostate cancer risk. J Natl Cancer Inst 2002; 94:391–398.

38. Hadley CW, Schwartz SJ, Clinton SK. Tomato-based beverages: implications for the prevention of cancer and cardiovascular disease. In: Wilson T, Temple NJ, eds. Beverages in Nutrition and Health. Humana Press, Totowa, NJ, 2003, pp. 107–123.

39. Ippolito PM, Mathios A. Health claims in food marketing: evidence on knowledge and behavior in the cereal market. J Pub Policy Marketing 1991; 10:15–32.

40. Levy A, Stephenson M. Nutrition Knowledge Levels About Dietary Fats and Cholesterol: 1983–1988. Draft Division of Consumer Studies, Food and Drug Administration, 1990.

41. Kane GC. How can the consumption of grapefruit juice and other beverages affect drug action? In: Wilson T, Temple NJ, eds. Beverages in Nutrition and Health. Humana Press, Totowa, NJ, 2003, pp. 93–105.

21 Use of Biotechnology to Improve Food Production and Quality

Travis J. Knight and Donald C. Beitz

KEY POINTS

- Current technology allows for detailed genetic manipulation of plants and animals.
- Adding or deleting genes in plants or animals can result in foods with improved nutritional or processing characteristics.
- Genetically modified plants or animals can be used to economically produce medicinal proteins or other compounds that can be used to treat or prevent disease in livestock or humans.
- There are no scientific data to support the idea that transgenic proteins could harm consumers or cause an increased chance of allergic reaction when compared with native proteins in common foods.
- The scientific hurdles of creating genetically modified organisms are diminishing rapidly because of sound research, but, unfortunately, the sociopolitical hurdles are currently preventing the widespread use of genetically modified organisms where they could be used to alleviate malnutrition and disease in humans.

1. INTRODUCTION

This chapter describes the use of biotechnology by the food industry to increase the efficiency of production and the quality of foods for use by humans. Selected examples are presented in which new technologies of food production by plants and animals are being used because of economic advantages to producers and because of nutritional or health benefits to human consumers. Some benefits of biotechnology can be summarized as follows (1):

1. Plant production.
   a. Higher yielding varieties and more nutritious foods and feeds.
   b. Improved resistance to diseases, pests, and adverse conditions.
   c. Decreased need for fertilizers and other chemical treatments.
   d. Production of novel products.

From: *Nutritional Health: Strategies for Disease Prevention, Second Edition*
Edited by: N. J. Temple, T. Wilson, and D. R. Jacobs © Humana Press Inc., Totowa, NJ

2. Animal production.
   a. Improved efficiency of converting feeds into useful animal products.
   b. Greater control of plant and animal diseases.
   c. Modified composition of foods derived from animals.

The remainder of the chapter amplifies on the potential benefits of using biotechnology to produce animal feed and human food by plants and animals.

2. USING BIOTECHNOLOGY TO IMPROVE FOOD PRODUCTION BY PLANTS

Modification of plants, animals, and microbes to produce more desirable traits began nearly 10,000 yr ago *(2)*. During the past 50 yr, tremendous success has been achieved in food production by plants through development of production systems and of varieties of crops. Major improvements in varieties have been made by traditional breeding practices of identifying and selecting strains of crops that exhibit specific valuable traits, such as yield, standability, composition, and resistance to pests and adverse conditions *(3)*. Biotechnological producers are catalyzing another revolution by allowing specific crops to be identified, selected, and even created that have desired traits. Generally speaking, new crop varieties are created by development of cell cultures of the plant under study, inserting new genes into the plant cells, and promoting the differentiation of plant cells in culture into plantlets that eventually are grown into mature plants.

2.1. Extent of Use of Genetically Modified Crops

Agricultural biotechnology companies, such as Monsanto, Dupont, Novartis, and Dow Chemical, have invested billions of dollars in the development of genetically engineered crops. Monsanto introduced "Roundup Ready" soybeans in 1996 as the first genetically modified crop available for commercial production. In 2004, the National Agricultural Statistics Service of the United States Department of Agriculture estimated that 85% of US soybean acreage is planted to soybeans that are genetically modified (GM) to be herbicide resistant. Corn has been modified to be insect resistant (27% of 2004 US acreage), herbicide resistant (13% of acreage), or both insect and herbicide resistant (5% of acreage). Nearly three-fourths of all cotton grown in the United States is GM to be insect or herbicide resistant. Globally, 167 million acres of GM crops were planted in 2003 according to the International Service of the Acquisition of Agri-Biotech Applications (www.isaaa.org). The global acreage of GM crops represents 7 million farmers in 18 countries. The acceptance of GM crops continues to grow because of continued safety testing *(4)* and economic advantages *(5)*, but scientific, moral, ethical, and emotional objections to, and support for, biotechnology are being expressed openly and vigorously as regulatory agencies, governments, and consumer groups debate the health, environmental, and commercial risks and benefits of technology. Research on the acceptance of foods resulting from GM crops has indicated that consumers are less likely to purchase those foods because of information supplied by environmental groups, but third-party, verifiable information usually completely dissipates the negative influences of the environmental groups *(6)*.

2.2. Modifying Plants to Change Nutrition Value

The health and well-being of humans are entirely dependent on foods derived directly from plants or indirectly when plants are consumed by food animals. Carbohydrates, lipids, and proteins make up the bulk of plants and supply energy for human life. Organic and inorganic micronutrients provide essential roles in life processes. Essential dietary micronutrients include 17 minerals and 13 vitamins *(7)*. Nonessential compounds include a variety of unique organic phytochemicals that are linked to promotion of good health (*see* Chapter 10). Modification of the content of macronutrients, micronutrients, and phytochemicals in plant foods is an urgent need worldwide, but especially in developing countries where people exist on a few staple foods that are deficient in essential nutrients *(7)*. For example, deficiencies of vitamin A, iron, and iodine are especially common. Even in developed countries where food is abundant and caloric intake is often excessive, deficiencies of micronutrients, such as iron, are prevalent because of poor eating habits. Hence, genetic modification of nutrient content of plants can have significant impact on nutritional status and human health.

In contrast to the situation with essential nutrients, primary evidence for health-promoting roles of phytochemicals is more difficult to prove because of their complex interaction with food constituents, and therefore, must come from epidemiological studies. In fact, the exact identity of many active phytochemicals still needs to be determined. Selected phytochemicals that are considered candidates for genetic modification of plants are *(7)*:

1. Carotenoids, such as lycopene in tomatoes and lutein in kale and spinach.
2. Glucosinolates, such as glucoraphanin in broccoli and broccoli sprouts.
3. Phytoestrogens, such as genistein and diadzein in soybeans, tofu, and other soy products.
4. Phenolics, such as resveratrol in red wine and red grapes.

Traditional breeding programs of plants have emphasized increased yields of foods; little emphasis, however, has been placed on micronutrient content. Variation in micronutrient content is known to exist and can be used by breeders to modify plant foods. Today, tools of biotechnology allow manipulation of plant food composition. Genes for synthesis of carotenoids, biotin, thiamin, vitamin E, and iron uptake have become available for transfer between different plants. Genes for other nutrients and phytochemicals are being isolated and studied as tools to improve human nutrition. Furthermore, unique plant systems, such as moss bioreactors and green alga, are being modified genetically to synthesize recombinant proteins and biomolecules *(8,9)*. The advantages of the moss and alga systems are that they can be highly contained, they are transformed readily, and they are relatively inexpensive to maintain.

2.3. Modification of Some Nonstaple Crops

Research is underway to improve resistance of potatoes to several viral, fungal, and bacterial diseases. Cassava that is resistant to the African cassava mosaic virus has been developed. Palm plants are being engineered to produce modified oils (e.g., more oleic acid) and possibly even biodegradable plastics. Bananas are being engineered for improved viral resistance and edible vaccines (e.g., against *Escherichia coli* diarrhea).

Creating a naturally decaffeinated coffee is the goal of some researchers. Two research groups have cloned genes for three of the key enzymes, all *N*-methyltransferases, in the caffeine biosynthetic pathway *(10,11)*. Ultimately, learning about the kinetics of each enzyme and now knowing the sequence of the cDNA for each gene will potentially lead to naturally decaffeinated coffee.

2.4. Other Engineered Traits of Economic Importance

Plant-derived vaccines may be the fastest growing research focus of plant genetic engineering because of the potential impact that this delivery system could have on improving health and saving lives of humans and food animals. In 2000, approx 55.7 million people died of a communicable disease, many of which could have been prevented by traditional or plant-derived vaccines *(12)*. Currently, most plant vaccines are focused on animal agriculture *(13)*, but some investigators have been studying plant vaccines of human interest, such as tetanus vaccine antigen *(14)*. As the inherent advantages of plant-based vaccines are realized, especially with respect to cost, scale-up, no need for refrigeration, and convenience of delivery, this technology has great potential to become a common technology that could save millions of human and animal lives each year *(15)*.

Nitrogen fixation by rice would be one approach to help increase rice production 60% over the next 30 yr, which is the expected need to maintain global food security *(16)*. To date, no transgenic plants have been converted to nitrogen fixers, but nitrogen deficiency in rice production systems is the greatest threat to future yields and will be the focus of research. Drought resistance in rice also has been addressed by Capell et al. *(17)* when they studied polyamine biosynthetic pathways in transgenic rice. For example, transgenic rice expressing arginine decarboxylase from *Datura stramonium* (jimson weed) had greater concentrations of putrescine when stressed by drought, which promoted spermidine and spermine synthesis and ultimate protection from drought.

Along with diseases, drought, and pests, plant growth is retarded by excesses of specific metals in soils. Recently, scientists have identified metal-resistant genes in plants and other organisms *(18)*. Now, the potential exists for making food-producing plants more tolerant to excess aluminum, mercury, copper, or cadmium in soil by introducing genes for phytochelatins that sequester the metal complexes in cells. This technology could improve the acreage of tillable land available for food production. Such modified plants may have greater use as cost-effective agents of environmental remediation. To perform such remediation, the plants could be harvested and incinerated to clean polluted soils. Soil cleaned of pollutants then might become available for the production of consumable foods. Similar mechanisms may be used to modify plants with respect to micronutrient content (i.e., micronutrient elements and vitamins) as an approach to help the estimated 3 billion people who are micronutrient malnourished *(19)*.

The production of ethanol from highly fermentable plant starches has become common in industry as a renewable fuel source. One argument against fermenting grain into ethanol is that potential human food sources are being used as an industrial fuel source. Alternatively, there are many byproducts of food processing that are now being explored as sources of ethanol if the cellulose could be efficiently saccharified. Fujita et al. *(20)* constructed a recombinant *Saccharomyces cerevisiae* that expressed endoglucanase II and cellobiohydrolase II from *Trichoderma reesei* and β-glucosidase I from *Aspergillus aculeatus*. Fermentation of amorphous cellulose with the recombinant organism resulted in 88.5% of theoretical yield of ethanol, but it required 40 h of fermentation. The next step is to develop a biocatalyst with improved ability to degrade and ferment cellulose.

GM plants that contain lactoferrin and lysozyme have been created and are ready for large-scale growth (www.checkbiotech.org). These antibacterial proteins have also been expressed and grown in barley; there are plans to decrease pathogens that cause severe diarrhea especially in developing countries where many people, including children, die because of this type of infection. This technology could be adapted for use in many stages of food processing to ensure improved food safety.

2.5. Modified Lipid Composition of Selected Plants

Vegetable oils comprise as much as 25% of the average caloric intake of humans *(3)*. Biotechnology has made it possible to tailor the composition of plant-derived lipids with respect to food functionality and human dietary needs. Plant breeders have taken advantage of the natural diversity in fatty acids that exists among plant varieties and closely related species in order to develop plants that produce unique oils. For example, soy oils that are low in linolenic acid and high in linoleic and low in palmitic acid have been made commercially available by traditional breeding *(21)*. Because of having less of the highly oxidizable linolenic acid, this modified soy oil has greater stability against development of rancidity. Directed genetic modifications of plant lipids depend on the availability of genes of interest. Fatty acyl desaturase genes are available for synthesis of both α- and γ-linolenate. A Δ^5-desaturase for synthesis of eicosapentaenate has recently been cloned *(22)*. Gene sequences for several thioesterases for production of medium-chain fatty acids are now available. Moreover, genes for fatty acid elongases for synthesis of eicosamonoenoate (20:1) and docosamonoenoate (22:1) from oleate also have been cloned. Thus, several genes to control chain length and degree of unsaturation are available for use in causing plants to produce unique and novel oils. Because plant oils may form potentially toxic oxidized products when exposed to oxidative stress, increasing monounsaturated fatty acids at the expense of polyunsaturated fatty acids may be desired for improved heat stability and shelf life. By using antisense technology (oleate desaturase), oleic acid-rich (>80%) canola oil has been produced *(23)*. Similar antisense technology has been used to produce soy oil with greater than 80% oleate and about 11% saturated fatty acids and to decrease linolenate in soy oil from 8 to 2% *(22)*. Investigators continue to study ways to change fatty acid composition of oils (e.g., increased stearate content) to decrease formation of trans-fatty acids during hydrogenation. This research is of clinical significance for decreasing the intake of the atherogenic trans-fatty acids by humans.

Another application is the increased synthesis of the very-long-chain fatty acids with 20 and 22 carbons by plants *(22)*. These acids are important constituents of animal cell membranes, and the 20-carbon acids serve as precursors for the biologically active eicosanoids such as prostaglandins, leukotrienes, and thromboxanes. Intake of these very-long-chain fatty acids, especially crucial for newborn infants, is beneficial for cardiovascular disease, renal function, and retinal and brain development. Investigations are being made to engineer plant oils to increase their content of α-tocopherol, the most active chemical form of vitamin E. Most promise seems related to causing plants to up regulate the biosynthetic pathway for vitamin E synthesis *(7)*. This achievement may be especially important because many studies show that supranatural amounts of vitamin E are beneficial and because these amounts cannot be attained by consumption of conventional foods.

2.6. Golden Rice With Modified Nutrient Content

Billions of people in developing countries depend on rice as a food staple. Many of these people suffer from deficiencies of vitamin A and iron. About 400 million people in the world are vitamin A deficient and up to 3.7 billion people, particularly women, are iron deficient. Hence, there is a motivation to genetically modify rice. To this end, Swiss scientists undertook research to introduce into rice the genetic capability of synthesizing β-carotene and of increasing iron content *(24)*. Development of this type of modified rice is potentially of major humanitarian importance. Ensuring consumer acceptance of the "yellow" rice and the efficient absorption of the additional iron remains a challenge to nutritionists. Rice plants synthesize no β-carotene but do synthesize geranylgeranyl pyrophosphate, which can be converted to β-carotene with four additional enzymes. The Swiss researchers used daffodil and the bacterium *Erwinia uredovora* as the source of the four required genes and the plant infecting microbe *Agrobacterium tumefaciens* to transfer the four genes into rice cells in culture. The result was rice plants that produce golden rice rich in β-carotene *(24)*. About 300 g of this modified rice will meet the daily needs for vitamin A for an adult human. The same scientists studied development of iron-enriched rice *(24)*. This development required introduction of three genes. Normally, iron in rice is unavailable for absorption because of phytate. One gene introduced was for a heat-stable phytase, which improves iron availability. Introduction of the ferritin gene into rice doubled the iron availability *(24)*. The gene for a third protein, metallothionein-like protein, increases the absorption of iron from the human digestive tract. Consumption of modified rice with these three genes has great potential to decrease iron malnutrition throughout the world. Hybrid rice that contains both significant β-carotene and increased iron content has been developed. All of these varieties are being met with resistance, but golden rice could be grown on a commercial scale sometime in the next few years if the last major stumbling block, radical opponents of GM organisms (GMOs) can be overcome *(25)*. As of 2003, most Philippine farmers and even community leaders did not know what golden rice was, but would be willing to raise it if the seed was distributed for free, if it had a similar yield compared with typical varieties, and if it was shown to be safe for human consumption *(5)*.

3. USE OF BIOTECHNOLOGY
TO IMPROVE FOOD PRODUCTION BY ANIMALS

For thousands of years people have attempted to improve animal genetics through selection of animals with desired or superior phenotypes. Success depends on identifying traits and transmissibility of traits to offspring. Improvements are limited by naturally occurring variations and mutations within the species of interest. With the advent of recombinant DNA technology, a variety of new technologies became available that allowed the acceleration and refinement of genetic manipulation of animals.

Insertion of modified gene constructs into livestock can be used to create "designer production animals" that possess improved disease resistance and, therefore, improved productivity of the modified animals. Furthermore, producing useful proteins, tissues, and organs for pharmaceutical and biomedical use is likely to be another future use of GM animals. In general, scientists hope to produce animals that are larger, leaner, grow faster and more efficiently, produce more healthful foods, and are more resistant to diseases. These improvements may be made by development of transgenic animals where a transgene (functional sequence of DNA) is integrated into the host genome. More recently, cloning of animals through the transfer of a nucleus into enucleated oocytes capable of differentiating into an intact animal in surrogate mothers has opened new opportunities. Thus, a generation of a large number of identical animals from a single donor with a desired genotype is possible.

An excellent review on commercializing animal biotechnology has been written by Faber et al. *(26)*. It outlines the merits and pitfalls of utilizing animals to produce biomedical products and the modification of food-producing animals. The review points out that there are three factors—economics, societal values, and regulatory agencies—that will drive the intensity in which animals will be modified genetically. The following examples illustrate the breadth of applications of animal transgenesis for improved food and even pharmaceutical production *(1,27,28)*:

1. Meat animals, including fish, with increased copy numbers of genes for somatotropin or insulin-like growth factor for improved growth efficiency.
2. Food-producing animals with greater resistance to viral and bacterial diseases for improved productivity.
3. Lactating cattle with specific genes that increase efficiency of milk production.
4. Lactating animals with capability of secreting novel proteins into milk, such as human albumin, α_1-antitrypsin, α-glucosidase, antibodies, antithrombin III, collagen, factor IX, fibrinogen, hemoglobin, lactoferrin, protein C, tissue plasminogen activator, and cystic fibrosis transmembrane conductance regulator.
5. Genetic modification of animals for use in human organ replacement.

3.1. Modification of Digestive Tract Micro-Organisms to Improve Efficiency of Food Production by Animals

An important application of biotechnology to animal agriculture is the genetic modification of microbes that inhabit the rumen and cecum of food animals. For example, development of a modified microbe population that could be maintained in the rumen and/or cecum and that increases lignin degradation in fibrous feeds would improve digestibility of dietary fibers *(29)*. Degradation of lignin would, in most cases, improve the digestion of cellulose and thus increase the quantity of useful nutrients and nutriceuticals absorbed from a given quantity of consumed feed. Another application is the modification of the rumen microbial population so that a greater amount of microbial protein is synthesized from a given amount of dietary protein. As a result, less of the feed protein would be degraded and excreted as urea in the urine. Genetic modifications for improvement of cellulose digestion and protein utilization by microbes merit greater research emphasis because feed represents a major cost of food production by animals and because there is sufficient margin for improvement in digestibility of dietary fibers and protein.

Recombinant phytase represents a unique application of biotechnology to animal agriculture. Depending on diet composition, a significant fraction of phosphate, especially in the cereal component of the diet, is linked covalently to inositol. This phosphate is unavailable to the nonruminant animal and is therefore excreted in the feces. Incorporation of recombinant phytase into the diet results in the hydrolysis of phosphate from the inositol; this released phosphate is then available for absorption. The phytase has two pH optima; one is similar to the pH of the stomach, and the other is similar to that of the small intestine. Use of phytase has proven practical in regions of the world where the amount of fecal phosphate spread on farm fields as manure is limited by regulations based on environmental concerns. The biotechnological applications of phytase in animal feed and food industries are reviewed by Vohra and Styanarayana (30).

S. cerevisiae has been studied as a means of delivering recombinant proteins or peptides to the gut. Blanquet et al. (31) studied two recombinant strains of S. cerevisiae in an in vitro simulated human digestive tract and found greater than 80% survival of both organisms after 270 min of simulated digestion. Engineered yeasts could be envisioned to secrete compounds into the digestive tract that act as oral vaccines, that correct metabolic disorders, or are biological mediators.

There are animal health and food safety problems that could be addressed by administering recombinantly derived antimicrobial peptides, such as alamethicin, cecropin, melittin, and magainin. Lazarev et al. (32) prevented mycoplasma infection in chickens by treating animals with a melittin-expressing plasmid, but other infectious pathogens, including common food pathogens such as E. coli O157:H7 or salmonella, also could be prevented with antimicrobial peptide technology. Nandiwada et al. (33) used colicin Hu194 to decrease and, in some cases, eliminate strains of O157:H7 from alfalfa seeds for use in growing alfalfa sprouts.

α1,4-Linked N-acetylglucosamine is a naturally occurring compound that has antimicrobial activity against H. pylori. Genetic modification of cows to produce milk containing this enzyme, or similar modification of plants, could prevent ulcers and even stomach cancer associated with H. pylori (34). The antibiotic properties of this enzyme were noted when Kawakubo et al. (34) realized that H. pylori usually cannot thrive in the deeper mucin layers of the stomach that are rich in this particular class of glycoproteins.

3.2. Production of Low-Lactose Milk

To assist lactose-intolerant humans with consumption of dairy foods, lactose-free dairy products can be made by treatment of milk with β-galactosidase (lactase). The capability of expressing a lactose-hydrolyzing enzyme in the mammary gland of mice has been developed (35). These transgenic female mice secreted lactase into milk that contained 50–85% less lactose and with no changes in fat and protein concentrations. Thus, milk with more desirable composition for lactose-intolerant humans can be developed through animal transgenesis.

3.3. Gene Farming With Cloned Animals

Sheep, cows, mice, and goats have been cloned by somatic cell nuclear transfer (36–38). In a recent development, nuclei from quiescent fetal cells of goats were transferred into enucleated oocytes and the manipulated embryos were implanted into surrogate mothers (39). The fetal cells were derived from a goat that had been mated to a transgenic male containing a human antithrombin transgene. One of the cloned offspring that began lactating produced milk with 3.7–5.8 g/L of antithrombin in her milk, which was similar to that of her female ancestors on her father's side. Cloned animals, therefore, still synthesized a foreign protein at the expected level. This technology indicates a potential method to produce a herd of lactating animals from one transgenic animal for production of a useful pharmaceutical compound.

3.4. Use of Recombinant Somatotropin for Production of Dairy Foods

In 1937 scientists documented that injections of crude extracts of pituitary glands stimulated milk production by dairy cows. This initial discovery led to a classic study at Cornell University in which dairy cows produced about 40% more milk during a 6-mo period when injected daily with purified bovine somatotropin *(40)*. Numerous follow-up studies at many research institutions demonstrated efficacy and safety of the technology to increase milk production with natural or recombinantly derived bovine somatotropin. The following list summarizes findings of these studies *(41–43)*:

1. Milk production increased.
2. Feed intake increased to compensate for increased milk production.
3. Amount of milk produced per unit of feed consumed increased.
4. Milk composition did not change.
5. Milk quality did not change.

Milk produced by cows treated with recombinant bovine somatotropin were considered safe because *(44)*:

1. The hormone is a protein and is degraded during normal digestive processes.
2. The hormone is species specific and thus is inactive in humans.
3. Milk from treated cows contains normal concentrations of the hormone.
4. The hormone is inactivated by the commonly used pasteurization process.
5. All animal-derived foods contain small amounts of natural somatotropin.

Monsanto of St. Louis, MO, received Food and Drug Administration approval in 1995 for commercialization of their product called Posilac®, which is an injectable and slow release preparation of recombinant bovine somatotropin. According to the company website, in 2004, approx 35% of the dairy cows in the United States are being treated with Posilac to improve profitability (www.monsantodairy.com). In a study of the use of recombinant somatotropin in the northeastern United States, scientists concluded that this technology improves lactation yield and persistency over the 4-yr postapproval period with no effects on cow stayability and herd life *(41)*.

3.5. Use of Recombinant Somatotropin for Meat Production

In 1934 scientists noted that injections of pituitary gland extracts into rats stimulated growth and produced carcasses with more protein and less fat. Hence, administration of exogenous somatotropin to meat-producing animals seemed to merit additional study. Subsequently, researchers demonstrated that injections of bovine somatotropin into growing beef cattle improved growth rates and slightly increased the lean-to-fat ratio of carcasses. Such improvements, however, have not yet proved economical, and thus, commercial adoption of this technology has not occurred. Similarly, injections of porcine somatotropin into young growing pigs caused marked increases in the lean-to-fat ratio of pig carcasses *(45)*. Efficiency of growth improved as well. The color of lean pork was slightly paler because of the treatment; firmness, juiciness, and flavor were not changed, but tenderness tended to be slightly decreased. Especially important for fat-conscious consumers, marbling or fat content of the pork was decreased markedly. To date, however, economics and injection protocol have not justified commercialization of administration of recombinant porcine somatotropin to growing pigs, even though the pork from treated pigs seems more desirable for human health. Administration of recombinant somatotropin does not show promise in poultry meat production because no significant improvements in growth efficiency or carcass composition were observed.

4. SAFETY OF GENETICALLY MODIFIED FOODS

4.1. The Assessment of GM Foods

The concept of substantial equivalence has been used for approval of GM foods by the FDA. In other words, if a GM food can be characterized as substantially equivalent to its "natural" antecedent, it can be assumed to pose no new health risks to consumers and hence to be acceptable for commercial use. The concept of substantial equivalence was introduced in 1993 by the Organization for Economic Cooperation and Development and was endorsed by the Food and Agricultural Organization and the World Health Organization in 1996 *(46)*. Use of this concept was made for approval of glyphosate-tolerant soybeans. These GM soybeans, although clearly different because of the newly acquired biochemical trait, are not different from their nonmodified counterparts in terms of amounts of protein, carbohydrates, vitamins, minerals, amino acids, fatty acids, fiber, isoflavones, and lecithins. Thus, the modified soybeans were deemed substantially equivalent and acceptable. More recent debate has questioned the use and definition of this concept and encouraged the use of more biochemical and toxicological testing before commercial use is allowed. Of principal concern is the presence of foreign proteins in the modified foods that cause human allergies. Allergenicity is a concern, but recombinant proteins should pose no more risk of being allergenic than would naturally occurring proteins *(4)*.

A great deal of energy has been put into testing the spread of recombinant DNA into non-GMOs after commercialization. Simple and complex polymerase chain reaction analysis have been developed to screen for the presence of the commonly used genes in cereal and oil crops *(47)*. A thorough review on detection and traceability of recombinant proteins and DNA in foods has been prepared by Miraglia et al. *(48)* as a summary of the Working Group IV discussions that were part of the ENTRANSFOOD Thematic Network on the Safety Assessment of Genetically Modified Food Crops. van den Eede et al. *(49)* reviewed the concern of horizontal gene transfer and summarized that horizontal gene transfer is the origin of the variety of life and that the consumption of transgenic food or feed adds no particular risk. Furthermore, whereas uptake of ingested DNA by mammalian somatic cells has been demonstrated, there is no evidence that such DNA may end up in germ line cells as a consequence of the consumption of GMOs.

The National Academy of Science has published a book entitled *Safety of Genetically Engineered Foods—Approaches to Assessing Unintended Health Effects (2)*. This book provides firm evidence for the safety of GMOs. However, it also discusses possible hazards that may result from this technology. First, here are examples where traditional plant breeding techniques led to health problems. Examples of unintended change described in this publication include selecting celery plants that have elevated concentrations of psoralens because this compound is associated positively with resistance to insects and disease. Farm workers harvesting celery are exposed to elevated psoralen concentrations and sometimes develop skin rashes. Another example is kiwi fruit. Originally, they were unpalatable and were domestic to China. Using traditional breeding programs they were developed into the tasty fruits that are currently available in grocery stores. Unfortunately, the appearance of this new fruit resulted in susceptible people suffering allergic reactions. Similar unintended changes can be predicted for recombinant organisms and thus testing and safety assurance programs need to be in place to evaluate the potential risk of both newly established "natural" foods and recombinant foods.

4.2. Perceptions and Concerns With Biotechnology

Biotechnology has been under scientific and lay scrutiny for more than 25 yr. Although some claims against any technology in general could be scientifically valid, others can only be "validated" by individuals' religious or moral belief system. However, scientists and politicians alike must be sensitive to those who choose not to partake of the obvious benefits and potential risks of consuming foods that have been modified by using biotechnology. To this end, traditional crops should remain available for those who wish to partake of foods generated by traditional breeding programs and raised by using traditional methods.

There are several grounds for objection to biotechnology. One is that it is bad to force genetic change to occur at a faster rate than, or in a direction other than, what nature intended. These rapid changes potentially could result in changes in micro- or macronutrient composition of foods, insertion of allergenic proteins, or the accumulation of toxic compounds to name a few. There are examples where all of these events have occurred because of biotechnology. Another objection is that large multinational companies will control the technology to efficiently produce crops by using genetic modification, and this control will put our food supply in the hands of a few powerful companies. Whereas all of the arguments presented here are potentially valid, our highly litigious society will do an efficient job at keeping the large corporations "honest" when it comes to introducing new products to the marketplace. Just as the argument that livestock producers sometimes "abuse" their animals is hard to understand because an abused animal does not provide as good of financial return to its owner, so too, the biotechnology companies want to continue to gain the consumer's trust and provide a safe and long-term product that will provide them with financial reward, which requires that they develop safe and acceptable products.

The use of biotechnology in producing food is an excellent example of where risk/benefit analysis should be employed. Some would argue that only foods produced and processed by using traditional methods should be consumed, even if they cost more and require a DNA analysis to detect any differences between modern and traditional crops. Others would want the most economical food within reasonable safety limits. In the end, both types of consumers should be accommodated; therefore, biotechnology has a place in food systems, but it should not be a mandate for the consumer.

5. CONCLUSION

Application of techniques of biotechnology has permitted the development of transgenic bacteria, plants, and animals that have a wide variety of new capacities. For example, new plant varieties have been developed that produce grains with more desirable composition for consumption by humans and animals and that are highly resistant to infectious diseases, insects, and adverse environmental conditions. Additionally, bacteria and yeast can be altered genetically to produce vaccines, dietary constituents, biologically active compounds such as insulin and somatotropin, and a variety of other protein products that are used directly by humans or are used in food production by animals. The only limit to what a microbe can be used to produce seems to be whether the corresponding specific gene can be isolated. Moreover, transgenic animals show promise of increased efficiency of production of foods and fiber and perhaps even of pharmaceutical compounds by the mammary gland of lactating transgenic animals. Scientific discoveries before modem biotechnology became available led to improved agricultural productivity and improved food composition. The use of biotechnology, however, has accelerated the rate of those improvements and will continue to do so in the future.

REFERENCES

1. Madden D. Food Biotechnology: An Introduction. ILSI Press, Washington, DC, 1995.
2. National Research Council and Institute of Medicine of the National Academies. Safety of genetically engineered foods—Approaches to assessing unintended health effects. National Academy of Science, Washington, DC, 2004.
3. Designing Foods. Animal Product Options in the Marketplace. National Academy Press, Washington, DC, 1988.
4. Helm RM. Food biotechnology: is this good or bad? Implication to allergic disease. Ann Allergy Asthma Immunol 2003; 90:90–98.
5. Chong M. Acceptance of golden rice in the Philippine "rice bowl." Nat Biotechnol 2003; 21:971, 972.
6. Huffman WE, Rousu M, Shogren JF, Tegene A. Controversies over the adoption of genetically modified organisms. J Agric Food Ind Organ 2004; 2:1–13.
7. DellaPenna D. Nutritional genomics: manipulating plant micronutrients to improve human health. Science 1999; 285:375–379.
8. Decker EL, Reski R. The moss bioreactor. Curr Opin Plant Biol 2004; 7:166–170.
9. Franklin SE, Mayfield SP. Prospects for molecular farming in the green alga *Chlamydomonas reinhardtii*. Curr Opin Plant Biol 2004; 7:159–165.
10. Uefuji H, Ogita S, Yamaguchi Y, Loizumi N, Sano H. Molecular cloning and functional characterization of three distinct *N*-methyltransferases involved in the caffeine biosynthetic pathway in coffee plants. Plant Physiol 2003; 132:372–380.
11. Mizuno K, Kato M, Irino F, Yoneyama N, Fujimura T, Ashihara H. The first committed step reaction of caffeine biosynthesis: 7-methylxanthosine synthase is closely homologous to caffeine synthases in coffee (*Coffea arabica* L.). FEBS Lett 2003; 547:56–60.
12. The World Health Report 2001—Mental health: new understanding, new hope. Geneva, 2001.
13. Lamphear BJ, Jilka JM, Kesl L, Welter M, Howard JA, Streatfield SJ. A corn-based delivery system for animal vaccines: an oral transmissible gastroenteritis virus vaccine boosts lactogenic immunity in swine. Vaccine 2004; 22:2420–2424.
14. Tregoning J, Maliga P, Dougan G, Nixon PJ. New advances in the production of edible plant vaccines: chloroplast expression of a tetanus vaccine antigen TetC. Phytochemistry 2004; 65:989–994.
15. Streatfield SJ, Howard JA. Plant-based vaccines. Int J Parasit 2003; 33:479–493.
16. Britto DT, Kronzucker HJ. Bioengineering nitrogen acquisition in rice: can novel initiatives in rice genomics and physiology contribute to global food security? BioEssays 2004; 26:683–692.

17. Capell T, Bassie L, Christou P. Modulation of the polyamine biosynthetic pathway in transgenic rice confers tolerance to drought stress. Proc Natl Acad Sci USA 2004; 101:9909–9914.

18. Moffatt AS. Engineering plants to cope with metals. Science 1999; 285:369, 370.

19. Welch RM, Graham RD. Breeding for micronutrients in staple food crops from a human nutrition perspective. J Exp Bot 2004; 55:353–364.

20. Fujita Y, Ito J, Ueda M, Fukuda H, Kondo A. Synergistic saccharification, and direct fermentation to ethanol, of amorphous cellulose by use of an engineered yeast strain codisplaying three types of cellulolytic enzymes. Appl Environ Microbiol 2004; 70:1207–1212.

21. Hidetoshi S, Pokorny J. The development and application of novel vegetable oils tailor-made for specific human dietary needs. Eur J Lipid Sci Technol 2003; 105:769–778.

22. Broun P, Gettner S, Somerville C. Genetic engineering of plant lipids. Annu Rev Nutr 1999; 19:197–216.

23. Hitz WD, Yadav NS, Reiter RS, Mauvais CJ, Kinney AJ. Reducing polyunsaturation in oils of transgenic canola and soybean. Kluwer, London, 1995.

24. Gura T. New genes boost rice nutrients. Science 1999; 285:994, 995.

25. Potrykus I. Nutritionally enhanced rice to combat malnutrition disorders of the poor. Nutr Rev 2003; 61:S101–S104.

26. Faber DC, Molina JA, Ohlrichs CL, Vander Zwaag DF, Ferre LB. Commercialization of animal biotechnology. Theriogenology 2003; 59:125–138.

27. Agricultural Biotechnology: Strategies for National Competitiveness. National Academy Press, Washington, DC, 1988.

28. Schnieke AE. Human factor IX transgenei sheep produced by transfer of nuclei form transfected fetal fibroblasts. Science 1997; 278:2130–2133.

29. Russell JB, Wilson DB. Potential opportunities and problems for genetically altered rumen microorganisms. J Nutr 1988; 118:274–279.

30. Vohra A, Satyanarayana T. Phytases: Microbial sources, production, purification, and potenatial biotechnological applications. Crit Rev Biotechnol 2003; 23:29–60.

31. Blanquet S, Antonelli R, Laforet L, Denis S, Marol-Bonnin S, Alric M. Living recombinant Saccharomyces cerevisiae secreting proteins or petpides as a new drug delivery system in the gut. J Biotechnol 2004; 110:37–49.

32. Lazarev VN, Stipkovits L, Biro J, et al. Induced expression of the antibicrobial peptide melittin inhibits experimental infection by Mycoplasma gallisepticum in chickens. Microbes Infect 2004; 6:536–541.

33. Nandiwada LS, Schamberger GP, Schafer HW, Diez-Gonzalez F. Characterisation of an E2-type colicin and its application to treat alfalfa seeds to reduce Escherichia coli 0157:H7. Int J Food Microbiol 2004; 93:267–279.

34. Kawakubo M, Ito Y, Okimura Y, et al. Natural antibiotic function of a human gastric mucin against Helicobacter pylori infection. Science 2004; 305:1003–1006.

35. Jost B, Vilotte JL, Duluc I, Rodeau JL, Freund JN. Production of low-lactose milk by ectopic expression of intestinal lactase in the mouse mammary gland. Nat Biotechnol 1999; 17:180–184.

36. Hammer RE, Pursel VG, Rexroad CE, et al. Production of transgenic rabbits, sheep, and pigs by microinjection. Nature 1985; 315:680–683.

37. Wilmut I. Viable offspring derived from fetal and adult mammalian cells. Nature 1997; 385:810–813.

38. Wilmut I, Schnieke E, McWhir J, Kind AJ, Colman A, Campbell KHS. Nuclear transfer in the production of transgenic farm animals. CABI Publishing, New York, 1999.

39. Baguisi A. Production of goats by somatic cell nuclear transfer. Nat Biotechnol 1999; 17:456–461.

40. Bauman DE, Eppard PJ, DeGeeter MJ, Lanza GM. Response of high producing dairy cows to long-term treatment with pituitary somatotropin and recombinant somatotropin. J Dairy Sci 1985; 1352–1362.

41. Bauman DE, Everett RW, Weiland WH, Collier RJ. Production responses to bovine somatotropin in Northeast dairy herds. J Dairy Sci 1999; 82:2564–2573.

42. McGuffy RK, Green HB, Easson RP, Ferguson TH. Lactation response of dairy cows receiving bovine somatotropin via daily injections or in a sustained-release vehicle. J Dairy Sci 1990; 73:763–771.

43. Soderholm CG, Otterby DE, Ehle FR, Linn JG, Hansen WR, Annerstad RJ. Effects of recombinant bovine somatotropin on milk production, body composition, and physiological parameters. J Dairy Sci 1988; 71:355–365.

44. Juskevich JC, Guyer CG. Bovine growth hormone: human food safety evaluation. Science 1990; 249:875–884.

45. Etherton TD, Wiggins JP, Chung CS, Evock CM, Rebhun JF, Walton PE. Stimulation of pig growth performance by porcine somatotropin and growth hormone releasing factor. J Anim Sci 1986; 63: 1389–1399.

46. Millstone E, Brunner E, Mayer S. Beyond substantial equivalence. Nature 1999; 401:525, 526.

47. James D, Schmidt AM, Wall E, Green M, Masri S. Reliable detection and identification of genetically modified maize, soybean, and canola by multiplex PCR analysis. J Agric Food Chem 2003; 51:5829–5834.

48. Miraglia M, Berdal KG, Brera C, et al. Detection and traceability of genetically modified organisms in the food production chain. Food Chem Toxicol 2004; 42:1157–1180.

49. van den Eede G, Aarts H, Buhk H, et al. The relevance of gene transfer to the safety of food and feed derived from genetically modified (GM) plants. Food Chem Toxicol 2004; 42:1127–1156.

22

Food Industry and Political Influences on American Nutrition

Marion Nestle, Ted Wilson,
and Audrey Balay-Karperien

KEY POINTS

- The US Department of Agriculture is the government organization responsible for promoting healthy eating habits, but it is also under pressure to maintain consumption of foods that lie within the sparing use part of the Food Pyramid.
- The dollars spent on advertising by private industry far outweigh the dollars spent on public service nutrition information.
- Our food consumption patterns are influenced by commercial activities such as advertising. This starts in childhood where we develop the eating patterns we carry with us as adults.
- Legal measures (lawsuits) can be used by either public advocacy groups or private industry to influence the formation and implementation of nutritional policy.

1. "INFLUENCE: A POWER INDIRECTLY OR INTANGIBLY AFFECTING A PERSON OR COURSE OF EVENTS"

Everyone eats. What we eat depends on what we buy, harvest, and acquire, and on what is available, on what tastes good, and on what we swallow. What we believe about nutrition shapes our decisions as to what foods to put in our mouths. A nutritionist's viewpoint with respect to eating is expected to be governed largely by objective, peer-reviewed science, but the beliefs of most people are insulated from that primary layer of information. In modern industrialized nations, most people's beliefs and behaviors about nutrition are influenced directly or indirectly by governmental nutritional policy. For all of us, appreciating the influence placed on our nutrition habits can be a tough pill to swallow.

For at least a century, nutrition-related consumer behavior in the United States has been shaped to some degree by governmental food policy, but in recent years both individual behavior and governmental policies have begun to be shaped by the pressures exerted by food companies. By exploring how this influence occurs, this chapter looks

From: *Nutritional Health: Strategies for Disease Prevention, Second Edition*
Edited by: N. J. Temple, T. Wilson, and D. R. Jacobs © Humana Press Inc., Totowa, NJ

at the general nature of nutritional policy and its practical application by consumers in the United States.

This chapter is based on the book *Food Politics: How the Food Industry Influences Nutrition and Health,* written by one of the coauthors of this chapter, Dr. Marion Nestle *(1)*. The reader is directed to that book for a more detailed description of this history and additional examples of how US food policy has been manipulated by the food industry.

2. THE FOOD INDUSTRY AND ITS INFLUENCE

Eating-related behavior, and purchasing in particular, occurs in a very complicated social context in which marketers play a huge part. Advertising is the most obvious tool by which the food industry attempts to manipulate consumer habits. But other marketing strategies are also employed and these are usually much more subtle.

2.1. Advertising and the Problem of Manufactured Food

Tremendous amounts of money are spent on advertising to boost the consumption of particular products. In 2003, direct media spending on promoting McDonald's, Burger King, Pepsi soft drinks, and Coca-Cola was $619 million, $524 million, $208 million, and $168 million, respectively *(2)*. In contrast, only about 2.2% of food advertising spending is used to promote consumption of unrefined foods, such as fruits, vegetables, whole grains, and beans *(3)*. Consider American TV advertising during the Super Bowl: corporations are willing to pay $1 million for each 30-s advertising slot.

The federal government has done, and perhaps can do, little to redress this imbalance. Of the $300 million budgeted by the US Department of Agriculture (USDA) for "nutritional education," relatively little is spent on truly promoting the food pyramid or encouraging people to eat more fruits and vegetables. Given their limited reserves, the USDA's Nutritional Education program and the many nonprofit consumer advocacy groups can do little more than act as spectators while the food habits of the consumer change. As a result the quality of the American diet worsens and the prevalence of "diseases of the waistline," such as diabetes, continues to grow.

To increase the palatability, appearance, marketability, and consumption of food products, they undergo increased amounts of processing. The cost of the raw materials ("farm cost") is about 55% for eggs, 13% for frozen peas, 10% for corn flakes, 9% for canned tomatoes, and 4% for corn syrup *(4)*. The remainder of the consumer cost (45–96%) is for such things as transportation, labor, and packaging, and, most importantly, advertising to promote demand. On average, 80% of the cost of a food product goes for these costs *(5,6)*.

For the manufacturer, it is enormously advantageous if the degree of food processing is increased because this allows huge price markups. This can be most easily seen by the following simple demonstration. The reader can check the cost of basic food ingredients, such as sugar, raisins, oil, and wheat, if purchased in the bulk section of a supermarket. Then check the price of the same foods, but this time after they have been mixed together and converted into a manufactured food. The price per kilogram will be about three times higher for the manufactured foods than for the basic ingredients. Food corporations therefore have an obvious incentive to concentrate their advertising on manufactured food.

We can look at this issue of "added value" another way. If 10% of the product price is used for advertising and a raw apple costs 20¢, then 2¢ would go to advertising the raw product. But if the apple is converted into a "Microwaveable Breakfast Apple Crisp" that sells for $1, then 10% means that 10¢ is now available for advertising. In other words, the funding available for advertising has jumped fivefold after the apple has been processed. And that, in brief, helps explain why so little money is spent on the advertising and promotion of raw food.

Advertising, therefore, serves mainly to promote manufactured products, and, in consequence, skews consumers' perceptions of which foods are healthy and convenient. When people consume manufactured food, they generally have little idea of the nutritional value of their food and how well their diets conform to the food pyramid or other nutrition guides. The content, convenience, and availability of these foods, and the money spent on their marketing, all hinder the implementation of healthful nutritional policy. The real nutritional value of food may be further obscured by the addition of supplemental vitamins and minerals ("fortification"). Recent relaxation of food label claims, such as "lowers cholesterol" and "reduces risk of cancer," can also be used to improve marketability.

2.2. Innocence by Association

One way the food industry influences people is through "image management." Consider, for example, a donation from a corporation that aggressively markets a product known to negatively affect the oral health of children. Should this act be judged as good for society or harmful?

Illustrating this, in 2003 Coca-Cola donated $1 million to the American Academy of Pediatric Dentistry (AAPD) for research (7). This was not done anonymously. Whereas at least some officials of the AAPD found the gift acceptable, many others—including consumer groups, such as the Center for Science in the Public Interest, and children's advocates, such as Dads and Daughters—did not. This type of donation can be considered a marketing ploy that has been dubbed "innocence by association." The action runs the risk of undermining the science incriminating sugar-rich soda in poor dental health. It can potentially confuse the message of the AAPD, which states that consumption of soft drinks may be harmful to dental health (8).

Coca-Cola also made a donation to the National Parent Teacher's Association. In addition, one of its executives gained a position on the Parent Teacher's Association board of directors for the 2003–2005 term. That person is John H. Downs, Jr., senior vice-president of public affairs for Coca-Cola Enterprises, "the world's largest Coca-Cola bottler with annual net operating revenues of $16.8 billion" (9). It has been suggested that such influences will curb the very active efforts of concerned parents trying to get soft drinks out of the schools. Downs became a board member coincident with a sociolegal movement that had started around 2000 and was gaining momentum. This movement involves lawsuits blaming food companies for obesity, the introduction of campaigns and bills to prevent advertising to young people (e.g., HeLP, or the Healthy Lifestyles and Prevention America Act of 2004), and schools banning soft drink sales and pulling out of "pouring rights" and similar deals (in sum, these were exclusive arrangements to market soft drinks in schools in return for a payment).

2.3. Schooling Kids to Become Adult Consumers

Pouring rights provide marketers with a valuable tool to influence brand name loyalty in children (9). Manufacturers often provide cash for exclusive pouring rights in an attempt to create brand loyalty and to boost sales. In 1998 a typical 10-yr agreement would reward an urban school district, which would have a student base of around 10,000, with 1.73 million dollars in exchange for exclusive pouring rights *(10)*. This money can be an important source of revenue for schools that can be applied to a variety of school needs *(1,11)*. But this form of marketing undermines sound nutritional teaching to children and has been criticized as being exceptionally unethical. To allay the concerns of school administrators and parents, companies often place apparently "healthy" choices in their machines. In a recent survey of schools in the Winona, MN, area, one of the authors (TW) found that approximately one-quarter of the beverage vending machines had "Fruitopia® with real fruit juice" or other healthy-sounding beverages. What many of these perceived healthy choices have in common is that fruit juice is only about 5% of the content, whereas the large majority of the calories come from corn syrup sweeteners.

Perhaps the most disturbing way the food industry influences consumer behavior is when it targets the nutrition behavior of children. Acknowledging that very young people need help to make sound nutrition choices, Coca-Cola, in November 2003, vowed to improve its corporate image by, among other moves, refraining from promoting the sale of soft drinks to elementary students during the day *(12)*. However, the company still claimed that it was appropriate to continue to promote the consumption of soft drinks by children in middle and high schools.

School students are often targeted by food companies. Campbell's Soup, Pizza Hut, and McDonalds are just a few of the many manufacturers who create special "educational" materials that highlight the "selective nutritional value" of their products. These materials may focus on, for example, the variety of food types in a slice of pizza, but neglect to mention how the fat content and refined grains may contribute to obesity and diabetes in children who consume too much of them. These companies sometimes distribute alternative food pyramids that include pictures of their products and marketing symbols.

Manufacturers know that children learn to recognize brand names, symbols, and cartoon/action figures as product advocates. The Keebler® elves, Tony the Tiger™, and Ronald McDonald™ are a few examples of cartoon personalities that carry a consumer from childhood products through to products marketed to adults.

Attempts to modify consumer activity include using children's peers as a marketing tool. The press statement that follows here, taken from the Cattlemen's Beef Promotion and Research Board website, provides an example of this *(13)*. The statement was made during the 2001 Cattle Industry Convention in San Antonio, TX, by the Cattlemen's Beef Board and the National Cattlemen's Beef Association.

A new program has been launched to teach youth about the benefits of eating beef. A checkoff-funded public relations campaign featuring figure skating sensation Sasha Cohen will target magazines and other information sources used by girls.

The NCBA and the United States Figure Skating Association have teamed up to promote the importance of a healthy diet and the role that beef plays in the development of girls ages eight to 12. Findings by the checkoff-funded Beef Industry Youth Task Force, released in 2000, revealed that girls of this age are the most important youth target audience.

At this age, girls are forming life-long attitudes about foods. What they eat before entering high school is often what they feed their own families when they become mothers," says Scott George, a beef producer from Wyoming and chairman of the NCBA Youth Education and Information Subcommittee. "We often think of youth only as a long-term audience. Through our task force research, we discovered just how influential youth are in determining what foods are eaten by families today."

3. PROBLEMS WITH THE FOOD SUPPLY

The United States has the ability to produce tremendous amounts of food, something that is perhaps both a blessing and a curse for health. Surplus agricultural commodities are purchased and distributed to needy persons in the United States by a series of programs supervised by the USDA. These programs also support farm income and land values. A large percentage of this food consists of butter, cheese, peanuts, and a variety of vegetable oils. Unfortunately, much of it lives in the top "sparing use" portion of the food pyramid.

The USDA is caught in the middle. On the one hand, it is responsible for promoting the food pyramid and therefore the sparing use of many empty-calorie foods, such as butter and sugar. But, at the same time, it is under political pressure from various lobby groups to boost sales of the products it purchases as part of its price-support programs. Surplus commodities are distributed, in large part, through school lunch programs and to persons of low income. This may partly explain why the prevalence of obesity in the United States is inversely related to income *(14)*. These programs may also lead to poor nutrition education: the school lunch programs are where many people learn their food preferences, and these poor nutritional habits may well continue into adulthood.

4. INFLUENCE OF SPECIAL INTEREST GROUPS AND POLITICAL ACTION COMMITTEES

There are a great number of special interest groups in the United States, and they exert a tremendous influence on nutritional health policy. Here is one example that implicitly makes this point. A press release from the Grocery Manufacturers of America (GMA) in 2002 reported that Health and Human Services Secretary Tommy Thompson "encouraged GMA members to 'go on the offensive' against critics blaming the food industry for obesity" and "said the industry is 'doing wonderful things' to educate people about proper diet and exercise, but that GMA member companies should tell more people about them and implement wellness programs for their own employees." *(15)*.

As explained previously in this chapter, the value added to food products during manufacturing and processing allows appreciably higher prices to be charged. The larger revenues generated this way allow food corporations to influence the direction of nutritional health policy in both obvious and less obvious ways. Advertising was discussed earlier. Corporate funds are used to sponsor lobbyists who influence the writing and enforcement of laws. Special interest groups support lobbyists who work at the state and national levels of government. By giving contributions to campaign funds, corporations help ensure that politicians are sympathetic to the needs and wants of their donors. It has been estimated that in 1998 $2.7 million dollars were spent lobbying each US senator and representative *(16)*. For instance, former senator and presidential candidate Robert Dole earned $17 million in 1997 alone for his lobbying activities *(1)*.

4.1. The Case of Sugar

The manipulation of policy is well-illustrated by looking at the activities of the sugar lobby. The question of sugar consumption was discussed in a series of recently published research reports sponsored by the National Cancer Institute. Federal nutritional policy guidelines for sugar consumption have changed in a clear direction of increasing obfuscation. In 1980 and 1985, the US Dietary Guidelines for sugar said, simply, and in just four words, "Avoid too much sugar." In 1990, it went to five words, "Use sugars only in moderation," and in 1995 to six: "Choose a diet moderate in sugars." In 2000, the scientific committee recommended that the guideline say, "Choose beverages and foods to limit your intake of sugars" (10 words), but even that was too strong. Under pressure from sugar lobbyists, the government agencies substituted the word "moderate" for "limit" so it read "Choose beverages and foods to moderate your intake of sugars." The committee working on the guidelines for 2005 dropped the sugar recommendation entirely, and discussed the issue under the heading, "Choose carbohydrates wisely....", comments made by the USDA and Department of Health and Human Services, 2005 Report of the Dietary Guidelines Advisory Committee (17).

These changes make little sense in the light of the rising sugar intake in the United States concurrent with rising obesity and diabetes, and of the well-established strong association between high sugar intake and poor dental health (18). The change in the guidelines can be readily understood when viewed from a market perspective. As several authors have noted, whereas health research has repeatedly told us that sugar consumption should decrease, the guidelines have evolved in a fundamentally different direction, one that is friendly to the wishes of the sugar industry. In this regard we see some disturbing echoes of the saga over the health hazards of tobacco, where the tobacco industry have spent decades in a rearguard action against the scientific evidence and policy initiative that sought to curb smoking.

The sugar industry's stated interpretation of the evidence has for many years stood in sharp contrast to the opinions of health professionals. A saga during 2003–2004 illustrates this well. The World Health Organzation issued guidelines recommending a limit on sugar consumption to 10% of total caloric intake. This is an old recommendation, one used by many countries that issue dietary advice and the precise level recommended in the booklet that accompanies the USDA Food Guide Pyramid. Nevertheless, in a campaign characterized by the media and consumer groups as tantamount to blackmail, the year between the initial release and ratification of these guidelines saw vigorous attempts by the sugar industry to prevent their adoption (19). The Sugar Association argued that the preponderance of evidence indicates that people can safely consume a quarter of their calories as sugar. The sugar lobby's efforts included demands that the report be removed from the internet and threats that the industry would be asking congressional appropriators to challenge the $406 million in US funding of the World Health Organization if the report was not withdrawn (20–22).

4.2. The Influence of TV

When these public service messages are played on TV, the TV station must be careful to avoid alienating their advertisers. Messages that promote moderation in calorie, fat, or sugar consumption can provide a valuable public health service, but airing these adds may negatively impact the station's relationships with the food and beverage companies that choose to advertise on the same TV airways. Profitability is required for the economic survival of private media outlets and the corporations they are part of. Predictably, therefore, a TV station in Iowa, "the Pork State," will be reluctant to air a public service message that says: "…. reduce your fat intake ….eat less pork…."

By sponsoring the production and presentation of programs on private and public television, corporations also exert influence on the content of our programming. The MacNeil/Lehrer News Hour on PBS is one such example, receiving generous underwriting by the large agribusiness firm, Archer Daniels Midland (ADM). It would be naïve to believe that public TV programs, underwritten by food manufacturers, would unhesitatingly air a news item that was clearly damaging to the interests of their sponsors. As with private TV, there is no surer way to lose one's funding than to alienate one's sponsors.

4.3. Influence of Farm and Corporate Interests on Research

A large number of commodity and farm/food product promotion boards and organizations exist in the United States. How do commodity groups generate the large amounts of money needed to influence nutritional health policy? Here is one example. The Beef Checkoff Program was established as part of the 1985 Farm Bill. The National Cattlemen's Beef Promotion and Research Board, which administers the national checkoff program, receives $1 per head on all cattle sold. Although subject to USDA approval, the organization is a nongovernmental body (23). Checkoff revenues may be used for promotion, education, and research programs to improve the marketing climate for beef (24). In the United States, this program has been very successful in promoting the popular and familiar "Beef: Its What's for Dinner" program.

Marketing boards and corporate interests tend to fund research projects that have the potential to improve the marketability of their products. This seed funding has generated a literal explosion of research studies in areas of corporate/marketing interest. The following example illustrates this. A search for publications with the word "soy" on PubMed (done on January 10, 2004) for the last 6 mo of 1992 found 66 hits, but 10 yr later this same 6-mo period yielded 667 hits. Industrial giant ADM (net sales of $30.7 billion in 2003) and others like it contribute millions of research dollars into selective projects related to soy proteins and isoflavones. By sponsoring advertisements in peer-reviewed journals, corporate soy advocates help ensure, directly or by indirect influence, that pro-soy publications will likely receive a more favorable passage through the peer-review process.

These selective projects generally have some features in common: if their findings are published, they will probably be positive, they will help ensure future grants, and the results will probably increase product marketability. The best evidence in support of this argument comes from the realm of medical research, especially research on drugs. A study of 332 randomized trials of drugs and other medical interventions published between 1999 and 2001 revealed that those that had received industry funding were 90% more likely to report statistically significant pro-industry findings (25). Another study confirmed this for biomedical research in general (26). Funding this type of research also places pressure on the USDA and other government sources to divert funds to validate and expand on what has already been done. This sequence of events means that the original grant, obtained from industry, has the potential to create an industry-friendly research agenda.

5. USING THE LEGAL SYSTEM
TO INFLUENCE NUTRITIONAL POLICY

Corporate giants, such as ADM and Monsanto, have gone to great lengths to ensure that food labels do not provide information that could hurt product marketing. If a corporation cannot influence nutrition, they can sometimes dictate it via the courts. The recent attempts to improve consumer acceptance of genetically engineered grains with improved insect resistance and meats produced with bovine growth hormone are classic examples. Another noteworthy episode concerns attempts to block the ability of the consumer to identify the source and methods used in the production of their food took the form of a lawsuit in Maine. Monsanto filed suit against Oakhurst Dairy, a small dairy company, which placed the words: "Our Farmer's Pledge: No Artificial Growth Hormones Used" on its packaging. A settlement was reached where Oakhurst was permitted to keep their original claim as long as their packaging also included this statement: "FDA states: No significant difference in milk from cows treated with artificial growth hormones" *(27)*. Small companies often find the threat of legal action by a corporate giant is tantamount to blackmail, just by considering the costs of a legal defense.

Lawsuits are a two-way street. A variety of public interest organizations, such as the Center for Science in the Public Interest, the Union of Concerned Scientists, and the Center for Food Safety, have turned to the US legal system as a way to influence nutrition and food quality policy. By initiating lawsuits, food producers or government organizations can be influenced. The impact often comes more from the bad press that can be associated with a lawsuit, in addition to any fines that may result. More recently groups with little history of involvement in nutrition have weighed in, groups such as the Sierra Club and their dispute with the use of genetically modified grains in the United States and other countries.

6. CONCLUSIONS

Today, Americans are locked into an ever-worsening spiral of obesity and diabetes, what are often called "diseases of the waistline." This tells us that American nutritional habits have become terribly misdirected. Vast amounts of money are now spent on advertising and other forms of marketing so as to generate consumer demand for products.

Lobbyists for the food industry have become entrenched in the political system; their primary function being to serve the narrow financial interests of particular farm and food industry interests. As a result, government food policy is often dictated by questions of economics rather than of health. Trade and political action groups also influence the availability of research funding and the direction of projects funded by otherwise "independent" universities and research centers. Finally, the legal system has become a tool where corporate interests can influence national health policy in such areas as food labeling. More recently, legal measures have also been implemented by consumer advocacy groups hoping to assert new policies for promoting consumer health.

A variety of voices will continue to influence the way our nutritional health is determined. What remains to be determined is how effective farm and industrial groups will be at influencing the formation of a policy that promotes economic success and profitability. What also remains to be determined is how effective consumer advocacy groups, such as the Center for Science in the Public Interest, can be at providing a counterbalance to corporate interests. What is most difficult to determine is the extent to which government organizations can be neutral with respect to setting nutritional health guidelines and legislation that ensures both the health of people and the economy.

Many people suppose that, knowing this, governments, like nutritionists, rely heavily on the best available health-related scientific evidence in formulating their nutrition policies. Alas, this is often far from the case. In practice, governmental nutritional policy translates nutrition science then tempers it within the current context of the relevant food market, which leaves it sometimes attempting to serve at once the disparate interests of individuals and economic interests of corporations. As such, the cart of nutritional policy oftentimes seems to be in the lead with the horse of scientific justification following some distance behind. This routinely seems to have been the case with how nutritional health policy was created, manipulated, and implemented in the United States.

REFERENCES

1. Nestle, M. Food Politics: How the Food Industry Influences Nutrition and Health. University of California Press, Berkeley, CA, 2002.
2. Advertising Age. 100 Leading National Advertisers: 49th Annual Report. June 28, 2004.
3. Gallo AE. Food advertising in the United States. In: Frazao E, ed. America's Eating Habits: Changes & Consequences. USDA, Washington, DC, 1999.
4. Dunham D. Farm costs from farm to retail in 1993. USDA, Washington, DC, Economic Research Service, 1994.
5. Meade B, Rosen S. Income and diet differences greatly affect food spending around the globe. Food Review 1996; 19;39–44.
6. Haung KS. Prices and incomes affect nutrients consumed. Food Review 1998; 21:11015.
7. American Academy of Pediatric Dentistry Foundation. Campaign Quarterly: Healthy Smiles-Healthy Children. Fall 2003. AAPDF, Chicago, IL.
8. Center for Science in the Public Interest. CSPI Urges AAPD to Put Kids' Teeth Ahead of Coke's Money. March 4, 2003. www.cspinet.org/new/ 200303041.html. Last accessed July 29, 2004.
9. National Parent Teacher Association. PTA Board Member Profiles. http://www.pta.org//aboutpta/board/downs.asp. Last accessed January 7, 2004.
10. North Syracuse School District. Agreement with Coca Cola Bottling Company of New York, July 1, 1998.
11. United States General Accounting Office Report to Congressional Requesters, September 2000. Public education: Commercial activities in schools GAO/HEHS-00-156.
12. The Coca-Cola Company. Model guidelines for school beverage partnerships. http://www2.coca-cola.com/ourcompany/hal_school_beverage_guidelines.pdf. Last accessed August 23, 2005.
13. National Cattlemen s Beef Promotion and Research Board. Beef industry launches youth public relations program with figure skating star. http://www.beefboard.org/dsp_content.cfm?locationId=1071&contentId=36&contentTypeId=2. Last accessed: January 7,2005.
14. Drewnowski A, Specter SE. Poverty and obesity: the role of energy density and energy costs. Am J Clin Nutr 2004; 79:6–16.
15. Grocery Manufcturers Association. Top administration officials brief GMA board: Thompson, Hubbard, McClellan give views. http://www.gmabrands.com/news/docs/NewsRealease.cfm?DocID=1028& Last accessed August 23, 2005.
16. Stout D. Tab of Washington Lobbying: $1.42 Billion. New York Times, July 29, 199:A14.
17. USDA and DHHS, 2005. Report of the Dietary Guidelines Advisory Committee. www.health.gov/dietaryguidelines. Last accessed January 7, 2005.

18. Jamel H, Plasschaert A, Sheiham A. Dental caries experience and availability of sugars in Iraqi children before and after the United Nations sanctions. Int Dent J 2004; 54:21–25.

19. The Sugar Association, letter addressed to Gro Harlem Brundtland, WHO, dated April 14, 2003. www.commercialalert.org/ sugarthreat.pdf. Last accessed January 7, 2005. 20. The Sugar Association. WHO report on diet, nutrition and prevention misguided. News Release. Washington, DC, March 3, 2003.

21. Boseley S. Sugar industry threatens to scupper WHO. April 21, 2003. Guardian Unlimited, The Guardian (UK).

22. Sibbald B. Sugar industry sour on WHO report. CMAJ 2003; 168:1585.

23. National Cattlemen s Beef Promotion and Research Board; Cattlemen s board approves fiscal 2006 budget. http:/www.beef.org/NEWSCATTLEMENSBEEFBOARDAPPROVESFISCAL2006 BUDGET23108.aspx.Last acccessed August 16, 2005.

24. National Cattlemen s Beef Promotion and Research Board. Checkoff Report Describes Beef Promotion Efforts. http://www.beef.org/NEWSCheckoffReportDescribesBeefPromotionEfforts3916.aspx. Last accessed August 16, 2005.

25. Bhandari M, Busse JW, Jackowski D. Association between industry funding and statistically significant pro-industry findings in medical and surgical randomized trials. CMAJ 2004; 170:477–480.

26. Bekelman JE, Li Y, Gross CP. Scope and impact of financial conflicts of interest in biomedical research: a systematic review. JAMA 2003; 289:454–465. 27. Oakhurst slogan settlement was no win for Monsanto. Portland Press Herald. December 29, 2003;10A.

23 Population Nutrition, Health Promotion, and Government Policy

Norman J. Temple and Marion Nestle

KEY POINTS

- Health promotion campaigns of various types have been conducted: in communities, at worksites, and in physician offices. The most common targets have been smoking, exercise, dietary fat, and intake of fruit and vegetables. The aim has most often been to reduce excess weight, lower the blood cholesterol and blood pressure, and prevent coronary heart disease (CHD). Results of these campaigns have been mixed. Some have achieved very little whereas others have met with moderate success. Typically, target outcomes have been improved by a few percentage points and this should reduce the risk of CHD by about 5–15%.
- In the light of this limited success we argue in support of government policy initiatives to improve population health. In particular, by use of taxes and subsidies the price of various foods can be changed so as to shift consumption patterns to healthier foods. Other policy measures can include restrictions on advertising of unhealthy food, especially to children, and improved food labeling.
- Policy measures along these lines are likely to meet with resistance from the food industry.
- Low socioeconomic status, such as low income and poor education, is a major risk factor for poor health. This may be mediated via unhealthy lifestyle choices, such as a poor diet, as well as by psychological factors. Therefore, attempts to improve the population health will require action in this area.

1. INTRODUCTION

It is now generally accepted that lifestyle—diet, tobacco use, exercise—have a major impact on health, especially the Western diseases. However, there is a world of difference between awareness of these facts and their translation into preventive action.

Although the focus of this chapter is on nutrition in relation to health promotion, we also examine other areas, especially smoking and exercise. This is necessary because most health promotion campaigns take a broad lifestyle approach and simultaneously tackle nutrition, exercise, and smoking.

From: *Nutritional Health: Strategies for Disease Prevention, Second Edition*
Edited by: N. J. Temple, T. Wilson, and D. R. Jacobs © Humana Press Inc., Totowa, NJ

Trends toward a healthier lifestyle during the last 20–30 yr have been inconsistent. There has been an impressive fall by about half in smoking rates in men in many Western countries for the last 30 yr. The percentage of Americans who smoke dropped from 37.4% in 1970 to 22.5% in 2002 *(1)*. In the United States deaths from coronary heart disease (CHD) have fallen by half since their peak in the late 1960s. Yet, at the same time, the United States has been struck by an epidemic of obesity. Between 1976 and 1980 and 1988 and 1994 obesity among adults jumped from 14.5 to 22.9% *(2)*. This then climbed to 30.5% in 1999–2000 *(3)*. A fast rising prevalence of overweight and obesity has also been reported from other Western countries *(4)*.

Between 1972 and 1998, Americans increased their consumption of fruit and vegetables (excluding potatoes) by about one serving per day *(5)*, an underwhelming rate of progress.

Moreover, half of Americans eat no fruit on any given day *(6)*. In the years 1985–2000, the available food energy in the United States increased by 300 kcal/d. This increased energy came largely from refined grains (46%), sugars (24%), and added fats (23%), but with a mere 8% coming from fruit and vegetables *(7)*.

This poor rate of progress in the area of diet should be seen as part of a more general problem that large sections of the population give a low priority to a healthy lifestyle. For instance, the proportion of middle-aged adults in England engaged in at least moderate exercise, such as a brisk walk for at least 30 min on 5 or more days each week, is no more than one-half of men and one-quarter of women *(8)*. In the United States about one third of adults achieve this level of exercise *(9)*, whereas another one-third report no leisure-time physical activity at all *(10)*.

2. HEALTH PROMOTION CAMPAIGNS

During the 1970s the intimate connection between lifestyle and health became increasingly apparent. As a result many people assumed that the next step was to disseminate this information to the public and exhort lifestyle changes, action deemed sufficient to bring about the necessary changes. However, a review of 24 evaluations of the effectiveness of using the mass media across a range of health topics found little evidence of behavior change as a result of education alone *(11)*. Here we look at various types of health promotion campaigns, most of them focused on risk factors for cardiovascular disease.

2.1. Campaigns in Communities

A number of community interventions have used the mass media combined with various other methods to reach the target population. Three major projects were carried out in the United States during the 1980s. Their aims were to lower elevated levels of blood cholesterol, blood pressure, and weight, to cut smoking rates, and to persuade more people to exercise. Each program lasted 5–8 yr and succeeded in implementing its intervention on a broad scale, involving large numbers of programs and participants. In the Stanford Five-City Project, conducted by Farquhar and colleagues *(12)* in California, two intervention cities received health education via TV, radio, newspapers, other mass-distributed print media, direct education, and schools. On average each adult was exposed to 26 h of education, achieved at the remarkably low per capita cost of $4/yr (i.e., about 800 times less than total health care costs). A similar project was the Minnesota Heart

Health Program, which included three intervention cities and three control cities in the upper Midwest *(13)*. A third project was the Pawtucket Heart Health Program in which the population of Pawtucket, RI, received intensive education at the grass roots level: schools, local government, community organizations, supermarkets, and so forth, but without involving the media *(14)*.

An analysis combined the results of the three studies so as to increase the sample size to 12 cities *(15)*. Improvements in blood pressure, blood cholesterol, body mass index, and smoking were of very low magnitude and were not statistically significant; the estimated risk of CHD mortality was unchanged. These results are mirrored by two other community projects: the Heart To Heart Project in Florence, SC *(16)*, and the Bootheel Heart Health Project in Missouri also showed little success *(17)*.

One factor contributing to the lack of effect may have been secular trends; the projects took place at a time when American lifestyles were becoming generally more healthy and CHD rates were falling. This suggests that when a population starts receiving health education, even if little more than reports in the mass media and government policy pronouncements, large numbers of people will decide to adopt a healthier lifestyle. A health promotion campaign superimposed on such secular trends may have little *additional* benefit. However, we cannot discount the possibility that different types of intervention might be successful, whereas those described earlier were not.

Fortunately, we have some examples of reasonably successful community projects for heart disease prevention. One of the earliest and most informative of such projects was conducted in North Karelia, a region of eastern Finland that had an exceptionally high rate of the disease *(18)*. The intervention began in 1972 before much health information had reached the population. Nutrition education was an important component of the intervention. During the next few years, CHD rates in North Karelia fell sharply. Later, an intensive educational campaign spread to the rest of the country leading to a national drop in CHD rates *(19)*.

Two other European studies also achieved some success. Positive results were seen in the German Cardiovascular Prevention Study *(20)*, which took place from about 1985 to 1992, when there was no particularly favorable trend in risk factors for the population as a whole. It was carried out in six regions of the former West Germany using a wide-ranging approach similar to that used in the American community studies. The intervention caused a small decrease in blood pressure and serum cholesterol (about 2%) and a 7% fall in smoking, but had no effect on weight. Action Heart was a community-based health promotion campaign conducted in Rotherham, England *(21)*. After 4 yr, 7% fewer people smoked and 9% more drank low-fat milk, but there was no change in exercise habits, obesity, or consumption of wholemeal bread.

Two recent community campaigns are of particular interest because each was narrowly focused on changing only one aspect of lifestyle and used paid advertising as a major intervention strategy. The 1% Or Less campaign aimed to persuade the population of two cities in West Virginia to switch from whole milk to low-fat milk (1% or less) *(22)*. Advertising in the media was a major component of the intervention (at a cost of slightly less than $1 per person) together with supermarket campaigns (taste tests and display signs), education in schools, as well as other community education activities. Low-fat milk sales, as a proportion of total milk sales, increased from 18 to 41% within just a few weeks. The intervention campaign was repeated in another city in West Virginia; this time only paid advertising was used *(23)*. Low-fat milk sales increased from 29 to 46% of total milk sales. An Australian intervention campaign also used paid advertising as a major component *(24)*. The campaign ran in the State of Victoria from 1992 to 1995 and aimed to increase consumption of fruit and vegetables. Significant increases in consumption of these foods was reported (fruit by 11% and vegetables by 17%).

Taken together, the community intervention studies indicate that small changes in cardiovascular risk factors can be made by the methods used to date. The evidence is suggestive that interventions focused on a small number of changes and using paid advertising can achieve much success.

2.2. Worksite Health Promotion

As an alternative to health promotion using a community intervention approach other interventions have focused on the worksite. A pioneering project of this type, which started in 1976, was carried out in Europe by the World Health Organization. The project was conducted for 6 yr in 80 factories in Belgium, Italy, Poland, and the United Kingdom with the aim of preventing CHD *(25,26)*. The trial achieved modest risk factor reductions (1.2% for plasma cholesterol, 9% for smoking, 2% for systolic blood pressure, and 0.4% for weight); these were associated with a 10% reduction in CHD.

At around the same time Live for Life was carried out by the Johnson & Johnson company in the United States. This comprehensive intervention was started in 1979 and lasted 2 yr. Employees exposed to the program showed significant improvements in smoking behavior, weight, aerobic capacity, incidence of hypertension, days of sickness, and health care expenses *(27)*.

Another worksite project took place in New England *(28)*. Employees were encouraged to increase their intake of fiber and to reduce their fat intake. Compared with the control sites, the program had no effect on fiber intake but fat intake fell by about 3%. A few years later the research team reported that they succeeded in increasing employees' intake of fruit and vegetables by 19% (0.5 serving/d) using an approach that targeted employees and their families *(29)*. A similar project in Minnesota offered employees weight control and smoking cessation programs *(30)*. The program had no effect on weight but the prevalence of smoking was reduced by 2% more than occured in the control worksites.

2.3. Health Promotion in the Physician's Office

In 1994 two British studies reported the effects of intervention carried out by nurses in the offices of family physicians. The aim was to improve cardiovascular risk factors. Each study was a randomized trial aimed at cardiovascular screening and lifestyle intervention. Both studies achieved only modest changes despite intensive intervention. The OXCHECK study reported no significant effect on smoking or excessive alcohol intake but did observe small significant improvements in exercise participation, weight, dietary intake of saturated fat, and serum cholesterol *(31,32)*. The Family Heart Study achieved a 12% lowering of risk of CHD (based on a risk factor score) *(33)*. Similar findings came from an American study. Patients were given mailed personalized dietary recommendations, educational booklets, a brief physician endorsement, and motivational counseling by phone. After 3 mo the intervention group had increased its consumption of fruit and vegetables by 0.6 serving/d but there was no change in intake of red meat or dairy products *(34)*.

Wilcox and colleagues *(35)* reviewed 32 intervention studies carried out in a medical setting. They concluded that:

> *Overall, these interventions tended to produce modest but statistically significant effects for physical activity or exercise, dietary fat, weight loss, blood pressure, and serum cholesterol... Whereas small by conventional statistical definitions, these findings are likely to be meaningful when considered from a public health perspective.*

A variation of the above trials is the targeting of patients at high risk of CHD, probably the most cost-effective form of intervention *(36)*. A study from Sweden exemplifies this approach. Subjects at relatively high risk of cardiovascular disease received either simple advice from their physician or intensive advice (five 90-min sessions plus an all-day session) *(37)*. The intensive advice had a modest impact; it reduced the risk of CHD by approx 6%. Two highly successful randomized, controlled trials, one in the United States and one in Finland, were carried out on overweight subjects with impaired glucose tolerance, the goal being to prevent the development of type 2 diabetes *(38,39)*. The interventions consisted of physical activity and dietary change. In both studies the estimated risk reduction was about 58%. These studies are more fully described in Chapter 5. In general, interventions focused on high-risk subjects have been more successful than other interventions *(40)*

The major deficiency of the high-risk approach, as Rose *(41)* has pointed out, is that it only affects a minority of future cases: the 15% of men at "high risk" of CHD account for only 32% of future cases. Therefore, to achieve a major effect on CHD it is necessary to target the entire population. This logic also applies to other diseases related to diet and lifestyle practices, such as stroke and cancer.

2.4. Health Promotion and the Individual

What these projects teach us is that appealing to individuals to change their lifestyles will be effective in some instances but not in others and can therefore be frustratingly difficult. Although some projects have achieved a moderate degree of success, typically progress has amounted to no more than a few percentage points. This might be expected to reduce the risk of CHD by about 5–15%. Although this is certainly beneficial, it will not, however, affect the majority of people at risk. Thus exhortations to the individual, whether via the media, in the community, at the worksite, or in the physician's office, are most unlikely to turn the tide of the Western diseases.

Myriad factors influence people's lifestyle behavior besides concerns about how to protect health. Social factors, such as housing, employment, and income also shape people's attitudes, as does education. Advertising directly affects what people want and prices determine whether they can afford it. We are also creatures of habit and custom; resistance may therefore be expected when lifestyle modification demands changes in longstanding behavior and goes against fashion or peer pressure. We must also bear in mind that individuals have little control over many aspects of their physical environment, such as pollution and food contamination. It is probably naïve, therefore, to expect dramatic results from interventions that merely exhort the individual to lead a healthier lifestyle. Indeed, this has sometimes been characterized as "victim blaming."

This is in no way to dismiss interventions aimed at encouraging people to improve their lifestyle. Quite the contrary, minor changes can make valuable contributions to public health that more than justify the expense and effort involved. For instance, Jeffery and associates *(30)* concluded that a smoking cessation program at a worksite costs about $100 to $200 per smoker who quits, whereas the cost to the employer for each employee who smokes is far greater. Similarly, Action Heart estimated that the cost per year of life gained was a mere 31 (British) pounds *(21)*.

Health promotion, therefore, can be a cost-effective way to improve lifestyles and thereby improve the health of large numbers of people *(42,43)*. This is emphasized by the fact that in the United States poor dietary practices cost an estimated $71 billion/yr in lost productivity, premature deaths, and medical costs *(44)*. More research is required to determine why different health promotion projects have achieved such varying levels of success. Would campaigns be more successful if the focus was on one lifestyle change rather than many? Is paid advertising the best means to use scarce resources?

3. GOVERNMENT POLICY

Effective interventions may need to tackle the factors that determine how people make food choices. Such interventions require the implementation of policies, especially by governments. In the words of Davey Smith and Ebrahim *(45)*:

> *"...even with the substantial resources given to changing people's diets the resulting reductions in cholesterol concentrations is disappointing. [Health promotion programs] are of limited effectiveness. Health protection—through legislative and fiscal means—is likely to be a better investment."*

Governments have a variety of powers at their disposal that can be put into service. One approach, which relies entirely on voluntary cooperation, is to issue statements of policy. However, these can easily amount to no more than hollow declarations as is illustrated by government policies on tobacco in many countries. On the other hand, policy statements can serve as a clarion call to action. For instance, British and American government policy on diet and disease, in conjunction with the media and medical science, helped change the climate of opinion so that it is now widely accepted that diets should preferably be much lower in fat and richer in fiber.

3.1. The Effect of Price on Sales

Prominent among available government powers are legislation and the use of taxation and subsidies. Action on tobacco control most graphically illustrates the necessity for placing these powers at the service of health promotion. Educational efforts over the last three decades have been enormously important in persuading millions of people to quit smoking. Nevertheless, smoking rates are still well more than half of their level of 30 yr ago. There is convincing evidence that price hikes are an effective means to reduce smoking rates (i.e., there is price elasticity) *(46)*. It has been estimated that a 10% increase in price reduces tobacco consumption by about 5%, especially among the lower socioeconomic groups *(47)*. The Canadian experience is particularly illuminating. The prevalence of smoking in young Canadians fell by half during the 1980s in tandem with a doubling of the price. This trend was reversed in the early 1990s when the price was slashed in an attempt to reduce smuggling from the United States *(48)*. Price increases appear to be a far more effective means of tobacco control than education or media campaigns *(49)*.

Alcohol intake shows a similar price elasticity to tobacco intake: a price rise of 10% causes a decrease in consumption by 3–8% (50). Studies in Eastern Europe, especially Poland and the former Soviet Union, have demonstrated that pricing, sometimes in combination with rationing, sharply reduces consumption and associated mortality (51).

The lesson we learn from tobacco and alcohol is, first and foremost, that price increases are an effective vehicle to lower consumption.

What applies to tobacco and alcohol also applies to food. By means of taxes and subsidies fruit, vegetables, and whole-grain cereals might become more attractively priced in comparison with less healthy choices. This would most likely induce many people to shift their diets in a healthier direction. Recommendations along these lines in the area of food and nutrition policy were advocated by the World Health Organization (52) at the Adelaide Conference in 1988. The policy recommendation given was: "Taxation and subsidies should discriminate in favor of easy access for all to healthy food and improved diet."

Jeffery, French, and colleagues in the United States carried out a series of studies that demonstrated the potential of policy interventions, especially of low prices, to increase the consumption of healthy food choices. In one study, investigators reduced by half the price of low-fat snacks sold in vending machines in worksites and secondary schools; purchases of these foods increased by 93% (53). In a worksite cafeteria the range of fruit and salad ingredients was increased at the same time as the price was halved. As a result purchases trebled (54). In a similar study conducted in a high school cafeteria, prices for fruit, carrots, and salads were halved. This led to a fourfold increase in sales of fruit, a twofold increase for carrots, and a slight increase for salads (55).

3.2. Advertising, Marketing, and Labeling of Food

Another area where policy interventions could positively affect food choices concerns food advertising. The annual advertising budget in 2003 for Coca-Cola, Burger King, and McDonald's were $473, $524 million, and $619 million, respectively (56). In stark contrast, the education component of the National Cancer Institute-sponsored five-a-Day campaign to promote fruit and vegetable consumption is under $1 million. Only about 2.2% of the food advertising budget is used to promote consumption of unrefined foods such as fruits, vegetables, whole grains, and beans (57). The extent to which these huge imbalances in advertising budgets affect people's actual diets is not known but is almost certainly significant (58). Common sense dictates that if advertising did not work, the advertisers would not be wasting their money.

A particular issue is food advertising on children's TV. A study of advertisements appearing on Saturday morning TV in the United States found that 44% were for fats, oils, and sugar, 23% were for highly sugared cereals, and 11% for fast-food restaurants (59). None were for fruit and vegetables. The authors concluded that: "The diet that is presented on Saturday morning television is the antithesis of what is recommended for healthful eating for children." Similar findings were reported for Canadian TV (60).

Advertising is but one part of the wider production and marketing strategy of the food industry. James and Ralph (61) pointed out that in response to demand, manufacturers sell foods with less fat but the missing fat often reappears in "added value" foods, which are often little more than concoctions of fat, sugar, and salt. James (62) made the compelling point that the food industry promotes high-fat food because it is so profitable, whereas at the same time food labeling is "completely confusing" (with particular reference to

Britain). The system is, in theory, based on "consumer choice" but, in reality, choices become largely uninformed decisions. Now, there have certainly been serious efforts in recent years to make food labels more user-friendly but there is still a long way to go. For example, large numbers of consumers no doubt fail to realize that beverages, such as "fruit nectar" and "fruit beverage," have only a small fraction of the fruit juice of a product labeled as "fruit juice." To make matters worse these beverages typically have images of fruit on their containers. We really don't know what proportion of consumers actually read the small print and deduce what they are really buying. A more honest label for such drinks would be "fruit-flavored sugar water."

3.3. Government Policy and Food

The discussion in Subheadings 3.1. and 3.2. suggests that government policies concerning food prices and, to a lesser extent, food advertising and labeling may be an effective means to induce desirable changes in eating patterns.

Here we offer some specific suggestions regarding how existing government policies could be modified along the above lines so as to encourage healthier diets (63,64).

1. Subsidies paid to milk producers could be changed to favor low-fat milk. Likewise, by the use of such means as subsidies, grading regulations, and labeling, and perhaps even taxation, the sale of low-fat meat could be encouraged over high-fat varieties.
2. There is always scope for improved food labels so as to facilitate purchase of foods with a low content of fat, especially saturated fat. In addition, labeling and nutrition information should be extended to areas presently outside the system, especially restaurant menus and fresh meat.
3. By means of regulations and rewards, schools could be encouraged to sell meals of superior health value while restricting the sale of junk food. Similar policies could be applied to other institutions under government control, such as the military, prisons, and cafeterias in government offices.
4. Television advertising could be regulated so as to control the content, duration, and frequency of commercials for unhealthy food products, especially when the target audience is children.

The approach discussed in Subheading 3.3. was well put by Blackburn (65):

...even the newer community-based lifestyle strategies continue to assign much of the burden of change to the individual. A shift of focus to reducing, by policy change, many widespread practices that are life-threatening, while enhancing life-supportive practices, should redirect the currently misplaced emphasis on achieving "responsible" behavior and its purported difficulty. For example, local communities may more appropriately be considered to have a "youth tobacco access problem," approachable in part by regulation, than a "youth smoking problem," approachable mainly by education. Policy interventions may also be designed to .... make preventive practice more economical, as well as to encourage the development of more healthy products by industry. They may be a partial answer to another major paradox: although unhealthy personal behavior is medically discouraged for individuals, the whole of society legalizes, tolerates, and even encourages the same practices in the population.

Schmid et al. *(66)* summed up the approach discussed here:

Health departments that support disincentives for high-fat foods, tax breaks for cafete-
rias that offer healthy food choices, policies that require zoning ordinances to include
sidewalks, or school facilities open to the public might be labeled radical or experimental
today; tomorrow, however, they may be considered prudent stewards of the public health.

We must at this point inject a note of caution. Although the policy proposals discussed here appear to make excellent sense, there is a lack of solid research evidence to demonstrate their effectiveness *(67)*.

The problem of lead pollution is an excellent illustration of what can be achieved by governmental action. In the 1970s regulations implemented by the American government forced major reductions or removal of lead from gasoline, paint, water, and consumer products. As a result by the early 1990s the blood level of the average American child was less than one-quarter of what it had been in the late 1970s *(68,69)*. Another remarkable success story concerns folic acid. After it was discovered that giving supplements of the vitamin to women during early pregnancy prevents neural tube defects, it became mandatory, starting in 1998, to add it to cereals in both the United States and Canada. This has apparently caused a reduction in the incidence of neural tube defects by approx 20–78% *(70–72)*.

3.4. Barriers Against Public Health Policies

Although many might consider the policies discussed here to be worthy of implementation, it must be appreciated that barriers exist. In particular, industry profits enormously from the sale of highly processed food and has often shown itself to be resistant to change. In this regard industry often secures government support.

The history of attempts to enact legislative control over tobacco illustrate how effective an industry can be when it uses a large budget in attempts to delay, dilute, or stop laws. There is clear evidence regarding the likely reason why the US Congress has been so lethargic when it comes to antismoking legislation. In 1991 and 1992 the average senator received $11,600 per year from the tobacco industry *(73)*. In the opinion of the researchers who carried out this study: "The money that the tobacco industry donates to members of Congress ensures that the tobacco industry will retain its strong influence in the federal tobacco policy process." Similarly, researchers looked at the California legislature and concluded: "Legislative behavior is following tobacco money rather than reflecting constituents' prohealth attitudes on tobacco control" *(74)*.

If the tobacco industry can achieve so many successes, then it will likely be much easier for the food industry to thwart interventions that threaten its profits. This is because the relationship between diet and disease is far less clear than is the case with tobacco. Indeed, there is ample evidence that governments are sympathetic to the wishes of the agricultural and food industries. Typically, although the health arm of governments encourages people to eat less fat, the departments responsible for the agricultural and food industries are largely concerned with maintaining high sales. James and Ralph *(61)* asserted that, "analysis of different policies suggest that health issues are readily squeezed out of discussion by economic and vested interests."

There is considerable evidence of how industry has successfully pressured governments to bow to their wishes on questions of nutrition policy. As discussed by Nestle *(75)*, the meat industry has been particularly effective in rewriting dietary guidelines. In the late 1970s the goal was "eat less meat." This then became "choose lean meat." By 1992 people were encouraged to consume at least two or three servings daily. There is also evidence that the 1992 version of Canada's Food Guide was similarly modified under pressure from the food industry *(76)*.

Discussing the question of salt, Goodlee *(77)*, assistant editor of the *British Medical Journal*, put it as follows:

> *...some of the world's major food manufacturers have adopted desperate measures to try to stop governments from recommending salt reduction. Rather than reformulate their products, manufacturers have lobbied governments, refused to cooperate with expert working parties, encouraged misinformation campaigns, and tried to discredit the evidence...The tactics over salt are much the same as those used by other sectors of industry. The Sugar Association in the United States and the Sugar Bureau in Britain have waged fierce campaigns against links between sugar and obesity and dental caries.*

The pressure exerted by the food industry in protection of its financial welfare is further explored in Chapter 22.

3.5. National Nutrition Policies: Examples

One pioneering project was the Norwegian Nutrition and Food Policy *(78)*. Implemented in 1976 it recognized the need to integrate agricultural, economic, and health policy. The policy included consumer and price subsidies, marketing measures, consumer information, and nutrition education in schools. Unfortunately, the policy clashed with policies aiming to stimulate agriculture. As a result subsidies went to pork, butter, and margarine rather than to potatoes, vegetables, and fruit. Despite these setbacks the policy has achieved some success in moving the national diet in the intended direction *(79)*.

Another noteworthy effort, which implemented several of the policies discussed here, was Heartbeat Wales carried out in Wales from 1985 to 1990 *(80)*. This project was carried out in Wales with the aim of preventing CHD. Specific measures included better food labeling, price incentives, and greater availability of healthier food. The active support was enlisted of catering departments and a food retailer. Unfortunately, the degree of success of this intervention is not known *(81)*.

3.6. Are Nutrition Policies Acceptable to the Public?

An important question concerns the extent to which the public would accept the suggested policies. The issues of seat belt use and drunk driving illustrate that when legislation is implemented and the public is educated regarding their importance, there is a high degree of acceptance. A study by Jeffery and colleagues *(82)* in the upper Midwest of the United States indicated widespread support for regulatory controls in the areas of alcohol, tobacco and, to a lesser extent, high-fat foods, especially with respect to children and youths. If such policies are acceptable to Americans, then they are also likely to be acceptable in other countries.

4. SOCIOECONOMIC STATUS AND HEALTH

One area of importance is the relationship between socioeconomic status (SES) and health. Low SES is strongly and consistently associated with a raised mortality rate. This applies to total mortality as well as to death from CHD and cancer. The risk ratios are in the range 1.5–4, clearly making SES a major determinant of health. Various measures of SES have been examined—income, social status of job, being unemployed, area of residence, and education—and each seems to manifest a similar relationship to mortality *(83–89)*.

Various studies have investigated why SES is associated with increased mortality. In general, lower SES is associated with higher rates of smoking and a diet of lower nutritional quality. Is SES merely a proxy measure of lifestyle? Or does SES affect health by a more direct mechanism? This question is of much more than mere theoretical importance and has a bearing on health strategies. If people of low SES are unhealthy because they lead an unhealthy lifestyle, then the solution lies in encouraging changes in their lifestyles. However, if a low SES is intrinsically unhealthy, then the solution lies elsewhere.

Our best evidence is that both possibilities are partially correct. After correcting for confounding variables, especially smoking, exercise, blood cholesterol, blood pressure, and weight, most studies have found that the strength of the association between SES and mortality is reduced by about one-quarter or one-half *(83,86,90,91)*. This indicates that people with lower SES tend to lead a less-healthy lifestyle and this partly explains their poorer health.

However, this still leaves half to three-quarters of the association between SES and mortality unexplained. In one study the relationship between diet and SES was investigated *(92)*.

This revealed that people of low SES tend to eat a less nutritious diet. Consistent with this, Drewnowski *(93)* showed in his cost analysis that energy-dense foods, such as sugar, oil, fried potatoes, and refined grains, provide energy at far lower cost than lean meat, fish, fresh vegetables, and fruit. This helps explain why such conditions as hypercholesterolemia, hypertension, and overweight are associated with low SES. Nevertheless, it appears that much of the association between SES and mortality cannot be explained by lifestyle and must therefore be a more direct consequence of low SES.

Psychological factors appear to play an important role in explaining the association between SES and mortality *(87,94)*. The psychological factor most closely associated with risk of poor health is lack of control at work *(94–96)*. We can speculate that other psychological factors, such as resentment, frustration, and a feeling of disempowerment, all contribute to poor health among low-income groups. Whatever the precise mechanisms, there is little doubt that structural elements of inequality within Western societies—economic, educational, social status—lead to reduced health.

But what should be done about this? An effective strategy to deal with the challenge of low SES may have to include efforts to reduce socioeconomic inequalities. If people of lower SES could be persuaded to adopt the same lifestyle, including diet, as those of higher SES, perhaps as much as half of the problem would likely disappear. Therefore, dietary advice is still worth the effort.

5. CONCLUSIONS

Based on the close association between various measures of SES and health, an essential component of enhancing a population's health must be measures to improve health-oriented policies, including the SES of the more deprived sections of the population. This means serious measures by the public health sector to counter such widespread problems as poverty and poor education. In countries where there is a strong tradition of social welfare, such measures can be undertaken by the government. Where more individualistic and business-oriented ideologies exist, implementing such measures are a greater challenge. The private sector would need to act, e.g., through charitable and other nongovernmental organizations and private schools. The goal to have both a healthy population and a healthy economy would seem more difficult to realize under such governmental systems; nevertheless, a healthy workforce and population is ultimately in the interest of business. Such societies must also find a way to public health.

This was well put by James *(62)* with specific regard to obesity:

The needed transformation in thinking on transport, environment, work facilities, education, health and food policies, and perhaps in social and economic policies is unlikely when governments are wedded to individualism, but without these changes to enhance physical activity and alter food quality, societies are doomed to escalating obesity rates.

This viewpoint applies to the relationship between nutrition and all diseases related to it. Where the primary force driving government policy is economics, governments and the public health sector must be encouraged to prioritize maintenance and improvement of the national health. The weight of evidence strongly suggests that when governments reorientate toward economic issues, they lose sight of nutrition policies, and national health can easily become a distant priority. In that case the failure of the government and business sectors to work together for the public health may lose great opportunities for the prevention of such diseases as cancer and CHD.

The philosophy discussed here need not stop at nutrition: what applies to nutrition certainly applies to other areas of lifestyle, especially to smoking. Exercise also lends itself to policy initiatives. What is the point in telling people to exercise if there is a lack of appropriate facilities? What is the point in telling people to cycle if the roads are too dangerous for bikes? What is needed is a comprehensive view of human health that takes all such factors into consideration.

As the century unfolds people may look back with incredulity on today's world where narrow commercial interests and government *laissez-faire* predominate while the national health flounders. More optimistically, an innovative marriage of business interests, individualism, and recognition of community health needs will emerge.

ACKNOWLEDGMENT

The work in this chapter done by NT was partly carried out at the Chronic Diseases of Lifestyle Programme, Medical Research Council, Cape Town, South Africa.

NOTE ADDED IN PROOF

Matson-Koffman et al. have recently published an extensive review on interventions for promoting physical activity and nutrition with the goal of the prevention of cardiovascular disease. *See* ref. *97*.

REFERENCES

1. National Center for Chronic Disease Prevention and Health Promotion. Smoking Prevalence Among U.S. Adults. www.cdc.gov/tobacco/research_data/adults_prev/prevali. Last accessed January 11, 2005.
2. Flegal, KM, Carroll MD, Kuczmarski RJ, Johnson CL. Overweight and obesity in the United States: prevalence and trends, 1960–1994. Int J Obesity 1998; 22:39–47.
3. Flegal KM, Carroll MD, Ogden CL, Johnson CL. Prevalence and trends in obesity among US adults, 1999-2000. JAMA 2002; 288:1723–1727.
4. Siedell JC. Obesity in Europe: scaling an epidemic. Int J Obesity 1995; 19(Suppl. 3):S1–S4.
5. Krebs-Smith SM, Kantor LS. Choose a variety of fruits and vegetables daily: understanding the complexities. J Nutr 2001; 131(2S-1):487S–501S.
6. Tippett KS, Cleveland LE. . In: Frazao E, ed. America's Eating Habits: Changes and Consequences. USDA/ERS, Washington DC, April 1999. Agricultural Information Bulletin Number 750, pp. 51–70.
7. Putnam J, Allshouse J, Kantor LS. U.S. per capita food supply trends: more calories, refined carbohydrates, and fats. Food Review 2002; 25:2–15.
8. Activity and Health Research. Allied Dunbar National Fitness Survey, a Report on Activity Patterns and Fitness Levels: Main Findings. Sports Council and Health Education Authority, London, 1992.
9. Jones DA, Ainsworth BE, Croft JB, Macera CA, Lloyd EE, Yusuf HR. Moderate leisure-time physical activity: who is meeting the public health recommendations? A national cross-sectional study. Arch Fam Med 1998; 7:285–289.
10. Anon. Self-reported physical inactivity by degree of urbanization—United States, 1996. MMWR Morb Mortal Wkly Rep 1998; 47:1097–1100.
11. Redman S, Spencer EA, Sanson-Fisher R. The role of the mass media in changing health-related behavior: a critical appraisal of two models. Health Prom Int 1990; 5:85–101.
12. Farquhar JW, Fortmann SP, Flora JA, et al. Effects of communitywide education on cardiovascular disease risk factors. The Stanford Five-City Project. JAMA 1990; 264:359–365.
13. Luepker RV, Murray DM, Jacobs DR, et al. Community education for cardiovascular disease prevention: risk factor changes in the Minnesota Heart Health Program. Am J Public Health 1994; 84:1383–1393.
14. Carleton RA, Lasater TM, Assaf AR, Feldman HA, McKinlay S, Pawtucket Heart Health Program Writing Group. The Pawtucket Heart Health Program: community changes in cardiovascular risk factors and projected disease risk. Am J Public Health 1995; 85:777–785.
15. Winkleby MA, Feldman HA, Murray DM. Joint analysis of three U.S. community intervention trials for reduction of cardiovascular risk. J Clin Epidemiol 1997; 50:645–658.
16. Goodman RM, Wheeler FC, Lee PR. Evaluation of the Heart To Heart Project: lessons from a community-based chronic disease prevention project. Am J Health Promot 1995; 9:443–455.
17. Brownson RC, Smith CA, Pratt M, et al. Preventing cardiovascular disease through community-based risk reduction: the Bootheel Heart Health Project. Am J Public Health 1996; 86:206–213.
18. Puska P, Nissinen A, Tuomilehto J, et al. The community based strategy to prevent coronary heart disease: conclusions from the ten years of North Karelia project. Ann Rev Public Health 1985; 6:147–193.
19. Valkonen T. Trends in regional and socio-economic mortality differentials in Finland. Int J Health Sci 1992; 3:157–166.

20. Hoffmeister H, Mensink GB, Stolzenberg H, et al. Reduction of coronary heart disease risk factors in the German Cardiovascular Prevention study. Prev Med 1996; 25:135–145.
21. Baxter T, Milner P, Wilson K, et al. A cost effective, community based heart health promotion project in England: prospective comparative study. BMJ 1997; 315:582–585.
22. Reger B, Wootan MG, Booth-Butterfield S, Smith H. 1% Or Less: a community-based nutrition campaign. Public Health Rep 1998; 113:410–419.
23. Reger B, Wootan MG, Booth-Butterfield S. Using mass media to promote healthy eating: A community-based demonstration project. Prev Med 1999; 29:414–421.
24. Dixon H, Boland R, Segan C, Stafford H, Sindall C. Public reaction to Victoria's "2 Fruit 'n' 5 Veg Day" campaign and reported consumption of fruit and vegetables. Prev Med 1998; 27:572–582.
25. World Health Organisation European Collaborative Group. European collaborative trial of multifactorial prevention of coronary heart disease: final report on the 6-year results. Lancet 1986; i:869–872.
26. World Health Organisation European Collaborative Group. Multifactorial trial in the prevention of coronary heart disease. Eur Heart J 1983; 4:141–147.
27. Breslow L, Fielding J, Herrman AA, Wilbur CS. Worksite health promotion: its evolution and the Johnson & Johnson experience. Prev Med 1990; 19:13–21.
28. Sorensen G, Morris DM, Hunt MK, et al. Work-site nutrition intervention and employees' dietary habits: the Treatwell program. Am J Public Health 1992; 82:877–880.
29. Sorensen G, Stoddard A, Peterson K, et al. Increasing fruit and vegetable consumption through worksites and families in the Treatwell 5-a-Day Study. Am J Public Health 1999; 89:54–60.
30. Jeffery RW, Forster JL, French SA, et al. The Healthy Worker Project: a work-site intervention for weight control and smoking cessation. Am J Public Health 1993; 83:395–401.
31. Imperial Cancer Research Fund OXCHECK Study Group. Effectiveness of health checks conducted by nurses in primary care: results of the OXCHECK study after one year. BMJ 1994; 308:308–312.
32. Imperial Cancer Research Fund OXCHECK Study Group. Effectiveness of health checks conducted by nurses in primary care: final results of the OXCHECK study. BMJ 1995; 310:1099–1104.
33. Family Heart Study Group. Randomised controlled trial evaluating cardiovascular screening and intervention in general practice: principal results of British Family Heart Study. BMJ 1994; 308:313–320.
34. Delichatsios HK, Hunt MK, Lobb R, Emmons K, Gillman MW. EatSmart: efficacy of a multifaceted preventive nutrition intervention in clinical practice. Prev Med 2001; 33(2 Pt 1):91–98.
35. Wilcox S, Parra-Medina D, Thompson-Robinson M, Will J. Nutrition and physical activity interventions to reduce cardiovascular disease risk in health care settings: a quantitative review with a focus on women. Nutr Rev 2001; 59:197–214.
36. Field K, Thorogood M, Silagy C, Normand C, O'Neill C, Muir J. Strategies for reducing coronary risk factors in primary care: which is most cost effective? BMJ 1995; 310:1109–1112.
37. Lindholm LH, Ekbom T, Dash C, Eriksson M, Tibblin G, Schersten B. The impact of health care advice given in primary care on cardiovascular risk. BMJ 1995; 310:1105–1109.
38. Tuomilehto J, Lindstrom J, Eriksson JG, et al. Prevention of type 2 diabetes mellitus by changes in lifestyle among subjects with impaired glucose tolerance. N Engl J Med 2001; 344:1343–1350.
39. Knowler WC, Barrett-Connor E, Fowler SE, et al. Reduction in the incidence of type 2 diabetes with lifestyle intervention or metformin. N Engl J Med 2002; 346:393–403.
40. Ammerman AS, Lindquist CH, Lohr KN, Hersey J. The efficacy of behavioral interventions to modify dietary fat and fruit and vegetable intake: a review of the evidence. Prev Med 2002; 35:25–41.
41. Rose G. The Strategy of Preventive Medicine. Oxford University Press, Oxford, 1992.
42. Aldana SG. Financial impact of health promotion programs: a comprehensive review of the literature. Am J Health Promot 2001; 15:296–320.
43. Golaszewski T. Shining lights: studies that have most influenced the understanding of health promotion's financial impact. Am J Health Promot 2001; 15:332–340.
44. Frazao E. High costs of poor eating patterns. In: Frazao E, ed. America's Eating Habits: Changes and Consequences. Washington, DC: USDA/ERS, April 1999. Agricultural Information Bulletin Number 750, pp. 5–32.
45. Davey Smith G, Ebrahim S. Dietary change, cholesterol reduction, and the public health—what does meta-analysis add? BMJ 1998; 316:1220.

46. Meier KJ, Licari MJ. The effect of cigarette taxes on cigarette consumption, 1955 through 1994. Am J Public Health 1997; 87:1126–1130.

47. Townsend J. Price and consumption of tobacco. Br Med Bull 1996; 52:132–142.

48. Stephens T, Pedersen LL, Koval JJ, Kim C. The relationship of cigarette prices and no-smoking bylaws to the prevalence of smoking in Canada. Am J Public Health 1997; 87:1519–1521.

49. Townsend J, Roderick P, Cooper J. Cigarette smoking by socioeconomic group, sex, and age: effects of price income, and health publicity. BMJ 1994; 309:923–927.

50. Anderson P, Lehto G. Prevention policies. Br Med Bull 1994; 50:171–185.

51. Zatonski W. Alcohol and health: what is good for the French may not be good for the Russians. J Epidemiol Commun Hlth 1998; 52:766, 767.

52. World Health Organisation Regional Office for Europe. The Adelaide Recommendations: Healthy Public Policy Regional Office for Europe. World Health Organisation, Geneva, 1988.

53. French SA, Jeffery RW, Story M, et al. Pricing and promotion effects on low-fat vending snack purchases: the CHIPS Study Am J Public Health 2001; 91:112–117.

54. Jeffery RW, French SA, Raether C, Baxter JE. An environmental intervention to increase fruit and salad purchases in a cafeteria. Prev Med 1994; 23:788–792.

55. French SA, Story M, Jeffery RW, et al. Pricing strategy to promote fruit and vegetable purchase in high school cafeterias. J Am Diet Assoc 1997; 97:1008–1010.

56. Advertising Age, Advertising Age. 100 Leading National Advertisers: 49th Annual Report. June 28, 2004.

57. Gallo AE. Food advertising in the United States. In: Frazao E, ed. America's Eating Habits: Changes & Consequences. USDA, Washington, DC, 1999.

58. Nestle M, Wing R, Birch L, et al. Behavioral and social influence on food choice. Nutr Rev 1998; 56:S50–S64.

59. Kotz K, Story M. Food advertisements during children's Saturday morning television programming: Are they consistent with dietary recommendations? J Am Diet Assoc 1994; 94:1296–1300.

60. Ostbye T, Pomerleau, White M, Coolich M, McWhinney J. Food and nutrition in Canadian "prime time" television commercials. Can J Public Health 1993; 84:370–374.

61. James WPT, Ralph A. National strategies for dietary change, In: Marmot M, Elliott P, eds. Coronary Heart Disease. From Aetiology to Public Health. Oxford University Press, Oxford, UK, 1992, pp. 525–540.

62. James WPT. A public health approach to the problem of obesity. Int J Obesity 1995; 19(Suppl 3):S37–S45.

63. Nestle M, Jacobson MF. Halting the obesity epidemic: a public health policy approach. Public Health Rep 2000; 115:12–24.

64. Jacobson MF, Brownell KD. Small taxes on soft drinks and snack foods to promote health. Am J Public Health 2000; 90:854–857.

65. Blackburn H. Community programmes in coronary heart disease prevention health promotion: changing community behaviour. In: Marmot M, Elliott P, eds. Coronary Heart Disease. From Aetiology to Public Health. Oxford University Press, Oxford, UK, 1992, pp. 495–514.

66. Schmid TL, Pratt M, Howze E. Policy as intervention: environmental and policy approaches to the prevention of cardiovascular disease. Am J Public Health 1995; 85:1207–1211.

67. Finkelstein E, French S, Variyam JN, Haines PS. Pros and cons of proposed interventions to promote healthy eating. Am J Prev Med 2004; 27(3 Suppl):163–171.

68. Pirkle JL, Brody DJ, Gunter EW, et al. The decline in blood lead levels in the United States. JAMA 1994; 272:284–291.

69. Brody DJ, Pirkle JL, Kramer RA, et al. Blood lead levels in the US population. JAMA 1994; 272:277–283.

70. Honein MA, Paulozzi LJ, Mathews TJ, Erickson JD, Wong LY. Impact of folic acid fortification of the US food supply on the occurrence of neural tube defects. JAMA 2001; 285:2981–2986.

71. Gucciardi E, Pietrusiak MA, Reynolds DL, Rouleau J. Incidence of neural tube defects in Ontario, 1986–1999. CMAJ 2002; 167:237–240.

72. Liu S, West R, Randell E, et al. A comprehensive evaluation of food fortification with folic acid for the primary prevention of neural tube defects. BMC Pregnancy Childbirth 2004; 4(1):20.

73. Moore S, Wolfe SM, Lindes D, Douglas CE. Epidemiology of failed tobacco control legislation. JAMA 1994; 272:1171–1175.

74. Glantz SA, Begay ME. Tobacco industry campaign contributions are affecting tobacco control policymaking in California. JAMA 1994; 272:1176–1182.

75. Nestle M. Food Politics. How the Food Industry Influences Nutrition and Health. University of California Press, Berkeley, CA, 2002.

76. Anon. Industry forced changes to food guide, papers show. Toronto Star, 1993 (January 15):A2.

77. Goodlee F. The food industry fights for salt. BMJ 1996; 312:1239, 1240.

78. Klepp K, Forster JL. The Norwegian Nutrition and Food Policy: an integrated approach to a public health problem. J Public Health Policy 1985; 6:447–463.

79. Norum KR, Johansson L, Botten G, Bjornboe G-EA, Oshaug A. Nutrition and food policy in Norway: effects on reduction of coronary heart disease. Nutr Rev 1997; 55:S32–S39.

80. Corson J. Heartbeat Wales: a challenge for change. World Hlth Forum 1990; 11:405–411.

81. Tudor-Smith C, Nutbeam D, Moore L, Catford J. Effects of the Heartbeat Wales programme over five years on behavioural risks for cardiovascular disease: quasi-experimental comparison of results from Wales and a matched reference area. BMJ 1998; 316:818–822.

82. Jeffery RW, Forster JL, Schmid TL, McBride CM, Rooney BL, Pirie PL. Community attitudes toward public policies to control alcohol, tobacco, and high-fat food consumption. Am J Prev Med 1990; 6:12–19.

83. Bucher HC, Ragland DR. Socioeconomic indicators and mortality from coronary heart disease and cancer: a 22-year follow-up of middle-aged men. Am J Public Health 1995; 85:1231–1236.

84. Lin RJ, Shah CP, Svoboda TJ. The impact of unemployment on health: a review. Can Med Ass J 1995; 153:529–540.

85. Sorlie PD, Backlund E, Keller JB. US mortality by economic, demographic, and social characteristics: The National Longitudinal Mortality Study. Am J Public Health 1995; 85:949–956.

86. Davey Smith G, Neaton JD, Wentworth D, Stamler R, Stamler J. Socioeconomic differentials in mortality risk among men screened for the Multiple Risk Factor Intervention Trial: I. White men. Am J Public Health 1996; 86:486–496.

87. Lynch JW, Kaplan GA, Cohen RD, Tuomilehto J, Salonen JT. Do cardiovascular risk factors explain the relation between socioeconomic status, risk of all-cause mortality, cardiovascular mortality, and acute myocardial infarction? Am J Epidemiol 1996; 144:934–942.

88. Morris JN, Blane DB, White IR. Levels of mortality, education, and social conditions in the 107 local education authority areas of England. J Epidemiol Commun Hlth 1996; 50:15–17.

89. Mackenbach JP, Kunst AE, Cavelaars AEJM, Groenhof F, Geurts JJM. Socioeconomic inequalities in morbidity and mortality in western Europe. Lancet 1997; 349:1655–1659.

90. Morris JK, Cook DG, Shaper AG. Loss of employment and mortality. BMJ 1994; 308:1135–1139.

91. Pekkanen J, Tuomilehto J, Uutela A, Vartiainen E, Nissinen A. Social class, health behaviour, and mortality among men and women in eastern Finland. BMJ 1995; 311:589–593.

92. Dubois L, Girard M. Social position and nutrition: a gradient relationship in Canada and the USA. Eur J Clin Nutr 2001; 55:366–373.

93. Drewnowski A. Obesity and the food environment: dietary energy density and diet costs. Am J Prev Med 2004; 27(3 Suppl):154–162.

94. Marmot MG, Bosma H, Brunner E, Stansfield S. Contribution of job control and other risk factors to social variations in coronary heart disease incidence. Lancet 1997; 350:235–239.

95. North FM, Syme SL, Feeney A, Shipley M, Marmot M. Psychosocial work environment and sickness absence among British civil servants: The Whitehall II Study. Am J Public Health 1996; 86:332–340.

96. Johnson JV, Stewart W, Hall EM, Fredlund P, Theorell T. Long-term psychosocial work environment and cardiovascular mortality and among Swedish men. Am J Public Health 1996; 86:324–331.

97. Matson-Koffman DM, Brownstein JN, Neiner JA, Greaney ML. Site-specific literature review of policy and environmental interventions that promote phyiscal activity and nutrition for cardiovascular health: what works? Am J Health Promot 2005; 19:167–193.

24 Dietary Intake, Cardiovascular Disease, and Sociodemographic Characteristics

Lyn M. Steffen

KEY POINTS

- African Americans (AAs) and Mexican Americans (MAs) are at higher risk than non-Hispanic whites (NHWs) for cardiovascular disease (CVD) and CVD risk factors—for example, obesity, the metabolic syndrome, and type 2 diabetes.
- Fewer AAs and MAs than NHWs meet the recommended US dietary guidelines for intakes of fruit, vegetables, and whole grains, likely in part because of their more limited resources.
- Low socioeconomic status typical of minority groups and acculturation of these groups are factors associated with increased risk of poor quality diets and, therefore, increased risk of disease.
- Independent of population subgroup membership, those who consume greater number of servings of fruit, vegetables, and whole grain products and fewer servings of meat are at lower risk of mortality and CVD.

1. INTRODUCTION

Risk of mortality and morbidity is influenced by behavioral and environmental factors, such as dietary intake, smoking, and physical activity *(1–3)*, genetic factors *(4)*, and socioeconomic determinants, such as income and education *(5–7)*. However, health disparities exist between different population groups, including a disproportionate burden of death and morbidity in minorities *(8)*, especially among African Americans (AAs) and Hispanics. Socioeconomic status (SES) often accounts for ethnic differences in risk factors for disease *(9)*. Roughly 11% of the US population is below the poverty threshold in income, but with a wide range between ethnic groups: 31.4% of AAs, 21.9% of Hispanics, and 7.5% of non-Hispanic whites (NHWs) *(10)*. Migration or acculturation is another factor that may influence the development of adverse risk factors, which ultimately lead to chronic disease. Less acculturation is defined in this chapter as those who

From: *Nutritional Health: Strategies for Disease Prevention, Second Edition*
Edited by: N. J. Temple, T. Wilson, and D. R. Jacobs © Humana Press Inc., Totowa, NJ

do not speak English, whereas acculturated individuals are those who speak English. This chapter will review the relations of dietary intake, acculturation, and SES with risk of developing cardiovascular disease (CVD), especially among (MAs), who make up the largest share of the US Hispanic population, a1nd AAs. First, the prevalence of CVD will be compared among NHW, AA, and MA populations, then the dietary intake of the US population for these groups will be described.

2. BURDEN OF DISEASE

Heart disease is the leading cause of death in the United States, despite substantial declines since the 1960s. This decline has plateaued, however, since 1990 *(11)*. In contrast, the prevalence of obesity, a modifiable CVD risk factor, increased by 75% since 1991 according to national surveys *(12,13)*. Increased body mass index (BMI) is a common factor in insulin resistance, a precursor for type 2 diabetes. Data from many studies have shown that insulin resistance is associated with the clustering of adverse cardiovascular risk factors, including increased levels of BMI or central adiposity, triglycerides, insulin, glucose, and systolic blood pressure, and low levels of high-density lipoprotein-cholesterol in children and adults of several race and ethnic groups *(14–21)*. Recently, the metabolic syndrome, defined as the clustering of these CVD risk factors, has been identified as a CVD risk factor as shown in Table 1 *(22)*.

Heart disease is also the leading killer across most racial and ethnic minority communities in the United States, accounting for approximately one-third of all deaths in 2001 *(11)*. AAs suffer the most from the disease; 41% of AA men and 44% of AA women have some form of heart disease, compared with 34% of NHW men, 32% of NHW women, and 30% of Hispanic men and women. AAs are also 29% more likely to die from the disease than NHWs.

Compared with NHWs, MAs and AAs suffer in greater numbers from obesity *(12,13)* and type 2 diabetes *(10)*, two of the leading risk factors for heart disease *(11)*. Minority women are at higher risk of both conditions than minority men and NHWs. However, MAs have less hypertension; the prevalence of hypertension was 18.4% for MAs, 27.9% for NHWs, and 33.5% for AAs *(23)*. The same pattern was seen in each sex group. Findings from the Third National Health and Nutrition Examination Surveys report the prevalence of the metabolic syndrome was 24 and 23.4% among men and women, respectively; and 31.9, 23.8, and 21.6% among MAs, NHWs and AAs, respectively *(24)*.

Recent findings from the Corpus Christi Heart Project, a population-based surveillance study of MA and NHW adults, observed that MAs are at higher risk of CVD mortality than NHWs *(25,26)*; moreover, MAs born in the United States and who speak English (acculturated) have a much higher risk of CVD mortality than do MAs born in Mexico (less acculturated) *(27)*. The discrepancy of findings between the national death certificate data and the Corpus Christi findings may relate to two factors: that many MAs return to Mexico to die, and that there may be bias in death certificate coding, e.g., MAs are more likely to be coded to diabetes than NHWs.

The relationship of income inequality with mortality and morbidity is complex and beyond the scope of this chapter. However, individual income and occupation grade, indicators of SES, are inversely related to mortality and morbidity, including CVD *(28,29)*. This is discussed in Chapter 23.

Table 1
CVD Risk Factors Defined by Adult Treatment Panel III as the Metabolic Syndrome [a]

Risk factor	Definition
Waist circumference	Men >102 cm
	Women >88 cm
HDL-cholesterol	Men <1.1 mmol/L (<40 mg/dL)
	Women <1.29 mmol/L (<50 mg/dL)
Fasting triglycerides	≥1.7 mmol/L (≥ mg/dL)
Fasting glucose	≥6.1 mmol/L (≥110 mg/dL)
Blood pressure	Systolic ≥130 mmHg
	Diastolic ≥85 mmHg

[a]Any combination of three cardiovascular disease risk factors defines the metabolic syndrome. HDL, high-density lipoprotein.
(Adapted from refs. *21* and *22*.)

3. FOOD INTAKE IN THE US POPULATION

In 1994–1996 the US Department of Agriculture Continuing Survey of Food Intakes by Individuals (CSFII) was administered. The prevalence of individuals meeting the 2000 US Department of Agriculture dietary guidelines for adults *(30)* is reported by race/ethnic and income group.

3.1. Fruit and Vegetables

The recommendation for adults is to consume a variety of fruit and vegetables, including two to four servings of fruit and three to five vegetable servings daily *(30)*. CSFII data show that only 28% of persons aged 2 yr and older consumed at least 2 daily servings of fruit, including 27% of NHWs, 29% of MAs, and 24% of AAs *(31)*. Only 23% of low-income individuals (defined by less than 130% of poverty threshold) consumed two or more servings per day of fruits compared with 29% with higher income. Fifty percent of NHWs and MAs consumed three or more servings per day of vegetables, whereas 43% of AAs consumed this amount. Of lower and higher income individuals, 42 and 50%, respectively, met this recommendation.

3.2. Grain Products

The dietary guidelines suggest adults choose a variety of grains each day, including 6–11 daily servings with at least 3 being whole grain. In 1994–1996, 51% of Americans consumed six or more servings per day of grains, of whom 7% met the recommendation for whole grain foods *(31)*. Fifty-four percent of NHWs consumed six or more servings per day of grains, whereas 46 and 40% of MAs and AAs, respectively, reached this goal. Twice as many NHWs than MAs or AAs met the whole grain recommendation (8% vs 4% vs 4%). According to income group, 44% of individuals in the low and 53% in the high-income groups met the recommendation for the grains; with 5 and 8% of low and high income, respectively, consuming three or more servings of whole grains.

3.3. Dairy Products

The dietary guidelines suggest choosing low-fat milk products to obtain essential nutrients without substantially increasing calorie and saturated fat intakes. The recommendation for adequate daily intakes of calcium is 1000–1200 mg for adults *(32)*. Less than 50% of the US adult population met this recommendation, including 49% of NHWs, 44% of MAs, and 30% of AAs, whereas 39% of low-income and 48% of high-income individuals met the recommendation for calcium.

3.4. Fast-Food Intake

Data from the 1994–1996 and 1998 CSFII surveys were used to describe the demographic characteristics and dietary intake of fast-food consumers *(33)*. Individuals with high school and some college education reported eating fast-food more frequently than college graduates. There were no ethnic differences between consumers and nonconsumers of fast-food. Adults who reported eating fast food ate considerably fewer servings of bread, cereals, grains, milk, legumes, and fruit and vegetables (except fried potatoes). Intake of soft drinks was two times greater among fast-food consumers than among nonconsumers.

3.5. Acculturation and Dietary Intake

Level of acculturation to American culture and values influences the dietary practices and health of MAs. Traditional Mexican foods include flour or corn tortillas, chilies, corn, tomatoes, tomatillos, beans and a variety of spices *(34)*. Fish and seafood are common in diets of MAs living on the coast. However, most Mexican families migrating to the United States have adopted some US dietary habits, including consumption of ready-to-eat cereals, peanut butter, hamburgers, pizza, high-sugar fruit drinks, and soft drinks *(35)*.

Dixon et al. *(36)* examined food intake from the Third National Health and Nutrition Examination Survey, 1988–1994, according to three migration and acculturation groups: Mexican born, US-born Spanish speaking, and US-born English speaking. The Mexican-born men and women had the lowest level of education, whereas the US-born English speakers had the highest level. The men and women born in Mexico consumed more fruit, fruit juice, vegetables, grains, and legumes than those born in the United States. US-born English-speaking men and women consumed more salty snacks, desserts, and added fats (salad dressing and margarine) than US-born Spanish speakers, who reported intermediate amounts, and MAs born in Mexico, who reported the lowest intake of snacks and desserts. Nutrient data were consistent with the reported food intake, where percent of total and saturated fat calories was lowest and fiber intake highest in those born in Mexico. In addition, more MAs born in Mexico met the dietary guidelines for total and saturated fat than the other MAs. These data suggest the need for nutrition education for second generation MAs to retain their native traditions.

Other studies have reported similar findings: based on the Healthy Eating Index (a rating system for having met the dietary guideline recommendations) first-generation MAs with lower incomes eat more healthy foods than higher income NHWs and second-generation MAs *(37)*. Older Hispanic adults living in the northeastern United States for a longer time tended to have nutrient intakes similar to those of NHWs. More acculturated Hispanics consumed fewer traditional ethnic foods than those who were less acculturated *(38)*.

Table 2
Amount Spent per Person on Food Categories by Income Level, 1998
(Approximate Amounts as Dollars per Year)

Food group	Low income	Middle income	High income
Total food expenditure	1750	2090	2770
Cereal and bakery	180	190	220
Meat, poultry, fish, eggs	300	300	370
Dairy	120	140	160
Fruit and vegetables	200	220	275
Sugar and sweets	45	50	55

Adapted from ref. *41*; Food and Rural Economics Division, Economic Research Service, USDA.

MAs living in Texas consumed a greater proportion of calories from saturated fat and cholesterol in meats than NHWs and AAs, although AAs reported consuming more meat products than MAs or NHWs *(39)*. MAs, however, consumed more calories from grain products, legumes, and vegetables than NHWs or AAs. Dairy consumption was greater in NHWs than AAs or MAs. Earlier studies of food pattern consumption of MAs revealed a diet consisting of more legumes, corn, and eggs and less meat, fat, and milk than was the case with NHWs *(40)*.

3.6. SES and Dietary Intake

3.6.1. FOOD SPENDING BY US HOUSEHOLDS

Income and household size are the factors that are most related to how and where Americans spend their food dollars *(41)*. In 1998, low-income households spent about 16 and 37% less per person on food compared to middle- or high-income households, respectively. This occurred despite the fact that low-income households spent 48% of their income on food, whereas middle- and high-income households spent only 13 and 8%, respectively (Table 2). The amount spent on food away from home was $638, $881, and $1301 per person per year for low-, middle-, and high-income households, respectively.

Food expenditures increased across all income groups between 1990 and 1998 and the trend is likely to continue given that disposable income increases faster than the inflation rate.

3.6.2. SES AND DIETARY INTAKE AMONG INDIVIDUALS

SES differences in health behaviors, such as dietary and alcohol intake, physical activity, and smoking, have been describes in population surveys *(42)*. Differences in health behaviors in different SES groups may be explained by determinants of behavior, such as attitudes, beliefs in health benefits, motivation, and perceived barriers to healthy choices. Expectation of a shorter lifespan in low-income individuals was associated with smoking and unhealthy dietary choices *(43)*. Breakfast patterns differ by SES and ethnicity *(44)*. Low-income individuals, as well as Hispanics and AAs, were more likely to not eat breakfast or eat an egg-based breakfast, whereas individuals with higher income or more education were more likely to choose healthier (lower fat and higher fiber) foods, including ready-to-eat and hot cereals, fruit, and juice.

4. DIETARY INTAKE, SES, AND CVD

The "diet–heart" hypothesis, that intake of dietary saturated fat and cholesterol increases risk and polyunsaturated fat decreases risk of coronary heart disease (CHD) through lipid mechanisms, is supported by many studies in adults regardless of race, ethnicity, or SES *(45)*. Population studies have also shown an increased risk of CHD with low intake of fiber. Beneficial effects of polyunsaturated fatty acids on inflammation markers have been demonstrated in animal and experimental studies *(46)*. There is much evidence that antioxidants, and therefore a diet rich in fruit and vegetables, reduce risk of CVD *(47)*.

4.1. Food Intake

More recent epidemiological studies provide evidence showing lower CVD mortality and morbidity with greater intakes of such foods as whole grains, fruit and vegetables, and fish. In prospective epidemiological studies, mortality from all causes and CVD is inversely related to intake of whole grain foods *(48–51)*. Feeding studies of increased whole grain consumption for 4–8 wk reported significantly reduced levels of fasting and 2-h insulin *(52)*, total and low-density lipoproteins-cholesterol levels *(53)*, systolic blood pressure *(54)*, and slightly reduced weight and BMI *(55)*. Intake of fruit and vegetables may offer protection from risk of death, CHD, and stroke *(51,56)*, for example, through modification of platelet activity *(57)*, homocysteine levels *(58,59)*, blood pressure *(60)*, and replacement of fatty acids in the diet, including reduced saturated fat intake. It is likely that these diet–disease relationships may apply to some extent to population subgroups, but whether they apply equally in all groups is not clear.

In the Atherosclerosis Risk in Community study of CVD in whites and AAs, risk of incident CHD was inversely associated with intake of fruit and vegetables; however, the relation was stronger in AAs *(51)*. Among AAs who consumed seven or more servings per day of fruit and vegetables, there was a 63% reduction in risk of incident CHD compared with those who consumed only 1.5 servings per day. In whites, the risk of incident CHD was lower with greater consumption of fruit and vegetables, but not as strong as in AAs. In subgroup analysis of refined grain products (such as white bread, rice, pasta, refined cereal, donuts, cookies, and cakes), AAs who consumed 5.5 servings of refined grain had two times the risk of CHD compared to AAs who consumed 0.5 serving per day. But, risk of CHD did not increase with greater intake of refined grains in whites. These multivariate models were adjusted for age, sex, energy intake, education, physical activity, alcohol intake, BMI, lipids, blood pressure, and vitamin supplement intake.

Lower blood pressure and risk of developing elevated blood pressure (defined as systolic blood pressure >135 mmHg or diastolic blood pressure >85 mmHg) is associated with higher intake of fruit, vegetables, and fish, and lower intake of meat products *(2,61,62)*. Numerous studies have shown that vegetarians have lower blood pressure than nonvegetarians *(2)*, and that adding meat to a vegetarian diet increases blood pressure *(63)*. Results from a study conducted in Hispanic Seventh Day Adventist vegetarians and Hispanic Catholic omnivores showed that the vegetarians had lower levels of several risk factors for CVD and type 2 diabetes than the omnivores *(64)*. The Hispanic vegetarians had lower BMI, systolic blood pressure, serum total cholesterol, and triglycerides than the Hispanic omnivores. In a study of white men aged 41–57 yr, consumption of 14–42 servings per month of vegetables vs less than 14 servings per month was associated with a lower increase in blood pressure, whereas consumption of beef, veal, lamb, and poultry was positively related to blood pressure during 7 yr of follow-up *(61)*. Among young AAs and white adults who were enrolled in the Coronary Artery Risk Development in Young Adults (CARDIA) study and were followed for 15 yr, plant food and dairy product consumption were inversely associated with risk of developing elevated blood pressure, whereas meat intake was positively related to risk *(62)*. Both AAs and whites were at the same risk of developing elevated blood pressure given the same intake of plant foods. However, a greater number of AA men and women developed elevated blood pressure because they consumed fewer servings of plant food, especially fruit, vegetables, and whole grains. Results from these studies are consistent; plant foods are beneficial to health and meat products increase the risk for chronic disease, regardless of race or ethnic group.

Dietary intake is correlated with the development of obesity and type 2 diabetes, two major risk factors for CVD. Clinical studies of weight management have shown that manipulation of energy and macronutrient intake, as well as intake of certain foods, may facilitate weight loss or gain in men and women of different ethnic groups *(65–68)*. Prospective studies in young white and AA adults have demonstrated inverse relations of fiber consumption with fasting insulin, weight gain, and other CVD risk factors *(69,70)* and development of type 2 diabetes in older women *(71)*. The association of fiber intake with 10-yr weight gain was examined among 2909 young white and AA adults aged 18–25 yr at baseline in CARDIA *(70)*. Fiber was inversely associated with weight gain and waist-hip ratio during 10 yr of follow-up, although this association was attenuated when adjusted for fasting insulin levels. The conclusion that may be drawn from the previous studies is that more plant food is beneficial for health, an effect seen in MAs, AAs, and NHWs, male and female.

4.2. Dietary Patterns

Although many studies have examined the role of nutrients and individual foods or food groups in the etiology of disease, few studies have reported on the effects of dietary patterns or quality of diet on health *(72)*. Recent prospective data suggest that eating patterns characterized by a diet including more plant foods and less meat products, a diet based on the US dietary guidelines, or a vegetarian diet, are related to decreased risk of mortality *(2,73,74)*. In a prospective study of 11,940 white and AA women and men enrolled in the Atherosclerosis Risk in Community study, risk of mortality was higher across increasing quintiles of intake of the "Western" diet pattern (an eating pattern characterized by more meat, whole milk, cheese, fried food, soft drinks, and fewer plant foods) *(74)*. Compared with individuals in the first quintile, those in the highest quintile had 1.5–2 times the risk of dying from all causes, CVD, and all cancers, even after adjustment for age, gender, race, education, energy intake, smoking, alcohol intake, physical activity, body mass, blood pressure, lipids, and hormone replacement therapy. In the Dietary Approaches to Stop Hypertension (DASH) trial, an 8-wk feeding study, investigators found in 459 moderately hypertensive white and AA men and women that a combination diet rich in fruit, vegetables, and low-fat dairy products, as well as reductions in saturated fat intake, substantially lowered systolic and diastolic blood pressure levels *(61)*. Results from all of these studies consistently show that a diet including more plant foods and fewer animal products is associated with a lower risk of mortality and morbidity in both white and AA black men and women. Considering the national survey data, that AA and MA consume fewer servings of fruit, vegetables, and whole grains than NHWs, this behavior may likely result in a higher risk of disease.

There is considerable evidence for an inverse relation of socioeconomic factors with all-cause mortality, CVD, and adverse CVD risk factors *(5–7)*. Analyses of data for 68,556 US adults in the National Health Interview Survey showed that the highest obesity rates were associated with low income and fewer years of education *(75)*. SES may influence health status through choices in lifestyle, including dietary intake, alcohol intake, smoking behavior, and physical activity *(9,76)*. Investigators from the Whitehall II study examined CVD risk factors in South Asian, Afro-Caribbean, and Caucasian civil servants. They observed higher levels of blood pressure and greater prevalence of diabetes among South Asians and Afro-Caribbeans compared with Caucasians, even after adjusting for grade of occupation, although these differences were not completely explained by SES *(77)*. However, dietary intake was not included in these analyses. Dietary intake and serum nutrients were examined among US adults who reported having insufficient or sufficient food *(78)*. Older adults who had insufficient food had lower dietary intakes of energy, vitamin B6, magnesium, iron, and zinc and lower serum levels of high-density lipoprotein-cholesterol, β-cryptoxanthin, and vitamins A and E. Clearly, lower intakes and concentrations of many nutrients in serum may compromise the immune system and promote the development of chronic disease.

5. CONCLUSIONS

Many health disparities are related to being a member of a minority group, especially AAs or MAs, or having a lower SES, including lower income, fewer years of education, or semi- or unskilled job classification. There is an epidemiological link between minority status and SES; a greater number of minority men and women have fewer years of formal education and less income than NHWs. Indeed, the prevalence of CVD and adverse CVD risk factors is greater among AAs and MAs than NHWs. Although there has been limited study of the role of diet in these health disparities, it is likely that differences in dietary intake across population subgroups plays a role. Epidemiological studies provide much evidence that dietary intake promotes health (or disease) given the quality of the diet. Consumption of both whole grain and fruit and vegetable intake is related to lower risk of dying or developing CHD, and that meat intake is related to higher risk among populations, regardless of race/ethnic groups. Dietary patterns that are plant based provide more health benefits than a meat- or animal-based diet. National survey data show that fewer AA and MA consume the recommended number of servings per day for fruit and vegetables or whole grain foods. For example, AA and MA are more likely to consume eggs for breakfast, rather than whole grain cereals. The few studies that directly address diet and health across population subgroups generally find the same diet–disease relations in AAs, MAs, and NHWs, but a less desirable diet in the minority groups.

The relatively poorer diet often found in minority group members may be a consequence of their generally lower SES. Low-income households spend less money annually for food, especially whole grains and fruit and vegetables, compared with those with moderate and high-incomes households. Food insecurity, one marker of poverty and more commonly found in minority group members, is related to lower levels of intakes or lower-quality diets and lower serum nutrients that may ultimately result in compromised health.

REFERENCES

1. U.S. Dept of Health and Human Services. The Health Consequences of Smoking- Cardiovascular Disease: A Report of the Surgeon General. DHHS publication PHS 84-50204. Public Health Service, Office on Smoking and Health, Rockville, MD, 1983.
2. Fraser GE. Diet, Life Expectancy, and Chronic Disease: Studies of Seventh-day Adventists and Other Vegetarians. Chapter 8. Vegetarianism and obesity, hypertension, diabetes, and arthritis. Oxford University Press, New York, 2003.
3. The President's Council on Physical Fitness and Sports. Physical Activity and Health: A Report of the Surgeon General. National Center for Chronic Disease Prevention and Health Promotion, Centers for Disease Control and Prevention, US Dept of Health and Human Services, Atlanta, GA, 1996.
4. Schull WJ, Hanis CL. Genetics and public health in the 1990's. Ann Rev Public Health 1990; 11: 105–125.
5. Fuhrer R, Shipley MJ, Chastang JF, et al. Socioeconomic position, health, and possible explanations: a tale of two cohorts. Am J Public Health 2002; 92:1290–1294.
6. Martikainen PT, Ishizaki M, Marmot MG, Nakagawa H, Kagamimori S. Socioeconomic differences in behavioral and biological risk factors: a comparison of a Japanese and an English cohort of employed men. Int J Epidemiol 2001; 30:833–838.
7. Martikainen PT, Marmot MG. Socioeconomic differences in weight gain and determinants and consequences of coronary risk factors. Am J Clin Nutr 1999; 69:719–726.
8. Hazuda HP, Haffner SM, Stern MP, Eifler CW. Effects of acculturation and socioeconomic status on obesity and diabetes in Mexican Americans: the San Antonio Heart Study. Am J Epidemiol 1988; 128: 1289–1301.
9. Kaplan GA, Keil JE. Socioeconomic factors and cardiovascular disease: a review of the literature. Circulation 1993; 88:1973–1998.
10. National Center for Health Statistics. Health, United States, 2004. Chartbook on Trends in the Health of Americans. Hyattsville, MD, 2004.
11. American Heart Association. Heart Disease and Stroke Statistics—2005 Update. American Heart Association, Dallas, TX, 2004.
12. Mokdad AH, Serdulea MK, Dietz WH, Bowman BA, Marks JS, Koplan JP. The continuing epidemic of obesity in the United States. JAMA 2000; 284:1650, 1651.
13. Hedley AA, Ogden CL, Johnson CL, Carroll MD, Curtin LR, Flegal KM. Prevalence of overweight and obesity among US children, adolescents, and adults, 1999–2000. JAMA 2004; 291:2847–2850.
14. Sinaiko AR, Jacobs DR, Jr., Steinberger J, et al. Insulin resistance syndrome in childhood: associations of the euglycemic insulin clamp and fasting insulin with fatness and other risk factors. J Pediatr 2001; 139:700–707.
15. Steffen-Batey L, Goff DC, Tortolero SR, et al. Summary measures of the insulin resistance syndrome are adverse among Mexican-American versus non-Hispanic white children: The Corpus Christi Child Heart Study. Circulation 1997; 96:4319–4325.
16. Svec F, Nastasi K, Hilton C, Bao W, Srinivasan SR, Berenson GS. Black-White contrasts in insulin levels during pubertal development: The Bogalusa Heart Study. Diabetes 1992; 41:313–317.
17. Ronnemaa T, Knip M, Lautala P, et al. Serum insulin and other cardiovascular risk indicators in children, adolescents and young adults. Ann Med 1991; 23:67–72.
18. Gray RS, Fabsitz RR, Cowan LD, Lee ET, Howard BV, Savage PJ. Risk factor clustering in the insulin resistance syndrome: The Strong Heart Study. Am J Epidemiol 1998; 148:869–878.
19. Reaven GM. Role of insulin resistance in human disease. Diabetes 1988; 37:1595–1607.
20. Kaplan NM. The deadly quartet: Upper-body obesity, glucose intolerance, hypertriglyceridemia, and hypertension. Arch Intern Med 1989; 149:1514–1520.

21. National Institutes of Health. Third Report of the National Cholesterol Education Program Expert Panel on Detection, Evaluation, and Treatment of High Blood Cholesterol in Adults (Adult Treatment Panel III). NIH Publication 01-3670. National Institutes of Health, Bethesda, MD, 2001.

22. Grundy SM, Brewer B, Cleeman JI, Smith SC, Lenfant C for the Conference Participants. Definition of Metabolic Syndrome Report of the National Heart, Lung, and Blood Institute/American Heart Association Conference on Scientific Issues Related to Definition. Circulation 2004; 109:433–438.

23. Fields LE, Burt VL, Cutler JA, Hughes J, Roccella EJ, Sorlie P. The burden of adult hypertension in the United States 1999 to 2000: a rising tide. Hypertension 2004; 44:398–404.

24. Ford ES, Giles WH, Dietz WH. Prevalence of the metabolic syndrome among US adults: Findings from the Third National Health and Nutrition Examination Survey. JAMA 2002; 287:356–359.

25. Pandey DK, Labarthe DW, Goff DC, Chan W, Nichaman MZ. Community-wide coronary heart disease mortality in Mexican-Americans equals or exceeds that in non-Hispanic whites: The Corpus Christi Heart Project. Am J Med 2001; 110:81–87.

26. Goff DC, Ramsey DJ, Labarthe DR, Nichaman MZ. Greater case-fatality after myocardial infarction among Mexican Americans and women than among non-Hispanic whites and men: The Corpus Christi Heart Project. Am J Epidemiol 1994; 139:474–483.

27. Sundquist J, Winkleby M. Cardiovascular risk factors in Mexican American adults: a transcultural analysis of NHANES III, 1988-94. Am J Publ Health 1999; 89:723–730.

28. Lynch JW, Smith GD, Kaplan GA, House JS. Income inequality and mortality: importance to health of individual income, psychosocial environment or material conditions. BMJ 2000; 320:1200–1204.

29. Colhoun H, Hemingway H, Poulter N. Socio-economic status and blood pressure: an overview analysis. J Hum Hypertens 1998; 12:91–110.

30. USDA and US Department of Health and Human Services. Dietary Guidelines for Americans, 5th edition. USDA Home and Garden Bulletin No. 232. USDA, Washington, DC, 2000.

31. USDA, Agricultural Research Service. Data from the 1994-96 Continuing Survey of Food Intakes by Individuals, February 1998.

32. Institute of Medicine. Dietary Reference Intakes for Calcium, Phosphorus, Magnesium, Vitamin D, and Fluoride. National Academy Press, Washington, DC, 1997.

33. Paeratakul S, Ferdinand DP, Champagne C, Ryan DH, Bray GA. Fast-food consumption among US adults and children: Dietary and nutrient intake profile. J Am Diet Assoc 2003; 103:1332–1338.

34. Algert SJ, Brzezinski E, Ellison TH. Mexican American Food Practices, Customs and Holidays. 2nd edition. American Dietetic Association, Chicago, 1998.

35. Dewey KG, Metallinos ES, Strokde MA, et al. Combining nutrition research and nutrition education for dietary change among Mexican American families. J Nutr Ed 1984; 16:5–7.

36. Dixon LB, Sundquist J, Winkleby. Differences in energy, nutrient, and food intakes in a US sample of Mexican-American women and men: findings from the Third National Health and Nutrition Examination Survey, 1988–94. Am J Epidemiol 2000; 152:548–557.

37. Aldrich L, Variyam JN. Acculturation erodes the diet quality of US Hispanics. Food Review 2000; 223: 51–55.

38. Bermudez OI, Falcon LM, Tucker KL. Intake and food sources of macronutrients among older Hispanic adults: association with ethnicity, acculturation, and length of residence in the US. J Am Diet Assoc 2000; 100:665–673.

39. Borrud LG, Pillow PC, McPherson RS, Nichaman MZ, Newell GR. Food group contributions to nutrient intake in whites, blacks and Mexican Americans in Texas. J Am Diet Assoc 1989; 89:1061–1069.

40. Center for Disease Control. Ten-State Nutrition Survey, 1968–70. Part V. Dietary. Department of Health, Education and Welfare, DHEW Publication No. (HSM) 72-8133, Atlanta, GA, 1972.

41. Blizard N. Food spending by US households grew steadily in the 1990s. Food Review 2002; 23:18–22.

42. Lantz PM, House JS, Lekowski JM. Socioeconomic factors, health behaviors, and mortality: results from a nationally representative prospective study of US adults. JAMA 1998; 279:1703–1708.

43. Wardle J, Steptoe A. Socioeconomic differences in attitudes and beliefs about healthy lifestyles. J Epidemiol Community Health 2003; 57:440–443.

44. Siega-Riz AM, Popkin BM, Carson T. Differences in food patterns at breakfast by sociodemographic characteristics among a nationally representative sample of adults in the United States. Prev Med 2000; 30:415–424.

45. Mensink RP, Katan MB. Effect of dietary fatty acids on serum lipids and lipoproteins: a meta-analysis of 27 trials. Arterioscler Thromb 1992; 12:911–919.

46. Calder PC. Polyunsaturated fatty acids, inflammation and immunity. Lipids 2001; 36:1007–1024.

47. Kromhout D, Menotti A, Kesteloot H. Prevention of coronary heart disease by diet and lifestyle: evidence from prospective cross-cultural, cohort, and intervention studies. Circulation 2002; 105:893–898.

48. Jacobs DR, Meyer KA, Kushi LH, Folsom AR. Whole-grain intake may reduce the risk of ischemic heart disease death in postmenopausal women: the Iowa Women's Health Study. Am J Clin Nutr 1998; 68:248–257.

49. Jacobs DR, Meyer KA, Kushi LH, Folsom AR. Is whole grain intake associated with reduced total and cause-specific death rates in older women? The Iowa Women's Health Study. Am J Public Health 1999; 89:322–329.

50. Liu S, Stampfer MJ, Hu FB, et al. Whole-grain consumption and risk of coronary heart disease: results from the Nurses' Health Study. Am J Clin Nutr 1999; 70:412–419.

51. Steffen LM, Jacobs DR Jr, Stevens J, Shahar E, Carithers T, Folsom AR. Associations of whole grain, refined grain, and fruit and vegetable consumption with all-cause mortality, incident coronary heart disease and ischemic stroke: The ARIC Study. Am J Clin Nutr 2003; 78:383–390.

52. Pereira MA, Jacobs DR, Pins JJ, et al. Effect of whole grains on insulin sensitivity in overweight hyperinsulinemic adults. Am J Clin Nutr 2002; 75:848–855.

53. Leinonen KS, Poutanen KS, Mykkanen HM. Rye bread decreases serum total and LDL cholesterol in men with moderately elevated serum cholesterol. J Nutr 2000; 130:164–170.

54. Saltzman E, Das SK. Lichtenstein AH, et al. An oat-containing hypocaloric diet reduces systolic blood pressure and improves lipid profile beyond effects of weight loss in men and women. J Nutr 2001; 131:1465–1470.

55. Poppitt SD, Keogh GF, Prentice AM, et al. Long-term effects of ad libitum low-fat, high carbohydrate diets on body weight and serum lipids in overweight subjects with metabolic syndrome. Am J Clin Nutr 2002; 75:11–20.

56. Ness AR, Powles JW. Fruit and vegetables, and cardiovascular disease: a review. Intl J Epidemiol 1997; 26:1–13.

57. Dutta-roy AK. Dietary components and human platelet activity. Platelets 2002; 13: 67–75.

58. Brattstrom LE, Israelsson B, Jeppsson JO, Hultberg BL. Folic acid: an innocuous means to reduce plasma homocysteine, Scan J Clin Lab Invest 1988; 48:215–221.

59. Rimm EB, Willett WC, Hu FB, et al. Folate and vitamin B6 from diet and supplements in relation to risk of coronary heart disease among women. JAMA 1998; 279:359–364.

60. Appel LJ, Moore TJ Obarzanek E, et al. A clinical trial of the effects of dietary patterns on blood pressure. DASH Collaborative Research Group. N Engl J Med 1997; 336:1117–1124.

61. Miura K, Greenland P, Stamler J, Liu K, Daviglus ML, Makagawa H. Relation of vegetable, fruit, and meat intake to 7-year blood pressure change in middle-aged men: The Chicago Western Electric Study. Am J Epidemiol 2004; 159:572–580.

62. Steffen LM, Kroenke CH, Yu X, et al. Associations of plant, dairy products, and meat consumption with fifteen-year incidence of elevated blood pressure in young black and white adults: The CARDIA Study. Presented at the Third Congress of Longitudinal Studies in Europe, September 24, 2004, UK.

63. Sacks FM, Donner A, Castelli WP, et al. Effect of ingestion of meat on plasma cholesterol in vegetarians. JAMA 1981; 246:640–644.

64. Alexander H, Lockwood LP, Harris MA, Melby CL. Risk factors for cardiovascular disease and diabetes in two groups of Hispanic Americans with differing dietary habits. J Am Coll Nutr 1999; 18:127–136.

65. Blundell JE, Cooling J. Routes to obesity: phenotypes, food choices and activity. Br J Nutr 2000; 83(Suppl 1):S33–S38.

66. Rolls BJ, Morris EL, Roe LS. Portion size of food affects energy intake in normal-eight and overweight men and women. Am J Clin Nutr 2002; 76:207–213.

67. Schrauwen P, Westerterp R. The role of high-fat diets and physical activity in the regulation of body weight. Br J Nutr 2000; 84:417–427.

68. Bray GA, Popkin BM. Dietary fat intake does affect obesity! Am J Clin Nutr 1998; 68:1157–1173.

69. Stevens J. Does dietary fiber affect food intake and body weight? J Am Diet Assoc 1988; 88:939–945.

70. Ludwig DS, Pereira MA, Kroenke CH, et al. Dietary fiber, weight gain, and cardiovascular disease risk factors in young adults. JAMA 1999; 282:1539–1546.

71. Meyer KA, Kushi LH, Jacobs DR, Slavin J, Sellers TA, Folsom AR. Carbohydrates, dietary fiber, and incident type 2 diabetes in older women. Am J Clin Nutr 2000; 71:921–930.

72. National Research Council. Committee on Diet and Health, Food and Nutrition Board, Commission on Life Sciences. Diet and Health: Implications for Reducing Chronic Disease Risk. National Academy of Sciences, Washington, DC, 1989.

73. Kant AK, Schatzkin A, Graubard BI, Schairer C. A prospective study of diet quality and mortality in women. JAMA 2000; 283:2109–2115.

74. Steffen LM, Wang L, Stevens J, Folsom AR. Consuming a western diet is associated with greater risk of mortality: The ARIC Study. Circulation 2004; 109:69.

75. Schoenborn CA, Adams PF, Barnes PM. Body weight status of adults: United States, 1997–98. Adv Data 2002; 330:1–15.

76. Winkleby MA, Kraemer HC, Ahn DK, Varady AN. Ethnic and socioeconomic differences in CVD risk factors: findings for women from the third National Health and Nutrition Examination Survey, 1988–94. JAMA 1998; 280:356–362.

77. Whitty CJM, Brunner EJ, Shipley MJ, Hemingway H, Marmot MG. Differences in biological risk factors for CVD between three ethnic groups in the Whitehall II study. Atherosclerosis 1999; 142: 279–286.

78. Dixon LB, Winkleby MA, Radimer KL. Dietary intakes and serum nutrients differ between adults from food-insufficient families and food-sufficient families: Third National Health and Nutrition Examination Survey, 1988–94. J Nutr 2001; 131:1232–1246.

25 Core Concepts in Nutritional Anthropology

Sera L. Young and Gretel H. Pelto

KEY POINTS

- Nutritional anthropology uses a holistic, biocultural approach to studying nutrition. It is fundamentally concerned with understanding the interrelationships of biological and social forces that shape human food use and the resulting nutritional status of individuals and populations.
- The ecological model provides a framework for understanding and modeling the human–food environment interactions that influence nutritional status.
- Attention to the adaptive process—how humans cope and adjust either genetically, physiologically, or socioculturally to meet material needs—is fundamental to research in nutritional anthropology.
- When describing nutrition-related practices, anthropologists try to present both the cultural insiders' ("emic") views of what people do and why as well as a more scientific, external ("etic") view. This is done because people's beliefs about food play a central role in their nutrition-related behavior.
- Methodologically, nutritional anthropological studies draw on research tools and techniques from multiple disciplines, ranging from nutritional biochemistry, physiology, genetics, and epidemiology to the social and policy sciences.

1. INTRODUCTION

In its development as a discipline whose aim is to understand the human animal and its place in the natural order of things, a hallmark of anthropology is that its practitioners often engage in research that has the effect of making the familiar strange, and the strange familiar. Nutritional anthropologists examine practices that are taken for granted as simply "normal" or "natural" and reveal how culture-bound they actually are. For example, the Euro-American organization of the structure of meals, in which foods are served sequentially with soup first and dessert last, strikes people in other parts of the world as quite peculiar. Looking outward beyond their own cultures, anthropologists seek to understand and "make sense" out of culinary practices that at first encounter

From: *Nutritional Health: Strategies for Disease Prevention, Second Edition*
Edited by: N. J. Temple, T. Wilson, and D. R. Jacobs © Humana Press Inc., Totowa, NJ

appear to be irrational, such as the prohibition of beef consumption in food-scarce, poor Hindu villages. On more careful study, this prohibition turns out to be ecologically sound because of the complex energetic relationships of animals, humans, fuel, and agricultural production in South Asia *(1)*.

Another objective of anthropology is to elucidate the variability across cultures in relation to human universals. Thus, nutritional anthropologists study food patterns, cultural practices related to food, and food production systems in various societies to understand how they meet or fail to meet nutritional requirements, and the health and social consequences of these nutritional decisions.

This chapter will outline the core concepts in nutritional anthropology that are used to accomplish these objectives.

2. NUTRITIONAL ANTHROPOLOGY: A BIOCULTURAL APPROACH TO UNDERSTANDING NUTRITION

For human beings, food has both sociocultural and biological dimensions. The symbolic meanings of food vary by society, as does the very definition of what is acceptable to consume. The analysis of food choice behavior, as well as its determinants and social consequences, involve the application of social science theories and methods. After it is consumed, the characteristics of food become the province of biological sciences, which are used to reveal how it is used for growth and maintenance of the body *(2)*. The field of nutritional anthropology attempts to integrate studies of human behavior and social organization (i.e., the sociocultural or "predental" aspects of food), with those of nutritional status, nutrient requirements, and growth (i.e., the biological or "postdental" aspects of food). Nutritional anthropology is "fundamentally concerned with understanding the interrelationships of biological and social forces in shaping human food use and the nutritional status of individuals and populations" *(3)*. Because it is focused particularly on the interactions of social and biological factors, nutritional anthropology is fundamentally biocultural in its approach.

The aim of much of the research conducted by nutritional anthropologists is to understand how the physical well-being of humans is affected by their food systems. This aim contrasts with the approach of cultural anthropologists, sociologists, and historians who use food as a vehicle for understanding how social and cultural systems work. Both orientations, however, yield knowledge about food and society, through time and across space.

3. AN ECOLOGICAL MODEL FOR NUTRITION

The ecological model was first introduced into nutritional anthropology by Jerome, Kandel, and Pelto *(4)*. It attempts to identify the multiple social and environmental factors that affect the nutrition of a population in a simple schematic but holistic manner. Although aspects of society are not as easily compartmentalized as Fig. 1 might imply, it is a heuristic tool that is useful for drawing attention to and organizing the complexities of the context of human nutrition. The model aims to encompass biological and cultural aspects of nutrition through their linkage with diet.

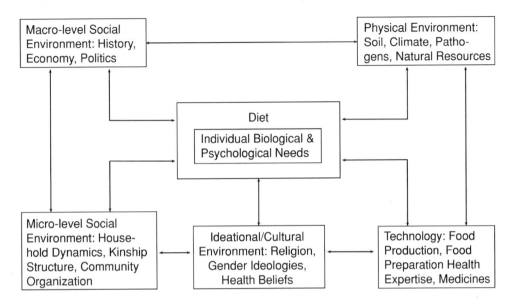

Fig. 1. An ecological model for Nutritional Anthropology. (Adapted from ref. *4*.)

The component labeled "physical environment" refers to the climate, soil characteristics, water resources, flora and fauna, land availability, pathogens, and other features that establish the conditions for food procurement and production. "Technology" includes the range of tools and techniques used for production, distribution, acquisition, storage, and preparation of all that is nutritionally valuable, including food and medicines. The "ideational environment" refers to cultural features, including beliefs about the role of food in well-being, cultural expectations related to health, definitions of food, gender ideologies, food taboos, and religious influences on diet. The "macro-level social setting" refers to politics, economics, and history, whereas the "micro-level social setting" refers to household dynamics, community organization, and kinship structure. All of these affect the diet of an individual, which, in turn, influences and is influenced by biological characteristics.

The ecological model can be considered a roadmap of a food system. "Food system" is a concept in nutritional anthropology that refers to the totality of activities, social institutions, material inputs and outputs, and cultural beliefs within a social group that are involved in the production, distribution, and consumption of food *(3)*. It is often a useful exercise to map out the food system that is being studied to identify the patterns of interaction among its components.

Methodologically, nutritional anthropological studies draw on research tools and techniques from multiple disciplines, ranging from nutritional biochemistry, physiology, genetics, and epidemiology to the social and policy sciences. Occasionally, nutritional anthropologists turn to humanistic scholarship as a source of insights into the cultural and historical aspects of food. Thus, multidisciplinary collaboration with scientists in other social and biological fields commonly occurs in anthropological research in nutrition. Typically, studies use open-ended interviews and participant observation to generate descriptive, qualitative data, as well as highly structured formats for interviews and physical measurements that yield data amenable to statistical analysis. Taken together, these complementary methodologies help to integrate multiple perspectives on human behavior and experience to explain nutritional conditions in a population.

4. THE ADAPTIVE PROCESS

Attention to the adaptive process—how humans cope and adjust to meet material needs—is fundamental to research in nutritional anthropology *(4)*. Three levels of adaptation are distinguished: (1) genetic adaptation, (2) physiological adaptation, and (3) sociocultural adaptation. Nutritional anthropologists tend to focus on the latter two because they are relatively more common and more rapid: humans are constantly responding to environmental change.

Examples of physiological adaptations are decreased basal metabolic rates during periods of starvation and expanded lung capacity when living at high altitudes. Sociocultural adaptations involve behavioral and technological innovations that improve people's ability to successfully exploit food resources. Examples of sociocultural adaptations include food prohibitions that serve to protect or regulate animal food sources and the development of methods for preparing foods that remove toxic substances and make them safe for human consumption.

When one finds long-standing food patterns, it is wise to investigate them to determine whether they represent positive cultural adaptations that optimize nutritional well-being. The traditional method of preparing maize in Mexico and Central America by soaking it in lime and water is a case in point. Examination of this practice revealed that the soak in an alkaline solution chemically frees up the niacin that would otherwise be metabolically unavailable, and therefore permits maize to be used as the primary food staple without putting the population at risk of pellagra *(5)*. In other parts of the world where this practice was not adopted, pellagra became a major public health problem when maize became a staple food.

5. DIFFERENTIATING EMIC AND ETIC PERSPECTIVES

"Emic" and "etic" are key concepts in the entire field of anthropology, not only in nutritional anthropology. Emic refers to the perspective of the "insiders" in a culture, the definitions and interpretations of reality as seen through local eyes and perceived through local ideas. The term etic is used to refer to the external, analytic perspective that is used by scientists when they are studying cultural and social phenomena. These concepts are important both methodologically and theoretically for nutritional anthropologists. With respect to description of nutrition-related practices, anthropologists try to obtain the emic perspectives of the people they are studying, to present the insiders' views of what they do and why. From a theoretical standpoint, etic analysis in nutritional anthropology depends heavily on concepts drawn from nutritional biochemistry, as well as on theories of biological and ecological adaptation.

From an etic perspective, some cultural features related to nutrition have negative consequences for health. For example, the cultural practice of restricting food intake during pregnancy, which is common in some South Asian communities, contributes to the widespread prevalence of dangerously low birth-weight. However, larger infant size at birth, for which greater food intake is a significant determinant, increases the risk of serious problems in delivery that threaten the life of both mother and baby. Thus, there appears to be some logic to the practice of restricting food intake during pregnancy, although it clearly has a negative component.

For the purpose of programmatic decisions, Jelliffe and Bennett (6) suggested that food practices could be classified into four categories from the perspective of their impact on health: practices that are harmful, those that are beneficial, neutral practices, and practices whose health impact is unknown. Although an emic explanation might be "wrong" from the current scientific point of view, in many situations there is not enough knowledge about a particular practice to determine whether it is beneficial, harmful, or neutral in that particular setting, a fact that was clearly recognized by Jelliffe and Bennett. The etic perspective is also incomplete and changes over time with the development of new theories and empirical findings.

The two perspectives, emic and etic, may not be mutually exclusive; there is room for both explanations in the ecological model outlined earlier. Taken together, the concepts of emic and etic help to better characterize food practices. Because people's beliefs about food play a central role in their nutrition-related behavior, understanding the emic perspective is usually an essential step in the design and development of interventions that aim to reduce the burden of human disease through improved nutrition.

6. APPLYING AN ECOLOGICAL PERSPECTIVE TO UNDERSTAND INGESTION PRACTICES: PICA ON PEMBA ISLAND, ZANZIBAR

To illustrate the utility of the concepts outlined thus far, we have modeled how the ecological perspective can be applied to understand a seemingly aberrant nutritional behavior that was encountered in the course of the fieldwork by one author (SLY):

SLY: What else do you eat when you're pregnant?

Pemban woman: Umm…every day, twice a day, I eat some earth scraped from the house walls.

6.1. What Is Pica?

Pica is broadly defined as the persistent eating of nonnutritive substances (7). The name comes from the magpie, *Pica pica*, a bird known for its indiscriminate appetite (8). Yet those who ingest pica substances do not consume them indiscriminately; only certain nonfood substances are craved and subsequently consumed, particularly earth, laundry starch, large quantities of ice (as much as an 8-lb bag per day), and uncooked rice. Pica has been observed in over 200 cultures, from the United States, Africa, Central America, South America, India, the Middle East, and Europe (9). It is not a habit that has disappeared with "modernity," as some researchers had predicted (10); the practice remains common in rural and urban settings around the world (11–13). Picas seem to be especially common among pregnant women, among whom prevalence rates have been documented to be as high as 66% in the United States (14) and even higher in developing countries (15,16). In some parts of the world the consumption of earth is even considered to be a "symptom" of pregnancy (17–19). In short, the consumption of substances few would consider as food is not an uncommon behavior.

6.2. Pica in Pemba

Pemba is the second biggest island in the Zanzibar archipelago, which lies in the Indian Ocean, just off the coast of Tanzania. It is a lush tropical island; clove and seaweed farming are the main economic activities. Swahili is the predominant language, Islam is the most commonly practiced religion, and the culture is similar to the rest of coastal East Africa. The social system is patriarchal, polygynous, and patrilineal.

In Pemba, nonfood substances are predominantly eaten by pregnant women. The three most commonly ingested nonfood items are *mchele* (husked but uncooked rice), *udongo* (soil, clay, or dirt), and ice. Soil is sought out from specific locations: a pit located outside the village, the foundations of houses, or termite mounds. It is sometimes dried in the sun and then eaten, or crushed into a powder and mixed with water. All of the soils consumed are notably smooth and are obtained from places not likely to be contaminated by human or animal excretions. Ice consumption is not always pica; a few chunks are not a nutritional aberration but rather a refreshing and rare treat. However, Pemban women who were nauseated during pregnancy ate as much as 12 glasses of ice per day. Less commonly mentioned substances were ash, dust, charcoal, powdered shells, chalk, and soil soaked with cow's urine, all of which women encountered in the course of their daily lives *(19)*.

6.3. The Emic Perspective on Pica in Pemba

There is an element of embarrassment or shyness about pica; most informants switched to the third person when beginning to discuss it. "*They* like it because they are pregnant." "*They* just like it too much." "*They* don't do it again after giving birth." But after some nonjudgmental conversation, women warmed to the subject and began to enjoy discussing the motivations for their cravings.

Pembans explained pregnant women's pica cravings in similar ways. "Everyone eats them when they are pregnant." "It is just a sign of pregnancy." "Eating that stuff is just a habit of pregnant women." When further probed about why pica was a habit, they could only explain that it is a *kileo*, a craving or addiction. Pica outside of pregnancy was seen as more problematic, less healthy, and even indicative of mental illness.

6.4. Etic Perspective: Pica as an Adaptation

Until recently, picas have been characterized as harmful, "depraved appetites," and held responsible for a long list of detrimental side effects including dental damage, intestinal blockage, constipation, peritonitis, caloric displacement, iron deficiency, fatigue, lead poisoning, geohelminth infection, lead poisoning, toxemia, hypertension, tetanus, and heightened susceptibility to infection *(14,20–23)*.

The way in which pica is practiced in Pemba makes it difficult to associate it with negative effects. The quantities of earth consumed have been estimated to be about 40 g/d; an amount unlikely to cause intestinal blockage. The soils that are eaten are chosen because of their soft texture and easy dissolvability; therefore they are not likely to harm the mouth. Furthermore, soils are usually collected far from contaminated sites.

Using the ecological model outlined previously, it becomes possible to hypothesize that pica is a positive sociocultural adaptation to the condition of pregnancy. Several useful effects of pica have been suggested. Many, but not all, ingested soils have biologically important quantities of minerals, especially iron and calcium *(24,25)*. Whether or not these minerals are bioavailable, and the extent to which the soil binds minerals that are already present in the diet so that dietary minerals are no longer biologically available, is not presently known and needs to be examined on a sample-by-sample basis. To that end, chemical analysis of pica substances on Pemba is currently being undertaken. Mineral supplementation of the diet may occur not only as a consequence of the mineral content of the earths that are consumed, but also because their consumption slows the motility of the gastrointestinal tract, thereby allowing more time for nutrients to be absorbed before being excreted *(26)*.

Pica in Pemba may also be useful for relieving gastrointestinal distress (i.e., nausea, vomiting, and diarrhea). Many clays contain kaolin, which has a soothing effect on the intestinal tract. (The commercial antidiarrheal medicine, Kaopectate®, originally contained kaolin.) Quelling nausea enables women to consume (more) food. Furthermore, preventing diarrhea and vomiting permits the nutrients that are consumed to remain in the digestive tract long enough to be absorbed.

Several researchers have proposed other adaptive benefits of geophagy, not related to the mineral content of soil, but to the earth's capacity as a detoxifier *(25,27–30)*. Based on their biochemical analyses of geophagous soils, Johns and Duquette *(30)* argue that although geophagy can be a source of nutrients, "detoxification broadly defined" is the most satisfactory explanation for this practice. The clays may form a protective coating on the mucous membrane of the digestive tract that protects the mucosal cells from damage by toxins. It may protect the vulnerable fetus from exposure to teratogens *(27,28)*. A change in gastric pH brought about by the clays may also destroy gastrointestinal parasites *(30)*.

There are a number of alternative adaptive and nonadaptive hypotheses for pica in general and for geophagia in particular. One of us (SLY) in company with a behavioral ecologist (Paul Sherman) has initiated an extensive exploration of the costs and benefits of pica and geophagia and thus the likelihood of these various possibilities.

Seen in the holistic context that the ecological model helps to delineate, our understanding of picas as a nutritional adaptation is beginning to emerge. For Pemban women, who have limited access to medicines and adequate health care, who are frequently undernourished and repeatedly exposed to environmental toxins that endanger the developing fetus, and who commonly experience pregnancy-related nausea and vomiting, pica begins to "make sense."

Finally, it should be noted that the emic and etic explanations of pica in Pemba are complementary. A Pemban husband explained his wife's geophagy as "a sign of her pregnancy;" an American dietitian attributed the expectant Pemban woman's consumption of earth to a mineral deficiency. There is a place for both types of explanation; the Pemban woman may be nutritionally deficient *because of* the added demands of pregnancy.

7. TYPES OF RESEARCH IN NUTRITIONAL ANTHROPOLOGY

The types of research undertaken by nutritional anthropologists can be classified into the following main categories: (1) sociocultural processes and nutrition; (2) social epidemiology of nutrition; (3) cultural/ideational systems and nutrition; (4) physiological adaptation, population genetics, and nutrition; and (5) applied research for nutrition programs *(31)*.

7.1. Sociocultural Processes and Nutrition

Investigations that can be categorized as studies of "sociocultural processes and nutrition" often focus on large-scale processes of change, such as globalization, modernization, urbanization, changing women's roles, and technological change. The studies are aimed at understanding how these processes affect food and nutrition. Although many investigators conduct studies in which they examine the effects of broad social processes in a specific location (e.g., rural to urban migration in a particular developing country), others are concerned with understanding how large-scale changes have affected nutritional conditions across many populations. The basic structure of the questions that nutritional anthropologists ask about the relationship of sociocultural processes to nutrition is: "What is the impact of X (a sociocultural process) on nutrition?"

Anthropological studies on the health and nutritional consequences of the historical and global shift from a foraging-hunting mode of subsistence to settled agriculture food systems are examples of research whose underlying aim is to understand the impact of a sociocultural process on nutrition. To accomplish this, investigators use a variety of biological techniques; they analyze skeletal and plant remains from archeological sites so as to evaluate changes in nutritional status and other health status indicators in relation to information on changes in diet and lifestyle. For example, Goodman and colleagues *(32)* made detailed studies of skeletal remains, comparing the types of lesions produced by malnutrition and disease before and after the adoption of agriculture. This was done in archeological sites in Illinois where agriculture spread into the region from Meso-America many centuries before the arrival of Europeans. Substantial evidence was found suggesting that the people who lived by foraging and hunting had fewer signs of disease and poor nutrition and greater longevity. Similar evidence has been obtained from many other parts of the world *(33)*. The differences cannot, of course, be attributed only to diet because other factors, including increasing population density and disease exposure, also played important roles.

7.2. Social Epidemiology of Nutrition

Nutritional anthropological research that falls into the category of "social epidemiology of nutrition" resembles other types of epidemiological studies in nutrition. Investigators examine relationships between sociodemographic factors, which are conceptualized as determinants of food intake and/or nutritional outcomes. When such studies are conducted by anthropologists, the emphasis is on cultural factors, as well as on other social and biological characteristics. The research question takes the general form: "What are the determinants or factors associated with X (dietary practice or nutritional condition) in a particular population group or between different populations?"

Among the topics that have attracted attention are social and ecological determinants of micronutrient deficiencies, interactions of socioeconomic and cultural factors in infant and young child growth faltering, and the role of cultural perceptions about health and beauty as predictors of obesity.

Anthropologist Daniel Sellen's work among the Datoga, a pastoral group in Tanzania, is illustrative *(34)*. He was interested in the determinants of nutritional status in children in a small-scale society whose economy depends on raising livestock. One of the factors he considered was the role of polygyny. In a culture in which having several wives is a social goal for men and indicates their relative economic superiority, one would expect that children of polygynous marriages would be better off nutritionally than children whose mother was the only wife. Contrary to this expectation, Sellen found that the anthropometric status of children in families with multiple wives was poorer than for single wife families, even when the overall wealth of the family was taken into account in his statistical models. This finding, an example of "social epidemiology of nutrition," led him to a further ethnographic examination of resource use in Datoga households.

Another way in which this type of research is practiced by nutritional anthropologists is by incorporating sociocultural factors in baseline epidemiological studies that are undertaken before the design of public health interventions. Research by Noel, Gittelsohn, and colleagues (35) is illustrative of this approach. In poor populations throughout the world, fatness is culturally valued because it indicates that the individual has enough to eat and is well provided for by his or her family. On the other hand, the fact that over-weight and obesity present serious threats to health is also becoming more and more widely known. Therefore, at the beginning of a project to prevent obesity and diabetes in a native American population in the southwestern part of the United States, the senior anthropologist in the research team, Joel Gittelsohn, felt it was important to assess beliefs about healthy body size before the intervention was designed.

Gittelsohn first conducted ethnographic research to develop an understanding of local people's perceptions about healthy body size and eating, including their views about how these applied to young children. This information was used to design questions for a large-scale survey that included data on food intake, body mass index (BMI), health status, sociodemographic characteristics, and cultural/ideational variables. Using epidemiological statistical methods, the investigators examined the relationship of caregivers' perceptions about the importance of controlling food intake of preschoolers and concerns about weight with the children's BMI, an indicator of child size and fatness. They found that caregivers who expressed greater worry about their children's weight and restricted their eating also had heavier children. This relationship remained statistically significant, even when parental BMI, sociodemographic variables, and the frequency of consumption of specific foods were taken into account. Thus, the epidemiological investigation shows that in spite of the poverty and history of hunger the community has experienced, many families are well aware of the dangers of being overweight and are trying to take steps to deal with it in their young children. What the community needs is better knowledge and behavioral strategies for managing the problem.

7.3. Ideational Systems and Nutrition

Studies in the area of cultural/ideational systems and nutrition are often aimed at understanding how particular beliefs relate to food selection, including food prescriptions and proscriptions, as well as responses to food and nutrient-related illness. The ways in which culturally structured food avoidances in pregnancy or in childhood illness affect health outcomes are among the topics investigated by nutritional anthropologists who link their work to public health issues. The general format of the basic research question that characterizes studies on "ideational systems and nutrition" is: "What is the relationship of X (beliefs) to Y (food practice, nutritional or health condition)?"

An investigation of vitamin A deficiency in two areas of Niger in West Africa by anthropologist Lauren Blum illustrates this type of research (36). The first phase of her study involved in-depth interviews with mothers and traditional healers. In an arid northern region where there was reason to expect people to be familiar with the signs of vitamin A deficiency, many people mentioned traditional cures for night blindness (a sign of vitamin A deficiency) that involved consuming liver (an ideal practice because it contains a high level of vitamin A). In-depth interviews led Blum to hypothesize that these home remedies were not the result of nutrition education by outside public health activities, but were indigenous practices that had been passed down through the generations. In another part of the country, where higher rainfall supported more fruit and vegetable varieties, the people whom she interviewed did not describe these traditional remedies.

The second phase of her study was designed to assess how people respond to signs and symptoms of vitamin A deficiency and where they would turn for help in managing these problems. To obtain the data she used a "scenario method" in which a sample of mothers was presented with several different scenarios illustrating different manifestations of vitamin A deficiency in children and pregnant women. As each "story" was presented, the respondent was asked a series of questions concerning the causes of the signs and symptoms and was asked to recommend treatment strategies. In the arid northern region, the majority of the mothers said that both the child and the pregnant woman with night blindness were suffering from a food-related malady and felt that home remedies that involved liver should be used to treat it. In the tropical region, some respondents felt that night blindness was caused by a disease, whereas others thought it was the result of witchcraft. Depending on their views of the etiology, they recommended that the afflicted person should be taken either to a medical doctor or to a traditional specialist who deals with witchcraft. From this example we see that in both communities the interpretations people make of a nutritional problem is highly influenced by local cultural knowledge.

7.4. Population Genetics and Nutrition

Another area of research in nutritional anthropology is the relationship between genetic variability in populations and food consumption patterns. Nutritional anthropologists who are interested in the relationship of nutrition to biological experiences of populations often conduct research to elucidate how the nutritional history of a population has shaped or influenced its physiological or genetic characteristics.

Studies on population distributions of lactose tolerance in adults are illustrative of this type of research. Anthropologists have sought to understand the genetic distribution of the trait that makes it possible for adults in some populations to consume milk when the common pattern is for humans to lose their capacity to digest lactose after childhood. The role of this genetic trait has been explored in relation to the development of dairy-based food economies in northern Europe and some regions of Africa (37). It is likely that there will be an expansion of this type of research with the development of new techniques and knowledge in nutritional genomics.

7.5. Applied Research for Nutrition Programs

In addition to conducting basic research, some nutritional anthropologists also engage in applied research, which is undertaken in direct support of public health activities. Often investigations that fall in this category involve community-level investigations, although applied nutritional anthropology may also be carried out for the purpose of informing national-level or international nutrition policy and planning. Community-level studies may focus on identifying the sociocultural factors that need to be taken into account in instituting intervention activities (i.e., "formative research") or in process evaluations to see how these factors are affecting the utilization of programs.

Another type of research activity that falls into this category is the development of tools that can be used by nutrition and health programs to quickly and efficiently collect and analyze data on local conditions to plan or reorganize intervention activities. The RAP (Rapid Assessment Procedures) Manual *(38,39)* and the guidelines for focused ethnographic studies of vitamin A *(40)* are examples of such tools; they have been used across a wide range of countries and situations.

8. CONCLUSIONS: IMPLICATIONS OF THE NUTRITIONAL ANTHROPOLOGICAL PERSPECTIVE

Nutritional anthropology is a discipline that approaches the analysis of nutritional conditions within and across populations in a holistic fashion, as exemplified by the ecological model. The ecological model provides a general framework for understanding and modeling the human–food environment interactions that influence nutritional status. The holistic, biocultural approach requires competency in several types of methodologies, and familiarity with both biological and cultural aspects of human nutrition. As a result, the studies that nutritional anthropologists conduct are usually multidisciplinary and collaborative, bringing together investigators from several scientific fields. The inclusion of cultural/ideational elements in their explanatory frameworks often requires researchers to step into the worldview of the people whom they are studying to obtain emic interpretations, as well as testing etic theories.

"Strategies for disease prevention" is the subject of this volume. In this chapter we have focused on nutritional anthropology as a research strategy that is useful for generating a holistic understanding of nutritional behaviors. We used the example of pica on Pemba to show how this perspective can lead to new ways of conceptualizing the analysis of cultural food practices. Once regarded with derision, pica is beginning to make sense as an adaptive strategy when contextualized in terms of the social and physiological burdens pregnant Pemban women face.

Finally, in addition to illustrating the range and types of research questions that nutritional anthropologists address, we have also attempted to indicate the value of incorporating anthropological approaches into research that is undertaken to help solve public health problems and facilitate the translation of basic nutrition knowledge into actions to improve people's health.

REFERENCES

1. Harris M. India's sacred cow. Human Nature 1978;2 Feb:28–36.
2. Quandt SA. Nutrition in medical anthropology. In: Sargent CF, Johnson TM, eds. Medical Anthropology. Praeger, Westport, CT, 1996, pp. 272–289.
3. Pelto GH, Goodman AH, Dufour DL. The biocultural perspective in nutritional anthropology. In: Goodman AH, Dufour DL, Pelto GH, eds. Nutritional Anthropology. Mayfield Publishing Company, Mountain View, CA, 2000, pp. 1–9.

4. Jerome NW, Kandel RF, Pelto GH. An ecological approach to nutritional anthropology. In: Jerome NW, Kandel RF, Pelto GH, eds. Nutritional Anthropology: Contemporary Approaches to Diet and Culture. Redgrave Publishing Company, New York, 1980, pp. 13–45.

5. Katz SH, Hediger ML, Valleroy LA. Traditional maize processing techniques in the New World. Science 1975;184:765–773.

6. Jelliffe DB, Bennett FJ. Cultural and anthropological factors in infant and maternal nutrition. Fed Proc 1961;20:185–188.

7. Cooper M. Pica. Charles C. Publisher, Springfield, Illinois, 1957.

8. Lackey CJ. Pica–a nutritional anthropology concern. In: Bauwens EE, ed. The Anthropology of Health. C.V. Mosby, St. Louis, MO, 1976, pp. 121–129.

9. Danford DE. Pica and Nutrition. Ann Rev Nutr 1982;2:303–322.

10. Horner RD, Lackey CJ, Kolasa K. Pica Practices of Pregnant Women. J Am Diet Assoc 1991;91:34–38.

11. Grigsby RK, Thyer BA, Waller RJ, Johnston GA. Chalk eating in middle Georgia: A culture-bound syndrome of pica. South Med J 1999;92:190–192.

12. Woywodt A, Kiss A. Geophagia, a forgotten diagnosis? S Afr J Surg 2000;38:42.

13. Kettaneh A, Sontag C, Fain O, Thomas M. Perception du pica et de ses relations avec la carence martiale par les medecins hospitaliers de la region parisienne. Presse Med 2001;30:155–158.

14. Sayetta RB. Pica: An overview. Am Fam Physician 1986;33:181–185.

15. Hooper D, Mann HH. Earth-eating and the earth-eating habit in India. Memoirs of the Asiatic Society of Bengal 1906;1:249–270.

16. Vermeer DE. Geophagy among the Ewe of Ghana. Ethnology 1971;10:56–72.

17. Vermeer DE. Geophagy among the Tiv of Nigeria. Ann Assoc Amer Geogr 1966;56:197–204.

18. Laufer B. Geophagy. Field Museum of Natural History, Chicago, Illinois, 1930:99–198.

19. Young SL. "Listen, Without blood there is no life": An ethnography of anemia during pregnancy. Nutr Anthrop 2004;26(1–2):10–19.

20. Rothenberg SJ, Manalo M, Jiang J, et al. Maternal blood lead level during pregnancy in south central Los Angeles. Arch Environ Health 1999;54:151–157.

21. Kirchner JT. Management of pica: A medical enigma. Am Fam Physician 2001;63:1117.

22. Halsted JA. Geophagia in man: Its nature and nutritional effects. Am J Clin Nutr 1968;21:1384–1393.

23. Key TC, Horger EO, Miller JM. Geophagia as a cause of maternal death. Obstet Gynecol 1982;60:525, 526.

24. Cronk L. From hunters to herders: Subsistence change as a reproductive strategy among the Mukogodo. Curr Anthrop 1989;30:224–234.

25. Wiley AS, Katz SH. Geophagy in pregnancy: A test of a hypothesis. Curr Anthrop 1998;39:532–545.

26. Oke OL. Rickets in developing countries. World Rev Nutr Diet 1972;15:86–103.

27. Profet M. Pregnancy sickness as adaptation: A deterrent to maternal ingestion of teratogens. In: Barkow JH, Cosmides L, Tooby J, eds. The Adapted Mind: Evolutionary Psychology and the Generation of Culture. Oxford University Press, Oxford, 1992, pp. 327–366.

28. Nesse RM, Williams GC. Why We Get Sick: The New Science of Darwinian Medicine. Vintage, New York, 1996.

29. Johns T. The chemical ecology of human ingestive behaviors. Ann Rev Anthrop 1999;28:27–50.

30. Johns T, Duquette M. Detoxification and mineral supplementation as functions of geophagy. Am J Clin Nutr 1991;53:448–456.

31. Pelto GH. Nutritional anthropology. Encyclopedia of Food and Culture. Vol. 2. Scribners, New York, 2002, pp. 595, 596.

32. Goodman AH, Lallo J, Armelagos GJ, Rose JC. Health changes at Dickson Mounds, Illinois (AD 950-1300). In: Cohen MN, Armelagos GJ, eds. Paleopathology at the Origins of Agiculture. Academic Press, New York, 1984, pp. 271–306.

33. Cohen MN. Health and the Rise of Civilizations. Yale University Press, New Haven, CT, 1989.

34. Sellen D. Polygyny and child growth in a traditional pastoral society: The case of the Datoga of Tanzania. Hum Nat 1999;10:329–371.

35. Noel J, Gittelsohn J, Ethelbah B, Caballero B. Caregivers' perceptions and feeding practices are related to weight status of American Indian preschool children. FASEB J 2003;17:4, 5. (abstract no. 445.9).

36. Blum L, Pelto G, Pelto P. Coping with a nutrient deficiency: Cultural models of vitamin A deficiency in northern Niger. Med Anthrop 2004;23:195–227.
37. McCracken RD. Lactase deficiency: An example of dietary evolution. Curr Anthrop 1971;12:479–517.
38. Scrimshaw N, Gleason G. Rapid Assessment Procedures: Qualitative Methodologies for Planning and Evaluation of Health Related Programmes. International Nutrition Foundation for Developing Countries, Boston, 1992.
39. Scrimshaw S, Hurtado E. Rapid Assessment Procedures for Nutrition and Primary Health Care: Anthropological Approaches to Improving Programme Effectiveness. Latin American Studies Center, Los Angeles, 1987.
40. Blum L, Pelto P, Pelto G, Kuhnlein H. Community Assessment of Natural Food Sources of Vitamin A: Guidelines for an Ethnographic Protocol. International Nutrition Foundation for Developing Countries and International Development Research Center, Boston, 1997.

26 Nutrition on the Internet

Tony Helman

KEY POINTS

- The defining characteristics of the Internet are its size and decentralized nature, allowing distance-independent communication, universal availability of information, and immediate interactivity.
- For health professionals seeking nutrition information, this has allowed vastly improved access to the current medical literature through resources such as PubMed and a number of nutrition e-journals. Practice guidelines, food nutrient analysis, and course material are other useful resources, examples of which are provided in this chapter.
- A huge variety of individuals and organizations publish nutrition material on the Internet. This means that web portal sites that catalogue and list other websites are an important starting point for finding relevant material.
- Individual judgment will always be required to assess the credibility and accuracy of any Internet resource.

1. INTRODUCTION

Over the last few years the Internet—the fastest growing communication medium in history—has fulfilled some of its promise to markedly impact our professional, educational, and personal lives. At the same time, it has created its own difficulties and challenges. In this chapter we examine some of those issues as they apply to the world of nutrition.

2. WHAT IS THE INTERNET?

The Internet is a network that connects computers globally. It is distinguished from other computer networks by two unique characteristics, namely its size and its decentralized organization:

2.1. Size

Nobody knows for sure how many computers are connected to the Internet, nor how many people have access to the Internet through those computers. The best guesstimate of the total number of Internet users globally in the year 2004 is more than 800 million

From: *Nutritional Health: Strategies for Disease Prevention, Second Edition*
Edited by: N. J. Temple, T. Wilson, and D. R. Jacobs © Humana Press Inc., Totowa, NJ

(1). This represents a high rate of growth compared to the figure of 260 million that appeared in the previous edition of this book. Usage was originally biased heavily towards the Western world, and in many Western countries more than two-thirds of the population now uses the Internet. But in recent years, Asia has also experienced phenomenal Internet growth with, for example, an estimated 87 million users in China and two-thirds of the population of South Korea going "on-line." Africa, however, remains far behind with a less than 2% of the population having Internet access *(1)*.

2.2. Decentralized

Because of its origins as a communication medium for institutions engaged in military research, the Internet was deliberately organized to be free of central administration as much as possible (by diffusing control, it is more protected from deliberate attack or malfunction). Thus there is no central controlling body to set or police standards of content, acceptable use, etc. This has created both benefits (exchange of information remains on the whole uncensored and free of taxes) and problems (an epidemic of unwanted emails, pornography, and cyber-crime).

3. IMPLICATIONS

Stemming directly from these two defining elements, the Internet as a medium has three striking characteristics:

1. Distance-independent communication.
2. Universal availability of information.
3. Immediate interactivity.

As you might expect, these characteristics can be applied both for our benefit and to our detriment.

3.1. Distance-Independent Communication

The Internet is the first communications medium in history for which the cost and ease of use is essentially independent of distance. In the case of email, for example, the unit cost of sending an email is essentially zero (i.e., it costs very little more to send an email to one thousand people than to one person). This has engendered a new form of communication called a mailing list. Sometimes known as a discussion list, this is a way in which large numbers of people can discuss topics of mutual interest by sharing emails among the whole group. There are many such nutrition mailing lists, both professional and lay.

These same factors can, however, create problems, an obvious example being the spawning of a large and rapidly increasing volume of spam (unsolicited communication, frequently with commercial or pornographic elements). Another problem of academic relevance is the greatly heightened potential to spread rumor and create libel by even a casually penned email sent to multiple recipients. Although the law on Internet libel remains not entirely clear, some recent legal precedents suggest that those who post content on the Internet carry potential liability over much wider territory than ever before *(2)*. This should certainly make any academic careful about what they say in any email that has multiple recipients, or on any website, mailing list discussion, or bulletin board posting.

3.2. "Universal" Availability of Information

Although "universal" in this context means "universal among those with Internet access," the ability of the Internet to make information available instantaneously across the globe is quite unparalleled in human history. The volume and diversity of websites currently available has continued to grow at a brisk pace—those search engines whose business is to catalog web pages count in the order of 6 billion such pages *(3)*, but nobody knows with any accuracy what proportion of the web this represents.

The web has effectively democratized the flow of information. In essence, it is a gigantic library, and indeed librarians themselves now use it as much as teachers, students, and anyone else who has access to the Internet as a major—if not the first—source for seeking information on just about any topic. "Look it up on the Internet" has become the catch-cry for the 21st-century information gatherer!

It is hard to quantify the impact this has had on global access to information, but it has certainly shortened from weeks to hours the time that it takes a new piece of information, or misinformation, to spread and become "common currency" throughout the world.

Newspapers from *The New York Times* to the *Zimbabwe Chronicle* have websites where up-to-the minute news can be read at any time *(4)*. If you are interested specifically in nutrition news—whether it be academic research, food or supplement business, or the latest fad diet—many media websites have sections or will send you emails specifically devoted to the subject (e.g., *The New York Times [5]* or CNN *[6]*). Medical textbooks can be kept up-to-date by having continuously fresh text placed on a companion website. *Harrison's Textbook of Medicine*, for example, provides daily content updates from its editors and contributors and information on the latest clinical trials *(7)*.

Even if many physicians do not avail themselves of such web resources, many of their patients probably do. In a recent survey of American urban primary care clinics, a third of the patients had used the Internet to obtain health information within the preceding 12 mo, and nutrition was one of the main topics they studied *(8)*. As health professionals throughout the world have discovered, this can affect the balance of knowledge in the consultation between themselves and their patients *(9)*.

Requiring health professionals to stay up-to-date with what their patients may be reading on the Internet has some advantages, but there are also a number of unquestionable challenges to such democratization of information. One problem that any Internet user will be familiar with is the difficulty in finding the specific information you are after. In essence, the Internet is a library without any cataloguing system. Although there are many websites that attempt to provide some semblance of organization (known as "web portals"), and search engines that ceaselessly trawl the web adding to their enormous database of web page content, it is still no easy task to find specific information.

The other closely related challenge is that the Internet is inherently incapable of vouching for the accuracy of the material within an apparently useful website. Indeed, a number of studies have shown that a significant proportion of the health information presented on the Internet lacks good scientific foundation *(10–12)*.

Search engines such as Google *(13)* attempt to get around this dilemma in its search listings by weighting websites according to the number of other websites that link to that site (and further weighting these weightings by the ranking of those linking sites themselves). In essence, they are working on the principle that if a lot of well-visited sites appear to like this website, it is probably a good site. Yet it remains very much the responsibility of the user to use their critical faculties to assess the accuracy and relevance on any information being presented.

3.3. Immediate Interactivity

The Internet allows immediate and, if desired, anonymous interaction. Direct on-line messaging and chatting, supplemented in many cases by a web-cam (a low-resolution video camera attached to the computer and thus feeding an image directly into the Internet) allows the creation of virtual communities, often with a specific common interest, which has enormous potential to facilitate teaching and learning.

Let us look at just a few examples of the academic and patient care applications of this immediate interactivity. On-line surveys can be conducted by email or directly from a web page, potentially allowing access to large and diverse samples while maintaining subject privacy (14). Such survey methods can also display the accumulating results in real time. Virtual seminars conducted on the Internet allow "delegates," not only to watch a conference paper as it is being presented half-way round the world, but to participate in the discussion (15). Doctors can be encouraged to report their mistakes via a web form that entirely maintains their anonymity (16), and students can learn at their own pace through interactive Internet-based courses (17).

In providing clinical care to patients, new forms of support can be provided via inter-active programs (18), particularly for situations, such as chronic disease or lifestyle change, where support may need to be ongoing (19,20). Patients can be helped by one of the innumerable patient support websites and mailing lists that exist on the Internet (21).

4. NUTRITION APPLICATIONS

There are nutrition applications paralleling all of the above features of the Internet. Broadly, these resources can be divided into those for the lay public and those for health professionals. This chapter will focus mainly on the latter, if only because the scope of lay nutrition resources is too large to cover. (The search engine Google lists more than 44 million "hits" under the key word "nutrition" as of January 2005 [22]).

4.1. Accessing Research

The ability to have rapid access to current, published, peer-reviewed research (along with expert and meta-analysis of that research) is the cornerstone of evidence-based medical practice. The Internet has made such access to the medical literature possible throughout the globe to an extent that could not even have been imagined 10 yr ago.

Perhaps the premier Internet resource for those seeking to check on the latest published research in nutrition is the US National Library of Medicine's Medline data base of published articles. Although there are many ways of accessing this on-line, the Library provides its own entirely free access points, such as PubMed (23). Medline Plus is an additional service that has more of a lay focus, but also offers health professional resources, and has a nutrition subset (24).

For those interested in learning about research trials still in their planning or recruitment phase a useful website from the National Institutes of Health is www.clinical trials.gov *(25)*.

Many nutrition journals now have an on-line presence, generally providing abstracts without charge but requiring per article payment or journal subscription to access the full text. Many also publish their tables of contents for distribution via email. Some provide on-line access to articles before their release in print form. For a partial list of some of the main nutrition journals with significant on-line presence *see* Table 1.

Some general medical journals, such as the *British Medical Journal (26)*, offer to provide email notification whenever an article relevant to a specific topic, such as nutrition, is published. Some journals offer to email you whenever a selected academic paper is referenced by a subsequent paper.

There are also third-party Internet resources that can help keep track of the latest nutrition research from a variety of journals. *Amedeo:Nutrition* sends weekly emails with a simple collated list of the new articles published in a range of nutrition journals selected by the user *(27)*. *Doctor's Guide* is a physician website with a section reporting news on nutrition and metabolism from a variety of sources, as well as having webcasts and case histories *(28)*.

The Arbor Clinical Nutrition Updates takes this one step further by summarizing each week several recent research papers on one specific clinical topic, and providing commentary on the meaning of that research for clinicians. As a measure of the impact of the Internet in promoting nutrition communication, this e-journal is the world's most widely read nutrition publication, having approx 110,000 readers (as of August 2005) and published in nine languages *(29)*.

Journals are increasingly using web-based platforms to allow authors to submit papers, and referees to review them, which usually results in a substantial decrease in the lead times between submission and publishing. The *Medical Journal of Australia* went several steps further in two pilot trials, in one of which their invited reviewers participated in on-line discussion about the papers under review, and in another of which any interested visitors to the website were invited to submit comments on selected papers under consideration for publishing *(30)*.

The obvious next step is to publish a journal entirely on-line, and there are at least two such nutrition journals—*Nutrition and Metabolism (31)* and *Nutrition Journal. (32)*. *Clinmed NetPrints (33)* is an on-line journal site with a nutrition section that allows articles to be published without peer review. The website Biomed Central *(34)*, which hosts the first two of the above two journals, is one of the leading websites in publishing journal articles for free on-line access.

These developments are just one part of a much broader movement of open-access publishing that seeks to make the full content of academic journals available to everyone at no charge, while also facilitating the publication of research papers. This movement is not restricted to the Internet, having been given impetus in late 2004 by the United States National Institutes of Health proposing that all research funded by it (which makes up nearly one-third of material published in biomedical journals) should be made freely avail-

Table 1
Some Nutrition Journals With On-Line Content

American Journal of Clinical Nutrition	www.ajcn.org/
Annals of Nutrition & Metabolism	www.karger.com/anm
Asia Pacific Journal of Clinical Nutrition	www.blackwell-synergy.com/Journals/member/institutions/issuelist.asp?journal=ajc
British Journal of Nutrition	www.cabi-publishing.org/Journals.asp?SubjectArea=&PID=63
Clinical Nutrition	www.harcourt-international.com/journals/clnu/
European Journal of Clinical Nutrition	www.nature.com/ejcn/
International Journal of Obesity	www.nature.com/ijo/
Journal of the American Dietetic Association	www.adajournal.org
Journal of the American College of Nutrition	www.jacn.org/
Nutrition	www.elsevier.com/wps/find/journaldescription.cws_home/525614/description
Nutrition and Metabolism	www.nutritionandmetabolism.com
Nutrition Research Reviews	www.cabi-publishing.org/Journals.asp?SubjectArea=&PID=65
Public Health Nutrition	www.cabi-publishing.org/Journals.asp?SubjectArea=&PID=10
Journal of Nutrition	www.nutrition.org/

For a comprehensive list of over 160 nutrition and food science journals websites, *see* the Arbor Nutrition Guide (select: Applied → Journals, newsletters, books) (From ref. 37).

able *(35)*. However, it has very much been driven by those unique characteristics of the Internet that we have been discussing. It is likely that this movement will bring about profound challenges and changes in the world of academic publishing during the next 5 yr.

4.2. Clinical Resources

A large range of web resources for nutrition professionals is available on the Internet. Obviously, only the tiniest sample can be mentioned here, so perhaps the first type of resource to mention is the nutrition portal sites.

4.2.1. PORTAL SITES

A web portal is a site that contains information about and links to other websites. It helps the user to find things. A portal specializing in nutrition sites is likely to be of more value than a general search engine or directory.

There are two leading nutrition portal sites on the Internet. For the lay public, Tufts University's Nutrition Navigator *(36)* is the one of choice, having independent reviews and a rating for each site. For the health professional, the best site is the Arbor Nutrition Guide, which has over 4000 listings across a wide range of topics *(37)*. Martindale "Virtual" Nutrition Center *(38)* is a web portal with more of a food science focus.

4.2.2. DIETARY ASSESSMENT

This is one area that lends itself well to the Internet medium. There are a number of sites through which individual foods and whole diets can be analyzed for nutrient content, based on US Department of Agriculture (USDA) or other dietary tables. The USDA's own website allows searching of this data base for individual foods *(39)*. NutritionData *(40)* offers a variety of ways to search for nutrition data, such as lists of foods that match user-specified nutrient criteria and nutrient data for many popular fast foods.

4.2.3. INSTITUTIONAL RESOURCES

Many institutions offer resources that derive from their own internal resources. These typically would come from government organizations, universities, nongovernmental organizations, book publishers, and, of course, a vast number of commercial entities. Material might include lay health information, practice guidelines, Extension newsletters, course content, and official reports.

The usefulness of these resources varies enormously. As mentioned earlier, one of the most important decisions that any website visitor must make is to decide what credibility to attach to what is being offered.

Good examples of websites maintained by universities are The Nutrition Source from Harvard University Department of Public Health *(41)* and the website of Tufts University Nutrition Department *(42)*. Colorado State University Extension website *(43)* exemplifies the offerings that are provided by many of the Extension departments that are such an integral part of lay nutrition outreach within the United States.

Websites that support university nutrition courses can offer a good source of nutrition material for health professionals; for example, those from Columbia and Pennsylvania State universities *(44,45)*. For those with responsibility for developing such courses, a comprehensive curriculum tailored for family physician education is available on the website of the Society for Teachers of Family Medicine *(46)*.

Government and professional associations are another good source of institutional websites with rich nutrition content; for example:

- USDA *(47)*, including two nutrition-specific websites, namely the Food and Nutrition Center *(48)* and www.nutrition.gov.
- Center for Food Safety and Applied Nutrition *(49)*.
- American Dietetic Association *(50)*. This offers position statements, a list of accredited dietetic training institutions, and lay material. For a listing of many of the dietetic associations globally, refer to the International Confederation of Dietetic Associations *(51)*.
- Nutrition Screening Initiative *(52)* provides resources for assessing nutritional status in the elderly, a project that has been developed by a number of health professional organizations acting in concert.

4.2.4. DIETITIAN RESOURCES

There are numerous sites belonging to individual dietitians, which generally feature some lay nutrition information along with advertisements for the owner's dietetic services. Cyberdiet *(53)* is a particularly good example of a website originally set up by an individual dietitian, which has now become part of a larger Internet health network, and has a focus on weight loss. Ask the Dietitian *(54)* is another of the best dietitian-authored websites, and has a particularly good question-and-answer section for the lay visitor.

4.2.5. MAILING LISTS AND NEWSGROUPS

There are numerous nutrition-related mailing lists and newsgroups, allowing discussion amongst small to large numbers of like-minded individuals. These include lay or patient mailing lists for people suffering from or interested in such nutrition issues as weight problems, eating disorders, diabetes, and vegetarianism. Topics of discussion can vary from patient support to the latest news on treatment and alternative therapies, through to philosophical debates. There are a number of mailing lists specifically for nutrition professionals. The easiest way to find such resources is through a website dedicated to cataloging mailing lists *(55)*.

4.2.6. DISEASE-SPECIFIC INFORMATION

Information on specific medical conditions is generally found on websites of the relevant health professional organizations. The American Society for Parenteral and Enteral Nutrition website *(56)*, for example, has guidelines and standards of practice documents on nutrition support. Useful nutrition resources are also available at such websites as the American Diabetes Association *(57)*, the American Heart Association *(58)*, the National Heart, Lung, and Blood Institute *(59)*, and the Canadian Pediatric Society *(60)*. The American Association of Clinical Endocrinologists website *(61)* has nutrition material related to osteoporosis and growth disorders.

A number of commercial entities provide nutrition information targeted at health professionals, and although the obvious caution regarding commercial bias is required, some of the better ones, such as Nestle Wound Nutrition *(62)*, offer good quality material.

4.2.7. MISCELLANEOUS RESOURCES

The variety of individuals and organizations producing nutrition related websites is so enormous that this can only be an almost random sample. The Obesity Forum is a UK-based organization with a focus on the role of medical and other health professionals in tackling the obesity epidemic. Its website *(63)* has a number of useful guidelines and tools. The subject matter of the website Food Psychology *(64)* is obvious from its name. The Path Guy *(65)* is a unique contribution from an individual pathologist who has placed an extended set of lecture notes on pathology of nutrition-related diseases on the web. For those looking to develop their own lecture material, Food Clipart *(66)* offers many free downloadable food drawings. If it is more anatomical pictures you are after, Feldman's Gastroatlas Online *(67)* is a good port of call. And finally, after all that academic effort, an excellent site to visit and contemplate the more traditional and pleasurable aspects of nutrition science is one devoted to the slow food movement *(68)*.

5. WHAT DOES IT MEAN?

What does all this mean for the nutrition professional and what of the future?

The Internet has already boosted the accessibility of nutrition information and fostered communication between nutrition professionals to a degree that few would have anticipated as recently as 1999. Nutritionists who want to keep up with the latest developments in their field have unprecedented opportunity to do so.

At the same time, the quest to efficiently find the needle of relevant information in the vast and unorganized haystack that is the web has become only marginally easier in recent years. The advent of sophisticated search engine technology has helped, such as that employed by Google *(13)*, but specialized nutrition portal sites will remain a valuable asset. Experience certainly helps the regular user to find what they are after more quickly, and hopefully it will become increasingly common to see librarians being given space in academic curricula to teach these skills to health professionals.

Knowledge has also been democratized—our patients and clients are now very likely to come to us with information they "looked up on the Internet." Essentially anyone with an inquiring mind and the determination to do so can now access the same information base as any health professional. There is evidence that this is already leading to subtle changes in the relationship between health professionals and their patients *(69)*.

To a large extent this is a good thing, but as has been pointed out several times, it is also important to remember that there is no quality control on the Internet. News about fad diets and new supplements spreads through the Internet at amazing speed. The rapid rise in popularity of the low-carbohydrate approach to eating and the recent appearance of a range of commercial lower-carbohydrate packaged foods in the supermarkets—surely one of the fastest "turn arounds" of dietary practice in history—has been largely attributed to the Internet.

We will have to help our patients to learn to distinguish reliable science-based information from unreliable nonscience-based, something that is not always easy to determine on the Internet even as a health professional.

On the other hand, the individual interaction offered by the Internet provides a chance for patients to receive much more personally tailored information and support resources from nutrition professionals. The concept is not new—some doctors already send their patients text message reminder notices of their next appointment via the patient's cell phone. But few clinical practices have used the interactive potential of the Internet to tailor support programs to individual patient needs. Current technology is, in fact, capable of facilitating this now, whether by emails reminding and encouraging patients to take their medication or maintain dietary or lifestyle change, or web pages with content personalized for each patient. Such a web page could, in theory, allow a diabetic patient to input their own dietary or glucose testing data onto a personalized website into which selected results from the laboratory were also posted, and then view their clinical progress on that site in a graphic and compelling way. Patients on restrictive diets could enter their dietary history into a web page that analyzes the diet and sends an immediate report back to their treating physician or dietitian.

There is some evidence that such tailored Internet-based approaches are likely to be not only more convenient but also at least as effective as more conventional methods of patient support *(70,71)*, although they are unlikely to replace the impact of personal contact *(72)*.

On the negative side, problems with security, fraud, and spam have risen sharply in the last few years to the point where they are threatening the practicality of using the Internet. We cannot assume that an email or a website is necessarily what it purports to be. The consequence of this is that responsible use of the Internet now necessitates appropriate protective measures, such as a virus checker and firewall. Nor is it practical to use it without having a pop-up blocker and spam filter. Not only do such measures protect the user from viruses, worms, and other infections, but it prevents these infections from spreading to others on their email contact list. The analogy with more conventional public health concepts is obvious.

There is little doubt that the innocent child that the Internet was in 1999 has turned into the troublesome adolescent that is still very much finding its feet. Resolution of security issues is an essential prerequisite to the continued growth of Internet use in health applications, including specifically its use in the sharing of confidential medical records between health providers.

At the same time as Internet security problems have escalated, shopping on the web has become commonplace. This is a mixed blessing. More items are available to purchase, including a vast array of nutrition supplements. But it has also meant that the ethos of providing and accessing information for free, simply for the sake of sharing, which characterized the early years of the Internet, has sharply diminished. For publishers of intellectual content this presents a paradox, faced as they are with a strong push towards open publishing. It will be a challenge for nutrition journals to find an economic model that will enable them to thrive in the Internet era.

The last few years have seen an increase in use of the Internet in nutrition and dietetic tertiary education; for example, in on-line courses and virtual seminars *(73,74)*, but not nearly to the extent and with not nearly as rich multimedia content as was predicted in the first edition of this book. This has been largely owing to bandwidth limitations. However, with the widespread adoption of broadband connections that is taking place in the developed world, this situation is likely to change by 2010.

Another benefit likely to flow from widespread adoption of broadband connectivity is the ability to use the Internet as a medium for real time health professional collaboration at remote distances, in applications ranging from remote patient consultation to remotely supervised or even activated medical and surgical procedures.

The Internet is already being used as the medium to allow medical records to be shared and updated in real time between geographically dispersed health care and practice locations *(75)*, and with patients themselves *(76)*. In some cases websites allow the patient to directly enter their own data into the medical record *(77)*.

This sharing of health records will be greatly helped by the newly introduced technology of wireless broadband. This is a system analogous to mobile phone networks that allows broadband connectivity while moving freely around in a wide geographical area. For example, a wireless broadband service is currently available throughout much of Sydney, Australia *(78)*.

6. CONCLUSIONS

Already, the Internet offers a wealth of resources in the field of nutrition, particularly in provision of nutrition information to the lay public, and giving health professionals a medium to communicate with each other and to access current medical literature and guidelines.

In the main, however, such nutrition resources tend to make use of the "lower tech" elements of the Internet, whereas health professional nutrition websites utilizing the "higher tech" elements, such as interactivity and multimedia, still tend to be rather lacking. The realities of commercial funding being what they are, such developments are likely to come initially within websites developed for the wider field of general medicine.

Web portal sites will remain an important tool in identifying the best of what is available, although they will never absolve the user from the need to make considered decisions about the independence of the source and the accuracy of the content for any Internet resource they come across.

REFERENCES

Note: all websites were accessed on January 6, 2005.

1. http://cyberatlas.internet.com/big_picture/geographics/article/0,1323,5911_151151,00.html.
2. http://www.rcfp.org/news/2002/1210dowjon.html.
3. http://www.caslon.com.au/metricsguide2.htm.
4. http://www.dailyearth.com/#directory.
5. http://www.nytimes.com/top/news/health/topics/diet/index.html.
6. http://www.cnn.com/HEALTH/diet.fitness/archive/.
7. http://www3.accessmedicine.com/public/learnmore_hol.aspx.
8. Dickerson S, Reinhart AM, Feeley TH, et al. Patient internet use for health information at three urban primary care clinics. J Am Med Inform Assoc 2004; 11:499–504.
9. van Woerkum CM. The Internet and primary care physicians: coping with different expectations. Am J Clin Nutr 2003; 77(4 Suppl):1016S–1018S.
10. Schmidt K, Ernst E. Assessing websites on complementary and alternative medicine for cancer. Ann Oncol 2004; 15:733–742.
11. Veronin MA, Ramirez G. The validity of health claims on the World Wide Web: a systematic survey of the herbal remedy Opuntia. Am J Health Promot 2000; 15:21–28.
12. Miles J, Petrie C, Steel M. Slimming on the Internet. J R Soc Med 2000; 93:254–257.
13. www.google.com.
14. Simmons RD, Ponsonby AL, van der Mei IA, Sheridan P. What affects your MS? Responses to an anonymous, Internet-based epidemiological survey. Mult Scler 2004; 10:202–211.
15. Kolasa K, Poehlman G, Jobe A. Virtual seminars for disseminating medical nutrition education curriculum ideas. Am J Clin Nutr 2000; 71:1403, 1404.
16. Suresh G, Horbar JD, Plsek P, et al. Voluntary anonymous reporting of medical errors for neonatal intensive care. Pediatrics 2004; 113:1609–1618.

17. Henly DC. Use of Web-based formative assessment to support student learning in a metabolism/nutrition unit. Eur J Dent Educ 2003; 7:116–122.

18. Womble LG, Wadden TA, McGuckin BG, Sargent SL, Rothman RA, Krauthamer-Ewing ES. Obes Res 2004; 12:1011–1018.

19. Anhoj J, Jensen AH. Using the Internet for life style changes in diet and physical activity: a feasibility study. J Med Internet Res 2004; 6:e28.

20. Ralston JD, Revere D, Robins LS, Goldberg HI. Patients' experience with a diabetes support programme based on an interactive electronic medical record: qualitative study. BMJ 2004; 328:1159.

21. http://www.drsref.com.au/support.html.

22. http://www.google.com/search?hl=en&lr=&as_qdr=all&q=nutrition&btnG=Search.

23. http://www.ncbi.nlm.nih.gov/entrez/query.fcgi.

24. http://www.nlm.nih.gov/medlineplus/nutrition.html.

25. http://clinicaltrials.gov.

26. http://bmj.bmjjournals.com.

27. http://www.amedeo.com/medicine/nut.htm.

28. http://www.docguide.com.

29. http://www.nutritionupdates.org.

30. http://www.mja.com.au/public/papers/papers.html.

31. http://www.nutritionandmetabolism.com.

32. http://www.nutritionj.com/articles/browse.asp.

33. http://clinmed.netprints.org/collections.

34. http://www.biomedcentral.com/.

35. http://www.washingtonpost.com/wp-dyn/articles/A64389-2004Sep5.html?referrer=.

36. http://navigator.tufts.edu/.

37. http://arborcom.com.

38. http://www.martindalecenter.com/Nutrition.html.

39. http://www.nal.usda.gov/fnic/foodcomp/search/.

40. http://www.nutritiondata.com/.

41. http://www.hsph.harvard.edu/nutritionsource/.

42. http://nutrition.tufts.edu/.

43. http://www.ext.colostate.edu/.

44. http://www.columbia.edu/itc/hs/medical/nutrition/.

45. http://www.med.upenn.edu/nutrimed/.

46. http://www.stfm.org/pdfs/GroupOnNutrition.pdf.

47. http://www.nal.usda.gov.

48 http://www.nal.usda.gov/fnic/.

49. http://vm.cfsan.fda.gov/.

50. http://www.eatright.org.

51. http://www.internationaldietetics.org/.

52. http://www.aafp.org/nsi.xml.

53. http://www.cyberdiet.com.

54. http://www.dietitian.com.

55. http://tile.net/.

56. http://www.nutritioncare.org/.

57. http://www.diabetes.org.

58. http://www.amhrt.org.

59. http://www.nhlbi.nih.gov/index.htm.

60. http://www.cps.ca.

61. http://www.aace.com/.

62. http://www.woundnutrition.com/.

63. http://www.nationalobesityforum.org.uk/.

64 http://www.foodpsychology.com/.

65. http://www.pathguy.com/lectures/nutr.htm#intro.

66. http://www.foodclipart.com/.

67. http://www.gastroatlas.com/login.aspx.

68. http://www.slowfoodusa.org/.

69. Hart A, Henwood F, Wyatt S. The role of the Internet in patient-practitioner relationships: findings from a qualitative research study. J Med Internet Res 2004; 30;6:e36.

70. Brug J, Oenema A, Campbell M. Past, present, and future of computer-tailored nutrition education. Am J Clin Nutr 2003; 77(4 Suppl):1028S–1034S.

71. Harvey-Berino J, Pintauro SJ, Gold EC. The feasibility of using Internet support for the maintenance of weight loss. Behav Modif 2002; 26:103–116.

72. Harvey-Berino J, Pintauro S, Buzzell P, et al. Does using the Internet facilitate the maintenance of weight loss? Int J Obes Relat Metab Disord 2002; 26:1254–1260.

73. Litchfield RE, Oakland MJ, Anderson JA. Improving dietetics education with interactive communication technology. J Am Diet Assoc 2000; 100:1191–1194.

74. Kolasa KM, Daugherty JE, Jobe AC, Miller MG. Virtual seminars for medical nutrition education: case example. J Nutr Educ 2001; 33:347–351.

75. Wiecha J, Pollard T. The interdisciplinary eHealth team: chronic care for the future. J Med Internet Res 2004; 6:e22.

76. Kim MI, Johnson KB. Patient entry of information: evaluation of user interfaces. J Med Internet Res 2004; 6:e13.

77. Ross SE, Moore LA, Earnest MA, Wittevrongel L, Lin CT. Providing a web-based online medical record with electronic communication capabilities to patients with congestive heart failure: randomized trial. J Med Internet Res 2004; 6:e12.

78. http://www.unwired.com.au/.

Index

A

Absorption,
  calcium, 326
  soy isoflavones, 354
Adequate intake (AI), 292
Adipocytes, 230
Adipose tissue
  deposition pattern, 230
Adiposity rebound, 270
Advertising, 388–389, 399–400, 403
Africans, 44, 50, 79, 121, 127
African-Americans, 79, 121, 125, 413–421
Age,
  calcium, 294
  blood pressure, 118
  diabetes, 80
  homocysteine, 215
Aging, 39, 68, 216, 265, 303
Albumin, 379
Alcohol, 211–218
  blood pressure, 111, 115, 125, 127, 215
  cancer, 151, 163–164, 212–213
  consumption, 211, 218
  cost, 218, 403
  coronary heart disease, 64, 213–214
  dementia, 215
  diabetes mellitus, 64, 85, 216
  drinking patterns, 217–218
  gallstones, 216
  harmful effects,
    accidents, violence, suicides, 211–212
    chronic alcohol abuse, 212
    fetal alcohol syndrome (FAS), 212
    folate, 213
    homocysteine, 214–215
  hearing loss, 215
  impotence, 215
  lung disease, 217
  mortality, 217
  obesity, 213
  osteoporosis, 216
  protective effects, 213–217
    genetic, 215
  prostatic hyperplasia, 216
  sports, effect on performance, 332
  stroke, 215

Aloe vera, 190, 198
Alzheimer's disease, 144–145, 173, 216
Amino acids, 304, 321, 322–324, 334, 337, 358
Animal source foods, 44–45
Anthocyanin, 177, 195
Anthropology, nutritional, 425–435
  adaptive process, 428
  biocultural approach, 426
  ecological model, 426–428
  emic and etic perspectives, differentiating,
    428–429
  objectives of, 425–426
  pica on Pemba Island, 429–431
    emic perspective, 430
    etic perspective, 430–431
      adaptive and non-adaptive processes, 431
  research in, 431–432
    applied research for nutritional programs,
      434–435
    epidemiology, social, 432–433
      determinants of nutritional status, 432–433
      sociocultural factors, 433
    ideational systems, 433–434
    population genetics, 434
    sociocultural processes, 432
Antioxidants, 160, 173, 179, 181, 182, 183,
  see also Phytochemicals,
  cancer, 182
  coronary heart disease, 134, 173
Arachidonic acid, 135, *see also* Polyunsaturated
  fatty acids
Arginine, 322, 334
Arjun, 195
Arrhythmia, 139
Arthritis, *see* Rheumatoid arthritis
Artichoke, 94, 122
Ascorbic acid, *see* Vitamin C
Asians, 44, 420, *see also* China and Japanese
Asparagine, 322
Assessment,
  dietary, 26–31
Astragalus, 192
Atherosclerosis, 96, 140–141, *see also* Coronary
  heart disease
Athletes, *see* Sports nutrition
Atkins diet, *see* Obesity
Autoimmunity, 52

B

Balance of Good Heath, 288–289
Barker hypothesis, *see* Fetal development
Basal metabolic rate (BMR), 11–12, 213, 428
Basil, holy, 195, 198
Beta cells, 72, 85
Bioactive peptides, 347, 356, 357
Biotechnology, food production/quality, 373–384
   food production by plants, 374–378
      engineered economic traits, 376–377
         ethanol production, 376–377
         food safety, 377
         metal resistance, 376
         nitrogen fixation, 377
         plant vaccines, 377
      genetically modified crops, 374
      golden rice, 378
      modification of,
         lipid composition, 377–378
           decrease formation of trans fat, 377
           increased synthesis of very-long-chain
              fatty acids, 377
           vitamin E content, 377
         nonstaple crops, 375–376
         nutrition value, 375
   food production by animals, 378–379
      cloned animals, 380–381
      low-lactose milk, 380
      modification of digestive tract micro-
         organisms, 379–380
         antimicrobial peptides, 380
         recombinant phytase, 380
         yeasts, 380
      recombinant bovine somatotropin, 381–382
         meat production, 381–382
         production of dairy foods, 381
      safety of genetically modified foods, 382–384
         assessment of, 382–383
         perceptions and concerns with biotech-
           nology, 383
Bitter melon, 192, 197
Bitter orange, 202
Blackcurrant seed oil, 192, 199
Blood lipids, control of, 91–107
   designer diets, 103–107
      DASH diet, 104, 106
      Lifestyle Heart Program, 104, 106
      Mediterranean Diet, 104, 105–106
      National Cholesterol Education Program/
         AHA Recommendations, 103–104
      Step I and Step II diets, 103–104
      Therapeutic Lifestyle Changes, 104
   Portfolio Diet, 104–105

   foods that modify lipids and lipoproteins, 97–103
      dairy products, 98
      fish, 100
      fruits, 97
      lean meat, 98–99
      nuts, 100, 101
      vegetable oils, 100, 102–103
      vegetables, 97
      whole grains, 97–98
   nutrients that modify lipids and lipoproteins,
      92–96
      cholesterol, dietary, 96
      fiber, dietary, 96
      monounsaturated fatty acids, 95
      polyunsaturated fatty acids, 95–96
         docosahexanoic acid (DHA), 95–96
         eicosapentanoic acid (EPA), 95–96
         linoleic acid (LA), 95
      saturated fatty acids, 92–93
      trans fatty acids, 93–95
Blood pressure, 111–127
   activity, 115, 126–127
   alcohol, 111, 115, 125, 127, 215
   body weight, 125–127
   caffeine, 202
   calcium, 111, 120, 127
   classification, 117
   diabetes, 54
   dietary interventions to prevent and manage,
      121–125
      DASH, 121–124, 419–420
      Diet, Exercise and Weight Loss Intervention
         (DEWIT), 124
      PREMIER study, 124–125
   magnesium, 111, 120–121, 127
   n-3 polyunsaturated fatty acids, 140
   potassium, 119, 127
   sodium, 111–116, 119, 127
      allcause mortality, 114
      end-organ damage, 113
      coronary heart disease risk, 114
      intake patterns, 119
      restriction, recommended levels, 114–116, 119
      salt sensitivity, 112, 119
Body mass index (BMI), 46, 80–81, 226
Body shape, 81
Body weight, *see also* Obesity,
   cancer, 152
   hypertension, 91, 97, 125–126
   type II diabetes, 70
Bone,
   calcium, 294, 330, 335, 356
   health, 216, 356
   mass/density, 216, 320, 365

osteoporosis, 326, 356, 368
reabsorption, 326
vitamin D and, 295, 326
Boron,
    ergogenic aids, 330, 337
Branched-chain amino acids (BCAA), 322, 323, 336
Brazil, 45–46
Breast cancer, *see* Cancer
Britain, *see* United Kingdom
Butyrate, 154

C

Caffeine, 338
    energy supplementation, 359
    ergogenic aids, 330, 332, 336, 338
    genetically modifed plants, 376
    weight loss, 202
Calcium, 294
    absorption of, 58, 326
    blood pressure, 111, 120, 294
    bone, 294, 330, 335, 356
    cancer, 159
    dietary intake, 294, 416
    ergogenic aids, 330
    excretion of, 120
    function of, 63
    obesity, 356
    osteoporosis, 294, 330, 335, 356, 368
    phosphate, 331
    polycystic ovary syndrome, 52
    recommended intake, 294
    vitamin D, 294, 326
Calcium D-glucarate, 318
Calories, *see* Energy intake
Canada's Food Guide to Healthy Eating, 287–288
Cancer, 151–152
    body weight, 151, 152
    breast, 144, 152, 153, 154, 155, 158, 164,
        200–201
    cervix, 155
    colorectal, 153–155, 164
    colosolic acid, 318, 329
    dietary factors,
        alcohol, 151, 163–164, 212–213
        butyrate, 154
        fat, 152–154
        fiber, 158
        fruits and vegetables, 155–158
        herbs, 189, 192, 200–201, *see also* Herbs
            and plant extracts
        micronutrients, 159–163
        phytochemicals, 159–163, 173, 181, 184
        n-3 polyunsaturated fatty acids, 153–154
        preparation/preservation, 164–165
        soy, 160

esophageal/oral, 155, 163, 201
etiology, 151–152
genetic susceptibility, 155–156
lifestyle, 152
liver, 155, 159, 164
lung, 155, 164
multiple myeloma, 155
non-Hodgkin's lymphoma, 155
obesity, 66, 68, 80–81, 86, 154–155
pancreas, 155, 159, 164, 181, 201
physical activity, 154–155
prostate, 153, 155, 158, 163, 164
stomach, 160, 181
Casein, 321, 325, 349, 355
Carbohydrates,
    counting, 69–71
    diabetes, 61–62
    low-carbohydrate diets, 231
    low-carbohydrate foods, 351–353
    obesity, 228–229
Carcinogens, 164
Cardiovascular diseases (CVD), *see* Coronary
        heart disease
L-Carnitine, 320, 334, 337, 358, 359
α-Carotene, 161, 180
β-Carotene, 161, 179, 180
    cancer, 64, 160–163, 174, 183–184, 201
    coronary heart disease, 64
    ergogenic aids, 328
    genetically modified foods, 378
Carotenoids, 174–175, 179–180, 201, *see also*
        β-Carotene
Case–control studies, 16–17
Cataract, 184
Catechin, 160, 163, 175, 196
Cat's claw, 192, 199
Centella, 201
Center for Food Safety and Applied Nutrition
        (CFSAN), 368–369
Cereals, *see* Grains
Cervix cancer, *see* Cancer
Chamomile, 190, 195
China, 41, 43–45, 79, 200, 289, 290, 440
Cholesterol, 91, 99
    blood level, 55, 91–107
    dietary cholesterol, 91, 93, 96, 99, 348
    high-density lipoprotein (HDL), 55, 61, 91,
        97, 98, 103–107
    LDL-oxidation, 143, 182–183, 191, 196
    low-density lipoprotein (LDL), 55, 61, 91, 96–98,
        103–107
Choline
    ergogenic aids, 332
Chondroitin, 347, 357

Chronic diseases, *see also* Cancer, Coronary heart disease, Diabetes mellitus
   countering chronic disease, 291–292
   developmental origins, 261–279
Chronic Obstructive Pulmonary Disease (COPD), *see* Lung disease
Chromium,
   diabetes, 72, 77, 84, 294
   ergogenic aids, 330, 335, 337
Cinnamon, 192, 199
Coagulation, 140, 196, 215
Cobalamin, *see* Vitamin B$_{12}$
Coenzyme Q, 196
   ergogenic aids, 332
Coffee, 163, 332, 338, 376, *see also* Caffeine
Cohort studies, 18–19
Colon adenomas, 158
Colorectal cancer, *see* Cancer
Colosolic acid, 318
Colostrum, 347, 349, 357
Committee on Medical Aspects of Food and Nutrition Policy (COMA), 292
Conjugated linoleic acid (CLA), 154, 320, 349, 358
Copper, 376
Coronary heart disease (CHD), 97–107
   alcohol, 64, 213–214
   antioxidants, 181–183
   body weight, 91, 97, 125–126
   dairy products, 98, 351
      intake of, 416
   diabetes, 56–58
   dietary fats, 92–96
   fetal development, 46, 273, 275–276
   fish, 95–96, 100, 133–145
   fruits and vegetables, 97
   herbs, 189, 191–196
   homocysteine, 215, 294, 327, 418
   meat, 98–99
   nuts, 100, 101
   phytochemicals, 173, 181–183
   prevention campaigns, 406
   risk factors, 118
   sodium, 114
   soy, 354
   whole grain, 97
Cranberry, 174, 190
Creatine, 318, 323, 334, 336, 339, 358
Creatinine, 164
Cross-sectional studies, 17–18
Cruciferous vegetables, 157, 159, 160
β-Cryptoxanthin, 179, 161
Center for Science in the Public Interest (CSPI), 389
   consumer advocacy group, 394–395

D

Daidzein, 353
DASH diet, 96, 104, 111, 115, 121–122, 419–420
Dementia, 216
Diabetes mellitus, 49–71
   blood glucose, 54–56
   blood lipids, 50, 54–56, 63
   blood pressure, 54–56
   body weight, 54, *see also* obesity
   coronary heart disease, 54–56
   diagnosis/screening, 50–51, 78
   dietary factors, 61–64
      alcohol, 64, 85, 216
      carbohydrate, 61–62, 81, 86
      chromium, 70, 84
      fat, 63, 81, 83–84, 86
      fiber, 62, 81–82, 86
      magnesium, 84
      n-3 polyunsaturated fatty acid, 145
      protein, 62–63, 72
      vitamin E, 63–64, 72
   euglycemia, 70
   fetal weight gain, 261
   genetics, 80
   gestational diabetes, 53
   glycemic index and load, 83
   glycated hemoglobin A1 (HbA1c), 56, 59–61
   herbs, 196–199
   impaired glucose control, 51, 53, 78–80
   ketoacidosis, 52, 56
   ketone test, 56
   lifestyle, 54–56, 69, 85–86
   management of, 53–71
      nutrition therapy, 59–65, 68–71
   medications,
      insulin, 56–58, 71
      oral glucose lowering medications, 58–59
   metabolic changes, 51–52, 79–80
   metabolic control, 53–54
   metabolic syndrome, 67, 80, 126
   mortality, 79
   obesity, 66, 68, 80–81, 86
   physical activity, 67, 81, 86
   prevalence, 50, 77–79
   prediabetes, 53, 67–68
   prevention, 77–87
Diet,
   speed of change, 39–41
Diet, Exercise and Weight Loss Intervention Trial (DEWIT), 124
Dietary Guidelines, 285–298
   adequate intake (AI), 292
   Balance of Good Heath, 288–289

Canada's Food Guide to Healthy Eating, 287–288
Committee on Medical Aspects of Food and
         Nutrition Policy (COMA), 292
countering chronic disease, 291–292
     United Kingdom, 292
     United States, 291
     World Health Organization, 291
dietary reference intakes (DRI), 292
dietary reference values (DRV), 293
differences between guides, 290
estimated Average Requirements (EAR), 292
food Guide Pyramid, 286–287
food Guides, 286–290
lower Reference Nutrient Intake (LRNI), 293
recommendations for nutrient intake,
     Canada, 292–293
     United Kingdom, 293
     United States, 292–293
recommended dietary allowances (RDA), 286
recommended nutrient intakes (RNI), 292–293
supplements, 293–296, see also Supplements
     antioxidants, 295
     calcium, 294
     chromium, 294
     fish oil, 295
     folate, 293
     selenium, 294
     vitamin D, 294–295
     vitamins, 295
tolerable upper intake levels (UL), 292
Dietary Reference Intakes (DRI), 292
Dietary Reference Values (DRV), 293
Diets, 239, see also Obesity
     DASH diet, 96, 104, 111, 115, 121–122
     Mediterranean diet, 104, 105–106
     Portfolio diet, 104–105
     Step I and Step II diets, 103–104
Dihydroxy-acetone phosphate (DHAP), 318
1,25-Dihydroxyvitamin D, see Vitamin D
DNA, 181, 378–379, 382
Docosahexanoic acid (DHA), 95–96, 134, see also
         Polyunsaturated fatty acids
Dutch, 276, 277
Dyslipidemia, 53, 70, 118

E

Echinacea, 190, 199, 202
Ecological model, 426–428
Ecological studies, 16–17
Edible oil, 43, see also Vegetable oils
Eicosapentanoic acid (EPA), 95–96, 134, see also
Polyunsaturated fatty acids
Emic perspectives, 428–429
Endothelial cells, 140

Energy,
     balance, 155, 156, 213, 225–226, 252
     energy density, 233–234
     expenditure, 253
     restriction, 247, 251, 252
     supplementation, 359
Ephedra, 202, 308–309, 336
Ephedrine, 202, 336, 337
Epidemiology,
     biological samples, 13–14
     confounding, 3–5
     nutritional, 1–22, 25–33
         designing a nutritional epidemiological
             study, 21–22
         dietary assessment, 6–7, 26–31
         dietary data error, assessing, 7–9
         energy adjustment, 13
     research challenges, 25–33
     types of studies, 14–19
         case–control studies, 16–17
         cohort studies, 18–19
         cross-sectional studies, 15–16
         ecological studies, 15
         experimental studies, 19
     under- and overreporting, 10–13
     validation, 9–10
Ergogenic acids, 329–338
Eskimos, see Inuit
Essential amino acids (EAA), 323, 334, 336, 339
Essential fatty acids, 320, 325, 142, see also
         Polyunsaturated fatty acids
Estimated Average Requirements (EARs), 292
Estrogen
     soy, 354, see also Phytoestrogens and Soy
Ethnic groups, diet, disease, African-Americans,
         Mexican-Americans, Native Americans
Etic perspectives, 428–429
Evening primrose oil, 195
Eye health, 357
Experimental studies, 19
Exercise, see Physical activity
Exercise for weight loss, 241, 253–257

F

Famine, 38
Fat cells, see Adipocytes
Fat, dietary, see also Cancer, Diabetes,
         Monounsaturated fatty acids, Polyunsatu-
         rated fatty acids, Saturated fatty acids,
         Trans fatty acids
     cancer, 152–154
     coronary heart disease, 92–96
     diabetes mellitus, 63, 81, 83, 86

food intake,
  control of, 91–107
  reduction, 348, 351
  obesity, 230–231
  substitutes, 233
Federal Trade Commission (FTC), 302, 303, 309
Fennel, 190, 191, 200
Fenugreek, 192, 194, 197
Ferritin, 378
Fetal alcohol syndrome (FAS), 212
Fetal development,
  alcohol, 212, 213
  chronic disease, 46, 261, 262
  folate, 213, 294
  developmental origins of chronic disease, 44,
    261–279
    biological basis, 262–265
    confounding variables, 262
Feverfew, 190, 202
Fiber, dietary, 81–82, *see also* Grains
  cancer, 158
  cholesterol, 93, 96
  diabetes, 62, 81–82
Finland, 37, 45, 399
Fish, fish oil, and marine origin foods, 100, 133–145,
    295, *see also* Polyunsaturated fatty acids
Flavonoids, 175–177, 195, *see also*
    Phytochemicals
Flaxseed, 194, 198, 200–201
Foam cells, 183, 193
Folate, 294
  alcohol, 212–214
  cancer, 161, 213, 215, 294
  coronary heart disease, 294
  ergogenic aids, 328
  fetal development, 294
  homocysteine, 294
Food additives, 116
FDA (Food and Drug Administration), 304–306
  calcium, 356
  dietary fiber, 355
  EPA and DHA, 143, 356
  n-3 fatty acids, 356
  fish, 144
  folate, 294
  functional foods, 363, 368
  genetically modified foods, 382
  herbal supplements, 202
  labeling, 368–370
  plant esters, 355
  soy, 354
Folic acid, *see* Folate
Food choices, 252, 285, 325, 402, 403, 405

Food Guides, 286–290
Food Guide Pyramid, 243, 254, 286–287
Food production,
  animal sources, 378–379
  plant sources, 374–378
Food safety/poisoning, 43, 380, 382–384
Fortification, food, 32, 294–295, 356, 375, 377,
    378, 389
Free radicals, 181, *see also* Phytochemicals
Fructose 1,6-diphosphate (FDP), 318
Fruit
  antioxidants, 173, 176, 179
  blood pressure, 115, 116, 121–122
  cancer, 181, 182, 184
  coronary heart disease, 97, 134, 173, 182–183
  intake, 398, 415
  phytochemicals, 173–186
Functional foods, 363–371
  definitions of, 363–365
  government interest, 368
  health claims, 365–367
  labeling for food health claims, 368–370
    benefits and problems, 370–371
    Center for Food Safety and Applied Nutri-
      tion (CFSAN) required labeling,
      368–369
    foods that may qualify in future, 369–370
  processed foods, 366
  public interest, 367–368
  raw foods, 366
  supplemented foods, 366–367

G

Gallstones, 216
Garlic, 190, 193, 200, 202
Genetically modified foods, *see* Biotechnology,
    food production/quality
Genistein, 176, 353, 375
Germany, 290, 399
Gestational diabetes, *see* Diabetes mellitus
Ginger, 191, 201, 202
Ginkgo biloba, 190, 195–196, 202
Ginseng, 190, 197–198, 201, 202
β-Glucan, 356
Glucaric acid, 318
Glucomannan, 198, 202
Gluconeogenesis, 62–63, 249, 334
Glucosamine, 347, 357, 380
Glucose,
  ergogenic aids, 318
  fasting blood, 51, 55
  monitoring, 54–56
Glucose tolerance test, 78

Glutamine, 323, 358–359
Glutathione, reduced (GSH), 182
Glutathione peroxidase, 331
Glycemic control, 55, 61
Glycemic index, 83, 248–250
Glycerol, 313, 320, 329, 336, 339, 352
Glycogen, 225, 242, 247, 316, 317, 320–322, 325
Glycomacropeptide, 321, 347, 359
Glycyrrhizin, 192, 196, 199, 352
Goldenseal, 190
Gotu kolu, 201
Government policy, 305–306, 365, 402–406,
    see also FDA
Grains, 415, see also Fiber, dietary
Grape seeds, 192, 195
Green tea, 162–163, 196
Growth, compensatory, 271–271
Growth hormone releasing peptides (GHRP),
    ergogenic aids, 332
Guarana, 202, 359
Guggul, 192, 194
Gugulipid, 192, 194
Gurmar, 192, 198

H

Hawthorn, 194–195
Health food stores, 301
Health promotion, 397–408
    advertising, 403
    coronary heart disease, 399–401, 407
    government policy, 402–406
        acceptability to public, 406
        barriers against public health policies,
            405–406
        labeling, 403–404
        marketing, 403
        modification of, 404–405
        national nutrition policies, 406
        price, 402–403
    health promotion campaigns, 398–402
        community, 398–400
        individual, 401–402
        paid advertising, 399–400
        physician's office, 400–401
        worksite, 400
    trends, 398
Hearing loss, 215
Heart disease, see Coronary heart disease
Hemoglobin A1 (HbA1c), see Diabetes
Herbs and plant extracts, 189–203
    aloe vera, 190, 198
    arjun, 195
    artichoke, 194
    basil, holy, 195, 198

bitter melon, 197
bitter orange, 202
black currant seed oil, 199
blood glucose, 189
cancer, 189, 192, 200–201
cat's claw, 199
chamomile, 190, 195
cinnamon, 199
cardiovascular disease, 189, 191–196
cranberry, 174, 190
culinary herbs and spices, 189, 190
diabetes, 196–199
Echinacea, 190, 199, 202
ephedra, 202
fennel, 190, 191, 200
fenugreek,194, 197
feverfew, 190, 202
flaxseed, 194, 198, 200–201
garlic, 190, 193, 200, 202
ginger, 191, 201, 202
ginkgo biloba, 190, 195–196, 202
ginseng, 190, 197–198, 201, 202
goldenseal, 190
gotu kolu, 201
grape seeds, 195
green tea, 196
guarana, 202
guggul, 194
gurmar, 198
hawthorn, 194–195
horse chestnut seeds, 195
immune system, effects, 189, 199–200
ivy gourd, 197
kava, 190, 202, 309
lemon grass oil, 195
licorice root, 191, 192, 195, 196, 199, 202, 352
milk thistle, 190, 195
ma huang, 202
mint, 195
onions, 193–195, 200
parsley, 195
peppermint, 191
pine, French maritime, 195
prickly pear, 198
psyllium, 198–199
red yeast rice, 194
safety issues, 189, 202–203
saw palmetto, 190
St. John's wort, 190
soy, 191
tumeric, 201
valerian, 190
weight reduction, 201–202
yarrow, 195
yerba mate, 202

Heterocyclic amines, 164
High-density lipoprotein (HDL), *see* Cholesterol
Hispanics and diet, 413–421
HMG-CoA reductase, 191, 194
Homocysteine,
    coronary heart disease, 214–215, 294, 327, 328
    hyperhomocysteinemia, 297
    vitamins, 328
Horse chestnut, 192, 195
Human growth hormone (HGH), 303–304
Hydrogenated fat, *see* Trans fatty acids
β-Hydroxy-β-methylbutyrate (HMB), 323
Hypercholesterolemia, 103, 193
Hypertension, *see* Blood pressure
Hypoglycemia, 54, 55, 64, 70, 249

I

Ideational systems, 433–434
Immune system, 199–200, 347, 357
Impaired glucose homeostasis, 53, 79–80,
    see also Diabetes mellitus
Impotence, 215
India, 43, 197, 262, 429
Indoles, 159, 160
Inflammatory bowel disease, 141
Inosine, 333, 337,
Insulin, 56–58, 70–71
Insulin-dependent diabetes mellitus (IDDM),
    see Diabetes mellitus, type 1
Intergenerational effects, 276
Internet, 303–304, 308, 439–449
    heath records, 448–449
    nutrition applications, 442–446
        dietary assessment, 445
        disease-specific information, 446
        mailing lists and newsgroups, 446
        portal sites, 445
    research access, 442–445
    search engines, 441–442
    size, 439–440
Inuit, Greenland and Alaskan, 133, 142
Iron,
    deficiency, 378
    ergogenic aids, 330
    genetically modified foods, 378
Islet cell, 52
Isoflavones, 157, 160, *see also* Phytoestrogens
    and Soy
    cholesterol, 192
    content in soy products,
    daidzein, 354
    ergogenic aids, 333, 337
    estrogen and, 354
    genistein, 176, 354, 375

menstrual cycle, 354
osteoporosis, 333
Ivy gourd, 192, 197

J–K

Japanese, 142, 226, 365, *see also* Asians
Kaolin, 431
Kava, 190, 202, 309
Ketoacidosis, 51, 52
α-Keto-glutarate, 304, 322, 337
α-Keto-isocaproate, 322, 323, 337,
Ketone test, *see* Diabetes
Kidney(s),
    blood pressure, 112, 117, 269
    calcium, 120
    disorders/diseases of, 118, 155, 156, 246,
        265, 365

L

Labeling, 368–371
Lactose, 42, 380
Lactoferrin, 349, 357, 377
Lactoperoxidase, 357
Lauric acid, 92, 93
Lecithin, *see* Choline
Legumes, 160, 290, 353, *see also* Soy
Lemon grass oil, 195
Leucine, 323, 334
Licorice root, 191, 192, 195, 196, 199, 202, 352
Lifestyle factors/behaviors,
    blood pressure, 54, 114–115
    cancer, 152
    coronary heart disease, 104, 107
    diabetes, 54–56, 67, 85–86
    smoking, 107, 214, 262, 402
    vegetarians, 17, 18, 104, 107
Lifestyle Heart Program, 104, 107
Linoleic acid, 93, 95, 135, *see also* Polyunsatu-
    rated fatty acids
α-Linolenic acid, 134, *see also* Polyunsaturated
    fatty acids
Lipids, *see* Arachidonic acid, Cholesterol, Coronary
    heart disease, Diabetes, Docosahexanoic
    acid, Eicosapentanoic acid, Fat, dietary, Fish,
    Linoleic acid, α-Linolenic acid,
    Monounsaturated fatty acids, Myristic acid,
    Oleic acid, Palmitic acid, Polyunsaturated
    fatty acids, Saturated fatty acids, Stearic acid,
    Trans fatty acids, Wheat germ oil
Lipoprotein, *see* Cholesterol
Low birth-weight, 261, 262, 265, 266
Lower Reference Nutrient Intake (LRNI), 293
Low-density lipoprotein (LDL), *see* Cholesterol

Lung cancer, *see* Cancer
Lung disease, 217
Lutein, 161, 179, 180, 357
Lycopene, 160–162, 179, 180
Lysine, 322, 334

M

Macrophage, 183, 199
Ma huang, 202
Magnesium, 84
    blood pressure, 120–121
    diabetes, 31, 77, 84
    dietary sources, 122
    ergogenic aids, 330, 333, 335, 337
Maternal influences, 274–275, 278
Meat, 98–99
Mediterranean diet, 104, 105–106
Medium-chain triglyceride, 320
Menopause, 353
Menstrual cycle, *see* Estrogen
Metabolic syndrome, *see* Diabetes
Methionine, 164, 231
Methyltetrahydrofolate, *see* Folate
Mexican-Americans, 50, 413–421
Microalbuminuria, 62, 113, 118
Milk,
    micronutrients, 357
    protein, 355
Milk thistle, 190, 195
Minerals, *see* Boron, Calcium, Chromium,
        Copper, Iron, Magnesium, Potassium,
        Selenium, Sodium, Vanadium, Zinc
Mint, 195
Monounsaturated fatty acids, 95, 102
Mycoprotein, 355
Myristic acid, 92, 95

N

National Cancer Institute, 152
    5-A-Day for Better Health, 403
National Health Products Directorate, 306
Native Americans, 79
Natural Health Products (NHP), 306
Netherlands (Dutch), 276, 277
Neural development, *see* Folate
Neural tube defect, 294, 405; *see also* Folate
Niacin, ergogenic aids, 327
Nitric oxide, 126, 196
Nitrate, 164
Nitrite, 164
N-nitroso compounds (NOCs), 164
Non-Hispanic white, 413, 414
Non-Hodgkin's lymphoma, 155
Non-insulin dependent diabetes mellitus
        (NIDDM), *see* Diabetes mellitus, type 2

Norway, 137
Novel foods, 347–359
    ingredient websites, 350
    product websites, 349
    reduction of nutrients, 248–253
        carbohydrates, 351–353,
            Atkins foods, 351–353
            dietary fibers, 352–353
            low glycemic foods, 353
            sugar alcohols, 352
            sweeteners, 352
        cholesterol, 348
        dairy foods, 351
        fat, 348, 351
Nutraceuticals, 353–359
    food supplements for,
        body fitness,
            amino acids, 358–359
            conjugated linoleic acid (CLA), 358
            glycomacropeptide, 359
        bone and joint health,
            calcium, 356
            chondroitin, 357
            glucosamine, 357
        coronary heart disease, 355–356
            bioactive peptides, 356
            n-3 fatty acids, 356
            β-glucan, 356
            stanol esters, 355
        energy, 359
        eye health,
            lutein, 357
        gut health,
            prebiotics, 358
            probiotics, 358
        immune system,
            milk ingredients, 357
        skin health, 359
        protein supplements, 353–355
        snack foods, 351
        sodium, 348
        soy, 354–355
Nutrient recommendations, *see* Dietary Guidelines
Nutrition labeling, 368–370
Nutrition transition, 37–46
    animal source foods, 42–43
    biological differences, 44
    fat, 41
    modification of program and policy issues, 45–46
    nutrition patterns, 38–39
    sedentarism, 43–44
    speed of change, 39
    sugar, 42
Nutritional anthropology, *see* Anthropology,
    nutritional

O

Obesity, 223–234
    alcohol, 213
    calcium, 356
    cancer, 66, 68, 80–81, 86, 154–155
    carbohydrate intake, 228–229
    diabetes, 66, 68, 80–81, 86
    dietary fat, 224–228, 250
    dietary treatment, 229–234, 240–253
        Atkins diet, 241–248, 254
        Eat More, Weigh Less diet, 243, 254
        energy density, 233–234
        fat reduction/low-fat diets, 230–233, 244–246,
            250–252
        fat substitutes, 233
        glycemic index, 248–250
        low-calorie diets, 252–253
        low-carbohydrate diets, 231, 241–250
        portion size, 230
        Weight Watchers, 243, 253, 254
        Zone diet, 243, 246, 248, 254
    exercise for weight loss/control, 241, 253–257
    fat oxidation, 225
    genetics, 257
    herbs, 201–202
    portion size, 224
    prevalence, 234, 239
Octacosanol, 192
Oleic acid, 93, 375, 377
Olestra, 233, 351
Onions, 193–194, 195, 200
Ornithine, 304, 322, 334
Ornithine-α-ketoglutarate, 324
γ-Oryzanol, 337
Osteoporosis, 326, 356, 368, *see also* Bone and
    Calcium
    alcohol, 216
    calcium, 294, 356
Overweight, *see* Obesity
Oxidative stress/damage, 173, 179, 181, 377

P

Palmitic acid, 92, 93, 95, 116
Pancreas, 50, 53, 54, 79, 83, 198
Pancreas cancer, *see* Cancer
Pantothenic acid,
    ergogenic aids, 328
Parsley, 195
Pemba Island, 429–431
Peppermint, 191
Phenolics, 174–176
Phenolic acids, 178; *see also* Phytochemicals
Phenols, 159

Phosphate, 331, 380
    ergogenic aids, 331, 336
Phosphorus, *see* Phosphate
Physical activity, 43, 45, 69, 81, 115, 126–127,
    154–155, 255, 256, 329; *see also* Sports
    nutrition
Phytochemicals, 174
    antioxidants, 173, 179
    cancer, 159, 173
        prevention of, 181, 184, 200–201
    carotenoids, 174–175, 179–180, 201
        β-Carotene, 179, 180
        lutein, 179, 180
        lycopene, 179, 180
    coronary heart disease, 173,
        prevention of, 181–183
    flavonoids, 175–177
        anthocyanidin, 176–177
        catechin, 176–177
        genistein, 176–177
    health benefits, 179
        food synergy, 183–185
    levels, 203
    phenolics, 174–176, 178
        hydroxycinnamic acid, 178
    phytosterols, 193
    whole foods, 173–186
Phytoestrogens, 354, *see also* Isoflavones and Soy
Phytosterols, 193
Pica, 429, *see also* Pemba Island
Pima Indians, 79, 198, 227
Pine bark, 192
Pine, French maritime, 195
Pinitol, 318
Placenta, 276–277
Plant sterols or phytosterols, 193
Policosanols, 191–193
Political influences on American nutrition, 378–395
    food industry and its influence, 388–391
        advertising of manufactured food, 388–389
        educating children, 389–390
    food supply problems, 391
    influences of,
        farm and corporate interests on research, 393
        legal system, 394
        special interest groups and political action
            committees, 391–393
        sugar industry, 392
        television, 392–393
Polycyclic aromatic hydrocarbons (PAH), 164
Polycystic ovary syndrome, 50
Polylactate, 319, 329
Polyphenolics, 195, 201

Polyunsaturated fatty acids (PUFA), 95–96, 102
   n-3 polyunsaturated fatty acids, 95–96
      Alzheimer's disease, 144–145
      arrhythmias, 139
      atherosclerosis, 140–141
      biochemistry, 133–134
      blood pressure, 140
      cancer, 144, 153
      coronary heart disease, 95–96, 100,
         133–145, 356
      diabetes, 145
      dietary intake, 136–137
      dietary sources, 134, 136, 141–142
      endothelial function, 140
      ergogenic aids, 320
      inflammatory response, 140–141
      metabolism, 135
      plant derived vs marine derived, 141–142
      recommended intake, 142–143
      rheumatoid arthritis, 145
      safety/contaminantss, 142–144
      stroke risk, 138
      sudden death, 138
      thrombosis and hemostasis, 140
      triglycerides, 139–140
   n-6 polyunsaturated fatty acids, 95, 99, 101, 102
      cancer, 153,
      coronary heart disease, 93, 95
      metabolism, 135
Population nutrition, *see* Health promotion
Portfolio diet, 104–105
Portion size, 224, 230
Potassium, 119, 120
   blood pressure, 111, 116, 119, 127
   dietary, 119–120
   ergogenic aids, 331
   plant foods, 122
Prebiotics, 358
Prediabetes, *see* Diabetes mellitus
Pregnancy,
   alcohol, 212
   diabetes, *see* Diabetes, gestational
   diet and body composition, 277–278
   folate, *see* Folate
   future chronic disease, 263–264
   pica, *see* Pica
   placental size, 276–277
PREMIER study, 124–125
Premenstrual syndrome (PMS), 189
Prickly pear, 198
Probiotics, 358
Prostate cancer, *see* Cancer
Prostatic hyperlasia, 216

Protein, dietary, 62–63
Psyllium, 194, 199, *see also* Fiber
Pycnogenol, 192, 195
Pyridoxine, *see* Vitamin B_6
Pyruvate, 318–319, 329, 336–337

R

Reactive oxygen species (ROS), 162, 179
Recombinant bovine somatotropin, 381–382
Recommended Dietary Allowances (RDA), 286
Recommended Nutrient Intakes (RNI), 292–293
Red clover, 192
Red yeast rice, 194
Renal, *see* Kidney
Renin, 119, 126
Renolithiasis, 246
Resistant starch, 352
Rheumatoid arthritis, 141, 145, 356
Riboflavin, *see* Vitamin B_2
Ribose, 319, 329, 337
Rice, 353–354
   golden, *see* Golden Rice
   production, 376
   red yeast, 194

S

Salt, *see* Blood pressure, Sodium
Saturated fatty acids, 92–93
Saw palmetto, 190
Schizophrenia, 278
Secondary diabetes, *see* Diabetes mellitus
Selenium,
   antioxidant enzymes, 331
   cancer, 157, 160–161, 163, 294
   ergogenic aids, 331
Sedentarianism, 43, 45–46
Smoking, 107, 214, 262, 402
Sociodemographic status, 413–421
   disease risk, 414–415
   food intake, 415–420
   risk of mortality, morbidity, 413
Socioeconomic status (SES), health, 407
   coronary heart disease, 418–420
   dietary intake, 417
   type 2 diabetes, 418–419
Sodium 114,
   ergogenic aids, 331
Sodium bicarbonate,
   ergogenic aids, 332, 338–339
Sodium phosphate, 313
   ergogenic aids, 331, 335, 336, 339
Somatotrophin, 304
Soy, 191

absorption and metabolism, 354
biotechnology/genetically modified, 375
cancer, 160
heart disease, 354
hot flash symptoms, 354
menstrual cycle, 354
products and food containing, 354–355
South Korea, 46
Sports drinks, 313, 329
Sports nutrition, 313–339
amino acids, 322–324
carbohydrate, 316, 317–319, 321, 329
energy, 315–317
ergogenic aids, various, 318–320, 323, 332–333
fat, 316, 320, 325, 329, 334
general macronutrient guidelines, 317–329
minerals, 330–331, 335
nutrient timing, 325, 329
protein, 316, 325, 334
vitamins, 326–328, 334
water, 335, 338
Stanol esters, 355
Stearic acid, 92–93, 95
Step I and Step II diets, 103–104
Sterols, 193
St. Johns wort, 190, 309
Stomach cancer, see Cancer
Stroke, 113, 115, 118, 121, 138–139, 193, 195,
202, 215, 217, 261, 295
Sugar, 42, 70, 228–229, 249, 290, 292, 389, 392,
403, 416–417
Sugar alcohols, 352
Superoxide dismutase, 182
Supplements, see also Diabetes mellitus, Minerals,
Sport nutrition, Vitamins
benefits, 293–296
evaluating health claims, 307–309
marketing strategies, 300–304
regulations, 304–306
Canada, 306
United States, 304–306
size of market, 300
Sweeteners,
obesity, 228–229
types, 352
Synergy, food, 183–185

T

Tea, 162–163, 195–196, 201
Technology,
food biotechnology, see Biotechnology, food
production/quality
internet and nutrition, see Internet, nutrition

Therapeutic Lifestyle Changes (TLC), 103–104
Thiamin, see vitamin B_1
Thrombosis, 140, see also Coagulation
Tobacco, see Smoking
α-Tocopherol, see Vitamin E
Tolerable Upper Intake Levels (UL), 292
Trans fatty acids, 93–95
Triglycerides, blood level, 55, 61
Tryptophan, 322, 324, 334
Tumor, see Cancer
Turmeric, 201

U

United Kingdom, 17, 54, 78, 288, 290, 292–293, 400
United States,
cancer, 173
coronary heart disease, 107, 173, 398
diabetes, 50, 78
diet, 114, 123, 225, 398, 415–420
functional foods, 367
government, 286, see also Political influences
on American Nutrition
obesity, 154, 239, 398
supplement use, 300
Unsaturated fatty acids, see Monounsaturated or
Polyunsaturated fatty acids

V

Valerian, 190
Vanadium,
ergogenic aids, 331, 335, 337
Vegetable oils, 41, 100, 102–103, 377, see also
Monounsaturated fatty acids, Polyunsaturated fatty acids
Vegetables,
antioxidants, 32
blood pressure, 115, 116, 121–122
cancer, 155–158
coronary heart disease, 97
intake, 398, 415
phytochemicals, 173–186
Vegetarian, 17–18, 103, 107, 418–419
Very-low-density lipoprotein (VLDL), see Cholesterol
Vitamin A (retinol), 162
deficiency, 378
ergogenic aids, 326
Vitamin B_1 (Thiamin),
ergogenic aids, 326
Vitamin B_2 (Riboflavin),
ergogenic aids, 327
Vitamin B_3, see Niacin
ergogenic aids, 327

Vitamin B$_6$, (Pyridoxine),
   ergogenic aids, 327
Vitamin B$_{12}$ (cobalamin),
   ergogenic aids, 327
Vitamin C, 334
   antioxidant action, 32, 184
   cancer, 159, 184, 369
   diabetes, 32
   ergogenic aids, 328, 334, 338
   immune system, 338
   recommended intake, 328
Vitamin D,
   calcium regulation, 159, 326
   cancer, 159
   ergogenic aids, 326, 328
   fortification, 294–295
   recommended intake, 328
Vitamin E (tocopherol),
   antioxidant action, 32, 295
   cancer, 159–160
   coronary heart disease, 64–65, 136–137, 184
   diabetes, 70
   ergogenic aids, 326
   genetically modified food, 377–378
   recommended intake, 326
Vitamin K,
   ergogenic aids, 326

W

Water, 112, 313, 335–336, 338–339, 364
Websites, 303–304, 308, 349–350

Weight, *see* Obesity
Weight Watchers, *see* Obesity
Wernicke-Korsakoff, 212
Western diet, 250
Wheat, *see* Grains and Fiber, dietary
Whey
   ergogenic aids, 323, 325
   protein, 321, 354–356, 358
Wine, *see* Alcohol
Women,
   bone health, 368
   cancer, 153, *see also* Cancer
   iron deficiency, 378
World Health Organization, 291

Y

Yarrow, 195
Yerba mate, 202, 359
Yohimbine, 337

Z

Zinc,
   cancer, 157
   coronary heart disease, 420
   ergogenic aids, 331, 333, 335
   immune system, 314, 331, 338
   magnesium, 333, 337
   recommended intake, 331
Zone diet, *see* Obesity

About the Editors

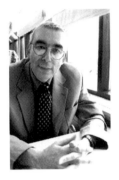

Dr. Norman J. Temple teaches nutrition at Athabasca University in Alberta, Canada, and develops distance education courses in nutrition and health. Dr. Temple's specialty is nutrition in relation to health, particularly the influence of dietary factors on heart disease and cancer. *Beverage Impacts on Health and Nutrition* is his sixth book on diet, health, and disease. He is coeditor with Denis Burkitt of *Western Diseases: Their Dietary Prevention and Reversibility* (Humana Press, 1994), which continued and extended Burkitt's pioneering work on the role of dietary fiber in Western diseases. He coedited with Dr. Ted Wilson the first edition of *Nutritional Health: Strategies for Disease Prevention* (Humana Press, 2001).

Dr. Ted Wilson received his PhD from Iowa State University; he then worked for several years in the Departments of Biology and Cardiac Rehabilitation at the University of Wisconsin–La Crosse, and currently works in the Department of Biology at Winona State University in Winona, Minnesota. Dr. Wilson has taught courses in nutrition, physiology, and cell biology. His research examines the impact of dietary components on human nutrition and physiology, cancer, cardiovascular disease, and cardiac rehabilitation. Dr. Wilson has been interested in the validation of food health claims, with regard to the promotion of measurable physiological effects. He has also examined dietary influences on platelet aggregation, lipoprotein oxidation, arterial vasodilation, mechanisms for urinary tract infection, and plant phenolic analysis. Specific dietary components 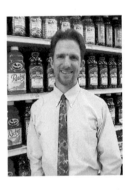 and supplements that he has studied include cranberry juice, apple juice, grape juice, wine, resveratrol, creatine phosphate, soy phytoestrogens, and tomatoes. Presently, Dr. Wilson conducts a USDA-sponsored study that investigates how cranberry juice consumption affects cardiovascular disease risk factors. *Beverages in Nutrition and Health* is the second book he has coedited with Dr. Norman Temple; the previous book is entitled *Nutritional Health: Strategies for Disease Prevention* (Humana Press, 2001).

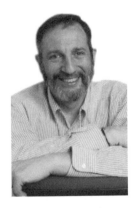

Dr. David R. Jacobs, Jr., holds a PhD in Mathematical Statistics (1971) from The Johns Hopkins University. He has been on the faculty of the School of Public Health, University of Minnesota since 1974, and has held the rank of Professor of Epidemiology since 1989. He concurrently holds a guest professorship at the Department of Nutrition at the University of Oslo, Norway (1999–present). He is a fellow of the American Heart Association and the American College of Nutrition. He serves on the editorial boards of the *British Journal of Nutrition, Clinical Chemistry, Current Nutrition Reviews,* and *Preventive Medicine.*

He has written over 400 articles on various topics concerning the epidemiology of chronic diseases and their risk factors, including the epidemiology of specific molecules, and particularly those relating to cardiovascular diseases. In recent years he has recognized a very important role of diet in chronic disease prevention and causation and, consequently, focused his research heavily on nutritional epidemiology. His work was influential in the 2000 decision of the USDA Dietary Guidelines Advisory Committee to add a specific guideline to "eat a variety of grains, especially whole grains," and in the strengthening of this message in the 2005 USDA Dietary Guidelines.

About the Series Editor

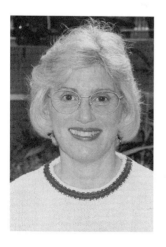

Dr. Adrianne Bendich is Clinical Director of Calcium Research at GlaxoSmithKline Consumer Healthcare, where she is responsible for leading the innovation and medical programs in support of several leading consumer brands including TUMS and Os-Cal. Dr. Bendich has primary responsibility for the coordination of GSK's support for the Women's Health Initiative (WHI) intervention study. Prior to joining GlaxoSmithKline, Dr. Bendich was at Roche Vitamins Inc., and was involved with the groundbreaking clinical studies proving that folic acid-containing multivitamins significantly reduce major classes of birth defects. Dr. Bendich has co-authored more than 100 major clinical research studies in the area of preventive nutrition. Dr. Bendich is recognized as a leading authority on antioxidants, nutrition and bone health, immunity, and pregnancy outcomes, vitamin safety, and the cost-effectiveness of vitamin/mineral supplementation.

In addition to serving as Series Editor for Humana Press and initiating the development of the 20 currently published books in the *Nutrition and Health™* series, Dr. Bendich is the editor of 11 books, including *Preventive Nutrition: The Comprehensive Guide for Health Professionals.* She also serves as Associate Editor for *Nutrition: The International Journal of Applied and Basic Nutritional Sciences,* and Dr. Bendich is on the Editorial Board of the *Journal of Women's Health and Gender-Based Medicine,* as well as a past member of the Board of Directors of the American College of Nutrition. Dr. Bendich also serves on the Program Advisory Committee for Helen Keller International.

Dr. Bendich was the recipient of the Roche Research Award, was a Tribute to Women and Industry Awardee, and a recipient of the Burroughs Wellcome Visiting Professorship in Basic Medical Sciences, 2000–2001. Dr. Bendich holds academic appointments as Adjunct Professor in the Department of Preventive Medicine and Community Health at UMDNJ, Institute of Nutrition, Columbia University P&S, and Adjunct Research Professor, Rutgers University, Newark Campus. She is listed in *Who's Who in American Women*.